Priorities in CRITICAL CARE NURSING

Priorities in CRITICAL CARE NURSING

3RD EDITION

LINDA D. URDEN, DNSc, RN, CNA
Associate Professor
Environments for Health
Indiana University
Indianapolis, Indiana

KATHLEEN M. STACY, MS, RN, CNS, CCRN
Critical Care Clinical Nurse Specialist
Veterans Administration San Diego Healthcare System
San Diego, California
and
Adjunct Faculty
San Diego State University School of Nursing
San Diego, California

With 267 illustrations

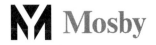 Mosby

St. Louis Baltimore Boston Carlsbad Chicago Minneapolis New York Philadelphia Portland
London Milan Sydney Tokyo Toronto

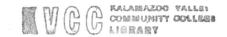

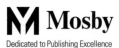 **Mosby**

Dedicated to Publishing Excellence

Executive Editor: *Barbara Nelson Cullen*
Developmental Editor: *Cindi Anderson*
Project Manager: *John Rogers*
Senior Production Editor: *Helen Hudlin*
Designer: *Kathi Gosche*

Third EDITION
Copyright © 2000 by Mosby, Inc.

Previous editions copyrighted 1992, 1996

NOTICE

Pharmacology is an ever-changing field. Standard safety precautions must be followed, but as new research and clinical experience broaden our knowledge, changes in treatment and drug therapy may become necessary or appropriate. Readers are advised to check the most current product information provided by the manufacturer of each drug to be administered to verify the recommended dose, the method and duration of administration, and contraindications. It is the responsibility of the appropriately licensed health care provider, relying on experience and knowledge of the patient, to determine dosages and the best treatment for each individual patient. Neither the publisher nor the editor assumes any liability for any injury and/or damage to persons or property arising from this publication.

Mosby, Inc.
A Harcourt Health Sciences Company
11830 Westline Industrial Drive
St. Louis, Missouri 63146

Printed in the United States of America

ISBN 0-323-01000-8

99 00 01 02 03 CL/KPT 9 8 7 6 5 4 3 2 1

CONTRIBUTORS

Jennifer N. Bloomquist, MN, RN
Cardiac Rehabilitation Clinical Nurse Specialist
Naval Medical Center
San Diego, California

Beverly Means Carlson, MS, RN, CCRN
Cardiac Research Project Director
Sharp Health Care
San Diego, California

JoAnn M. Clark, MSN, RN, CGNP, CFNP
Assistant Clinical Professor
Coordinator, Gerontological Nurse Practitioner
  Program
School of Medicine
Division of Graduate Nursing Education
University of California, San Diego
San Diego, California

Joni Dirks, MS, RN, CCRN
Clinical Nurse Specialist, Critical Care
Veterans Administration Health Care System
Palo Alto, California

Lorraine Fitzsimmons, DNS, RN, FNP, CS
Chair, Advanced Practice Nursing of Adults and
  Elderly, Graduate Program
San Diego State University School of Nursing
San Diego, California

Jeannine Forrest, PhD, RN
Clinical Instructor
University of Illinois
Chicago School of Nursing
Chicago, Illinois

Judith K. Glann, MSN, RN, CCRN
Cardiovascular/Critical Care Clinical Nurse
  Specialist
Emergency and Critical Care Departments
Lovelace Health Systems
Albuquerque, New Mexico

Ruth N. Grendell, DNSc, RN
Professor of Nursing
Point Loma Nazarene University
San Diego, California

Lynne Jett, MSN, RN, C
Professional Development Specialist
Tri-City Medical Center
Oceanside, California
Instructor, BSN Program
California State University
Dominiquez Hills, California

Karen L. Johnson, PhD, RN, CCRN
Clinical Nurse Specialist
University Medical Center
Tucson, Arizona

Martha J. Love, MN, RN
Staff Nurse
Intensive Care Unit
Veterans Administration San Diego Healthcare System
San Diego, California

Jeanne M. Maiden, MS, RN, CCRN
Professional Developmental Specialist
Tri-City Medical Center
Oceanside, California

Nancy McLaughlin, MSN, RN, CCRN
Nurse Manager
Surgical Intensive Care Unit
University of Alabama—Birmingham University
  Hospital
Birmingham, Alabama

Kathleen A. Mendez, MS, RN, CCRN
Neuroscience Clinical Outcomes Manager
Tri-City Medical Center
Oceanside, California

Mary Courtney Moore, PhD, RD, RN
Research Assistant Professor
Vanderbilt University School of Nursing
Nashville, Tennessee

Mimi O'Donnell, MS, RN, CS
Clinical Nurse Specialist
Cardiac Surgical Nursing
Massachusetts General Hospital
Boston, Massachusetts

Mary Schira, PhD, RN, CS, ACNP
Director, Acute Care Nurse Practitioner Program
The University of Texas at Arlington School of Nursing
Arlington, Texas

*To student nurses, practicing nurses, and educators who seek knowledge
to provide excellence in nursing practice for the critically ill.*

LDU

*To my fabulous family,
James, Sherrie-Anne, Meniko, and Jack
To my wonderful parents,
Robert and Rosemary
To my incredible in-laws,
Ed and Jo
Thank you for your love and encouragement.*

KMS

PREFACE

We are grateful to the many students, nurses and educators who made the first two editions of this book successful. We actively solicited input from users of the second edition and incorporated their comments and suggestions regarding format, content, and organization for this book. The emphasis continues to be on priorities for the critical care nurse. We believe that prioritizing conditions and issues will assist critical nurses in quickly assessing and intervening in the most efficient and effective manner

Organization

The book is again organized around alterations in dimensions of human functioning that span the biopsychosocial realms. We have gone beyond the traditional psychologic focus of critical care and incorporated the following chapters:

Nursing Process and Collaborative Care
Legal and Ethical Issues
Patient and Family Education
Psychosocial Alterations

Organizationally, the book comprises ten major units. The chapter content of Unit One, *Foundations of Critical Care Nursing Practice*, forms the basis of practice regardless of the physiologic alterations of the critically ill patient. Although chapters in this book may be studied in any sequence, we recommend that Chapter 1, *Nursing Process and Collaborative Care*, be studied first because it clarifies the major assumptions on which the book is based.

Unit Two, *Common Problems in Critical Care*, examines potential critical care practice problems and is divided into five chapters: *Psychosocial Alterations, Sleep Alterations, Nutritional Alterations, Gerontologic Alterations*, and *Pain Management*.

Unit Three, *Cardiovascular Alterations*, Unit Four, *Pulmonary Alterations*, and Unit Five, *Neurologic Alterations*, are each organized by the following three chapter formats:

Assessment and Diagnosis

Disorders

Therapeutic Management

This organization permits easy retrieval of information for students and clinicians and provides flexibility for the educator to individualize teaching methods by assigning chapters that best suit student needs.

Unit Six, *Renal Alterations*, Unit Seven, *Gastrointestinal Alterations*, and Unit Eight, *Endocrine Alterations*, are each organized by the following two chapter formats:

Assessment and Diagnostic Procedures

Disorders and Therapeutic Management

Unit Nine, *Multisystem Alterations*, addresses disorders that affect multiple body systems and necessitate discussion as a separate category. Unit Nine is organized by two chapter formats:

Trauma

Shock and Multiple Organ Dysfunction Syndrome

Unit Ten, *Nursing Management Plans of Care*, contains the core of critical care nursing practice in a nursing process format: signs and symptoms, nursing diagnosis, outcome criteria, and nursing interventions. The Nursing Management Plans of Care are referenced throughout the book within the *Nursing Diagnosis Priorities* boxes.

Finally, two appendices are included that contain useful information for all students and practitioners of critical care. Appendix A, *Advanced Cardiac Life Support (ACLS) Guidelines*, presents selected decision trees from the American Heart Association for use in treating life-threatening emergencies. Appendix B, *Physiologic Formulas for Critical Care*, features commonly encountered hemodynamic and oxygenation formulas and other calculations presented in easily understood terms.

Nursing Diagnosis and Management

The power of research-based critical care practice has been incorporated into nursing interventions. To foster critical thinking and decision-making, a boxed menu of nursing diagnoses complete with specific etiologic or related factors accompanies each medical disorder and major medical treatment discussion and directs the learner to the section of the book where appropriate nursing management is detailed.

In keeping with the emphasis on priorities in critical care, *Nursing Diagnosis Priorities* boxes list the most urgent potential nursing diagnoses to be addressed. To facilitate student learning, the nursing management plans of care incorporate nursing diagnoses, etiologic or related factors, clinical manifestations, and interventions with rationales. The nursing management plans of care are liberally cross-referenced throughout the book for easy retrieval by the reader.

New to Edition

New to this edition are the following chapters:

Nursing Process and Collaborative Care
Pain Management

A second feature new to this edition are diagnostic tables accompanying each diagnostic procedure discussion. The tables summarize the most commonly used diagnostic procedures for that disorder and include the purpose for the procedure along with pertinent comments that will assist the nurse in providing care. Also new to this edition is the inclusion of the average length of stay (LOS) for each disorder. The LOS is important to the nurse and health care team in planning care for patients within the designated projected hospital length of stay.

Learner Enhancements

To accompany the *Priorities in Critical Care Nursing* textbook, a comprehensive *Instructor's Resource Manual* is available, featuring the following elements: chapter issues, adopted course outlines, revised student worksheets (text and answers), a newly revised 400-item test bank with answers, and 30 transparency masters taken from this new, third edition.

ACKNOWLEDGMENTS

The talent, hard work, and inspiration of many people have produced *Priorities in Critical Care Nursing.* We appreciate the assistance of our Acquisition Editors, Barry Bowlus and Barbara Nelson Cullen; Developmental Editor, Cindi Anderson; and Editorial Assistants, Brooke Bagwill and Emily Frye. We are also grateful to our Production Editor, Helen Hudlin, for her scrupulous attention to detail.

We would like to acknowledge contributors to the third edition of *Critical Care Nursing: Diagnosis and Management:* Jacqueline Kartman and Bobbie Monroe.

We also would like to express our thanks to Mary E. Lough, coauthor to the second edition of *Priorities in Critical Care Nursing,* for her contribution.

CONTENTS

FOUNDATIONS OF CRITICAL CARE NURSING PRACTICE

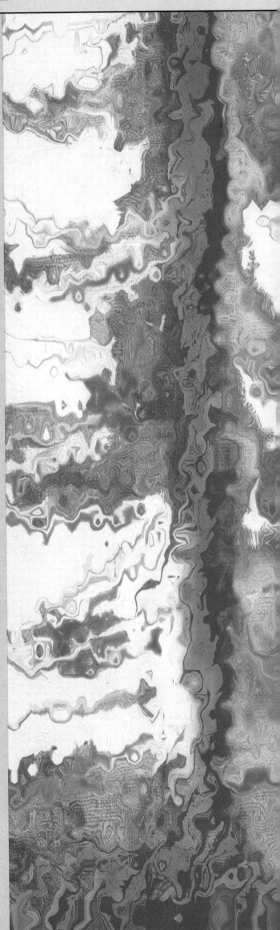

1

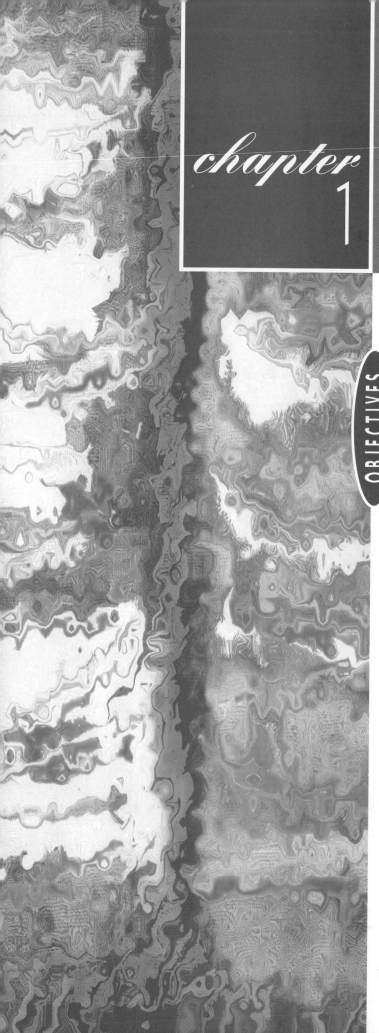

chapter 1

The Nursing Process and Collaborative Care

Linda D. Urden

OBJECTIVES

- Define nursing diagnosis.
- Formulate nursing diagnosis statements from the North American Nursing Diagnosis Association's taxonomy of approved diagnoses, etiologic/related factors, and defining characteristics.
- Describe three types of collaborative care models.
- Discuss four types of tools used to collaboratively coordinate and manage care.

THE NURSING PROCESS

The nursing process is a method for making clinical decisions. It is a way of thinking and acting in relation to the clinical phenomena of concern to nurses. Classically, the nursing process comprises five phases or dimensions: assessment, nursing diagnosis, planning, implementation, and evaluation. *Outcome identification* was added as a separate step, which follows after nursing diagnosis but comes before the planning stage (Fig. 1-1). The six phases constitute a continuous cycle throughout the nurse's moment-to-moment data interpretation and management of patient care.

Assessment

By virtue of nursing's unique orientation and commitment to holism, nurses collect an enormous amount of data about a patient's biopsychosocial health status. And by virtue of an array of technophysiologic monitoring devices, critical care nurses process an additional layer of data in the form of physiologic parameter measurements.

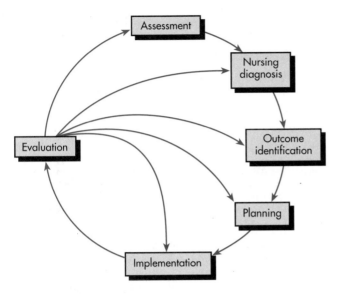

Fig. **1-1** Cyclical nature of the nursing process. (Modified from Fortinash K, Holoday-Worret P: *Psychiatric nursing care plans,* ed 2, St Louis, 1995, Mosby.)

TABLE **1-1** COMMONLY IDENTIFIED NURSING DIAGNOSES IN CRITICAL CARE*	
Nursing Diagnosis	**Percent of Time Identified**
Pain	93
Risk for Infection	92
Impaired Gas Exchange	92
Decreased Cardiac Output	91
Risk for Impaired Skin Integrity	90
Fluid Volume Excess	89
Altered Cardiopulmonary Perfusion	88
Ineffective Airway Clearance	87
Anxiety	84
Ineffective Breathing Pattern	81
Sleep Pattern Disturbance	81
Risk for Fluid Volume Deficit	81
Fluid Volume Deficit	78
Sensory Overload	75
Risk for Injury	74
Impaired Skin Integrity	73
Risk for Activity Intolerance	73
Activity Intolerance	73
Knowledge Deficit	70
Bathing/Hygiene Self-Care Deficit	70

*Top 20 diagnoses based on nurses' ratings in their critical care practice of "nearly always" and "frequently present."

Nursing Diagnosis

The North American Nursing Diagnosis Association (NANDA) endorsed the following working definition of nursing diagnosis[1]:

A nursing diagnosis is a clinical judgment about individual, family, or community responses to actual or potential health problems/life processes. Nursing diagnoses provide the basis for selection of nursing interventions to achieve outcomes for which the nurse is accountable.

The most essential and distinguishing feature of any nursing diagnosis is that it describes a health condition *primarily resolved by nursing interventions or therapies.*

Nursing diagnoses most commonly identified in critical care[2] are listed in Table 1-1. All approved diagnoses have accompanying definitions to better explain the health state they represent. These definitions are important because they clarify more about the health state than is apparent from the label alone.

Some nursing diagnoses need accompanying qualifiers or specifiers based on the characteristics of the health problem as it manifests itself in a particular patient. For example, the diagnosis *Fear* needs specification as to the object of the patient's particular fear, such as death, pain, disfigurement, or malignancy. See Box 1-1 for examples of the format for nursing diagnoses.

Outcome Identification

The emphasis on patient outcomes has become increasingly important in the provision of quality care and services. It is important that nurse-sensitive outcomes are delineated so that nursing care and services can be described and understood by all health care professionals,

consumers, and payors.[3,4] Outcome statements consist of highly specific indicators that will be used by the nurse in the evaluation phase as criteria that either (1) the actual diagnosis has been resolved or reduced or (2) the risk diagnosis has not occurred. An outcome statement is a projection of the expected influence that the nursing intervention will have on the patient in relation to the identified diagnosis.

Outcome criteria should be measurable, desirable, and, given full consideration to the resources of the patient and those of the nurse, attainable.

Measurable outcome criteria consist of patient behaviors, statements, and/or physiologic parameters that are recognizable on their occurrence. Many of the phenomena critical care nurses diagnose and treat are readily measurable, such as adequacy of spontaneous ventilation, cardiac output, and tissue perfusion. Outcome statements are made further measurable by indicating the date and time of anticipated attainment. Individual patient baseline and patterns and nurse and patient resources are the dominant considerations given to a projection of desired outcome versus normative values.

Planning

During the planning phase, comprehensive planning of all care and services for the patient is done. The process consists of collaboration by the nurse with all appropriate health care providers, patients, and family members/significant others.

BOX 1-1

FORMAT FOR NURSING DIAGNOSES

ACTUAL PROBLEM (THREE-PART STATEMENT)
Part 1: Nursing diagnosis

Altered Tissue Perfusion: Myocardial

Part 2: Etiologic factors (related to):

Acute myocardial ischemia secondary to coronary artery disease (CAD)

Part 3: Defining characteristics

Angina >30 min but <6 hr
ST-segment elevation on 12-lead ECG
Elevation of CK and CK-MB enzymes
Apprehension

RISK PROBLEM (TWO-PART STATEMENT)
Part 1: Nursing diagnosis

Risk for Aspiration

Part 2: Etiologic factors (related to):

Impaired laryngeal sensation or reflex
Impaired laryngeal peristalsis or tongue function
Impaired laryngeal closure or elevation
Increased gastric volume
Increased intragastric pressure
Decreased lower esophageal sphincter pressure
Decreased antegrade esophageal propulsion

CAD, Coronary artery disease; *CK,* creatine kinase; *CK-MB,* MB isoenzyme of creatine kinase.

Implementation

Implementation is the action component of planning. It is the phase of the nursing process in which the nursing treatment plan is carried out. Assessment and evaluation are continuous throughout this phase.

Nursing interventions

Also known as *nursing orders* or *nursing prescriptions,* nursing interventions constitute the treatment approach to an identified health alteration. Interventions are selected to satisfy the outcome criteria and prevent or resolve the nursing diagnosis. Interventions have the greatest impact when they are directed at the etiologic/related factors of the diagnosis, or, in the case of a risk diagnosis, the risk factors. This stipulates that the etiologic factors of a problem be modifiable by nursing management.

Nursing interventions classification

A research team at the University of Iowa has developed and refined a classification system of nursing interventions that is research-based and clinically driven. The Nursing Interventions Classification (NIC) framework contains 433 nursing interventions that are categorized into 27 classes and 6 domains.[5] Interventions consist of both direct care and indirect care nursing intervention (Box 1-2). Many nursing interventions are directly linked

BOX 1-2

ACID-BASE MANAGEMENT

DEFINITION:

Promotion of acid-base balance and prevention of complications resulting from acid-base imbalance

ACTIVITIES:

Maintain patent IV access
Maintain a patent airway
Monitor ABG and electrolyte levels, as available
Monitor hemodynamic status, including CVP, MAP, PAP, and PCWP levels if available
Monitor for loss of acid (e.g., vomiting, nasogastric output, diarrhea, and diuresis), as appropriate
Monitor for loss of bicarbonate (e.g., fistula drainage and diarrhea), as appropriate
Position to facilitate adequate ventilation (e.g., open airway and elevate head of bed)
Monitor for symptoms of respiratory failure (e.g., low Pao_2 and elevated $Paco_2$ levels and respiratory muscle fatigue)
Monitor respiratory pattern
Monitor determinants of tissue oxygen delivery (e.g., Pao_2, Sao_2, and hemoglobin levels and cardiac output), if available
Provide oxygen therapy, if necessary
Provide mechanical ventilatory support, if necessary
Monitor determination of oxygen consumption (e.g., Svo_2 and $avDo_2$ levels), if available
Obtain ordered specimen for laboratory analysis of acid-base balance (e.g., ABG, urine, and serum levels), as appropriate
Monitor for worsening electrolyte imbalance with correction of the acid-base imbalance
Reduce oxygen consumption (e.g., promote comfort, control fever, and reduce anxiety), as appropriate
Monitor neurologic status (e.g., level of consciousness and confusion)
Administer prescribed alkaline medication (e.g., sodium bicarbonate) as appropriate, based on ABG results
Provide frequent oral hygiene
Instruct the patient and/or family on actions instituted to treat the acid-base imbalance
Promote orientation

From McCloskey JC, Bulechek GM: *Nursing interventions classification,* ed 3, St Louis, 2000, Mosby (in press).
ABG, Arterial blood gas; *CVP,* central venous pressure; *MAP,* mean arterial pressure; *PAP,* pulmonary arterial pressure; *PCWP,* pulmonary capillary wedge pressure.

with NANDA nursing diagnoses. *Nurse-initiated treatments* are those interventions initiated by the nurse in response to a nursing diagnosis.[5] The use of the NIC framework facilitates clinical decision-making and provides a standardized language that describes the core of essential nursing interventions. In addition, the research base provides a method to link diagnoses with outcomes in the evaluation of care and services.[5] An example of how NANDA nursing diagnostic categories link with NIC interventions is presented in Box 1-3.

BOX 1-3

LINKING NANDA DIAGNOSIS WITH NIC INTERVENTIONS

NANDA NURSING DIAGNOSIS:

Sleep pattern disturbance

DEFINITION:

Disruption of sleep time causes discomfort or interferes with desired lifestyle

NIC INTERVENTIONS:
Suggested nursing interventions for problem resolution:

Dementia Management
Environmental Management
Environmental Management: Comfort
Medication Administration
Medication Management

Medication Prescribing
Security Enhancement
Simple Relaxation Therapy
Sleep Enhancement
Touch

Additional optional interventions:

Anxiety Reduction
Autogenic Training
Bathing
Calming Technique
Coping Enhancement
Energy Management
Energy Promotion
Exercise Therapy: Ambulation
Kangaroo Care

Meditation
Music Therapy
Nutrition Management
Pain Management
Positioning
Progressive Muscle Relaxation
Self-Care Assistance: Toileting
Simple Massage
Urinary Incontinence Care: Enuresis

Modified from McCloskey JC, Bulechek GM: *Nursing interventions classification,* ed 3, St Louis, 2000, Mosby (in press).

Evaluation

Evaluation of attainment of the expected patient outcomes occurs formally at intervals designated in the outcome criteria. Informal evaluation occurs continuously. The evaluation phase and the activities that take place within it are perhaps the most important dimensions of the nursing process.

Collaborative Care

The managed care environment has forced emphasis on examining methods of care delivery and processes of care by all health care professionals. Partnerships have been formed or strengthened, with a focus on increasing quality of care and services while containing or decreasing costs.[6-9] Coordination of care in critical care units has been demonstrated to significantly influence patient outcomes.[10] It is now more important than ever to create and enhance partnerships because the resulting interdependence and collaboration among disciplines is essential to achieve positive patient outcomes.

Collaborative Care Management Models

There are several different models of care delivery and care management used in health care. The reader is encouraged to seek additional resources and consultation for a more in-depth explanation of the models.

Care management

Care management is a system of integrated processes designed to enable, support, and coordinate patient care throughout the continuum of health care services. Care management takes place in many different settings; care is delivered by various professional health care team members and nonlicensed providers, as appropriate. Actual coordination of care and services may be done by health care staff or insurance/payor staff. Care management must be patient-focused, continuum-driven, based on a team approach, and results-oriented. Another term associated with this model of care is *disease state management,* which connotes the process of managing a population's health over a lifetime. In disease state management, however, there is a focus on managing complex and chronic disease states, such as diabetes or congestive heart failure, over the entire continuum.

Case management

Case management is the process of overseeing the care of patients and organizing services in collaboration with the patient's physician or primary health care provider. The case manager may be a nurse, allied health care provider, or the patient's primary care provider. Case managers are usually assigned to a specific population group and facilitate effective coordination of care services as patients move in and out of different settings. Ideally, the case manager oversees the care of the patient across the continuum of care.

Spectrum Health Downtown Campus

CONGESTIVE HEART FAILURE CLINICAL PATH
(DRG 127)

Ejection Fraction: _____
NYHA Functional Class:
Admit _____ **Discharge** _____
I-no limits   II-Limit w/activity
III-SOB w/ADLs   IV-symptoms@ rest

This pathway is only a guideline. Patient care will vary on their individual needs. Please refer to CPM Guidelines of Care and Education Record for the Congestive Heart Failure Patient.

Please fill in dates and check all boxes that apply, write NA over boxes that do not apply.

Length of stay will vary for each patient. Pathway is based on average stay. Less complicated and younger patients may have shorter than average length of stays. Some patients may stay longer than the average if their condition is more severe.

Stamp with addressograph

	ER	DAY 1	DAY 2	DAY 3	DAY 4	OUTCOMES
Consults (*see criteria on back)	☐ Consider cardiology NP ☐ Consider cardiology ☐ Consider MSW	☐ Consider Cardiac Rehab ☐ Consider cardiology NP ☐ Consider cardiology ☐ Consider Dietary ☐ Consider Pharmacy				☐ Follow up established with PCP/cardiology
Assessment & Interventions	☐ VS/strict I & O ☐ Consider BiPAP/CPAP ☐ Assess oxygen/O2 protocol ☐ Bronchodilator protocol ☐ Old records/echos ☐ Cardiac monitor ☐ Foley/Inter. Infusion Device	☐ VS/strict I & O ☐ Daily weight ☐ Continue O2 assessment	☐ VS/strict I & O ☐ Patient weighs self and logs their weight ☐ Use same scale if possible ☐ Consider d/c monitor, foley	☐ VS/strict I & O ☐ Patient weighs self and logs their weight ☐ Use same scale if possible	☐ VS/strict I & O ☐ Patient weighs self and logs their weight ☐ Use same scale if possible	☐ Patient keeps log of their weight daily and notifies MD/NP with weight gain as per education record teaching. ☐ F & E status WDL for this patient
Medications	☐ Pre-admission meds ☐ IV diuretics ☐ Consider digoxin, ACE inhibitors, nitrates, inotropes	☐ Adjusting of meds ☐ Consider ACE inhibitor ☐ Sq heparin if not on coumadin ☐ Consider pneumovax vaccine	☐ Change to po meds ☐ Consider adjusting ACE inhibitor ☐ D/C sq heparin if OOB	☐ Stabilization of meds ☐ Consider adjusting ACE inhibitor ☐ D/C sq heparin if OOB		☐ Patient verbalizes purpose of medications, doses, side effects, etc., per ed record
Diet	☐ Fluid restriction ☐ NPO except ice chips	☐ Fluid restriction ☐ Sodium restriction	☐ Fluid restriction ☐ Sodium restriction	☐ Fluid restriction ☐ Sodium restriction	☐ Fluid restriction ☐ Sodium restriction	☐ Patient verbalizes understanding of cardiac diet and fluid restriction
Activity	☐ Bedrest with BRP	☐ Bedrest with BRP ☐ Physical therapy prn	☐ OOB	☐ OOB		☐ Cardiac rehab or exercise program in place prn
Tests	☐ CXR, EKG, U/A ☐ CPK/MB, SMA + lytes, Mg++, plts, CBC, TSH - if a-fib/new onset CHF ☐ PT/PTT if on coumadin/hep ☐ Digoxin level if on digoxin	☐ Chem 7	☐ Consider repeat CXR ☐ Chem 7	☐ Chem 7	☐ Consider CXR prior to d/c ☐ Chem 7	☐ Diagnostic studies WDL for pt
Education (see Ed Record)	☐ See CHF Ed Record	☐ Reinforce CHF Ed Record ☐ Smoking counseling/**Smoking cessation program initiated prn** ☐ **Provide copy of CHF book/CHF kit - review w/pt**	☐ See Ed Record ☐ Smoking counseling ☐ **Review CHF book w/pt**	☐ See Ed Record ☐ Smoking counseling ☐ **Review CHF book w/pt**	☐ See Ed Record ☐ Smoking counseling ☐ **Review CHF book w/pt**	☐ Patient d/c with copy of the CHF book/kit and verbalizes understanding as per ed record ☐ **Smoking cessation program initiated prn**
Discharge Planning	☐ Assess support systems/home environment ☐ Identify pot. barriers to d/c	☐ Assess support systems/home environment ☐ Identify pot. barriers to d/c ☐ Assess need for cardiac rehab after d/c	☐ Assess need for home care ☐ Assess need for assistive devices (i.e. O2)	☐ RN review discharge plan. ☐ Assess need for assistive devices (i.e. O2)	☐ Discharge plans per preprinted d/c instruction sheet ☐ Support services in place (i.e.: O2, rehab, home nursing)	☐ Patient has home care and assistive devices in place prn ☐ Able to verbalize d/c plan ☐ Document d/c NYHA Functional class
Signatures (Name/Time)	_____	_____	_____	_____	_____	_____

Criteria for Medical Social Work Referral
Increased anxiety
Depressed Mood/Affect
Caregiver of a dependent spouse
Socially Isolated/limited support system
Inadequate financial resources to meet needs

Criteria for Dietary Consult
Serum albumin < 3.0
Diet for discharge is new to patient or different from diet prior to admission
Admission weight gain of ten pounds or greater over last discharge weight

Criteria for Cardiac Rehab Referral/PT
Decreased mobility/lack of ability to perform ADLs
Lack of knowledge of ways/activities to decrease tissue oxygen demands
New diagnosis
History of smoking/smoking cessation referrals
Secondary diagnosis of Ischemic Heart Disease

Criteria for Cardiology NP Consult
New onset CHF
Readmission within 30 days
NYHA function class III or IV
Needs CHF education

Criteria for Pharmacy Consult
Patient on 7 or more medications
Patient on two medications of same class
Serum Creatinine > 2.5 mg/dl excluding admission creatinine
Serum potassium > 5.6 or < 3.0 mEq/liter
Medication related admission (eg: Digoxin toxicity)

Instructions: Please indicate any significant variances that may prolong the stay in the boxes to the right. Write in the variance code, the date the variance occurred, comments and your initials. Your comments for improving the care for this population or the pathways format are appreciated.

CODES FOR COMMON VARIANCES:

Code	Issue
300.0	Anxiety
427.9	Arrhythmia
427.5	Cardiac arrest
786.50	Chest pain
298.9	Confusion
780.6	Fever/FUO
401.9	Hypertension
458.9	Hypotension
277.8	Metabolic instability
787.02	Nausea
997.3	Pulmonary complication
787.01	Vomiting

Code	Issue
P1	Lives alone/lack of home support
P2	Pt education not complete
P6	Unexpected transfer to ICU
P8	Abnormal lab values
P9	Activity intolerance
P16	Concurrent complex med card.
P21	Patient noncompliance
P39	Patient expired
P50	Patient taken to OR

Code	Issue
S1	Pathway documentation incomplete
S2	Imprinted Orders not used
S3	Discharge instructions not used
S5	Discharge facility delay
S6	Delay in PT consult
S8	Delay in MSW consult
S9	Delay in dietitian consult
S10	Other
S18	Physician discretion
S19	Late consult or test
S45	Outcomes not recorded

Pathway Variance/ Exception Code	Date	Comments	Initials

Ideas for improving care for this population:

Ideas for improving format of this pathway:

Fig. **1-2** Congestive heart failure pathway.

Outcomes management

Outcomes management refers to a model aimed at managing the outcomes of care by the use of various tools, quality improvement processes, and interdisciplinary team involvement and action. Specifically, there is an emphasis on consistent standards of care; measurement of disease-specific clinical outcomes, as well as patient functioning and well-being; and assessment of clinical and outcome data for the specific conditions.[11,12] Outcomes management also takes place in multiple settings across the continuum of care. Professional nurse outcomes managers ensure that variances from the plan of care are addressed in a timely manner, and they also examine aggregate information with the team for quality improvement in the interdisciplinary plan of care.

Care Management Tools

There are many quality improvement tools available to providers for care management. Four tools are addressed in this chapter: clinical pathways, algorithms, practice guidelines, and protocols.

Clinical pathway

The *clinical pathway* presents an overview of the entire multidisciplinary plan of care for routine patients.[13] It focuses on the critical elements in the care of certain patient populations and may track variances from the pathway. Pathways are developed by a multidisciplinary team, based on a specific diagnosis or condition, and integrated with latest research and best practices from the literature.

Clinical pathways have been demonstrated to decrease patients' length of stay and overall costs, while maintaining or increasing quality of care.[14-19] Fig. 1-2 is an example of a congestive heart failure (CHF) pathway.

Algorithm

An *algorithm* is a step-wise decision-making flowchart for specific care process(es). Algorithms are more focused than clinical pathways and guide the clinician through the "if, then" decision-making process, addressing patient responses to particular treatments.[18] Well-known examples of algorithms are the Advanced Cardiac Life Support (ACLS) algorithms published by the American Heart Association (Appendix A).

Practice guideline

Practice guidelines are usually developed by professional organizations (e.g., American Association of Critical Care Nurses, Society of Critical Care Medicine, American College of Cardiology, or government agencies such as the Agency for Health Care Policy and Research [AHCPR]). Practice guidelines are generally written in text prose style rather than in the flowchart format of pathways and algorithms. Practice guidelines are used as resources in formulating the pathway or algorithm. Of particular interest to the critical care practitioner is the AHCPR clinical practice guideline, *Heart Failure:*

Evaluation and Care of Patients with Left Ventricular Systolic Dysfunction.[20,21]

Protocol

A *protocol* is a very common tool in research studies. Protocols are more directive and rigid than pathways or guidelines, and providers are not supposed to vary from a protocol. Patients are screened carefully for specific entry criteria before being started on a protocol.

References

1. Kim MJ, McFarland GK, McLane AM: *Pocket guide to nursing diagnoses,* ed 7, St Louis, 1997, Mosby.
2. Gordon M, Hiltunen E: High frequency: treatment priority nursing diagnoses in critical care, *Nurs Diagn* 6(4):143-154, 1995.
3. Brooten D, Naylor M: Nurses' effect on changing patient outcomes, *Image J Nurs Sch* 27(2):95-99, 1995.
4. Himali U: A unified nursing language: the missing link in establishing nursing-sensitive patient outcomes, *Am Nurs* 27(2):23, 1995.
5. McCloskey JC, Bulechek GM, editors: *Nursing interventions classification (NIC),* ed 3, St Louis, 2000, Mosby (in press).
6. White KR, Begun JW: Profession building in the new health care system, *Nurs Adm Q* 20(3):79-85, 1996.
7. Society of Critical Care Medicine and American Association of Critical Care Nurses: *Essential provisions for critical care in health care system reform (joint position statement),* Anaheim, Calif, Aliso Viejo, Calif, 1994, The Associations.
8. Lumsdon K, Hagland M: Mapping care, *Hosp Health Netw* 67(20):34-40, 1993.
9. Grady G, Wojner A: Collaborative practice teams: the infrastructure of outcomes management, *AACN Clin Issues Crit Care Nurs* 7(1):153-158, 1996.
10. Knaus W, et al: An evaluation of outcomes from intensive care in major medical centers, *Ann Intern Med* 104:410-418, 1986.
11. Wojner A: Outcomes management: an interdisciplinary search for best practice, *AACN Clin Issues Crit Care Nurs* 7(1):133-145, 1996.
12. Zander K: Historical development of outcomes-based care deliver, *Crit Care Clin North Am* 10(1):1-11, 1997.
13. Price BJ, et al: Impact of a critical care pathway for unstable mechanically ventilated patients, *Crit Care Clin North Am* 10(1):75-85, 1997.
14. Redick E, Stroud A, Kurack T: Expanding the use of critical pathways in critical care, *DCCN* 13(6):316-321, 1994.
15. Capuano T: Clinical pathways, practical approaches, positive outcomes, *Nurs Manag* 26(1):34-37, 1995.
16. Rudisill P, Phillips M, Payne C: Clinical paths for cardiac surgery patients: a multidisciplinary approach to quality improvement outcomes, *J Nurs Care Qual* 8(3):27-33, 1994.
17. Philibin, et al: Does QI work? The management to improve survival in congestive heart failure (MISCHF) study, *Jt Comm J Qual Improv* 22(11):721-733, 1996.
18. Schriefer J: The synergy of pathways and algorithms: two tools work better than one, *Jt Comm J Qual Improv* 20(9):485-499, 1994.
19. Burns SM, et al: Design, testing, and results of an outcomes-managed approach to patients requiring prolonged mechanical ventilation, *Am J Crit Care* 7(1):45-57, 1998.
20. Dunbar S, Dracup K: Agency for health care policy and research: clinical practice guidelines for heart failure, *J Cardiovasc Nurs* 10(2):85-88, 1996.
21. Agency for Health Care Policy and Research: *Heart failure: evaluation and care of patients with left-ventricular systolic dysfunction,* Rockville, Md, 1994, US Department of Health and Human Services.

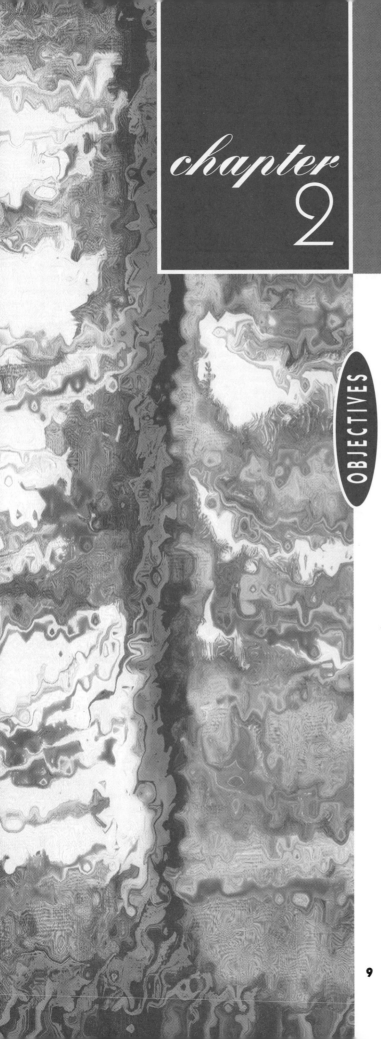

chapter 2

Legal and Ethical Issues

Linda D. Urden

OBJECTIVES

● Discuss ethical principles as they relate to critical care patients.

● Discuss the concept of medical futility.

● Describe what constitutes an ethical dilemma.

● List steps for making ethical decisions.

● Identify legal and professional obligations of critical care nurses.

● Describe the elements of certain torts that may result from critical care nursing practice.

● Identify and discuss specific legal issues in critical care nursing practice.

MORALS AND ETHICS

Morals Defined

The word *moral* is derived from the Latin *moralis*, which is defined as "good or right in conduct or character . . . making the distinction between right and wrong . . . principles of right and wrong based on custom."[1] Morals are the "shoulds," "should nots," "oughts," and "ought nots" of actions and behaviors and have been related closely to sexual mores and behaviors in Western society. Religious and cultural values and beliefs largely mold one's moral thoughts and actions. Morals form the basis for action and provide a framework for evaluation of behavior.

Ethics Defined

The word *ethics* is derived from the Greek *ethos*, which is defined as "the system or code of morals of a particular person, religion, group, or profession . . . the study of

9

standards of conduct and moral judgment."[1] The term *ethics* is sometimes used interchangeably with the word *morals*. However, ethics is more concerned with the "why" of the action rather than with whether the action is right or wrong, good or bad.[2] Ethics implies that an evaluation is being made that is theoretically based on or derived from a set of standards. *Normative ethics* is the division of ethics that focuses on "norms or standards of behavior and value and their ultimate application to daily life"[3] with an emphasis on evaluation for purposes of guiding moral action. *Bioethics* incorporates all aspects of life but most often refers to health care ethics and the application of ethical principles to individual cases.

ETHICAL PRINCIPLES

There are certain ethical principles that were derived from classic ethical theories that are used in health care decision-making.[4] Principles are general guidelines that govern conduct, provide a basis for reasoning, and direct actions. The six ethical principles that are discussed in this chapter are autonomy, beneficence, nonmaleficence, veracity, fidelity, and justice/allocation of resources (Box 2-1).

Autonomy

The concept of autonomy appears in all ancient writings and early Greek philosophy. In health care, autonomy can be viewed as the freedom to make decisions about one's own body without the coercion or interference of others. Autonomy is a freedom of choice or a self-determination that is a basic human right. It can be experienced in all human life events.

The obligation for health care professionals is to respect the values, thoughts, and actions of patients and not to let their own values or morals influence treatment decisions.[5]

The critical care nurse is often "caught in the middle" in ethical situations, and promoting autonomous decision-making is one of those situations. As the nurse works closely with patients and families to promote autonomous decision-making, another crucial element becomes clear. Patients and families must have all of the information about a certain situation to make a decision that is best for them. Not only should they be given all of the information and facts, but they must also have a clear understanding of what was presented. This is where the nurse is a most important member of the health care team—that is, as patient advocate, providing more information, clarifying points, reinforcing information, and providing support during the process.[5]

Beneficence

The concept of doing good and preventing harm to patients is a *sine qua non* for the nursing profession. However, the ethical principle of beneficence—which requires that one promote the well-being of patients—points to the importance of this duty for the health care professional. The principle of beneficence presupposes that harms and benefits are balanced, leading to positive or beneficial outcomes.

In approaching issues related to beneficence, there is commonly conflict with another principle, that of autonomy. Paternalism exists when the nurse or physician makes a decision for the patient without consulting or including the patient in the decision process. *Paternalism* is "making people do what is good for them" and "preventing people from doing what is bad for them."[6] Jameton[6] described two types of paternalists: strong paternalists who make decisions for obviously competent persons and weak paternalists who make decisions for persons who are mentally or physically unable to make their own decisions.

Nonmaleficence

The ethical principle of nonmaleficence, which dictates that one prevent harm and remove harmful situations, is a *prima facie* duty for the nurse. Thoughtfulness and care are necessary, as is balancing risks and benefits, which was discussed earlier with beneficence. Beneficence and nonmaleficence are on two ends of a continuum and are often carried out differently, depending on the views of the practitioner.

Veracity

Veracity, or truth-telling, is an important ethical principle that underlies the nurse-patient relationship. Veracity is important in soliciting informed consent, so that the patient is aware of all potential risks and benefits from specific treatments or their alternatives. Once again, the critical care nurse can be in the middle of a situation where all of the facts and information about a particular treatment option are not disclosed. Sometimes information has been given accurately but has been delivered with bias or in a way that is misleading. In this case and other instances with veracity, the ethical principle of autonomy has been violated.[7] Veracity must guide all areas of practice for the

---

BOX 2-1

ETHICAL PRINCIPLES IN CRITICAL CARE

- Autonomy
- Beneficence
- Nonmaleficence
- Veracity
- Fidelity
    Confidentiality
    Privacy
- Justice/allocation of resources

nurse, that is, colleague relationships and employee relationships, as well as the nurse-patient relationship.

Fidelity

Another ethical principle that is closely related to autonomy and veracity is fidelity. Fidelity, or faithfulness and promise-keeping to patients, is also a *sine qua non* for nursing. It forms a bond between individuals and is the basis of all relationships, both professional and personal. Regardless of the amount of autonomy that patients have in the critical care areas, they still depend on the nurse for a multitude of types of physical care and emotional support.

As do all the other principles, fidelity extends to the family of the critical care patient. When a promise is made to the family that they will be called if an emergency arises or that they will be informed of other special events, the nurse must make every effort to follow through on the promise.

Confidentiality is one element of fidelity that is based on traditional health care professional ethics. Confidentiality is described as a right whereby patient information can only be shared with those involved in the care of the patient. An exception to this guideline might be when the welfare of others is at risk by keeping patient information confidential. Again in this situation, the nurse must balance ethical principles and weigh risks with benefits. Special circumstances, such as mandatory reporting laws, will guide the nurse in certain situations.

Privacy has also been described as inherent in the principle of fidelity. It may be closely aligned with confidentiality of patient information and a patient's right to privacy of his or her person, such as maintaining privacy for the patient by pulling the curtains around the bed or making sure that he or she is adequately covered.

Justice/Allocation of Resources

The principle of justice is often used synonymously with the concept of allocation of scarce resources. With escalating health care costs, expanded technologies, an aging population with its own special health care needs, and (in some instances) a scarcity of health care personnel, the question of health care allocation becomes even more complex.

The application of the justice principle in health care is concerned primarily with divided or portioned allocation of goods and services, which is termed *distributive justice*.[8] According to Jameton, distributive justice appears at three levels of health care: national policies and budget, state or local distribution of resources, and distribution in the individual health care settings.[6]

As health care resources become increasingly more scarce, allocation of resources to certain programs and rationing of resources within certain programs will become more evident.[9] Allocation of resources brings ethical challenges to the daily clinical realities facing health care practitioners.[10]

MEDICAL FUTILITY

The concept of medical futility has resulted in various discussions and proposed criteria or formulas to predict outcomes of care.[11-14] Medical futility has both a qualitative and a quantitative basis and can be defined as "any effort to achieve a result that is possible but that reasoning or experience suggests is highly improbable and that cannot be systematically reproduced."[15]

Therapy or treatment that achieves its predictable outcome and desired effect is, by definition, effective. But effect must be distinguished from benefit. If that predictable and desired effect is of no benefit to the patient, it is therefore futile. It is suggested that when physicians conclude from either personal or colleague experiences or from empiric data that a particular treatment in the most recent 100 cases in which it has been used has been useless, the treatment should be considered futile.[15] It is incumbent on physicians to make optimal use of health-related resources in a technically appropriate and effective manner. Therefore in this era of escalating health care costs and limited resources, the physician has a particular responsibility to avoid futile treatment.[15]

ETHICS AS A FOUNDATION FOR NURSING PRACTICE

Traditional theories of professions include a code of ethics as the basis for the practice of professionals. The moral foundation of nursing is discussed in the literature by various authors who describe the unique relationship of the professional nurse with the patient, which establishes a caring, trusting approach.[16,17] It is by adherence to a code of ethics that the professional fulfills an obligation of quality practice to society.

Nursing Code of Ethics

The American Nurses' Association (ANA) provides the major source of ethical guidance for the nursing profession.[17] According to the preamble of the *Code for Nurses,* "When individuals become nurses, they make a moral commitment to uphold the values and special moral obligations expressed in their code."[17] The 11 statements of the Code are found in Box 2-2. They are based on the underlying assumption that nursing is concerned with protection, promotion, and restoration of health; prevention of illness; and the alleviation of suffering of patients.[17]

ETHICAL DECISION-MAKING IN CRITICAL CARE

As discussed earlier in this chapter, the critical care nurse encounters ethical issues on a daily basis. Because the nurse is on the "front line" with such issues as do not re-

CODE OF ETHICS FOR NURSES

1. The nurse provides services with respect for human dignity and the uniqueness of the client, unrestricted by considerations of social or economic status, personal attributes, or the nature of health problems.
2. The nurse safeguards the client's right to privacy by judiciously protecting information of a confidential nature.
3. The nurse acts to safeguard the client and the public when health care and safety are affected by the incompetent, unethical, or illegal practice of any person.
4. The nurse assumes responsibility and accountability for individual nursing judgments and actions.
5. The nurse maintains competence in nursing.
6. The nurse exercises informed judgment and uses individual competence and qualifications as criteria in seeking consultation, accepting responsibilities, and delegating nursing activities to others.
7. The nurse participates in activities that contribute to the ongoing development of the profession's body of knowledge.
8. The nurse participates in the profession's efforts to implement and improve standards of nursing.
9. The nurse participates in the profession's efforts to establish and maintain conditions of employment conducive to high quality nursing care.
10. The nurse participates in the profession's effort to protect the public from misinformation and misrepresentation and to maintain the integrity of nursing.
11. The nurse collaborates with members of the health professions and other citizens in promoting community and national efforts to meet the health needs of the public.

From the American Nurses Association: *Code for nurses with interpretive statements,* Washington, DC, 1985, The Association.

STEPS IN ETHICAL DECISION-MAKING

1. Identify the health problem.
2. Define the ethical issue.
3. Gather additional information.
4. Delineate the decision maker.
5. Examine ethical and moral principles.
6. Explore alternative options.
7. Implement decisions.
8. Evaluate and modify actions.

Before the application of any decision model, a decision must be made about the existence of a true ethical dilemma. Thompson and Thompson[22] delineated the following criteria for defining moral and ethical dilemmas in clinical practice: (1) an issue with different options, (2) an awareness of the different options, (3) two or more of the options have true or "good" aspects and the choice of one over the other compromises the option not chosen.

Steps in Ethical Decision-Making

To facilitate the ethical decision process, a model or framework must be used so that all involved will consistently and clearly examine the multiple ethical issues that arise in critical care. Steps in ethical decision-making are listed in Box 2-3.

Step one

First, the major aspects of the medical and health problem must be identified. In other words, the scientific basis of the problem, potential sequelae, prognosis, and all data relevant to the health status must be examined.

Step two

The ethical problem must be clearly delineated from other types of problems. Systems problems—that is, those resulting from failures and inadequacies in the organization and operation of the health care facility and the health care system as a whole—are often misinterpreted as being ethical issues. Occasionally, a social problem that stems from conditions existing in the community, state, or country as a whole is also confused with ethical issues. Social problems can lead to a systemic problem, which can constrain responses to ethical problems.

Step three

Although categories of necessary additional information will vary, whatever is missing in the initial problem presentation should be obtained. If not already known, the health prognosis and potential sequelae should be clarified. Usual demographic data—such as age, ethnicity, religious preferences, and educational and economic status—may be considered in the decision process. The

suscitate (DNR) orders, response to treatments, and application of new technologies and new protocols, he or she may be the one who best knows the patient's and/or family's wishes about treatment prolongation or cessation. Therefore it is important that the nurse be included as part of the health care team that determines ethical dilemma resolution.[18,19]

What is an Ethical Dilemma?

In general, ethical cases are not always clear-cut or black and white but rather arise in settings and circumstances that involve innumerable side issues and distractions.[20,21] The most common ethical dilemmas encountered in critical care are foregoing treatment and allocating the scarce resource of critical care. But how does one know that a true ethical dilemma exists?

role of the family or extended family and other support systems needs to be examined. Any desires that the patient may have expressed either in writing or in conversation about treatment decisions are essential to obtain.

Step four

The patient is the primary decision maker and autonomously makes these decisions after receiving information about the alternatives and sequelae of treatments or lack of treatments. However, in many ethical dilemmas, the patient is not competent to make a decision, such as when he or she is comatose or otherwise physically or mentally unable to make a decision. It is in these situations that surrogates are designated or court appointed because the urgency of the situation requires a quick decision. Although the decision process and ultimate decision are more important than who makes the decision, delineating the decision maker is an important step in the process.[22]

Others who are involved in the decision also need to be identified at this time, such as family, nurse, physician, social worker, clergy, and any other members of disciplines having close contact with the patient. The role of the nurse must be examined. There may not be a need for a nurse decision; rather the nurse may provide additional information and support to the decision maker.

Step five

Personal values, beliefs, and moral convictions of all involved in the decision process need to be known. Whether actually achieved through a group meeting or through personal introspection, values clarification facilitates the decision process.

General ethical principles need to be examined in relation to the case at hand. For instance, are veracity, informed consent, and autonomy promoted? Beneficence and nonmaleficence will be analyzed as they relate to the patient's condition and desires. Close examination of these principles will reveal any compromise of ethical or moral principles for either the patient or the health care provider and assist in decision-making.

Step six

After the identification of alternative options, the outcome of each action must be predicted. This analysis helps one to select the option with the best "fit" for the specific situation or problem. Both short-range and long-range consequences of each action must be examined, and new or creative actions must be encouraged. Consideration also must be given to the "no action" option, which is also a choice.[22]

Step seven

When a decision has been reached, it is usually after much thought and consideration and rarely does complete agreement occur among all interested persons.[22]

Step eight

Evaluation of an ethical decision serves to both assess the decision at hand and use it as a basis for future ethical decisions. If outcomes are not as predicted, it may be possible to modify the plan or to use an alternative that was not originally chosen.

Legal Issues

When a nurse commences employment in a critical care facility and assumes the care of a patient, a relationship is created between patient and nurse and between employer and nurse. Every state has a law mandating entry-level educational requirements to become licensed to practice nursing. Thus the act of licensing creates a legal relationship between the nurse and the state.

These relationships impose legal obligations. For example, the nurse owes a patient the duty of reasonable and prudent care under the circumstances. The nurse owes the employer the duty of competency and the ability to follow policies and procedures; other contractual duties may exist as well. The nurse owes the state and public the duty of safe, competent practice as legally defined by practice standards.

The critical care nurse's legal duties are enforceable, and the nurse can be held legally accountable for breach or violation through a variety of laws and legal processes. The scope of legal issues in nursing is broad. Nurses need to seek their own legal advice and counsel for any questions and concerns and not rely on the overview of material provided in this chapter.

TORT LIABILITY

The area of civil law is divided into many categories, two of which are *contracts* and *torts*. The law of contracts contains a set of rules governing the creation and enforcement of an agreement between two or more parties (entities or individuals). A tort is a type of civil wrong, meaning that a dispute resulted from an occurrence between the parties. Tort law is generally divided into intentional and unintentional torts, specific torts, and strict liability. Box 2-4 classifies torts and lists examples within each category.

Intentional torts involve (1) intent and (2) an act. Intent exists when the actor intends to achieve a particular outcome and consequence. Assault, battery, false imprisonment, trespass, and infliction of emotional distress are all examples of intentional torts. In each of these torts, a specific act is required, and there is intentional interference with a person or property.

In *assault,* the act is behavior that places the plaintiff (the one being wronged who later sues) in fear or apprehension of offensive physical contact. In civil law the person being sued for wronging another is referred to as the *defendant. Battery* is the unlawful or offensive touching of or contact with the plaintiff or something attached to the plaintiff. *False imprisonment* is detaining, confining, or re-

BOX 2-4

CLASSIFICATION OF TORTS

INTENTIONAL TORTS
Assault
Battery
False imprisonment
Trespass
Infliction of emotional distress

UNINTENTIONAL TORTS
Negligence
Medical/nursing treatment torts
 Professional malpractice
Abandonment

SPECIFIC TORTS
Defamation
 Slander
 Libel
Invasion of privacy

STRICT LIABILITY
Products liability

straining another against his or her will. There are two types of *trespass:* one type involves a person's land, and the other involves his or her personal property. These acts are defined as unauthorized entry onto land of another or unauthorized handling of another's personal property. In addition, the law protects a person's interest in peace of mind through the tort claim of *infliction of mental or emotional distress.* The act here, however, must be one of extreme misconduct or outrageous behavior.

Unintentional torts involve failures or breach of nursing duties that lead to harm, including negligence, malpractice, and abandonment. *Negligence* is the failure to meet an ordinary standard of care, resulting in injury to the patient or plaintiff. *Malpractice* is a type of professional liability based on negligence and includes professional misconduct, breach of a duty or standard of care, illegal or immoral conduct, or failure to exercise reasonable skill, all of which lead to harm. A more complete discussion of the elements of these torts is found later in this chapter. *Abandonment* is a type of negligence in which a duty to give care exists, is ignored, and results in harm to a patient. It is the absence of care and the failure to respond to a patient that may give rise to an allegation of abandonment.

Specific torts involve privacy interests and interests one has in his or her reputation. Defamation and invasion of privacy are both examples of such torts. *Defamation* is composed of two torts, *slander* (oral defamation) and *libel* (written defamation). Defamation is not the mere statement or writing of words that injures one's reputation or good name; the words must be communicated to another. If the words are true, this may provide a defense against a defamation claim. *Invasion of privacy* involves the violation of a person's right to privacy. Nurses can invade another's privacy by revealing confidential information

without authorization or by failing to follow the patient's health care decisions.

ADMINISTRATIVE LAW AND LICENSING STATUTES

A second type of law and legal process in which nurses are involved is administrative law and the regulatory process. This area of law governs the nurse's relationship with the government, either state or federal. Administrative law involves the rules of the government's activities in regulating health care delivery and practice, and the rules of investigation, procedure, and evidence differ from the civil and criminal law. Several government health care agencies are involved in such regulation.

A state has the power to regulate nursing because the state is responsible for the health, safety, and welfare of its citizens. Therefore establishing minimal entry-level requirements, standards of nursing practice, and educational requirements are acceptable state actions. State legislatures create laws governing nursing practice (generally termed *nurse practice acts*), and a unit of the state government within the executive branch is responsible for the enforcement of nursing laws. This unit is often called the State Board of Nursing or Board of Nurse Examiners; however, names vary by states. Standards also vary by state, which is another important reason that nurses seek advice from counsel licensed to practice law in their own state.

NEGLIGENCE AND MALPRACTICE

As defined earlier, negligence is an unintentional tort involving a breach of duty or failure (through an act or an omission) to meet a standard of care, causing patient harm. Malpractice is a type of professional liability based on negligence in which the defendant is held accountable for breach of a duty of care involving special knowledge and skill. These torts have several elements, all of which the plaintiff has the burden of proving.

Definition of Elements

The law recognizes the following four elements of negligence and malpractice (Box 2-5). The first element is *duty,* or legal obligation, that requires the actor to conform to a certain standard of conduct for the protection of others against unreasonable risks.[23] The critical care nurse's legal duty is to act in a reasonable and prudent manner, as any other critical care nurse would act under similar circumstances. The standard is that of a critical care nurse—one with special knowledge and skill in critical care. The standard is one that is owed at the time the incident or injury occurred, not at the time of litigation. In most jurisdictions, the standard of care is a national standard, as opposed to a local or community standard.

Breach of duty, the second element, involves a failure on the actor's part to conform to the standard required. *Causation,* the third element, involves proving that the ac-

---

BOX 2-5

ESSENTIAL ELEMENTS OF NEGLIGENCE AND MALPRACTICE

- Duty and standard of care
- Breach of duty
- Causation
- Injury or damages

BOX 2-6

EXAMPLES OF CRITICAL CARE NURSING ACTIONS INVOLVED IN NEGLIGENCE LAWSUITS

GENERAL

- Failure to advise physician and/or supervisor of change in patient's health status
- Failure to monitor patients at requisite intervals
- Failure to adhere to established institutional protocols
- Failure to adequately assess clinical status
- Failure to respond to alarms
- Failure to maintain accurate, timely, and complete medical records
- Failure to properly carry out treatment and evaluate results of treatment
- Failure to use safe, functional equipment

SPECIFIC

- Failure to provide supplemental oxygen when the ventilator cannot be promptly reattached
- Failure to properly use intravenous infusion equipment, causing extensive extravasation of fluid
- Failure to monitor intravenous infusions, recognize infiltration, and discontinue intravenous therapy
- Failure to recognize signs of intracranial bleeding
- Failure to investigate patient's complaint of pain and discover hematoma under blood pressure cuff

---

tor's breach was reasonably close or causally connected to the resulting injury. This is also referred to as *proximate cause.* The fourth element, *injury or damages,* must involve an actual loss or damage to the plaintiff or his or her interest. A plaintiff may claim different types of damages, such as compensatory and/or punitive. Patient injury can range in value, depending on what happened to the patient. The plaintiff must produce evidence of the damages and their value. If the nurse breaches a standard of care that leads to injury, the plaintiff must show what amount of money will compensate for his or her injuries. The goal of the compensation is to provide the amount of money that will place the plaintiff back in the position he or she was in before the injury occurred.

Res ipsa loquitur is a rule of evidence used by plaintiffs in negligence or malpractice litigation. It literally means "the thing speaks for itself." It is a rebuttable presumption or inference of negligence by the defendant, which arises on plaintiff's proof that (1) the injury is one that ordinarily does not happen in the absence of negligence and (2) the instrumentality causing the injury was in the defendant's exclusive management and control. The burden then shifts to the defendant to prove absence of negligence. For example, negligence can be inferred when muscle ischemia and necrosis occur as a result of improper body positioning and the application of splints or restraints. Negligence can also be inferred from a foreign object left in a patient's body cavity after surgery.

Because critical care nurses deal with life-threatening situations, patient injury is potentially severe or may result in death. Should this occur as a result of negligence, the nurse may be held liable for the patient's death and also for the resulting loss to surviving family members.

Box 2-6 illustrates specific examples of critical care nursing actions that have resulted in litigation. In cases such as these, the nurse's action is central to the lawsuit. However, nurses are named as sole or codefendants in a comparatively small percentage of cases. Although this pattern is changing, physicians and hospitals are generally named as defendants.

Legal Doctrines and Theories of Liability

In tort law there are several theories of liability under which the nurse's action may be examined and legal duties defined:

- Personal
- Vicarious: *respondeat superior*
- Corporate
- Other doctrines (e.g., temporary or borrowed servant; captain of the ship)

Under the theory of *personal liability,* each individual is responsible for his or her own actions. This includes the critical care nurse, the supervisor, the physician, the hospital, and the patient. Each has responsibilities that are uniquely his or her own. In contrast to personal liability, one may be afforded the protection of personal immunity.

Vicarious liability is indirect responsibility—for example, the liability of an employer for the acts of the employee. Under the doctrine of *respondeat superior,* a master is liable for certain wrongful acts of a servant, as is a principal for those of an agent. An employer may be liable for an employee's acts that are performed within the legitimate scope of employment. In critical care, the nurse typically is an employee of a hospital. However, nurses may be independent contractors with the hospital through critical care nursing agencies or businesses. If the latter is the case, the nurse is not an employee of the hospital and the hospital is not vicariously liable for the nurse's action.

Corporate liability is the liability attached to the corporate entity (e.g., the hospital) for its own corporate activities and decisions.

Other doctrines, such as *temporary or borrowed servant* and *captain of the ship,* may apply to the critical care nurse and the critical care unit. These doctrines are used when the plaintiff argues that the physician is responsible for the nurse's actions, even though the nurse is an employee of the hospital, not of the physician. If it can be shown that the nurse acted under the direction and control of the physician, it is possible that the physician may be accountable for the nurse's actions. However, these doctrines are becoming increasingly uncommon. What viability remains is typically found in cases involving nurse anesthetists and operating room nurses.

NURSE PRACTICE ACTS

The practice of nursing is regulated by the state. As a general rule, the state's police power to regulate prevails as long as the state's actions are not arbitrary or capricious. All nurses must be licensed to practice under their individual state's licensure statutes. Licensure authorizes (1) the right to practice and (2) access to employment. Therefore licensure is a property right that is constitutionally protected.[24] Every state has legislation that defines the legal scope of nursing practice and defines unprofessional and illegal conduct that may lead to investigation and disciplinary action by the state and sanctions on the right to practice. The state nurse practice act establishes entry requirements, definitions of practice, and criteria for discipline. Although licensure is mandatory for registered nurses, statutory content varies among the states.

Generally, state law contains two definitions of nursing: one for the registered (or professional) nurse and one for the licensed practical (or vocational or technical) nurse. These definitions determine titles that may be used by nurses, the scope of nursing practice, and requirements for entering the nursing profession. In some states, advanced registered nursing practice, prescriptive authority for certain nurses, and third-party reimbursement are also defined by statute. Mandatory continuing education requirements are also defined by statute in most states. The state authorizes its board of nursing to monitor practice, implement standards of care, enforce rules and regulations, and issue sanctions. Sanctions include additional education, restricted practice, supervised practice, license suspension, and license revocation. Some form of disciplinary action generally occurs as a result of unauthorized practice, negligence or malpractice, incompetence, chemical or other impairment, criminal acts, or violations of specific nurse practice act provisions.

Because it is afforded constitutional protection, the right to practice cannot be violated without due process of the law. The amount of due process in administrative law differs from other legal processes. Due process involves notice to the nurse that a complaint has been filed (voluntarily or by mandate); the notice is written and contains the charges against the nurse. Nurses in this situation should seek independent legal counsel immediately; the state will not provide it. The nurse must be given an opportunity to be heard, often in more than one forum, and be given the right to present his or her own evidence.

BOX 2-7

DELEGATION DECISION-MAKING TOOLS

THE FIVE RIGHTS OF DELEGATION[26]
- Right task
- Right circumstances
- Right person
- Right direction/communication
- Right supervision

DECISION GRID FOR DELEGATION[25]
- Potential for harm
- Complexity of task
- Problem solving and innovation necessary
- Unpredictability of outcome
- Level of interaction required with patient

Chemical impairment is a common reason for disciplinary action. In some states, the impaired nurse may avoid serious sanctions by voluntarily suspending practice and entering a rehabilitation program. This must be done with the advice of counsel (the nurse's own lawyer). Generally, this option is available as long as no patient has been harmed because of the nurse's impairment.

Delegation Issues

In order to provide quality, efficient, and effective health care, nurses have developed various assistive care-provider roles to support the delivery of nursing care. Questions and concerns have been voiced by individual nurses and professional nursing organizations regarding the appropriateness of types of care activities that the professional nurse may delegate to the non-licensed assistive personnel.[25-28]

Delegation has been defined by the National Council of State Boards of Nursing as "Transferring to a competent individual the authority to perform a selected nursing task in a selected situation. The nurse retains accountability for the delegation."[26] Additionally, "Inappropriate delegation by the nurse and/or unauthorized performance of nursing tasks by unlicensed assistive personnel may lead to legal action against the licensed nurse and/or unlicensed assistive personnel."[26]

The act of delegation must ensure that the professional registered nurse coordinates safe, effective patient care. Delegation allows the registered nurse to perform functions that only registered nurses can perform and utilizes the full potential of the whole health care team. Much has been published regarding what and how to delegate and how to assist professional registered nurses with the ability to delegate.[25-30] Box 2-7 delineates two methods to facilitate delegation.[25-26] Readers are referred to the published citations for in-depth description of delegation.

SPECIFIC PATIENT CARE ISSUES

Myriad legal issues and controversies exist in the field of critical care. Concerns commonly arise in the areas of (1) informed consent and authorization for treatment and (2) the patient's right to accept or refuse medical treatment.

Informed Consent and Authorization for Treatment

Intrinsic to the doctrine of informed consent is the physician's legal duty to disclose certain information to the patient and the patient's legal right to *informed consent* and to subsequently refuse or accept medical treatment. Central to critical care nursing is the issue of the extent to which the nurse is involved in obtaining consent. As a general rule, the physician cannot delegate this function entirely to a registered nurse, and the nurse's exposure to liability increases if the nurse accepts full responsibility for obtaining the patient's consent. It is common nursing practice to witness and document the procedure and to obtain the patient's signature after the physician has disclosed the required information.

There are two types of consent: *express* and *implied*. *Express consent* may be written or verbal and is the consent given specifically for nonroutine procedures. *Implied consent* may be implied in fact, an assumption based on patient behavior (e.g., the patient extending an arm for venipuncture or nodding approval), or it may be implied in law (e.g., an unconscious, hemorrhaging patient in the emergency department). The following discussion summarizes the elements of valid informed consent, the adequacy of consent and negligent nondisclosure, and exceptions to consent requirements and the duty to disclose.

Valid consent must be (1) voluntary, (2) obtained, and (3) informed. Although consent can be either verbal or written, most hospital policies require that informed, voluntary consent to nonroutine procedures be obtained and confirmed in writing: signed and dated by the patient, physician, and witness (if required). Most informed consent statutes provide that a consent, in writing, to a medical or surgical procedure that meets the consent and disclosure requirements of the statute creates a legal presumption that informed consent was given.

In the vast majority of jurisdictions the decision maker (the one giving the consent) must be a legally competent adult (i.e., having reached majority or, in most states, the age of 18 years). Competence is a legal judgment, and, as a general rule, there is a legal presumption of patient competence.[31] One is mentally incompetent (thereby rendering a consent invalid) if adjudicated incompetent. One must likewise have the capacity (a medical and nursing judgment) to give consent: the patient must be oriented and understand what he or she has been told; medications the patient is taking must be documented. In those adults legally adjudicated incompetent, the guardian may give consent if the guardian has been given this authority.

Minors are legally incompetent, and consent is obtained from the parent or guardian. However, in many jurisdictions there are two important exceptions to this rule: (1) mature minors may consent to treatment for substance abuse, sexually transmitted disease, and matters involving contraception and reproduction; and (2) emancipated minors may consent to treatment in general (minors are considered emancipated if married or divorced before the age of majority, if in the military service, or if living independently with parental consent).

Consent must also be informed and timely. The physician has a duty to disclose the following: diagnosis, condition, prognosis, material risks and benefits associated with the treatment or procedure, explanation of the treatment, providers of the treatment (who is performing, supervising, and/or assisting in the procedure), material risks and benefits of alternative therapy, and the probable outcome (including material risks and benefits) if the patient refuses the treatment or procedure. Failure to disclose such information or inadequate disclosure with resultant injury may constitute negligence and give rise to tort claims of malpractice, battery, negligent nondisclosure, and abandonment. Consent is generally valid for 7 to 30 days. However, the time at which consent expires must be explicitly stated in the institutional policy and procedure manual.

There are many exceptions to consent requirements and the duty to disclose, and clearly the exceptions vary according to jurisdiction. Emergencies constitute one exception unless the patient refuses treatment or has previously made a competent and informed refusal. States vary significantly in the following treatment situations: endangered fetal viability, alcohol or other drug detoxification, emergency blood transfusions, caesarean sections, and substance abuse during pregnancy. Jurisdictions also vary on the issue of sources of consent (informal directives) for the incompetent patient or the patient in an emergency who has no legal guardian. Alternatives include consensus from as many next of kin as possible, with evidence that (1) the treatment is reasonable and necessary and (2) the family's decision would not be contrary to the patient's wishes (this is known as substituted judgment made by a surrogate decision maker). Another alternative is a court order for treatment. In the absence of substituted judgment, many courts use what is known as the *best interests standard*.

Lawsuits involving informed consent and the duty to disclose generally require three elements: (1) proof that the health care provider failed to disclose an existing material risk unknown to the patient or alternatives to the proposed treatment, (2) proof that the patient would not have consented if the risk had been disclosed (in other words, that disclosure of the risk would have led a reasonable patient in the plaintiff's position to refuse the procedure or choose a different course of treatment), and (3) proof of injury occurring as a result of the failure to disclose.[32,33]

The Right to Accept or Refuse Medical Treatment and the Law of Advance Directives

The right to consent and informed consent includes the right to refuse treatment. In most cases a competent adult's decision to refuse even life-sustaining treatment is honored.[34-38] The underlying rationale is that the patient's right to withdraw or withhold treatment is not outweighed by the state's interest in preserving life.

There are some situations in which the right to refuse treatment is not honored. These include, but are not limited to, the following situations:

- The treatment relates to a contagious illness that threatens the health of the public.
- Innocent third parties will suffer (e.g., a parent's wish to refuse a blood transfusion most likely would be overruled to save the life of a child).
- The refusal violates ethical standards (e.g., a Massachusetts court held that a hospital was not required to compromise its ethical principles by following a patient's decision but must cooperate in the transfer of the patient to a hospital that is willing to cooperate).
- Treatment must be instituted to prevent suicide and to preserve life.

Withholding and Withdrawing Treatment

As indicated earlier, an adult has the right to refuse treatment, even treatment that sustains life. This right means that the critical care nurse may participate in the withholding or withdrawing of treatment. Historically, the distinction between withholding and withdrawing treatments was considered the issue of importance but that is no longer the case. Health care decisions become most complex when patients lose competency and capacity to personally make their own decisions.

Orders Not to Resuscitate and Other Orders

Hospital policies that address orders to withhold or withdraw treatment should exist in all critical care units. For example, orders not to resuscitate—commonly referred to as do-not-resuscitate (DNR) orders—should be governed by written policies, including, but not limited to, the following:

- DNR orders should be entered in the patient's record with full documentation by the responsible physician about the patient's prognosis and the patient's agreement (if he or she is capable) or, alternatively, the family's consensus.
- DNR orders should have the concurrence of another physician designated in the policy.
- Policies should specify that orders are reviewed periodically (some policies require daily review).

- Patients with capacity must give their informed consent.
- For patients without capacity, that incapacity must be thoroughly documented, along with the diagnosis, prognosis, and family consensus.
- Judicial intervention before writing a DNR order is usually indicated when the patient's family does not agree or there is uncertainty or disagreement about the patient's prognosis or mental status. As a general rule, however, in the absence of conflict or disagreement, DNR orders are legal in a majority of jurisdictions if executed clearly and properly.
- Policies should specify who is to be contacted and notified within the hospital administration.

Other orders to withhold or withdraw treatment may involve mechanical ventilation, dialysis, nutritional support, hydration, and medications such as antibiotics. The legal and ethical implications of these orders for each patient must be carefully considered. Hospitals should have written policies on all orders to withhold and withdraw treatment. Policies must cover how decisions will be made: who will decide and what the roles of patient, family, health care providers, and the institution will be. Policies must be developed that consider state laws and judicial opinions.

Advance Directives

Rarely has a case so galvanized public opinion as the case of Nancy Cruzan.[40-47] In *Cruzan* the issue before the U.S. Supreme Court was to consider whether Cruzan had a federal constitutional right that would require the hospital to withdraw life-sustaining treatment from her. The court rejected the request for authority to withdraw artificial nutrition and hydration and held that the U.S. Constitution did not prohibit the state of Missouri from requiring clear and convincing evidence of Cruzan's wishes before treatment withdrawal.

The court stated that when a person is incompetent and unable to exercise the right to refuse treatment and a surrogate must act on his or her behalf, the state may institute procedural safeguards to ensure that the surrogate honors the wishes expressed by the person while competent. The court also held that the U.S. Constitution does not require a state to accept the substituted judgment of the family; the state may recognize only a personal right to make such health care decisions. A state may choose to defer only to the person's express wishes, rather than relying on the family's decision.

The Cruzan decision quickly mobilized the U.S. Congress to pass landmark legislation known as the Patient Self-Determination Act/Omnibus Budget Reconciliation Act of 1990.[48-57] The statute requires that all adults must be provided written information on an individual's rights under state law to make medical decisions, including the right to refuse treatment and the right to formulate advance directives.

The 1990 law mandates that providers of health care services under Medicare and Medicaid must comply with requirements relating to patient advance directives, which are written instructions recognized under state law for provisions of care when persons are incapacitated. Providers may not be reimbursed for the care they provide unless the requirements of this provision are met.

Providers must have written policies and procedures to (1) inform all adult patients at the time treatment is initiated of their right to execute an advance directive and of the provider's policies on the implementation of that right, (2) document in medical records whether an individual has executed an advance directive, (3) not condition care and treatment or otherwise discriminate on the basis of whether a patient has executed an advance directive, (4) comply with state laws on advance directives, and (5) provide information and education to staff and the community on advance directives.

Patients themselves can provide clear direction by preparing in advance written documents that specify their wishes. These documents are termed *advance directives* and include the *living will* and *durable power of attorney for health care.* To be effective in a jurisdiction, both of these directives must be statutorily or judicially recognized. The living will specifies that if certain circumstances occur, such as terminal illness, the patient will decline specific treatment, such as cardiopulmonary resuscitation and mechanical ventilation. The living will does not cover all treatment. For example, in some states nutritional support may not be declined through a living will. The durable power of attorney for health care is a directive through which a patient designates an agent—someone who will make decisions for the patient if the patient becomes unable to do so.

References

1. Guralnik D, editor: *Webster's new world dictionary of the American language,* New York, 1981, Simon & Shuster.
2. Catalano JT: Systems of ethics: a perspective, *Crit Care Nurs* 14(6):91, 1992.
3. Fowler M: Introduction to ethics and ethical theory: a road map to the discipline. In Fowler M, Levine-Ariff J, editors: *Ethics at the bedside,* Philadelphia, 1987, JB Lippincott.
4. Krekeler K: Critical care nursing and moral development, *Crit Care Nurs* 10(2):1, 1987.
5. Singleton KA, Dever R: The challenge of autonomy: respecting the patient's wishes, *DCCN* 10(3):160, 1991.
6. Jameton A: Duties to self: professional nursing in the critical care unit. In Fowler M, Levine-Ariff J, editors: *Ethics at the bedside,* Philadelphia, 1987, JB Lippincott.
7. Aroskar M: Fidelity and veracity: questions of promise keeping, truth telling and loyalty. In Fowler M, Levine-Ariff J, editors: *Ethics at the bedside,* Philadelphia, 1987, JB Lippincott.
8. Omery A: A healthy death, *Heart Lung* 20(3):310, 1991.
9. White J: Rationing health care resources, *Nurs Connect* 4(1):22, 1991.
10. Terry P, Rushton CH: Allocation of scarce resources: ethical challenges, clinical realities, *Am J Crit Care* 5(5):326, 1996.
11. Miles S: Health-care reform and clinical ethics: old values for new times, *AACN Clin Issues Crit Care Nurs* 5(3):299, 1994.
12. Noland LR: Medical futility: a bedside perspective, *AACN Clin Issues Crit Care Nurs* 5(3):366, 1994.
13. Montague J.: A futile-care formula may ease end-of-life issues, *Hosp Health Netw* 4:176, August, 1994.
14. Taylor C: Medical futility and nursing, *Image J Nurs Sch* 27(4):301, 1995.
15. Schneiderman LJ, Jecker NS, Jonsen AR: Medical futility: its meaning and ethical implications, *Ann Intern Med* 112(12):949, 1990.
16. Curtin L: Collegial ethics of a caring profession, *Nurs Manag* 25(8):28, 1994.
17. American Nurses Association: *Code for nurses with interpretive statements,* Kansas City, Mo, 1985, The Association.
18. (No author listed): Nurses bring holistic view to ethical decision making, *Med Ethics Advisor* 9(5):49, 1993.
19. Holly C, Lyons M: Increasing your decision-making role in ethical situations, *DCCN* 12(5):264, 1993.
20. Broom C: Conflict resolution strategies: when ethical dilemmas evolve into conflict, *DCCN* 10(6):354, 1991.
21. Wicclair MR: Differentiating ethical decisions from clinical standards, *DCCN* 10(5):280, 1991.
22. Thompson J, Thompson H: *Bioethical decision-making for nurses,* Norwalk, Conn, 1985, Appleton-Century-Crofts.
23. Prosser WL, et al: *The law of torts,* ed 5, St Paul, Minn, 1988, West.
24. Walker DJ: Nursing 1980: new responsibility, new liability, *Trial* 16(12):43, 1980.
25. American Association of Critical Care Nurses: *Delegation of nursing and nonnursing activities in critical care,* Aliso Viejo, CA, 1990, The Association.
26. National Council of State Boards of Nursing, Inc: *Delegation: concepts and decision making process,* Chicago, IL, 1995, The Council.
27. Canavan K: Combating dangerous delegation, *AJN* 97(5):57-58, 1997.
28. Boucher MA: Delegation alert, *AJN* 98(2):26-33, 1998.
29. Johnson SH: Teaching nursing delegation: analyzing nurse practice acts, *J Contin Educ Nurs* 27(2):52-58, 1997.
30. Parsons LC: Delegating decision making, *JONA* 27(2):47-52, 1997.
31. Northrop CE: Nursing practice and the legal presumption of competency, *Nurs Outlook* 36(2):112, 1988.
32. Murphy EK: Informed consent doctrine: little danger of liability for nurses, *Nurs Outlook* 39(1):48, 1991.
33. Pauscher v. Iowa Methodist Med Center, 408 N.W.2d 355 (Iowa 1987).
34. Bouvia v. Superior Court, 225 Cal. Rptr. 297; 179 C.A.3d 1127, review denied (Cal. App. 1986).
35. In Re Farrell, 529 A.2d 404 (N.J. 1987).
36. McKay v. Bergstedt, 801 P.2d 617 (Nev. 1990).
37. State v. McAfee, 385 S.E.2d 651 (Ga. 1989).
38. Wilson-Clayton ML, Clayton MA: Two steps forward, one step back: McKay v. Bergstedt, *Whittier L Rev* 12:439, 1991.
39. Brophy v. New England Sinai Hosp., 497 N.E.2d 626 (Mass. 1986).
40. Cruzan v. Director, Missouri Dept. of Health, 110 S. Ct. 2841 (U.S. S. Ct. 1990).
41. Cruzan v. Director, Missouri Dept. of Health and the right to die: a symposium, *Ga I Rev* 25:1139, 1991.
42. Cruzan v. Missouri, USLW 58:4916, 1990.
43. Guarino KS, Antoine MP: The case of Nancy Cruzan: the Supreme Court's decision, *Crit Care Nurs* 11(1):32, 1991.
44. Kyba F: Decisions at the end of life: implications following Cruzan, *Tex Nurs* 65(2):13, 1991.
45. Morgan RC: How to decide: decisions on life-prolonging procedures, *Stetson L Rev* 20:77, 1990.
46. Quill T: Death and dignity, *N Engl J Med* 324(10):691, 1991.
47. Right to die symposium, *Issues Law Med* 7:169, 1991.

48. Iowa Hospital Association, Iowa Medical Society, Iowa State Bar Association: *Advance directives for health care: deciding today about your care in the future,* 1991, author.

49. American Hospital Association: *Put it in writing: a guide to promoting advance directives,* American Hospital Association, 840 North Lake Shore Drive, Chicago, Ill, 60611, 800-242-2626.

50. Cate FH, Gill BA: *The Patient Self-Determination Act: implementation issues and opportunities,* Washington, DC, 1991, The Annenberg Washington Program.

51. Choice in Dying: *Advance directive protocols and the Patient Self-Determination Act: a resource manual for the development of institutional protocols,* Choice in Dying, 200 Varick Street, New York, NY, 10014, 212-366-5540, 1991 (formerly Society for the Right to Die/Concern for Dying, 250 West 57th Street, New York, NY, 10107, 212-246-6962).

52. Emanuel L, Emanuel E: The medical directive: a new comprehensive advance care document, *JAMA* 261(22):3, 288, 1989.

53. Iowa Hospital Association: *The Patient Self-Determination Act of 1990: implementation in Iowa hospitals,* Iowa Hospital Association, 100 East Grand, Suite 100, Des Moines, Ia, 50309, 515-288-1955, 1991.

54. National Hospice Organization: *Advance medical directives,* National Hospice Organization, 1901 North Moore Street, Suite 901, Arlington, Va, 22209, 703-243-5900, 1991.

55. National Health Lawyers Association: *The patient self-determination directory and resources guide,* National Health Lawyers Association, 1620 Eye Street NW, Suite 900, Washington, DC, 20006, 202-833-1100, 1991.

56. *Patient Self-Determination Act/Omnibus Budget Reconciliation Act of 1990,* Pub L No 101-508, Sec. 4206; 42 U.S.C. Sec. 1395cc(a)(1) (1990).

57. Unisys Corp: *Advance directives, informational release general no 122,* Unisys Corp, PO Box 10394, Des Moines, Ia 50306, 800-776-6045, 1991.

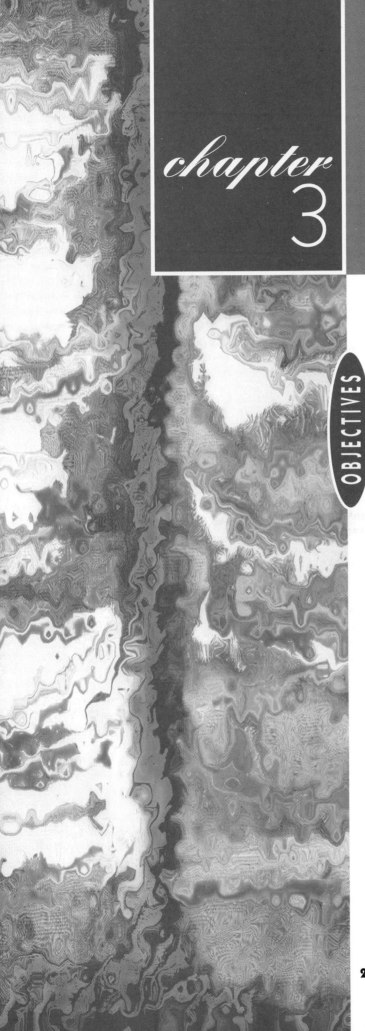

chapter 3

Patient and Family Education

Linda D. Urden

OBJECTIVES

● Adapt and apply teaching-learning theory to the critical care setting.

● Perform a learning needs assessment.

● Construct a teaching plan for patients in the critical care unit.

● Discuss four methods of instruction and the appropriateness of each to the critical care setting.

● Describe informational needs of families of critically ill patients.

CRITICAL CARE EDUCATION CHALLENGES

As the result of earlier hospital discharge, plans of care have more complicated treatment regimens and require new approaches to providing information for life-style changes.[1-3] Because of these changes, it is even more important that patients and families are provided with the information needed to make informed decisions and choices about health care alternatives.[4]

Priorities set by the critical care nurse must place maintenance of immediate physical and psychologic safety above the health promotion and educational needs. However, when the patient's clinical condition allows, the education plan can be initiated with continuation across the hospital stay into discharge. Box 3-1 delineates information that all patients and families must receive. Time constraints and the necessity to set priorities of care may limit the actual amount of time available for educating patients and families.

Along with a belief in the patient's right to know, the patient's right not to know must also be recognized in some cases. The patient's right not to know must be respected in those cases in which patients prefer not to

WHAT EVERY PATIENT NEEDS TO KNOW

- Orientation to room/environment: call light, bed controls, etc.
- Orientation to unit routines: visiting hours, frequency of monitoring and nurse assessments, lab draws, daily weights, special shift routines, etc.
- Explanations regarding reasons for equipment, monitors and associated alarms (e.g., cardiac monitor, ventilator, intravenous [IV] lines, IV pumps, pacemaker, pulse oximetry, etc.)
- Orientation to the various care providers and services that they deliver
- Explanation of all procedures, both in the unit and off the unit
- Medications: names, and why the patient is receiving them
- Transition to next level of care: reason for transfer, environment, staffing, availability of care providers
- Discharge plan: medications, diet, activity, pathophysiology of disease, symptom management, special procedures and associated equipment, when to call health care provider, community resources

THE TEACHING-LEARNING PROCESS

- Assess learning needs and readiness to learn
- Formulate teaching plan
- Implement teaching plan
- Evaluate attainment of learning objectives

The learner must be both physically and emotionally ready and able to learn.[6] The volume and complexity of information needed by persons facing new health challenges can be very confusing. In addition, there can be a significant loss of the capacity to focus and concentrate during periods after treatment and physiologic changes.[7] Patients and families may have different perceptions regarding the importance of information and whether that information was effectively communicated.[8,9] Box 3-2 delineates steps of the teaching-learning process.

Assessment

The assessment step in patient teaching involves gathering a data base to assist the nurse in meeting the patient's and family's learning needs.[6] It is a vital part of any successful educational plan. Among the components of this assessment in the critical care unit are identification of the various physiologic, psychologic, environmental, and sociocultural stressors present; the patient's response to these stressors and adaptation to illness; and an examination of motivation and readiness to learn. In reality, these issues are often related to one another and cannot be assessed as separate entities.

Readiness to Learn

Assessment of motivation and readiness to learn is an important part of the teaching-learning process. This assessment incorporates an analysis of multiple factors that have previously been discussed. These include an appreciation of multiple stressors and their response and the patient's stage of adaptation to illness. In addition, an examination of motivation theory is helpful. One well-known and important theory describing human behavior motivation is Maslow's hierarchy of needs, which provides background for the discussion of motivation to learn.

Maslow described a number of needs that were postulated as motivating all behavior. According to this theory, human beings have a number of needs that are interrelated and hierarchic. In other words, the lower-level needs must be met before higher-level needs can emerge and be satisfied.

The need to know and understand are among the highest-level needs. During a time of critical illness, a pa-

learn about their illnesses. Simple basic information about monitors and unit policy, for example, usually suffices in these cases. Indeed, more information than can be processed and integrated can greatly increase anxiety and may result in slower recovery. Individuals have the right to accept, adopt, or reject the information provided in educational encounters.

ADULT LEARNING THEORY

Central to successful implementation of an educational plan in the critical care and telemetry environment is the incorporation of the principles of adult learning theory.[5] Adult learners differ from children in several areas.[5] Adults must be ready to learn, having moved from one developmental or educational task to the next. They need to know why it is important to learn something before they can actually learn it. Inherent in their attitudes is a responsibility for their own decisions. Consequently, they may resent when others try to force different beliefs on them. Adults bring a wealth of experience to the learning environment that must be recognized and promoted in educational techniques. Their orientation to learning is life-centered, so that tasks being taught should focus on current problem resolution. Finally, motivation for the adult learner arises out of internal pressures such as self-esteem and quality of life.

TEACHING-LEARNING PROCESS

The teaching-learning process used in the health care setting incorporates the dynamics of adult learning theory.

tient's energy is often consumed by the lower-level physiologic and safety needs, and it would be impossible for the patient to attend to learning interactions. Attempting to teach a patient who fears for his or her life and safety is of little use unless the patient is being taught that he or she is safe and in no immediate danger of dying. Once the lower-level needs are met and the patient feels out of danger, he or she will be more ready to learn and higher-level needs can be addressed. Therefore if the assessment discloses significant needs in lower areas, the nurse must address those needs before attempting any teaching. Once met, these needs cease to be the primary motivators of behavior, and the patient can attend to his or her learning and other higher-level needs.

Formulate the Teaching Plan

The assessment of the multitude of factors that have been discussed assists the critical care nurse in the establishment of an adequate data base from which to formulate nursing diagnoses and devise an educational plan of care. In this plan of care, expected outcomes and behavioral objectives are identified. Refer to the Nursing Management Plan of Care for Knowledge Deficit on p. 442. Box 3-3 provides a sample education plan for patients undergoing coronary bypass surgery.

Implement the Teaching Plan

The teaching-learning experience

Patients in the critical care environment are educated in many informal interactions with the nurse, and the knowledge gained fosters patient understanding and well-being. Educational opportunities can be present during various nursing care activities, such as bathing and administration of medication. Each encounter with the patient and family must be viewed as a teaching opportunity. There are times, however, during the hospitalization when more formal or structured educational experiences are in order. Structured educational approaches have been found to be beneficial for immediate knowledge gain.[10]

The learning environment

Patient barriers to learning related to physiologic, emotional, and motivational factors have been discussed. To structure a successful teaching-learning experience in a critical care area, the nurse must also carefully assess the environmental and iatrogenic barriers that affect the interaction. Bright lights, unpleasant odors, unfamiliar noises, and untidy surroundings can distract patients and add to cognitive impairment. Control of these factors can facilitate the learning process. Factors that cannot be controlled must be explained to the patient to alleviate anxiety and facilitate a trusting relationship between patient and nurse.

Teaching methods

There are three basic methods of teaching: lecture, discussion, and demonstration. The selection of the methods will be determined by various factors, including patient clinical status, readiness to learn, cognitive abilities, learning style, instructional time, and availability of teaching materials and resources. In addition, innovative methods of teaching and presentation of educational materials must be developed and used efficiently to maximize existing resources.[11]

Lecture. Lecture is the presentation of information in a highly structured format to a group. In this method the teacher provides a great deal of material but may not provide ample opportunities for teacher-learner interaction. This style of teaching is inappropriate for acutely ill individuals in the critical care unit. However, it may be useful in the telemetry unit. Optimally, the group size should be arranged to enable the learners to ask questions and get appropriate feedback on content presented.

Discussion. Discussion is less structured than is lecturing and allows an exchange and feedback between the teacher and learner. The teacher can adapt the material to meet the needs of the individual or group. Discussion groups can be effective with hospitalized patients when a group with similar problems and at similar stages of adaptation can be gathered. Individual discussion with patients and families is appropriate and valuable during the acute phase of illness because it allows them to express their feelings and interpretations.

Demonstration. Demonstration involves acting out a procedure while giving appropriate explanations to provide the learner with a clear idea of how to perform a task. The patient can then practice the skill and be given feedback about his or her performance. This method is often used in the acute care setting, such as when coughing and deep breathing or taking one's own pulse is taught.

Other methods of instruction

In addition to the three basic methods just presented, several other approaches to delivering or augmenting information in a patient teaching program are available. They include commercially prepared or custom-designed printed materials, bedside videotape programs, and computer-assisted patient education programs.

Written materials can be very useful tools in patient and family education. They allow repetition and reinforcement of content and provide basic information in printed form for reference at a later time. To be useful, however, the content must be accurate and current, and the patient and family must be able to read and understand it.[12]

It is estimated that the median literacy level of the U.S. population is at the tenth grade level, with about 20% of the population having reading skills at the fifth grade level or lower.[13] Other research indicates that approximately 50% of health care clients have serious difficulty reading instructional materials written at the fifth grade level, and only 62% read materials given to them.[14,15] The

BOX 3-3

TEACHING PLAN FOR THE PATIENT UNDERGOING CORONARY ARTERY BYPASS SURGERY

PREOPERATIVE PHASE

During preoperative educational interactions, the nurse should assess the patient's and family's levels of anxiety and their effect on the ability or desire to learn. Preoperative education should be individualized to prepare the patient appropriately for the surgery, to provide education about postoperative care, and to minimize anxiety. Before the teaching-learning experience, the nurse should do the following:

- Assess the patient's level of anxiety and desire to learn about the upcoming surgery
- Individualize the preoperative teaching plan based on assessment findings

The following content may be included in the preoperative teaching session:

- Review of the coronary artery bypass graft (CABG) procedure
- Time leaving room for surgery, length of surgery
- Location of family waiting area
- Surgical preparation and shave
- Nothing by mouth after midnight
- What to expect when awakening from anesthesia
- Sights and sounds of the recovery room and/or critical care unit
- Tubes and drains: chest tubes, hemodynamic monitoring lines, Foley catheter, intravenous lines, pacemaker wires (if appropriate), endotracheal tube
- Inability to speak with endotracheal tube in place
- Discomfort to expect from incisions, availability of pain medication
- Coughing and deep breathing practice
- Use of incentive spirometer
- When family can visit, how long, how often
- Usual length of critical care unit stay

In addition to this content, the nurse needs to do the following:

- Reassure patient that many staff members and much activity around bedside is normal and does not indicate complications
- Elicit and answer any specific questions the patient and family have at that time
- Determine specific needs and desires for day of surgery (e.g., patient needs hearing aid or glasses as soon as possible)
- Meet with the family alone to offer support and address concerns they may not wish to voice to the patient

CRITICAL CARE UNIT PHASE

During the critical care unit phase, patient and family education is designed to meet immediate needs and reduce anxiety. The following are examples of content appropriate for this time:

- Basic explanation of bedside equipment
- Review of tubes and drains
- Turning, coughing, deep breathing
- Use of incentive spirometer
- Use of oxygen equipment

- Orientation to time, place, situation
- Explanation of procedures
- Basic purpose of medications
- Explanation of normal progression in early postoperative period
- Basic range-of-motion exercises (e.g., ankle circles, point and flex)

During this phase, the nurse also does the following:

- Reassures patient and family of normal progression
- Repeats and reinforces information as necessary
- Answers questions as they arise
- Begins early to prepare patient for transfer to prevent transfer anxiety
- Determines family learning needs and addresses them together with patient or in separate teaching sessions as appropriate

STEP-DOWN UNIT PHASE

After transfer from the critical care unit, the patient's and family's educational needs increase. Short daily educational sessions should be planned to cover the following content:

- Basic pathophysiology of coronary artery disease
- Review of surgical procedure
- Risk factors for coronary artery disease
- Upper extremity range-of-motion exercises
- Dietary recommendations (salt- and fat/cholesterol-modified diet)
- Taking of own pulse
- Recognition and treatment of angina (use of nitroglycerin)

During this phase, the nurse also does the following:

- Uses audiovisual materials in teaching sessions or as reinforcement of content
- Provides printed take-home materials outlining important content
- Answers questions as they arise

DISCHARGE TEACHING

Before discharge, the following content should be covered with the patient and family:

- Activity guidelines
- Lifting restrictions
- Incision care
- Possibility of patient being extremely fatigued or depressed after discharge
- Guidelines for return to work, driving, sexual activity
- Medication safety and administration

Before discharge, the nurse also does the following:

- Reassures patient that ups and downs are normal
- If necessary, reassures patient and family that likelihood of cardiac emergencies at home is small
- Provides printed material for further study by patient and family
- Answers questions as they arise
- Provides phone number for patient or family to call when further questions arise

---

BOX 3-4

SAMPLES OF DIFFERENT READING LEVELS

COLLEGE READING LEVEL

Consult your physician immediately with the onset of chest discomfort, shortness of breath, or increased perspiration.

TWELFTH GRADE READING LEVEL

Call your physician immediately if you experience chest discomfort, shortness of breath, or increased sweatiness.

EIGHTH GRADE READING LEVEL

Call your doctor immediately if you start having chest pain or shortness of breath or feel sweaty.

FOURTH GRADE READING LEVEL

Call your doctor right away if you start having chest pain, can't breathe, or feel sweaty.

BOX 3-5

TEACHING TIPS

- Assess patient and family learning needs
- Assess patient and family readiness to learn
- Set realistic and measurable goals
- "Clump" information together in the most simple and understandable manner
- Provide opportunity for demonstration and practice of new skill(s)
- Provide written, simple, clear instructions; consider videotape or other alternative presentation format as appropriate to patient/family learning style and teaching material
- Provide feedback and opportunity for review of information
- Individualize regimen to patient life-style and preferences
- Reinforce new knowledge and behaviors
- Ensure appropriate followup (e.g., community resources, support groups, home health care, etc.)

---

vast majority of patient education materials are written at or above the eighth grade level.[14] To ensure that the reading level of the educational material and the learner are well-matched, the patient needs to be questioned about the last grade level completed in school. Because this level may not equal the grade level in reading ability, written material two to four grade levels below that must be selected.[14] Box 3-4 depicts examples of an instruction written at various reading levels.

Videotapes can be used to address the basic and repetitive aspects of patient education for short-term knowledge gain.[16] The use of videotapes, however, is not a substitute for individualized patient teaching, and it is most effective when it is promoted by staff as reinforcing other educational activities.[16,17] It is essential that the nurse realize that audiovisual accessories are an adjunct to teaching but do not replace the central role of the nurse in objective accomplishment.

Closed-circuit television (CCTV) is becoming a common service in many health care settings. It also is best used as one component of a comprehensive educational program and is not intended to be used alone. CCTV allows for the viewing of the session to take place at the time that best suits the patient and family and can be stopped, restarted, or repeated as necessary. It ensures a consistent standard in presentation of routine educational topics.[18]

Evaluate Attainment of Learning

Evaluation of the educational plan of care focuses on the ability of the plan to attain the objectives and outcomes developed in the planning phase. This includes the documentation of the effectiveness of the teaching-learning process with measurement of the knowledge gain and behavior changes identified.[19]

In addition to the traditional evaluation of the educational plan based on objectives, other subtle effects of patient education can be identified. Less concrete but equally valuable outcomes, such as signs of relaxation when the information provided decreases anxiety or increases participation in self-care, also document beneficial effects of the educational plan. This does not negate the fact that in many situations written, measurable objectives are necessary and useful, but it does mean that they must not be the sole measures of educational success.[20] A good example of this is the interaction that occurs when a patient is taught about the cardiac monitor on admission to the critical care unit. In teaching the reason for and function of this equipment, the nurse not only increases the patient's knowledge about cardiac monitoring but may also decrease the patient's anxiety about the critical care setting, thereby promoting rest and healing. Strategies for successful teaching are summarized in Box 3-5.

Informational Needs of Families in Critical Care

Family members and significant others of critically ill patients are integral to the recovery of their loved ones. When planning for the overall care of patients, nurses and other caregivers need to consider the informational and emotional support needs of this group.[19-21] According to Henneman et al,[22] families of critically ill patients report their greatest need is for information. Flexible visiting hours and informational booklets regarding the critical care experience were recommended as ways to meet this need. Important specific information for families identified by Miracle and Hovenkamp[21] are listed in Box 3-6.

BOX 3-6

IMPORTANT INFORMATIONAL NEEDS OF FAMILIES

- To have questions answered honestly
- To know the facts about the patient's prognosis
- To know the results of procedures as soon as possible
- To have staff inform them of the patient's status
- To know why things are being done
- To know about possible complications
- To have explanations that can be understood
- To know exactly what is being done
- To know about the staff providing care
- To have directions about what to do during a procedure

TEACHING TOWARD TRANSFER FROM CRITICAL CARE

Transfer from the critical care unit to a telemetry or another acute care area can be an anxiety-producing time for patients. During the stay in the critical care unit, constant interaction with the nurse, monitoring devices, and controlled environment has offered security to the patient. To avoid anxiety, nurses prepare patients for imminent or eventual transfer—that is, teaching toward transfer. To do this, the nurse points out early in the stay that the patient will be there only temporarily until his or her condition improves and stabilizes, and these improvements will be made known to the patient on an ongoing basis. As the time for transfer approaches, careful explanations can reassure patients and families that close observation and monitoring are no longer necessary. When possible, tubes, machines, and equipment used in the critical care unit—which the patient may see as important to survival—need to be removed gradually rather than discontinued all at once. This will alleviate feelings of dependence on equipment. Transfer anxiety for patients in critical care may also be present in family members.[23]

At the time of transfer, patients and families can be told how care will change and what changes in activity, self-care, and visiting hours to expect. It is helpful to emphasize that the transfer represents an improvement in patient condition, and, contrary to common references to a "step-down" unit, telemetry units are, in fact, a "step-up." The critical care unit nurse accompanies the patient to the new floor and introduces the new staff members to the patient. The patient can be told that a complete report on his or her condition will be given and that nursing management needs at this stage of recovery will be met in the new setting. Family members should be contacted and informed of the transfer. The management plan and educational plan developed in the critical care area must accompany the patient to the floor, and the new nurses are informed about current short-term and long-term goals and the patient's progress.

Although careful preparation and planning for transfer are always desirable, a patient may be transferred unexpectedly to make room for a more critically ill patient. When this situation occurs, the patient to be moved from the unit must be notified and prepared for the possibility of a quick transfer. Tangible evidence of improvement, such as more favorable vital signs or need for fewer medications or tubes, can be helpful in pointing out advances in condition before unplanned transfers.

References

1. Seley JJ: 10 strategies for successful patient teaching, *Am J Nurs* 10:63-65, 1994.
2. Baranson S, Zimmerman L: A comparison of patient teaching outcomes among postoperative coronary artery bypass graft (CABG) patients, *Prog Cardiovasc Nurs* 10(4):11, 1995.
3. Katz JR: Back to basics—providing effective patient teaching, *Am J Nurs* 97(5):33, 1997.
4. Alberti LC: Managing patient education: a perspective for the 1990s, *Gastroenterol Nurs* 12:148, 1991.
5. Hansen M, Fisher JC: Patient-centered teaching from theory to practice, *Am J Nurs* 98(1):56, 1998.
6. Moss VA: Assessing learning abilities, readiness for education, *Semin Periop Nurs* 3(3):113, 1994.
7. Cimprich B: A theoretical perspective on attention and patient education, *ANS Adv Nurs Sci* 14(3):39, 1992.
8. Reiley P, et al: Discharge planning: comparison of patients' and nurses' perceptions of patients following hospital discharge, *Image* 28(2):143, 1996.
9. Duryee R: The efficacy of inpatient education after myocardial infarction, *Heart Lung* 21(2):217, 1992.
10. Murphy MC, et al: Education of patients undergoing coronary angioplasty: factors affecting learning during a structured educational program, *Heart Lung* 18(1):36, 1989.
11. Barnes LP: The illiterate client: strategies in patient teaching, *MCN Am J Matern Child Nurs* 17(3):127, 1992.
12. Bernier MJ: Developing and evaluating printed education materials: a prescriptive model for quality, *Orthop Nurs* 12(6):39, 1993.
13. Redman BK: *The process of patient teaching in nursing,* ed 7, St Louis, 1993, Mosby.
14. Albright J, et al: Readability of patient education materials: implications for clinical practice, *J Appl Nurs Res* 9(3):139, 1996.
15. Dowe MC, Lawrence PA, Carlson J, Keyserling TC: Patients' use of health-teaching materials at three readability levels, *Appl Nurs Res* 10(2):86, 1997.
16. Neilson E, Sheppard MA: Television as a patient education tool: a review of its effectiveness, *Patient Educ Couns* 11:3, 1988.
17. Durand RP, Counts CS: Developing audio-visual programs for patient education, *Am Neph Nurs Assoc* 13(3):158, 1986.
18. Chan V: Closed-circuit TV: an effective patient education tool, *Can J Nurs Admin,* Sept/Oct:20, 1992.
19. Weaver J: Patient education: an innovative computer approach, *Nurs Manag* 26(7):78, 1995.
20. Billie DA: Process oriented patient education, *DCCN* 2:2, 1983.
21. Miracle VA, Hovenkamp G: Needs of families of patients undergoing invasive cardiac procedures, *Am J Crit Care* 3(3):155, 1994.
22. Henneman EA, McKenzie JB, Dewa CS: An evaluation of interventions for meeting the information needs of families of critically ill patients, *Am J Crit Care* 1(3):85, 1993.
23. Leith BA: Transfer anxiety in critical care patients and their family members, *Crit Care Nurs* 18(4):24, 1998.

COMMON PROBLEMS IN CRITICAL CARE

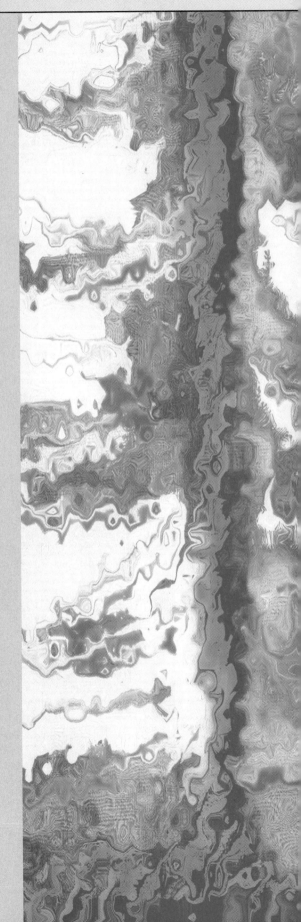

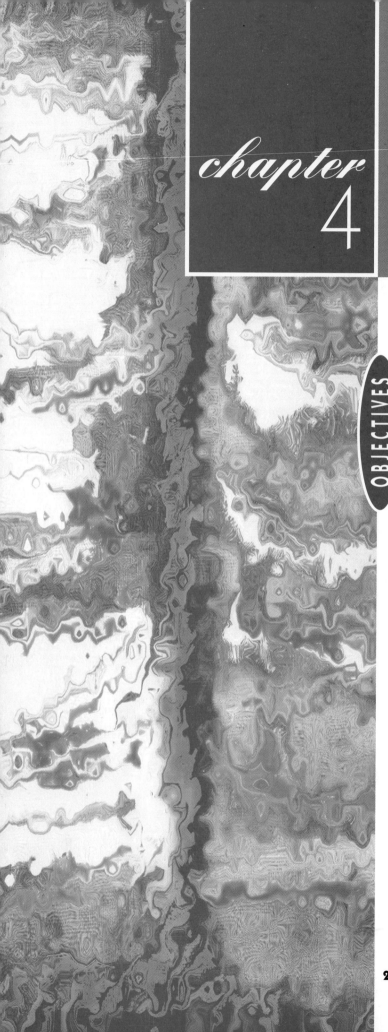

chapter 4

Psychosocial Alterations

Ruth N. Grendell

OBJECTIVES

- Explain the following coping strategies as they relate to critically ill patients: regression, suppression, denial, trust, religious beliefs, and family support.

- Describe the needs and coping mechanisms of families of critically ill patients.

- Explain interventions and nursing management for patients with coping alterations.

- Identify situations that increase the risk of disturbances of self-concept.

Patients requiring critical care must cope with a variety of stressors. A patient's response to these stressors depends on individual differences, such as age, gender, social supports, cultural background, medical diagnosis, current hospital course, and prognosis. Other major factors include stress, pain, past experiences with illness, and previous contact with the health care system, all of which influence the person's total response and use of coping strategies in a new crisis situation. The person's perception of self and relationships with others, spiritual values, and self-competency in social roles also play a major role in responses to stress and illness.

The human self-concept is a major concern for nurses because nursing interventions that do not consider the individual in his or her wholeness—including the self-concept—will probably not be effective. The self-concept comprises attitudes about oneself; perceptions of personal abilities, body image, and identity; and a general sense of worth. The stressors imposed by physical illness, trauma, and surgical procedures can cause disturbances in self-concept (Box 4-1).

BOX 4-1

STRESSORS IN THE CRITICAL CARE SETTING

Patients' experience of critical illness and care varies. However, each patient must cope with at least some of the following stressors:
- Threat of death
- Threat of survival, with significant residual problems related to the illness/injury
- Pain or discomfort
- Lack of sleep
- Loss of autonomy over most aspects of life and daily functioning
- Loss of control over environment, including loss of privacy and exposure to light, noise, and general activity of the critical care unit, including the care of other patients
- Daily hassles or common frustrations
- Loss of usual role and, with that, the arena in which usual coping mechanisms serve the patient
- Separation from family and friends
- Loss of dignity
- Boredom, broken only by brief visits, threatening stimuli, and frightening thoughts
- Loss of ability to express self verbally when intubated

Effects and response to the stressors are dependent on the individual's perception of the intensity of the stress and the following:
- Acute/chronic duration of stressors
- Cumulative effect of simultaneous stressors
- Sequence of stressors
- Individual's previous experience with stressors and coping effectiveness
- Amount of social support

Patients in critical care units usually do not have time to adjust to the illness and may exhibit signs of shock and numbness, avoidance of reality, and lack of understanding of the implications of the situation.

SELF-CONCEPT

Self-concept is what one believes about oneself; self-report is what one is willing to share about oneself. When assessing the self-concept of the critically ill patient, an understanding of the stages of illness and a person's behavioral responses is useful. The various stages of illness have been described by a number of scientists.[1-5] There is general agreement on three to four major stages. The initial, or impact stage, consists of the person experiencing symptoms, an interpretation of what they might mean, and an emotional response such as fear or anxiety. The person may attempt some sort of self-care, consult family or another nonprofessional for advice, or contact a physician. The next stage consists of diagnosis and assumption of the dependent sick role that may be marked by denial, frustration, anger, increased anxiety, hostility, and passive behavior. On the other hand, the person may seek information and do everything possible to assist in recovery. Patients in critical care units usually do not have

time to adjust to the illness and may exhibit signs of shock and numbness, try to avoid reality, and be unable to clearly understand the implications of the situation. Usually, only after patients have been transferred to an intermediate unit, does a true acknowledgment phase occur. The final stage encompasses recovery or rehabilitation, transition to chronic illness, or death.

These stages are complex, highly individualized, and require adjustments in the self-concept, including changes in body image and interpersonal relationships and the limitations imposed by the person's condition. An individual with an acute problem, such as a heart attack, may panic if he or she believes that help will not arrive in time and may exhibit excessive demands or be suspicious of motives and methods of the caregivers. Depression and anxiety are common reactions as the person experiences a loss of control and worries about outcomes. During the illness acceptance stage, the individual may be preoccupied with symptoms and their treatment or be resistant to dependency on caregivers and express anger and resentment. In the convalescent stage, the person must relinquish the dependent role and, perhaps, make major changes in life-style and role performance. The disturbances of self-concept and their adaptations are examined individually in this chapter. It must be remembered, however, that although each subcomponent has unique characteristics, some characteristics are shared with several or all the other subcomponents.

Body Image Disturbance

Changes to the body's appearance, structure, and/or function may be caused by disease, trauma, or surgery. Disturbances in body image arise when the person fails to perceive or adapt to the changes. A disturbance may have a biophysical, cognitive-perceptual, cultural, or spiritual basis. In some instances, the person may feel betrayed by the body, which no longer seems "normal." Such disturbances are manifested by verbal or nonverbal responses to the actual or perceived changes.[6] Some patients must extend their body image to incorporate environmental objects.[7] For example, the patient temporarily requiring assisted respirations must extend his or her body image to include the ventilator and its accessories. In this situation explanations to patient and family of the equipment being used and their purpose are helpful.

Another example is when a patient admitted to a surgical critical care unit after a traumatic amputation awakes to find his or her leg missing with no prior knowledge of the cause for the loss. Reliving the accident and receiving explanations about the need for the amputation are priorities for such a patient. Similar interventions are necessary after any disfiguring trauma or surgery, such as severe burns, a radical neck dissection, a mastectomy, or a colostomy. Body image may also be altered by the need to incorporate a prosthetic device or a donated body part.[8,9] The disease or problem may be corrected by surgery and treatments; however, whenever the result is visible to the patient and others, the change in body image can arouse intense feelings of anger, frustration, depression, and powerlessness. Refer to the Nursing Management Plan of Care for Body Image Disturbance on p. 450 for nursing interventions.

Self-Esteem Disturbance

Self-esteem, or self-measurement of one's worth, develops as a part of self-concept through the reflected appraisals of significant others.[8-11] The way such information is interpreted is probably more important than is the content. Self-esteem is only partly related to material, economic, or social conditions. The need for self-esteem is a part of the hierarchy of human needs postulated by Maslow.[12] Having high self-esteem helps one deal with the environment and face more easily the maturational and situational crises of life. Overall, the goal is to maintain a high positive regard for oneself in the midst of everchanging views of oneself. This goal, when met, contributes to the quality of life of the individual. Persons with a well-developed sense of self-esteem are at less risk for disturbances than those with poorly developed self-esteem.[13] Illness can rob a person of perspective and shrink both the familiar world and the one of possibility, often leading to low self-esteem, powerlessness, helplessness, and depression.[6,13] A low self-regard impairs one's ability to adapt. The person may refuse to participate in self-care, may exhibit self-destructive behavior, or may be too compliant—asking no questions and permitting others to make all decisions.[8]

In old age a person faces loss of autonomy; losses related to changes in health status and sensory impairment (e.g., vision/hearing); loss of work role through retirement; and death of loved ones, all of which may lower self-esteem. Changes in the expectations of others for one's behavior and capacity may occur. The elderly patient may feel inadequate and guilty when caregivers become impatient with the slowed responses and performance deficits. If patients are treated as children, they may believe themselves burdens and react with resentment. Failure to include them in decision-making may cause them to feel useless and rejected. On the other hand, people with a strong sense of self-worth are likely to be adjusted, happy, and competent.[13,14] Defensive self-esteem is used to defend against the person's perception of a gap between his or her real self and an ideal self. High self-esteem is associated with a low need for social approval, comfort with intimacy and self-disclosure, and the ability to acknowledge personal failures.

Powerlessness

Powerlessness as a nursing diagnosis is defined as the perception of the individual that one's own action will not significantly affect an outcome.[15-17] Unrelieved powerlessness may result in hopelessness, which is discussed in the next section.

The causes of powerlessness include factors in the health care environment, interpersonal interactions, one's cultural and religious beliefs, illness-related regimen, and a life-style of helplessness. A severe level of powerlessness may be manifested by a person's verbal expression of having no control or influence over a situation, its eventual outcome, or over self-care. Powerlessness can also be manifested by depression over physical deterioration that occurs despite the patient's compliance with a strict regimen or by passivity and apathy. The range in levels of powerlessness varies[14-16] and depends on the person's perceived control of a situation, the amount of loss experienced, and the availability of social support. Powerlessness can be manifested by refusal to participate in self-care, delayed decision-making or refusal to make decisions, and expressions of self-doubt in role performance. Frustration, anger, and resentment over dependency on others often occurs, with verbal expressions regarding dissatisfaction with care.

Most people expect to have the power to participate in making decisions that affect them. Both actual and perceived control over present or impending events are important.[17,18] When patients feel their choices are limited, they may act against their own best interests.[17-22] Given enough frustration, any exercise of control—even one with negative outcomes, such as signing out of the hospital against medical advice (AMA)—can become attractive.

Individuals vary in the amount of control they prefer. Important variables in this regard are the illness; values, traits, attitudes, and experiences; the hospital setting; and social displacement. Personality, age, religion, occupation, income, residence, and race may all be pertinent factors also. Apparently there is an increase in variability in the amount of control preferred as people age.[23-24] The critical care unit routines may oppose or preclude any control by the patient. The person to whom control is important should be helped to continue to control as many areas of life as possible. On the other hand, a patient must be given the opportunity to choose not to control.[22]

Another aspect of powerlessness is *learned helplessness*, or *excessive dependence*.[1,6] This occurs when a person who repeatedly experiences uncontrollable situations loses the motivation for making decisions about life events. Some people assume a martyr role and accept the illness state as their fate, thus doing nothing to improve their status. Others may find the sick role a gratifying means for gaining control over others by using their symptoms to gain attention.[2] Setting limits on these behaviors, encouraging independence and participation in self-care, counseling, and involving family members in establishing realistic goals are helpful strategies in assisting the person to abandon this manipulative behavior.

The patient's perception of control is affected by the interaction of the environment and limitations imposed by the disease process on the patient's physical and psychologic status. Critically ill patients generally experience a rapid onset of illness without time to acquire the illness role. A sense of powerlessness in such situations is not unexpected. If control is defined as the ability to determine the use of time, space, and resources, admission to a critical care unit strips away control of this power. Upon admission, persons lose their independent status; they become patients. Use of clothes and other personal belongings is usually restricted in a critical care unit. Patients cannot decide who enters the room, who provides personal care, or who intrudes with painful treatments. Hospital rules usually are not open to modification. Patients may feel anxious because they are separated from a familiar environment and have restrictions on visitors.

Poor interaction with the health care providers may make the situation worse. Patients may react aggressively, may try bargaining, or may refuse to comply with diagnostic and treatment regimens. They may resent the close scrutiny of the nurses and physicians and the invasion of their privacy. They may fear death or permanent loss of function and may feel guilty if they have contributed to the cause of their illness or injury. By virtue of their experiences of critical illness and care and because so much control is taken from them, these patients may lose sight of areas of influence they do retain over themselves. Nursing should emphasize this intact influence on control and thus help to preserve it.[18,27,28]

Procedures take priority over psychosocial needs in the ICU. The family feels powerless, uninformed, and uninvolved. Nurses must learn to recognize this anguish of waiting. The presence of family members can provide support to the patient and family, can bring a sense of reality to a situation, and can facilitate the grieving process, when necessary.[25]

Although liberal visiting in the ICU is still strongly opposed, a recent study indicated greater patient and family satisfaction when patients had greater control over access to visitors.[26] Patients participated in decisions regarding family member presence during painful procedures and established guidelines for visits. The nurses helped patients to anticipate causes of stress and to identify strategies to relieve stress as well as assisting family in providing effective support to the patient and themselves.

COPING MECHANISMS

When a patient copes effectively, what he or she is doing to cope may often go unnoticed. Emotionally the patient seems relatively comfortable, is a cooperative recipient of care, and exhibits nonproblematic behavior. The patient may be using multiple appropriate coping mechanisms that help manage a problem or stressful situation. Refer to the Nursing Management Plan of Care for Powerlessness on p. 455 for nursing interventions. The following discussion covers several coping mechanisms that may or may not be effective, depending on the degree that they are used.

Regression

Regression is an unconscious defense mechanism that involves a retreat, in the face of stress, to behavior char-

acteristic of an earlier developmental level.[5,28] Regression allows the patient to give up his or her usual role, autonomy, and privacy to become the passive recipient of medical and nursing management. In fact, the patient who does not regress jeopardizes his or her own care. For example, a patient may insist on conducting business from the bedside or demand bathroom privileges when getting out of bed would be unsafe. Conversely, the patient who becomes too regressed may become childlike in interactions with staff, whine, cling to staff, and attempt to keep the nurse at the bedside constantly. In both cases, the patient requires the setting of limits on behavior to receive essential care. The patient is best served when limits are set in a supportive manner.

Although the behavior of these patients can provoke confrontations or reprimands, these responses must be avoided. Such responses from staff may only worsen a situation in which a patient is already struggling with issues of dependence and autonomy.

Suppression

Suppression is a conscious, intentional process in which patients push ideas, problems, or desires out of their conscious thoughts.[5,29,30] Patients often use suppression when their problems are overwhelming and they are in no position to resolve them. Strategic suppression can be used as a conscious attempt to focus only on problems patients can solve in the present.[8]

Denial

According to NANDA, *denial* includes both conscious and unconscious attempts to disavow knowledge or the meaning of an event.[31] In this text, the psychoanalytic definition of denial, "an unconscious defense mechanism that reduces anxiety by eliminating or reducing the seriousness of the perceived threat," is used to allow for the distinction between denial and suppression. When used by a critically ill patient, denial reduces the anxiety and the threat of the illness.[6] Patients may deny different aspects of an illness. The degree to which denial is used varies among patients and may vary in the same patient at different times.

Trust

Trust manifests itself in the critical care patient as the belief that the staff will get him or her through the illness, managing any untoward event that might occur. Trust is an unconscious process in which the patient transfers the trust learned in early significant relationships onto caregivers in the present.[2,5]

Hope

Although hope has long been recognized as a significant factor in patient recovery and survival, the phenomenon receives little attention until the patient becomes hopeless. Hopelessness is often expressed as a feeling of doom and inability to help self or anticipate a positive outcome. The patient who is hopeless may verbalize the inability to cope, use inappropriate defense mechanisms, and cannot problem solve, meet basic needs, or meet role expectations. The person may also express feelings of anxiety and report that life is stressful but does not ask for help. *Hope* is a multidimensional life force that is future-oriented, empowering, and directs one energies. It is the expectation that a desire will be fulfilled. It can exist even in the face of a realistic appraisal of a grim situation. Hope supports the patient and helps him or her endure the physical and psychologic insults that are a part of the daily experience.[29,32,33]

Religious beliefs and practices

Religious beliefs and practices may provide the patient with some measure of acceptance of an illness, a sense of mastery and control, a source of hope and trust beyond the limits the staff can provide, and the strength to endure the current stress. A patient may discuss religious beliefs and concerns openly or view the subject as a private and personal matter. Patients who rely on religious beliefs benefit from the nurse who is accepting and respectful of those beliefs and who remains sensitive to the patient's willingness or reluctance to discuss those beliefs.[32-35]

Use of family support

The patient can use the presence of a supportive family to cope with critical illness. The patient with a supportive family knows that family members share a past and hope for a future with the patient. They love the patient as a person and member of the family. The patient also realizes that family members know him or her in ways the staff cannot. With them, the patient may know that his or her experience is truly understood, even when little is said. Family members can also be involved in the patient's personal care and can attend to the practical problems the patient cannot, such as managing finances.[9,25,26,36]

Sharing concerns

Sharing concerns with a caring and understanding listener can relieve some of the patient's emotional distress. The patient is consoled knowing that he or she is not alone and that someone knows and cares about what is being experienced.[8] The patient may share concerns with family members. On the other hand, the patient may be reluctant to upset loved ones further or may have a family in which such communication is not the norm. Such a patient, if he or she relies on this coping mechanism, will benefit from a nurse who recognizes when a patient needs to talk and who knows how to listen.

HIGH-RISK PATIENTS

Persons with chronic illness, trauma injuries, illnesses involving multiple systems, the elderly, persons on several drugs, and those who lack a social support network are considered to be at greater risk for the inability to cope with the stressful environment of the ICU. The elderly represent the largest population with chronic illnesses

and complications resulting from the use of multiple drugs or "polypharmacy." Other patient symptoms include those with acute burn injury, spinal cord injury, diabetes, and congestive heart failure. High-risk patients are more subject to complications, longer stays, and greater mortality. Case management is frequently used to assist in the care of these individuals. The taxonomy of nursing interventions (NIC) provides a valuable resource for therapeutic nursing interventions.[37-41] Refer to Box 4-2 for general assessment of coping and coping enhancement nursing interventions.

Coping Assessment

Ineffective coping may be suggested in patient behaviors. Overt hostility, severe regression, or noncompliance with treatment may suggest ineffective coping. The patient may also report problems such as severe anxiety or despondence. The nurse who suspects that coping is ineffective needs to review the patient's medical history, mental status, and associated psychosocial factors.

It is not always clear whether coping is truly ineffective or whether intervention is indicated. Witnessing problematic behavior can be very uncomfortable, especially when that behavior is directed at the caregiver(s). Careful evaluation of one's reaction to the behavior is needed to discover whether patient care can continue to be provided objectively, or whether consultation with others on the team is needed to alleviate the problem.[5,8]

Coping Enhancement

Although the delivery of physical care is essential for patient survival and recovery, "caring for patients' psychological and social needs can be one of the most challenging aspects of nursing."[5,8] Several essential techniques for effective interventions include having an attitude of caring, openness, and warmth and withholding judgment until you "know" the patient—have an understanding of the individual's perception about self, the current illness or problem, and the type of social support available. Assessment skills are essential as well as a willingness to become involved when there is the potential or actual use of ineffective coping mechanisms.

A patient's trust in the nurse's competence in the physical and technical aspects of care aids in the patient's participation. Hope is instilled when the nurse and other caregivers display a sense of optimism regarding the patient's progress. It is essential that patients receive honest feedback, for patients are keen observers of their caregivers, and they read them well. Patients have reported remembering the caring attitudes and competence of health care workers who anticipated their needs.[42] Trust and hope are easily lessened when inappropriate information is given. Refer to the Nursing Management Plan of Care for Anxiety on p. 448 and Ineffective Individual Coping on p. 453 for nursing interventions.

BOX 4-2

SELECTED STRATEGIES FOR COPING ASSESSMENT AND THERAPEUTIC NURSING INTERVENTIONS

ASSESSMENT

- Assess coping strategies used by patient. Determine what successful strategies were used previously.
- Appraise patient's adjustment to changes in body image, impact on self-concept and esteem, and understanding or misconceptions of disease process.
- Note patterns of subtle or sudden changes in patient's behaviors, attitudes, and mental status.
- Perform holistic assessment of patient. Gather information from a variety of sources.
- Determine persons at increased risk for depression and acute confusion (i.e., chronically ill, elderly, those on multiple medications, the malnourished, those with fluid and electrolyte imbalances, persons with multisystem health problems, trauma victims, those with lack of social support systems).

THERAPEUTIC NURSING INTERVENTIONS

- Reinforce effective coping strategies.
- Confront patient's ambivalent (angry/depressed) feelings. Set limits for persons using inappropriate coping mechanisms and manipulative behavior. Foster constructive outlets for anger and hostility.
- Remain calm. Present a caring, reassuring, and open nonjudgmental attitude. Avoid confrontation. Establish a trusting relationship.
- LISTEN—"know" the patient.
- Provide patient-centered/family-centered holistic care.
- Inform the patient and family of condition, procedures, etc. in understandable terms that are based on patient/family needs.

- Facilitate patient's control and participation in making decisions within capabilities.
- Involve members of patient's support system in personal care, in serving as resource of information, as appropriate. Instruct them in skills as needed.
- Facilitate patient's realistic hope as means for dealing with feelings of helplessness.
- Be sensitive to signs of patient's spiritual distress. Enlist aid from a spiritual advisor or respect patient's reluctance to express spiritual concerns.
- Include the spiritual counselor as member of health care team in ethical life/death decision-making.
- Use strategies to promote patient's own personal spiritual health and coping with stressful situations in critical care environment.
- Seek assistance from other personnel on the health care team in managing specific problems. Monitor patient/family progress and document findings.
- Remain current in technical skills to promote patient's trust in your capability in providing care.
- Administer medications as appropriate to promote healing, decrease pain and anxiety, and prevent confusion and depression.
- Minimize environmental stressors (e.g., noise, distractions). Schedule procedures to avoid frequent interruptions in sleep/rest periods. Allow patient to have some control over care, family visits, food choices, etc.
- Monitor patient's response to medications that may contribute to ineffective coping.

Modified from Stuart and Sundeen[5], Briones[37], Byers[38], Wirtz[39], Titler[40], McCloskey[41].

Supporting family members

Patient-centered care is also family-centered care. Consideration of nonbiologic or nonlegal partners of the patient as members of the patient's support system is also necessary in providing holistic care. The nurse's support of family members at the bedside can enhance the value of the visits for the patient.[25,43-45] Patients often look to the family for love, understanding, support, and care of matters to which they cannot attend themselves. Interventions to support family members[44] are outlined in Box 4-3. Refer to the Nursing Management Plan of Care for Ineffective Family Coping on p. 452 for additional nursing interventions.

Supporting spiritual care

Spiritual distress has been defined as the disruption in the life principle that pervades a person's entire being and that integrates and transcends one's biologic and psychosocial nature.[17] Separation from religious rituals and ties and intense suffering can induce spiritual distress for patients and their families.

BOX 4-3

INTERVENTIONS TO SUPPORT FAMILY MEMBERS

- Identify a family spokesperson and support persons
- Identify a primary nursing contact for the family
- Establish a mechanism for family access to the patient
- Promote access to the patient and ensure consistency in adhering to unit routines
- Establish a mechanism to contact the family and to update on changes in patient status
- Provide information based on family needs
- Ensure support services are available and refer to specialized services as needed
- Explain all procedures using understandable terms
- Include family in providing care
- Provide a comfortable environment for the family
- Include family in end-of-life planning and provide palliative care and support for terminally ill patients and families

Patients easily succumb to feelings of helplessness and powerlessness in the technologic impersonalized environment of the critical care unit. Standards from the Joint Commission for Accreditation of Healthcare Organizations (JCAHO) dictate patient care that considers personal dignity and respect for spiritual values. Seven major characteristics of spiritual distress have been identified:

- A feeling of emptiness
- No reason for living
- Request for spiritual assistance
- Concern over meaning of life
- A questioning and doubting of beliefs
- An inability to practice rituals
- A feeling of being detached from self and others

Interventions include the use of active listening, therapeutic touch, joining the patient in prayer or reading of scriptures, aiding with access to other rituals, and including family/significant others in providing spiritual care.[29,47,48] Including a pastor or chaplain on the health care team is also an important aspect of holistic care. The chaplain may be the best person to assess spiritual needs and to assist patients and their families in coping with the crisis. Providing access to religious rituals, prayer, and scriptures are meaningful strategies in alleviating stress. The religious leader is also a valuable asset in ethical decisions such as termination of life support and can be of great assistance to health care team members as their personal resources are drained from sustained or cumulative assistance to others in crisis.[46]

ACUTE CONFUSION

Acute confusion, which encompasses global cognitive impairment, has not been clearly or consistently defined.[49,50] Synonyms include *delirium* (the medical term), *critical care unit psychosis, postcardiotomy delirium,* and *acute brain failure.*[16] Additional terms are *acute mental status change, acute organic reaction, metabolic encephalopathy,* and *reversible cognitive dysfunction.* There is loss of orientation to person, time, or place and the ability to reason, follow directions, process incoming stimuli, or maintain concentration.[51] Confused persons may be aware of these disturbances and fear that they are "losing their minds." The confused state is a secondary response to organic causes (e.g., hypoxia, drugs, or fluid and electrolyte imbalances) or to inorganic causes (e.g., stress or sleep deprivation). Onset is abrupt, and duration can be shortened if early diagnosis and treatment are initiated. It is estimated that confusion develops in 50% of hospitalized elderly patients; however, it is often misdiagnosed because of inaccurate assessment and assumptions that a mental deterioration is a result of the effects of aging.[16,42] More than 80% of acute confusion status for the elderly can be attributed to organic causes. Behavioral symptoms may be subtle and varied. Prodromal symptoms include insomnia, distractibility, drowsiness, anxiety, and nightmares. Symptoms of acute confusion resemble those of dementia, which makes differentiation between the two conditions more difficult. However, dementia, which cannot be reversed, has a gradual onset and is of long duration.

Approximately 10% to 15% of all hospitalized medical-surgical patients experience symptoms of acute confusion. This percentage is increased by 30% to 40% in the critical care setting. Hospital stays are prolonged for this population, with the average increase in stay of 13 days.[49,50]

Etiology

There are many causes or contributors to acute confusion, which can occur for anyone at any given time. Three predisposing contributors to development of acute confusion are age 60 years or older, presence of brain damage, and presence of a chronic brain disorder, such as Alzheimer's.[49,50] Cognitive dysfunctions are believed to occur when "there is a widespread reduction of cerebral oxidative metabolism and an imbalance of neurotransmission."[49,50]

Drugs that are commonly used in the critical care unit are contributing factors to acute confusion. Some of these are digitalis, antibiotics, steroids, beta-blockers, anticholinergics, CNS-acting drugs, and respiratory stimulants. Additional causes include sleep deprivation, sensory underload or overload, fluid-electrolyte imbalance, immobilization, and infection, all of which are common events encountered in the critical care unit.

The patient in the critical care unit is robbed of the restorative benefits of deep sleep and the rapid eye movement (REM) phase because of frequent interruptions by equipment noises, voices, and procedures. Constant bright overhead lights, the absence of day-night cycles, immobility, pain, and medications contribute to the patient's disorientation to time and place. Daytime napping, complaints of fatigue, slurred speech, depression, cognitive impairment, and hallucinations can result. Delayed recovery, increased length of stay, and the seriousness of sleep deprivation are closely related.[4]

Assessment

Three forms of acute confusion have been identified: hyperactive, hypoactive, and a mixture of both forms.[16,49,50] The patient with the hyperactive form may remove intravenous lines, dressings, and catheters; be extremely restless and try to get out of bed; pick at things in the air; and call out to persons who are not there. Sympathetic nervous system responses of tachycardia, dilation of pupils, diaphoresis, and facial flushing are evident. In the hypoactive form, persons complain of extreme fatigue, are slow to respond, and have hypersomnolence that can progress to loss of consciousness. At times, these individuals are absorbed in a dreamlike state, mumble to themselves, experience vivid hallucinations, and make inappropriate gestures. The third form is a mixture of agitation and hypoactive behaviors that can vary throughout the day. Symptoms and hallucinations seem to worsen during nighttime hours, with more lucid intervals occurring during the day.

Mental status examination

The mental status examination is a full, criteria-based assessment of the patient's cognitive function and thought processes. Although the examination is rarely conducted in its entirety in the critical care setting, knowledge of its main components will enhance the nurse's effectiveness in collecting data to document findings by using accepted terminology and identifying issues that need further assessment. Refer to Box 4-4 for mental status examination considerations.

Medical management

Sedation is prescribed for patients with hyperactive delirium. Neuroleptic drugs such as haloperidol, droperidol, and chlorpromazine commonly used for neurotic and personality disorders are also useful in the treatment of delirium. Currently, haloperidol is considered to be the drug of choice, and a regular dosing schedule is preferred rather than waiting until symptoms reoccur. A combination of haloperidol and lorazepam, a benzodiazepine drug, allows lower doses of each drug to be given, is very effective, and produces fewer side effects. When delirium is considered to be secondary to pain, narcotics can be administered. However, the paradoxic effects of depressed respirations and cardiac output can exacerbate the delirium. The use of barbiturates is no longer recommended as routine treatment, but they can be used in the treatment of barbiturate withdrawal–induced delirium. Finally, neuromuscular blocking agents are sometimes used for severely agitated patients who are receiving mechanical ventilation; these agents decrease oxygen consumption, promote synchrony with the ventilator, and increase tissue oxygenation. These complex drugs can be dangerous and do not affect consciousness, cognition, or pain levels, thus necessitating the addition of sedatives or analgesics.[49,50]

Nursing management

Refer to the Nursing Management Plan of Care for Acute Confusion on p. 444 for nursing interventions.

References

1. Benner P, Wrubel J: *The primacy of caring: stress and coping in health and illness,* Menlo Park, Calif, 1989, Addison-Wesley.
2. Kozier B, Erb G, Blais K: *Professional nursing practice: concepts and perspectives,* ed 3, Menlo Park, Calif, 1997, Addison-Wesley.
3. Lee J: Emotional reactions to trauma, *Nurs Clin North Am* 5(4):577, 1970.
4. Smeltzer S, Bare B, editors: *Brunner and Suddarth's textbook of medical-surgical nursing,* ed 8, Philadelphia, 1996, JB Lippincott.
5. Stuart G, Sundeen S: *Principles and practice of psychiatric nursing,* St. Louis, 1995, Mosby.
6. Benner P, Tanner C, Chesla C: *Expertise in nursing practice,* New York, 1996, Springer.
7. Smith S: Extended body image in the ventilated patient, *Intensive Care Nurs* 5(1):31, 1989.
8. Barry P: *Psychosocial nursing: assessment and intervention in care of the physically ill,* ed 2, Philadelphia, 1989, JB Lippincott.
9. Barry P: *Care of physically ill patients and their families,* ed 3, Philadelphia, 1996, JB Lippincott.
10. Wright J, Skelton B: *Desk reference for critical care nursing,* Boston, 1993, Jones & Bartlett.
11. Norris J, Kunes-Connell M: Self-esteem disturbance, *Nurs Clin North Am* 20(4):745, 1985.
12. Maslow H: *Motivation and personality,* New York, 1954, Harper & Row.
13. Hirst SP, Metcalf BJ: Promoting self-esteem, *J Gerontol Nurs* 10(2):72, 1984.
14. Isaacs A: Depression and your patient, *AJN* 98(7):26-31, 1998.
15. Herr K, Mobily P: Geriatric mental health, chronic pain and depression, *J Psychosoc Nurs* 30(9):7-12, 1992.
16. Stanley M, Gauntlett-Beare P: *Gerontological nursing,* Philadelphia, 1995, FA Davis.
17. Kim M, McFarland GK, McLane AM: *Pocket guide to nursing diagnoses,* ed 7, St Louis, 1997, Mosby.
18. Canaille L, et al: A place to be yourself: empowerment from the client's perspective, *Image J Nurs Sch* 25(4):297-303, 1993.
19. Roberts SL, White BS: Powerlessness and personal control model applied to the myocardial infarction patient, *Progress Cardiovasc Nurs* 5(3):84, 1990.
20. Janis IL, Rodin J: Attribution, control, and decision-making: social psychology and health care. In Stone GC, Adler NC, editors: *Health psychology—a handbook,* San Francisco, 1979, Jossey-Bass.
21. Rotter JB: Generalized expectancies for internal versus external control of reinforcement, *Psych Monogr* 80(609):1, 1966.
22. Seligman ME: *Helplessness: on depression, development and death,* San Francisco, 1975, WH Freeman.
23. Janelli L: Are there body image differences between older men and women? *West J Nurs Res* 15(3):327-329, 1993.
24. Wolinsky F, Stump T: Age and the sense of control among older adults, *J Gerontol* 51B:217-220, 1996.

25. Eckel N: Family presence: where would you want to be? *Crit Care Nurs* 16(1):102, 1996.
26. Lazure L: Strategies to increase patient control of visiting, *Dimen Crit Care Nurs* 16(1):11-19, 1997.
27. Radwin L: Knowing the patient: a process model for individualized interventions, *Nurs Res* 44(6):364-370, 1995.
28. Reiley P, et al: Discharge planning: comparison of patients' and nurses' perceptions of patients following hospital discharge, *Image J Nurs Sch* (2):143-147, 1996.
29. Twibell R, et al: Spiritual and coping needs of critically ill patients: validation of nursing diagnoses, *Dimen Crit Care Nurs* 15(5):245-263, 1996.
30. Beck AT, et al: The measurement of pessimism: the hopelessness scale, *J Couns Clin Psych* 42(6):861, 1974.
31. North American Nursing Diagnosis Association: Nursing Diagnosis: *Definitions and Classifications,* St Louis, 1995-1996, The Association.
32. Johnson L, et al: Supporting hope in CHF patients, *Dimen Crit Care Nurs* 16(20):65-78, 1997.
33. Morse J, Doberneck B: Delineating the concept of hope, *Image J Nurs Sch* 27(4):277-278, 1995.
34. Millette B: Client advocacy and the moral orientation of nurses, *West J Nurs Res* 15(5):617-618, 1993.
35. Armentrout D: Heart cry: a biblical model of depression, *J Psychol Christianity* 14(2):101-111, 1995.
36. White N, Richter J, Fry C: Coping, social support and adaptation to chronic illness, *West J Nurs Res* 14(2):211-224, 1992.
37. Briones J, et al: Case management of patients with chronic critical illnesses, *Crit Care Nurs* 16(4):38-54, 1996.
38. Byers J, Flynn M: Acute burn injury: a trauma case report, *Crit Care Nurs* 16(4):55-67, 1996.
39. Wirtz K, et al: Managing chronic spinal cord injury: issues in critical care, *Crit Care Nurs* 16(4):24-35, 1996.
40. Titler M, Bulechek G, McCloskey J: Use of NIC by critical care nurses, *Crit Care Nurs* 16(4):38-44, 1996.
41. McCloskey J, Bulechek G: *Nursing interventions classification (NIC),* ed 2, St. Louis, 1996, Mosby.
42. Holland C, et al: Patients' recollections of critical care, *Dimen Crit Care Nurs* 16(30):132-141.
43. Hupcey JE: Establishing the nurse-family relationship in the intensive care unit, *W J Nurs Res* 20(2):180-194, 1998.
44. Twibell RS: Family coping during critical illness, *Dimen Crit Care Nurs* 17(2):100-112, 1996.
45. Leske JS: Interventions to decrease family anxiety, *Crit Care Nurs* 18(4):92-95, 1998.
46. Gillman J, et al: Pastoral care in a critical care setting, *Crit Care Nurs Q* 19(1):10-20, 1996.
47. Sumner C: Recognizing and responding to spiritual stress, *AJN* 98(1):26-31, 1998.
48. Carson V, Green H: Spiritual well-being: a predictor of hardiness in patients with acquired immunodeficiency syndrome, *J Prof Nurs* 8(4):209-220, 1992.
49. Geary S: Intensive care unit psychosis revisited: understanding and managing delirium in the critical care setting, *Crit Care Nurs Q* 17(1):51-63, 1994.
50. Foreman M, Zane D: Nursing strategies for acute confusion in elders, *AJN* 96(4):44-52, 1996.
51. Strachan G, Glenner G: Delirium, dementia, amnestic and other cognitive disorders. In Fortinash K, Holloday-Worrett P, editors: *Psychiatric-mental health nursing,* St Louis, 1996, Mosby.

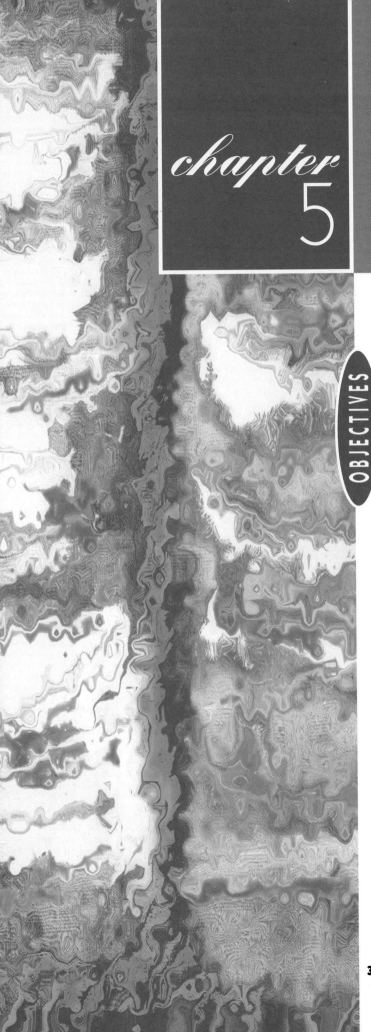

chapter 5

Sleep Alterations

Linda D. Urden

OBJECTIVES

- State the stages of sleep.
- Explain the three physiologic effects that occur during rapid eye movement (REM) sleep.
- Describe circadian desynchronization and its primary effects.
- Describe changes in sleep resulting from the aging process.
- Define *dysfunctional sleep.*
- Name three commonly prescribed critical care medications that decrease REM sleep.
- Describe common symptoms of sleep deprivation.

Because critical illness requires frequent treatments and 24-hour intensive monitoring, patients admitted to critical care units often suffer an altered sleep pattern. The inability to rest and sleep is one of the causes, as well as one of the outcomes, accompanying illness. A lack of sleep can have disastrous results for the critically ill patient. The nurse can promote recovery and healing through facilitating sleep for patients by controlling environmental noise and formulating individualized interventions.[1-2]

PHYSIOLOGY OF SLEEP

Sleep has been defined as "a state of unconsciousness from which a person can be aroused by appropriate sensory or other stimuli."[3] Adults normally spend approximately one third of their lives asleep. Research involving simultaneous monitoring using the electroencephalogram (EEG), electrooculogram (EOG), and electromyogram (EMG) has shown that there are two distinct stages of sleep: *non-rapid eye movement (NREM)* and *rapid eye movement (REM).*

NREM Sleep

NREM sleep is divided into four stages (NREM 1 through 4), which are associated with progressive relaxation. NREM stage 1 is a transitional state, with the EEG pattern being similar to that seen in the awake stage (Fig. 5-1). Stage 1 is the lightest level of sleep, lasting only 1 to 2 minutes. This stage is characterized by aimless thoughts, a feeling of drifting, and frequent myoclonic jerks of the face, hands, and feet. The individual is easily awakened during this stage.

NREM stage 2 differs from stage 1 in that the background wave frequency on the EEG is slower, with *sleep spindles* (characteristic waveforms) superimposed and high-voltage spikes known as *K-complexes.*[4] This stage lasts from 5 to 15 minutes, during which the individual becomes more relaxed but is still easily awakened. Stages 1 and 2 in the average young adult constitute 50% to 60% of the total sleep time.

Stages 3 and 4 are characterized by large, slow-frequency delta waves on the EEG and are primarily differentiated by the relative percentage of these waves. Random stimuli do not arouse the individual from these deepest levels of sleep. The time spent in stages 3 and 4 varies from 15 to 30 minutes and constitutes approximately 20% of the total sleep time. During NREM sleep, the EOG gradually slows and eye movements cease. EMG patterns also decline, indicating profound muscle relaxation; however, they do not reach the low levels that they do in REM sleep (Fig. 5-2). The parasympathetic nervous system predominates during NREM sleep. Cardiac and respiratory rates, metabolic rate, and blood pressure decreases to basal levels. Thus the supply/demand ratio

of coronary blood flow is likely to improve.[5] NREM sleep may, however, have antidysrhythmic properties.

In addition, during slow wave sleep, growth hormone (GH) is secreted by the anterior pituitary gland and functions to promote protein synthesis while sparing catabolic breakdown. Elevated GH and other anabolic hormones, such as prolactin and testosterone, imply that anabolism is taking place during NREM stage 4, particularly in tissues with a high protein content. Thus activities associated with NREM stage 4 include protein synthesis and tissue repair, such as the repair of epithelial and specialized cells of the brain, skin, bone marrow, and gastric mucosa.[6] NREM dreams are often realistic and thoughtlike, rarely in color, and often similar to a recent activity. These dreams are generally more difficult to remember than are REM dreams. NREM sleep, then, is a time of energy conservation and renewal.

REM Sleep

REM, or *paradoxical, sleep* constitutes 20% to 25% of the total sleep time in the young adult. This type of sleep is paradoxical in that some areas of the brain are quite active during REM sleep, while other areas are suppressed. During REM sleep, bursts of eye movements are seen on the EOG that are often associated with periods of dreaming. EMG patterns become essentially flat, indicating immobility and functional paralysis of the skeletal muscles. The cerebral cortical activity increases during REM so that the EEG patterns resemble those recorded during the waking state. During REM sleep, the individual is more difficult to awaken than in any other stage of sleep.[4] In this regard, REM sleep can be thought of as a "dissociative state."

The sympathetic nervous system predominates during REM sleep. Oxygen consumption increases, and cardiac output, blood pressure, heart rate, and respiratory rate may become erratic. An increase in premature ventricular

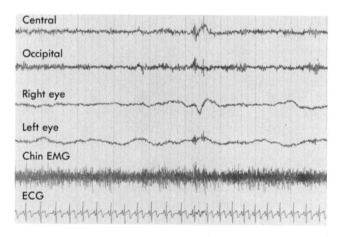

Fig. **5-1** Awake.

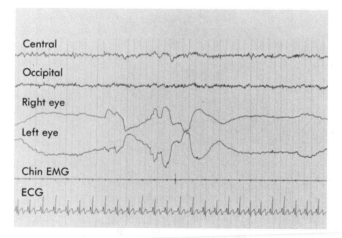

Fig. **5-2** REM sleep.

contractions (PVCs) and tachydysrhythmias associated with respiratory pauses may occur during REM sleep.[5] Evidence suggests that the adrenalin surge that more than doubles during REM sleep may be responsible for episodes of ischemia, sudden cardiac death, and strokes in the early morning hours.[6,7] Arterial pressure surge and increases in heart rate, coronary arterial tone, and blood viscosity could cause the combination of plaque rupture and hypercoagulability.[8] Serum cholesterol and antidiuretic hormone levels increase, and perfusion to the gray matter in the brain doubles. The dreams of REM sleep tend to be colorful, vivid, and implausible, often containing an element of paralysis. REM sleep filters information stored from the day's activities, sifting the important from the trivial, helping to psychologically integrate activities such as problem solving. REM sleep seems to facilitate emotional adaptation to the physical and psychologic environment and is needed in large quantities after periods of stress or learning. The adequacy of sleep is judged by the relative periods spent in each of the stages of sleep.[9]

REM sleep, like the other stages of sleep, is essential to physiologic and psychologic well-being. REM sleep is of great importance to nurses because as the patient is entering this stage of sleep, the nurse may notice a change in vital signs and become concerned that the patient's condition is worsening. If the nurse increases the monitoring of the patient, adjusts drips, and measures vital signs in response to this perceived change in condition, he or she may awaken the patient. Thus the patient may not get the sleep he or she needs. Further research must address the ways in which the nurse can assess sleep and all of its stages without unnecessarily disrupting the patient from the much-needed sleep. An accurate knowledge of sleep will assist nurses in monitoring patients safely while ensuring that they achieve optimal quality of sleep.

Cyclic Aspects of Sleep

At the onset of sleep, the individual normally progresses through repetitive cycles beginning with NREM stages 1 through 4 and then backward again to stage 2. From stage 2, the individual enters REM. Stage 2 is then reentered, and the cycle repeats (Fig. 5-3). These cycles occur at approximately 90-minute intervals, so that four or five cycles are normally completed in the sleep period. Early in the sleep period, NREM predominates. During the end of the sleep period, REM periods tend to be longer than those of NREM sleep.

The rhythmic nature of sleep is not unique. The body experiences rhythms in temperature, blood pressure, heart rate, respiratory rate, and hormone secretion. This cyclic 24-hour rhythm has been termed the *circadian rhythm*. Within the central nervous system, the bilaterally paired suprachiasmatic nuclei are the major endogenous pacemaker for the circadian rhythms. Sleep normally oc-

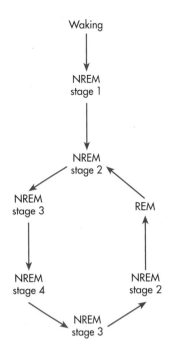

Fig. **5-3** Cyclic nature of sleep.

cupies the low phase of the circadian rhythm, whereas wakefulness and activity normally occupy the higher phase. Although regular nighttime sleep is synchronized with other circadian rhythms such as hormone levels, temperature, and metabolic rate, the major determinants of human sleeping are external time cues, light/dark changes, and particular social events such as meal times.[10]

SLEEP CHANGES WITH AGE

As the biologic systems change during the aging process, stress is placed on the human system, and the delicate mechanism of sleep is altered.[11] The number of daytime naps and nighttime awakenings and variability in sleep behaviors increase with age. By age 75, the number of naps and length of naptime increase, resulting in a gradual increase in the total sleep time.[9] These changes—along with more fragmentation, increased sleep-onset problems, and frequent long periods of wakefulness at night—cause elderly persons to perceive an impairment in their quality of sleep. In caring for older persons, it is important to remember that individuals differ widely in terms of both the age of onset of these changes and individual adaptations.

PHARMACOLOGY AND SLEEP

Patients hospitalized in critical care units often receive pharmacologic therapy, which may affect their quality of sleep and compound sleep disturbances. The critical care nurse must be aware of the effects that commonly used

TABLE 5-1

COMMON DRUGS THAT AFFECT SLEEP

Drug	Effect on Sleep	Comments
BARBITURATES		
Amobarbital	Increases NREM 2	Not considered drug of choice because of toxicity and long-lasting effects
Pentobarbital Secobarbital	Suppresses REM	Often patients experience rebound insomnia, restless sleep, and frequent dreaming and nightmares when drugs are discontinued
Phenobarbital	Decreases REM in doses greater than 200 mg	REM rebound (increased REM in subsequent sleep) after withdrawal of phenobarbital
BENZODIAZEPINES		
Diazepam	Increases NREM 1 Decreases NREM 3 and 4 Decreases REM	NREM suppression is not dose related REM suppression is dose related May increase sleep apnea episodes
Flurazepam	Increases total sleep time Decreases NREM 2, 3, and 4 Decreases REM	Conflicting reports about effects on sleep Long half-life may produce daytime drowsiness
Triazolam	Decreases sleep latency (time it takes to get to sleep) Decreases awakenings Increases total sleep time	Drug has a short half-life; should not be used for a prolonged time because of decreased effectiveness; use decreased doses with elderly patients
MISCELLANEOUS		
Chloral hydrate	Thought to be an effective sedative that does not disrupt sleep	Drug has a short half-life and some reports of nightmares; increased daytime drowsiness
Chlordiazepoxide	Minimally disrupts sleep	
Morphine	Decreases NREM 3 and 4 Decreases REM	Results in increased spontaneous arousals and overall lighter sleep

drugs have on sleep. In fact, hypnotic drugs have been found to promote the lighter stages of sleep (i.e., NREM stage 2) and may, paradoxically, be the cause of night terrors, hallucinations, and agitation in the elderly.[9] This area has great potential for nursing research. Common drugs that affect sleep are described in Table 5-1.

The prolonged half-life of medications, coupled with altered metabolism or decreased excretion of the drug resulting from renal or liver disease that may occur in elderly persons, can cause the effects of sedatives to continue into the daytime, leading to confusion and sluggishness. Sedative and analgesic medications must not be withheld, but, rather, decreased dosages of drugs that minimally disrupt sleep are to be used to complement comfort measures, with dosages reduced gradually as the medication is no longer necessary.

SLEEP DEPRIVATION

Much of what is known about the function of sleep has been learned from observations made when persons are deprived of sleep in the laboratory setting. Both physiologic and psychologic symptoms of sleep deprivation have been reported[12] (Box 5-1). These symptoms may be, but are not always, associated with the length of sleep

BOX 5-1

EFFECTS OF SELECTIVE SLEEP DEPRIVATION

SYMPTOMS OF NREM SLEEP DEPRIVATION

Fatigue
Anxiety
Increased illness

SYMPTOMS OF REM SLEEP DEPRIVATION

Restlessness
Disorientation
Combativeness
Delusions
Hallucinations

deprivation. The symptoms vary among individuals given such factors as age, premorbid personality, motivation, and the environment.[13]

Selective *REM deprivation* leads to irritability, apathy, decreased alertness, and increased sensitivity to pain. Continued loss of REM sleep may lead to perceptual distortion and significant disturbance in mental-emotional function, often within 72 hours of REM deprivation.

Manifestations of sleep deprivation range from disorientation and restlessness to frank auditory and visual hallucinations, with personality changes, including withdrawal and paranoia.[13]

Selective *NREM deprivation* is less well-studied, but it appears that fatigue is the primary result of NREM deprivation.[14] Because of the renewal, repair, and conservation functions of NREM sleep, deprivation may impair the immune system and depress the body's defenses, rendering the individual more vulnerable to disease and complications.

RECOVERY SLEEP

When an individual has been sleep deprived, the changes in physiologic and psychologic performance can be reversed through recovery sleep. Rosa and others[15] found that recall returned to baseline with 4 to 8 hours of recovery sleep after 40 to 64 hours of total sleep deprivation.

Deprivation of REM and NREM stage 4 results in rebounds in an attempt to compensate for "debts." The phenomenon of *REM rebound* occurs after selective REM deprivation. In an attempt to make up for lost REM and NREM stage 4 sleep, REM and NREM stage 4 periods quantitatively increase in the sleep periods after the deprivation. NREM stage 4 sleep is preferentially restored first, presumably because of its anabolic function. Because REM sleep is replenished last, it is more likely that REM debts will occur. REM rebound can exacerbate angina, dysrhythmias, duodenal ulcer pain, or sleep apneic episodes.[16] When a patient is exhibiting any of these symptoms and has had a period of sleep deprivation, REM rebound should be considered when determining the cause. Although the symptoms of angina, dysrhythmias, duodenal ulcer pain, and sleep apnea are treated as usual, further REM deprivation should be avoided.

SLEEP DISORDERS

Sleep Apnea Syndromes

Sleep apnea syndromes (SAS), or sometimes called *sleep-disordered breathing,* can be further differentiated into periodic cessation of breathing that results from upper airway obstruction *(obstructive sleep apnea),* lack of respiratory muscle activity *(central sleep apnea),* or a combination of both *(mixed apnea).*[17] It has been shown that an apnea index (the number of apneas per hour) exceeding 20 results in greater mortality. Treatment is recommended for patients with an apnea index of 5 to 20 if additional risk factors, such as smoking, hypercholesterolemia, or high blood pressure, are present. An apnea index less than 20 complicated by daytime sleepiness also requires treatment. SAS results in daytime somnolence, systemic or pulmonary hypertension, arterial blood gas abnormalities, life-threatening dysrhythmias, chronic respiratory failure, sexual dysfunction, and mental insufficiency. Hence it is clearly a life-threatening disorder that requires proper diagnosis and treatment.[18]

Obstructive Sleep Apnea

Description and etiology

Obstructive sleep apnea (OSA) is the most common form of sleep apnea. OSA is characterized by cessation of air flow resulting from upper airway obstruction although respiratory effort is exerted. Manifestations can range from a few mild symptoms to very severe symptoms that often constitute the pickwickian syndrome. This syndrome most commonly affects men older than 50 years and postmenopausal women, with predominant symptoms being snoring and excessive daytime sleepiness. Patients often have associated obesity, large jowls, and thick necks.[19] Other symptoms include systemic and pulmonary hypertension, arterial blood gas abnormalities, life-threatening cardiac dysrhythmias, chronic respiratory failure, sexual dysfunction, and mental insufficiency.

The cause of obstructive sleep apnea is not entirely understood; however, upper airway structure, hormonal balance, and neural control are implicated. Factors that contribute to OSA are (1) anatomic narrowing of the upper airway, (2) increased compliance of the upper airway tissue, (3) reflexes affecting upper airway caliber, and (4) pharyngeal inspiratory muscle function.[20]

Upper airway patency is also affected by upper airway function, which is under the control of the respiratory motor neurons. During sleep, this control varies and causes decreased neural activity, thereby narrowing the airway. This effect is especially prevalent during REM sleep when the motor neurons are hypotonic. Unstable control of the respiratory nerves of the diaphragmatic, intercostal, and upper airway muscles can cause sleep apneas.[20] Hypothyroidism can alter respiratory controls and therefore contribute to obstructive sleep apnea. Other contributing disorders are exogenous obesity, kyphoscoliosis, and autonomic dysfunction.

Pathophysiology

The patient with obstructive sleep apnea develops cycles of hypoxemia, hypercapnia, and acidosis with each episode of apnea until he or she is aroused and air flow resumes. Alveolar hypoventilation accompanies each episode of apnea and results in hypercapnia. Between episodes, alveolar ventilation improves so that overall there is no retention of CO_2. Morning headaches may result from lingering hypercapnia.

All types of sleep apnea are accompanied by arterial desaturation and potentially by hypoxemia, which may cause pulmonary vasoconstriction and an increased systemic vascular resistance. However, desaturation and hypoxemia are most severe in the obstructive type. With obstruction, inspiratory subatmospheric intrathoracic pressures are abnormally elevated. This leads to a tendency for airways to collapse, resulting in both hemodynamic and electrocardiographic changes.

The extremely elevated pressures that occur in individuals with obstructive sleep apnea who have apneic spells in both REM and NREM stages cause systemic and pulmonary hypertension. Systemic pressures of 200/120 mm Hg (awake control: 130/80 mm Hg) and pulmonary artery pressures of 80/54 mm Hg (awake control: 30/20 mm Hg) have been reported.[21] Cardiac dysrhythmias associated with obstructive apnea include bradycardias, sinus arrest, and occasionally, second-degree heart blocks. After resumption of air flow, tachycardias commonly occur. Thus bradycardia-tachycardia syndrome is associated with obstructive sleep apnea.

Assessment and diagnosis

The classic features of obstructive sleep apnea syndrome are daytime sleepiness and nocturnal snoring. Often the patient's sleep partner originally reports the disrupted sleep because of episodes of apnea and loud, abrupt sounds as breathing resumes. Patients become excessively sleepy during the day because of sleep fragmentation. Daytime napping and dozing at inappropriate times may be reported. Morning headaches are a complaint of many patients with OSA. The headache is frontal and diffuse, disappearing in several hours. Patients with OSA have increased motor activity during sleep. Memory loss, poor judgment, decreased attention span, irritability, personality changes, exercise intolerance, and impotence often lead to employment difficulties and marital problems for sleep apnea patients. Examination of the throat typically reveals enlarged tonsils, uvula, tongue, or excessive pharyngeal tissue.

Diagnosis of obstructive sleep apnea syndrome is made by polysomnogram (PSG), a sleep study. The polysomnogram is used to determine the number and length of apnea episodes and sleep stages, number of arousals, air flow, respiratory effort, oxygen desaturation, and vital signs.

After OSA is diagnosed, the patient's hematocrit (Hct) levels are checked for signs of hypoxia-induced polycythemia. Arterial blood gases are checked to assess for daytime hypoxia or hypercapnia. Thyroid function and the pharynx are evaluated for causes of sleep apnea that can possibly be medically or surgically corrected.

Medical management

Medical management includes mechanical and surgical approaches as well as the use of medication. Treatment varies depending on the type and extent of the patient's illness. Weight loss for those who are overweight is extremely important in the treatment of obstructive sleep apnea. Alcohol should be avoided, particularly before bedtime.

Nasal continuous positive airway pressure (CPAP) has been the most exciting development in recent years in the treatment of obstructive sleep apnea and is currently the treatment of choice.[18] Positive pressure is delivered via a mask placed over the nose, splinting the airway open. This improves oxygenation and stimulates afferent impulses from the upper airways, resulting in reflex dilation of the upper airways and stimulation of ventilation. Obstructive sleep apnea is improved by nasal CPAP, which in turn improves the sleep pattern and decreases daytime hypersomnolence.

Uvulopalatopharyngoplasty (UPPP) is a surgical approach to the treatment of obstructive sleep apnea. This procedure is used when anatomic abnormalities are the cause of the obstruction, and a surgical approach is indicated. Essentially, a large tonsillectomy is performed and redundant tissue is removed. After this procedure most patients no longer snore; however, only 50% experience sleep apnea improvement.[22] Because of the extensive resection of the posterior pharynx, regurgitation may be a problem for as many as 33% of patients. Patient selection by means of cephalometry or pharyngoscopy to identify the specific site of airway obstruction is important to the success of UPPP and other pharyngeal reconstructive surgeries.

Tracheostomy is rarely used in the treatment of obstructive sleep apnea since the development of nasal CPAP. Fewer than 5% of patients currently require tracheostomy.[18] It is indicated for severe apnea with life-threatening dysrhythmias, cor pulmonale, hypersomnolence, and failure of conservative treatment. The complications of tracheostomy are significant, including infection, bleeding, bronchitis, and granulation tissue as well as the psychosocial complications of an altered body image.

Because obstructive sleep apnea is so well treated by nasal CPAP, drug therapy is used only if CPAP is ineffective or unavailable. Protriptyline (Vivactil), a nonsedating tricyclic antidepressant, has been shown to decrease the number of apnea episodes and reduce daytime hypersomnolence by suppressing REM sleep, which is when apneic episodes occur. Oxygen may be used to relieve hypoxemia and nocturnal desaturations. In general, drug therapy has been disappointing in the treatment of obstructive sleep apnea.

Nursing management

Nursing management for patients diagnosed with OSA includes educating the patient, monitoring the effects of drug therapy, providing preoperative teaching, and monitoring for and preventing postoperative complications of UPPP or tracheostomy (Box 5-2).

Central Sleep Apnea

Description and etiology

Central sleep apnea (CSA) is not a single disease but rather a heterogenous group of disorders in which breathing ceases momentarily during sleep because of transient withdrawal of central nervous system (CNS) drive to the muscles of respiration.[23] Central sleep apnea is characterized by decreased respiratory output along with the absence of thoracic and abdominal muscle movements. Patients complain of disrupted sleep and of waking with a choking feeling. Snoring may be present. Central sleep apnea is a relatively rare disorder, occurring

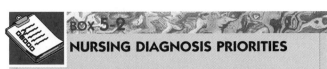

BOX 5-2

NURSING DIAGNOSIS PRIORITIES

Status Post-Uvulopalato-Pharyngoplasty (UPPP)

- Risk for Aspiration risk factors: impaired laryngeal sensation or reflex; impaired laryngeal closure or elevation; decreased lower esophageal sphincter pressure, p. 477
- Pain: related to transmission and perception of cutaneous, visceral, muscular, or ischemic impulses, p. 461
- Sleep Pattern Disturbance: related to fragmented sleep, p. 458
- Anxiety: related to threat to biologic, psychologic, and/or social integrity, p. 448
- Knowledge Deficit: reportable symptoms related to lack of previous exposure to information, p. 442

at perhaps 10% the rate of OSA. Patients tend to be older and have less pronounced oxygen desaturation and hemodynamic effects.

Pathophysiology

The mechanisms involved in central sleep apnea include defects in the respiratory control mechanism or muscles, transient instabilities in respiratory drive, and reflex inhibition of central respiratory drive. Central sleep apnea can be viewed clinically by hypercapnic and nonhypercapnic responses. Hypercapnic CSA arises in the situation of central alveolar hypoventilation or respiratory neuromuscular disease. This type of CSA is associated with encephalitis, brainstem neoplasm or infarction, spinal cord injury, muscular dystrophy, myasthenia gravis, bulbar poliomyelitis, and postpolio syndrome. Nonhypercapnic CSA occurs most often in patients with Cheyne-Stokes respiration secondary to other medical disorders or as an idiopathic disorder.[23]

Assessment and diagnosis

Because the underlying mechanisms are heterogenous, the presenting symptoms are variable as well. Patients with hypercapnic CSA characteristically have symptoms of chronic respiratory failure. Patients with nonhypercapnic CSA demonstrate a pattern of breathing characterized by a waxing and waning of tidal volume. This type of CSA can occur in patients with congestive heart failure and in patients with renal/metabolic disturbances.

Medical management

Central sleep apnea associated with central alveolar hypoventilation is managed generally by noninvasive measures—such as advice not to use sedative medications—and supplemental O_2 at nighttime after an assessment has been made of gas exchange during both sleep and wakefulness. Respiratory stimulants such as

medroxyprogesterone can improve ventilation during sleep in selected patients. If noninvasive and pharmacologic measures fail, consideration is given to a phrenic nerve pacemaker for nocturnal diaphragmatic stimulation or some form of assisted ventilation. Assisted ventilation may be intermittent positive pressure ventilation via a snug-fitting nasal mask or may require a tracheostomy. When there is associated neuromuscular weakness, supplemental O_2 and assisted ventilation with a nasal mask are generally very effective.[23]

Nursing management

The nursing management of the patient with central sleep apnea involves careful nighttime observation and assessment of breathing pattern. Anxiety about or fear of sleep because of apneic episodes is common and needs to be confronted. Patient reassurance of continuous nursing observation and monitoring is helpful.

References

1. Topf M, Bookman M, Arand D: Effects of critical care unit noise on the subjective quality of sleep, *J Advanced Nurs* 24:545-551, 1996.
2. Richards KC: Effect of a back massage and relaxation intervention on sleep in critically ill patients, *Am J Crit Care* 7(4):288-299, 1998.
3. Guyton AC: *Medical physiology,* ed 8, Philadelphia, 1991, WB Saunders.
4. Rechtschaffen A, Kales A: *A manual of standardized terminology, techniques and scoring systems for sleep stages of human subjects,* Washington DC, 1968, US Department of Health, Education and Welfare.
5. Verrier RL, Kirby DA: Sleep and cardiac arrhythmias, *Ann N Y Acad Sci* 533:238, 1988.
6. Somers VL, et al: Sympathetic/nerve activity during sleep in normal subjects, *N Engl J Med* 328(5):303, 1993.
7. Closs SJ: Assessment of sleep in hospitalized patients: a review of methods, *J Adv Nurs* 13:501, 1988.
8. Muller JE, Tofler MB, Stone PH: Circadian variation and triggers of onset of acute cardiovascular disease, *Circulation* 79(4):733, 1989.
9. Hayter J: Sleep behaviors of older persons, *Nurs Res* 32(4):242, 1983.
10. Hodgson L: Why do we need sleep: relating theory to nursing practice, *J Adv Nurs* 16:1503, 1991.
11. Wilse WB: Age-related changes in sleep, *Clin Geriatr Med* 5(2):275, 1989.
12. Brewer MJ: To sleep or not to sleep: the consequences of sleep deprivation, *Crit Care Nurs* 5(6):35, 1985.
13. Fordham M: In Wilson Bennett J, Butemp L, editors: *Patient problems: a research base for nursing care,* London, 1988, Scutain Press.
14. Wotring K: Using research in practice, *Focus Crit Care* 9(5):34, 1982.
15. Rosa R, Bonnet M, Warm J: Recovery of performance during sleep following sleep deprivation, *Psychophysiology* 20:152, 1983.
16. Sanford S: Sleep and the cardiac patient, *Cardiovasc Nurs* 19(5):19, 1983.
17. Noureddine S: Sleep apnea: a challenge in critical care, *Heart Lung* 25(1):37, 1996.
18. Kryger MH, Roth T, Dement W: *Principles and practice of sleep medicine,* Philadelphia, 1994, WB Saunders.

19. Katz I, et al: Do patients with obstructive sleep apnea have thick necks? *Am Rev Resp Disorders* 141:1228, 1990.

20. Hudgel DW: Mechanisms of obstructive sleep apnea, *Chest* 101:541, 1992.

21. Bjurstrom R, Schoene R, Pierson D: The control of ventilatory drives: physiology and clinical applications, *Respir Care* 31(11):1128, 1986.

22. Sanders M, et al: The acute effects of uvulopalatopharyngoplasty on breathing during sleep in sleep apnea patients, *Sleep* 11(1):75, 1988.

23. Bradley TD, Phillipson EA: Central sleep apnea, *Clin Chest Med* 13(3):493, 1992.

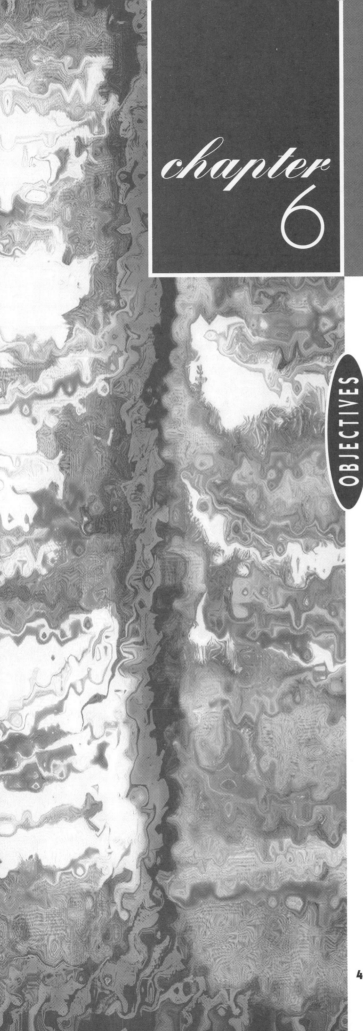

chapter 6

Nutritional Alterations

Mary Courtney Moore

OBJECTIVES

● Describe the adverse effects of nutritional impairments on critically ill patients

● Assess the nutritional status of critically ill patients with cardiovascular, pulmonary, neurologic, renal, gastrointestinal, and endocrine alterations.

● Recognize nutritional alterations commonly associated with cardiovascular, pulmonary, neurologic, renal, gastrointestinal, and endocrine alterations.

● Collaborate with a multidisciplinary team in designing a nutrition program for critically ill patients.

● Identify complications of nutrition support and nursing interventions for prevention and management of these complications.

METABOLIC RESPONSE TO STARVATION AND STRESS

To understand the development of malnutrition in the hospitalized patient, the nurse must understand the metabolic response to starvation and physiologic stress. Changes in endocrine status and metabolism work together to determine the onset and extent of malnutrition. Nutritional imbalance occurs when the demand for nutrients is greater than the exogenous nutrient supply. The major difference between one who is starved and one who is starved and injured is that the latter relies more heavily on endogenous protein breakdown to provide precursors for glucose production to meet increased energy demands.[1] (*Glucogenesis* refers to the process of forming glucose from amino acids and other noncarbohydrates). Therefore, although carbohydrate and fat metabolism are also affected, the main concern is with protein metabolism and homeostasis.

During an acute, nonstressed fast, blood levels of glucose and insulin fall, and glucagon levels rise. Glucagon promotes the use of glycogen reserves, which quickly become exhausted. Glucagon also stimulates gluconeogenesis for which skeletal muscle provides a large amount of the substrates required. As fasting progresses, triglycerides are mobilized from fat deposits, and free fatty acids and ketones derived from the triglycerides become the primary source of fuel. Consequently the blood ketone levels begin to increase. Once the circulating ketone level rises, the brain is able to use ketones for 70% of its energy, thereby decreasing the total body's reliance on glucose as a major energy source. As gluconeogenesis from protein precursors decreases, protein breakdown and nitrogen excretion also slow. Obligatory glucose users such as blood cells, the renal medulla, and 30% of brain cells still require a small amount of amino acids because they continue to rely on glucose as their preferred source of fuel. However, endogenous protein stores are spared from use for gluconeogenesis to a major extent, and protein homeostasis is partially restored.

Of concern to those caring for critically ill patients is the combination of starvation and the physiologic stress resulting from injury, trauma, major surgery, and/or sepsis. This physiologic stress results in profound metabolic alterations that persist from the time of the stressful event until the completion of wound healing and recovery. Stress normally causes an increased metabolic rate (hypermetabolism) that necessitates a rise in oxygen consumption and energy expenditure.

Hormonal changes that occur at the initiation of the stressful event begin the hypermetabolic process. With stimulation of the sympathetic nervous system, the adrenal medulla releases catecholamines (epinephrine and norepinephrine). These in turn, stimulate the body's metabolic response to stress. Also released in response to stress are adrenocorticotropic hormone (ACTH) and antidiuretic hormone (ADH) as well as glucocorticoids and mineralocorticoids. These hormonal changes tend to stimulate nutrient substrates, primarily amino acids, to move from peripheral tissues (e.g., skeletal muscle) to the liver for gluconeogenesis. Unfortunately, this mobilization of substrates occurs at the expense of body tissue and function at a time when the needs for protein synthesis (e.g., for wound healing and acute phase proteins) also are high. Hyperglycemia results from the effects of increased catecholamines, glucocorticoids, and glucagon. Again the body relies on its protein stores to provide substrates for gluconeogenesis because glucose now becomes the major fuel source. Loss of protein results in a negative nitrogen balance and weight loss. The classic response to metabolic stress is the use of protein for fuel.[1]

IMPLICATIONS OF UNDERNUTRITION FOR THE SICK OR STRESSED PATIENT

Malnutrition is widespread among hospitalized patients. For example, recent reports indicate that as many as one third of patients hospitalized for major abdominal surgery and one half of general medical patients show evidence of malnutrition.[2-5] Although illness or injury is the major factor contributing to development of malnutrition, other possible contributing factors include lack of communication among the nurses, physicians, and dietitians responsible for the care of these patients; frequent diagnostic testing, which causes patients to miss meals or to be too exhausted for meals; medications and other therapies that cause anorexia, nausea, or vomiting and thus interfere with food intake; or inadequate use of tube feedings or total parenteral nutrition to maintain the nutritional status of these patients. Nutritional status tends to deteriorate during hospitalization unless appropriate nutritional support is started early and continually reassessed.[4]

Malnutrition is an ominous finding among very ill patients. Wound dehiscence, decubitus ulcers, sepsis, and pulmonary infections are more common among undernourished patients. Medical patients with evidence of undernutrition at hospital admission have longer hospital stays as well as a trend toward greater mortality.[5]

ASSESSING NUTRITIONAL STATUS

A nutrition screening should be conducted on every patient admitted to a hospital or skilled nursing facility. A brief questionnaire completed by the patient or significant other, the nursing admission form, or the physician's admission note usually provides enough information to determine whether the patient is nutritionally at risk (Box 6-1). Any patient judged to be nutritionally at risk needs a more thorough nutrition assessment.

Biochemical Data

A wide range of laboratory tests can provide information about nutritional status. Those most often used in the clinical setting are described in Table 6-1. As the table emphasizes, there are no perfect diagnostic tests for evaluation of nutrition, and care must be taken in interpreting the results of the tests.

Clinical or Physical Manifestations

A thorough physical examination is an essential part of a nutrition assessment. Box 6-2 lists some of the more common findings that may indicate an altered nutritional state. It is especially important for the nurse to check for manifestations of muscle wasting, loss of subcutaneous fat, skin or hair changes, and impairment of wound healing.

BOX 6-1

PATIENTS WHO ARE AT RISK FOR MALNUTRITION

Adults who exhibit any of the following:
- Involuntary loss or gain of a significant amount of weight (>10% of usual body weight in 6 months, >5% in 1 month), even if the weight achieved by loss or gain is appropriate for height
- Weight 20% more or less than ideal body weight, or body mass index < 19 or > 27*
- Chronic disease
- Chronic use of a modified diet
- Increased metabolic requirements
- Illness or surgery that may interfere with nutritional intake
- Need for enteral tube feeding or parenteral nutrition
- Inadequate nutrition intake for >7 days
- Regular use of three or more medications
- Poverty

Infants and children who exhibit any of the following:
- Low birth weight
- Small-for-gestational age
- Weight loss of 10% or more
- Weight-for-length or weight-for-height <10th percentile or >90th percentile
- Increased metabolic requirements
- Impaired ability to ingest or tolerate oral feedings
- Inadequate weight gain or a significant decrease in an individual's usual growth percentile
- Poverty

*Body mass index (BMI) = weight in kg ÷ (height in m)^2; 1 kg = 2.2 lb, 1 m = 39.37 inches.

BOX 6-2

CLINICAL MANIFESTATIONS OF NUTRITIONAL ALTERATIONS

Manifestations that may indicate protein-calorie malnutrition:
- Hair loss; dull, dry, brittle hair; loss of hair pigment
- Loss of subcutaneous tissue; muscle wasting
- Poor wound healing
- Hepatomegaly
- Edema

Manifestations often present in vitamin deficiencies:
- Conjunctival and corneal dryness (vitamin A)
- Dry scaly skin; follicular hyperkeratosis, in which the skin appears to have gooseflesh continually (vitamin A)
- Gingivitis; poor wound healing (vitamin C)
- Petechiae; ecchymoses (vitamins C or K)
- Inflamed tongue; cracking at the corners of the mouth (riboflavin [vitamin B_2], niacin, folic acid, vitamin B_{12}, or other B vitamins)
- Edema; congestive heart failure (thiamin [vitamin B_1])
- Confusion; confabulation (thiamin [vitamin B_1])

Manifestations often present in mineral deficiencies:
- Blue sclerae; pale mucous membranes; spoon-shaped nails (iron)
- Hypogeusia, or poor sense of taste; dysgeusia, or bad taste; eczema; poor wound healing (zinc)

Manifestations often observed with excessive vitamin intake:
- Hair loss; dry skin; hepatomegaly (vitamin A)

Diet and Relevant Health History

Information about dietary intake and significant variations in weight is a vital part of the history. Dietary intake can be evaluated in several ways, including a diet record, a 24-hour recall, and a diet history. Information to include in a nutrition history is included in Table 6-2.

Evaluating Nutritional Assessment Findings

It is rare for a patient to exhibit a lack of only one nutrient. Usually nutritional deficiencies are combined, with the patient lacking adequate amounts of protein, calories, and possibly vitamins and minerals. A common form of combined nutritional deficit among hospitalized patients is protein-calorie malnutrition (PCM). Two types of PCM are kwashiorkor and marasmus.

Kwashiorkor is evidenced by low levels of the serum proteins albumin, transferrin, and prealbumin; low total lymphocyte count; impaired immunity; loss of hair or hair pigment; edema resulting from low plasma oncotic pressure caused by a loss of plasma proteins; and an enlarged, fatty liver. The person with kwashiorkor may have had little or no weight loss. Marasmus is recognizable by weight loss, a decrease in skinfold measurements, loss of subcutaneous fat, muscle wasting, and low levels of creatinine excretion (an indicator of loss of muscle mass). Because PCM weakens musculature, increases vulnerability to infection, and can prolong hospital stays, the health care team should diagnose this serious disorder as quickly as possible so that appropriate nutritional intervention can be implemented.

NUTRITION AND CARDIOVASCULAR ALTERATIONS

Diet and cardiovascular disease may interact in a variety of ways. In one situation, excessive nutrient intake—manifested by overweight or obesity and a diet rich in cholesterol and saturated fat—is a risk factor for development of arteriosclerotic heart disease. Conversely, the consequences of chronic myocardial insufficiency can include malnutrition.[6]

Nutrition Assessment

A nutrition assessment provides the nurse and other members of the health care team with the information necessary to plan the patient's nutrition care and teach-

TABLE 6-1

DIAGNOSTIC TESTS USED IN NUTRITION ASSESSMENT

Area of Concern	Possible Deficiency	Comments
SERUM PROTEINS		
Decrease of serum albumin, transferrin (iron transport protein), or thyroxine-binding prealbumin*	Protein	These proteins are produced in the liver, are depressed in hepatic failure, and are falsely low in fluid volume excess and elevated in volume deficit. Albumin has a long half-life (14-20 days) and is slow to change in malnutrition and repletion; transferrin has a half-life of 7-8 days, but levels increase in iron deficiency, and prevalence of iron deficiency limits usefulness in diagnosing protein deficits; prealbumin half-life is 2-3 days, and levels fall in trauma and infection.
HEMATOLOGIC VALUES		
Anemia (decreased Hct, Hgb)		Hct and Hgb are falsely low in fluid volume excess and falsely high in fluid volume deficit.
Normocytic (normal MCV, MCHC)	Protein	
Microcytic (decreased MCV, MCH, MCHC)	Iron, copper	
Macrocytic (increased MCV)	Folate, vitamin B_{12}	
Total lymphocyte count (TLC = WBC × % lymphocytes) <1200/mm^3	Protein	TLC is decreased in severe debilitating disease.
URINARY CREATININE		
Creatinine excretion of <17 mg/kg/day (women), <23 mg/kg/day (men)	Protein (reflects lean body mass)	It is difficult to collect accurate 24-hr urine; creatinine excretion varies widely from day to day; levels decline with age as percentage of lean body mass declines.
NITROGEN BALANCE†		
Negative values	Protein, calories (during calorie deficit, protein is metabolized to provide calories)	Negative values occur when more nitrogen is excreted than is consumed (reflects inadequate intake or increased needs); positive values occur when more is consumed than lost (e.g., during nutrition repletion, growth, or pregnancy); normal healthy adults excrete exactly what they consume. Limitations: it is difficult to collect accurate 24-hr urine; retention of nitrogen does not necessarily mean that it is being used for tissue synthesis.

*Evaluation of at least one of these is a part of almost every nutritional assessment.
†Protein is 16% nitrogen. Thus nitrogen balance = [24-hr protein intake (g) × 0.16] − [24-hr urine urea nitrogen (g) + 4 g]. The 4 g is an estimate of fecal, skin, and other minor losses.
Hct, Hematocrit; *Hgb,* hemoglobin; *MCV,* Mean corpuscular volume; *MCHC,* mean corpuscular hemoglobin concentration; *MCH,* mean corpuscular hemoglobin.

ing. Key points of the nutrition assessment of the cardiovascular patient are summarized in Table 6-3. The major nutritional concerns relate to appropriateness of body weight and the levels of serum lipids and blood pressure.

Nutrition Intervention

Myocardial infarction

The following guidelines will assist the nurse in providing appropriate nutritional care for the patient in the immediate postmyocardial infarction (MI) period:

- Limit meal size for the patient with severe myocardial compromise or postprandial angina.

- Monitor the effect of caffeine on the patient, if caffeine is included in the diet.
- Use caution in serving foods at temperature extremes.

Hypertension

A substantial number of individuals with hypertension are "salt sensitive," with their disorder improving when sodium intake is limited. Consequently restriction of sodium intake, usually to 2.5 g or less/day, is often advised to help control hypertension.[7] The primary sodium source in the American diet is salt (sodium chloride) added during food processing and preparation or at the

TABLE 6-2

NUTRITION HISTORY INFORMATION

Area of Concern	Significant Findings	Nutrients of Special Concern
Inadequate intake of nutrients	Avoidance of specific food groups because of poverty or poor dentition	Protein, iron
	Alcohol abuse	Protein, vitamin B$_1$, niacin, folate
	Anorexia, nausea, vomiting	Most nutrients, particularly protein, electrolytes
	Confusion, coma	All nutrients
Inadequate absorption or utilization of nutrients	Previous GI surgeries:	
	Gastrectomy	Vitamin B$_{12}$, minerals, calories (if the patient experiences dumping syndrome)
	Ileal resection	Vitamins B$_{12}$, A, E; minerals; calories (in extensive small bowel resection)
	Certain medications:	
	Antacids, cimetidine (reduce upper duodenal acidity)	Minerals
	Cholestyramine (binds fat-soluble nutrients)	Vitamins A, D, E, K
	Corticosteroids	Protein
	Anticonvulsants	Calcium
Increased nutrient losses	Chronic or acute blood loss	Iron
	Severe diarrhea	Fluid, electrolytes
	Fistulas, draining abscesses, wounds	Protein, zinc
	Nephrotic syndrome	Protein, zinc
	Peritoneal dialysis or hemodialysis	Protein, zinc, water-soluble vitamins
Increased nutrient requirements	Fever*	Calories
	Surgery, trauma, burns, infection	Calories, protein, zinc, vitamin C
	Neoplasms (some types)	Calories, protein
	Physiologic demands (pregnancy, lactation, growth)	Calories, protein, iron

*Each 1° C (1.8° F) elevation in temperature increases caloric needs by approximately 13%.

TABLE 6-3

NUTRITION ASSESSMENT OF THE CARDIOVASCULAR PATIENT

Area of Concern	Significant Findings		
	History	Physical Assessment	Laboratory Data
Overweight/obesity	Excessive kcal intake Sedentary life-style	Weight >120% of desirable, or BMI >27	
Protein-calorie malnutrition (cardiac cachexia)	Chronic cardiopulmonary disease, causing: Decreased food intake related to angina, respiratory embarrassment, or fatigue during eating Malabsorption of nutrients caused by hypoxia of the gut Medications that impair appetite (e.g., digitalis, quinidine)	Weight <85% of desirable, or BMI <19 Muscle wasting Loss of subcutaneous fat	Serum albumin <3.5 g/dL (or low transferrin or prealbumin level) Negative nitrogen balance Creatinine excretion of <17 mg/kg/day (women), <23 mg/kg/day (men)
Altered serum lipid levels	Frequent or daily use of foods high in cholesterol and saturated fat Sedentary life-style Family history of hyperlipidemia Overweight or obesity	Xanthomas, or yellowish plaques, deposited in the skin (uncommon)	Serum cholesterol >200 mg/dL Low-density lipoprotein cholesterol >100 mg/dL High density lipoprotein (HDL) cholesterol <35 mg/dL
Elevated blood pressure	Daily use of high-sodium foods and salt at the table Consumption of >2 alcoholic drinks/day		

Modified from Moore MC: *Pocket guide to nutritional care,* ed 3, St Louis, 1996, Mosby.

table. One teaspoon of salt provides about 2.3 g of sodium. Most salt substitutes contain potassium chloride and may be used with the physician's approval by the patient who has no renal impairment. Litesalt is about half sodium chloride and half potassium chloride. If used, it must be used very sparingly to maintain an adequate restriction of sodium intake.

Heart failure

Nutrition intervention in heart failure (HF) is designed to reduce fluid retained within the body and thus reduce the preload. Because fluid accompanies sodium, limitation of sodium is necessary to reduce fluid retention. Specific interventions include (1) limiting sodium intake, usually to 2 g/day or less, and (2) limiting fluid intake as appropriate. If fluid is restricted, the daily fluid allowance is usually 1.5 to 2 L/day, to include both fluids in the diet and those given with medications and for other purposes.

Cardiac cachexia

The severely malnourished cardiac patient often suffers from CHF.[6] Therefore sodium and fluid restriction, as previously described, are appropriate. It is important to concentrate nutrients into as small a volume as possible and to serve small amounts frequently, rather than three large meals daily, which may overwhelm the patient. The patient also can be given calorie-dense foods and supplements.

Because the patient is likely to tire quickly and to suffer from anorexia, enteral tube feeding may be necessary. Most commonly used tube feeding formulas provide 1 calorie/ml, but more concentrated products (1.5 to 2 calories/ml) are available to provide adequate nutrients in a smaller volume.

The nurse must monitor the fluid status of these patients carefully when they are receiving nutrition support. Assessment of breath sounds, presence and severity of peripheral edema, and changes in body weight are performed daily or more frequently. A consistent weight gain of more than 0.11 to 0.22 kg (0.25 to 0.5 lb) a day usually indicates fluid retention, rather than gain of fat and muscle mass.

NUTRITION AND PULMONARY ALTERATIONS

Malnutrition has extremely adverse effects on respiratory function, decreasing surfactant production, diaphragmatic mass, and vital capacity.[8] Patients with acute respiratory disorders find it difficult to consume adequate oral nutrients and can rapidly become malnourished. Ventilator dependency not only interferes with nutrient intake but can also increase energy expenditure.

Nutrition Assessment

Nutrition assessment is summarized in Table 6-4. The patient with respiratory compromise is especially vulnerable to the effects of fluid volume and carbohydrate excess and must be assessed continually for these complications.

Nutrition Intervention

Prevent or correct undernutrition and underweight

The nurse and dietitian work together to encourage oral intake in the undernourished or potentially undernourished patient who is capable of eating. Small frequent feedings are especially important because a very full stomach can interfere with diaphragmatic movement. Mouth care needs to be provided before meals and snacks to clear the palate of the flavors of sputum and medications. Administering bronchodilators with food can help to reduce gastric irritation caused by these medications.

Avoid overfeeding

Overfeeding of total calories or of carbohydrate or lipid alone can impair pulmonary function. This is unlikely to be significant in the patient who is eating foods. Instead, it is an iatrogenic complication of TPN, the predominant calorie source, or of tube feeding. Excessive calorie intake can raise $PaCO_2$ sufficiently to make it difficult to wean a patient from the ventilator. A balanced regimen with both lipids and carbohydrates providing the nonprotein calories is optimal for the patient with respiratory compromise, and the patient needs to be reassessed continually to ensure that caloric intake is not excessive.[8]

Excessive lipid intake can impair capillary gas exchange in the lungs, although this is not usually sufficient to produce an increase in $PaCO_2$ or decrease in PaO_2.[9-10] However, the patient with severe respiratory alteration may be further compromised by lipid overdose. If lipid intake is maintained at no more than 2 g/kg/day, lipid excess is rarely a problem. Lipids are available as 20 g/100 ml (20% lipid emulsion) and 10 g/100 ml (10% emulsion). Serum triglyceride levels greater than 150 mg/dL may indicate inadequate lipid clearance and a need to decrease the lipid dosage.

Prevent fluid volume excess

Pulmonary edema and failure of the right side of the heart, which may be precipitated by fluid volume excess, further worsen the status of the patient with respiratory compromise. Strict intake records must be maintained to allow for accurate totals of fluid intake. Usually the patient requires no more than 35 to 40 ml/kg/day of fluid. For the patient receiving nutrition support, fluid intake can be reduced by using 20% lipid emulsions as a source of calories, by using tube feeding formulas providing at least 2 calories/ml (the dietitian can recommend appropriate formulas) and by choosing oral supplements that are low in fluid. Some examples are cottonseed oil (Lipomul [Upjohn]), an oral lipid supplement providing 6 calories/ml, and powdered glucose polymers, which in-

TABLE 6-4

NUTRITION ASSESSMENT OF THE PULMONARY PATIENT

Area of Concern	Significant Findings		
	History	Physical Assessment	Laboratory Data
Protein-calorie malnutrition	Chronic lung disease: poor intake of protein and calories because of the following: Breathing difficulty from pressure of a full stomach on the diaphragm Unpleasant taste in the mouth from chronic sputum production Gastric irritation from bronchodilator therapy Increased energy expenditure from increased work of breathing	Muscle wasting Loss of subcutaneous fat Recent weight loss, weight measurement of <85% of desirable, or BMI <19	Serum albumin <3.5 g/dL, or low transferrin or prealbumin level Total lymphocyte count <1200/mm^3 Creatinine excretion <17mg/kg (women) or <23 mg/kg (men)
	Acute respiratory alterations: inadequate intake of protein and calories because of the following: Upper airway intubation Altered state of consciousness Dyspnea Increased protein and calorie requirements caused by increased work of breathing or acute pulmonary infections Catabolism resulting from corticosteroid use	Same as for chronic disease	Same as for chronic disease
Overweight/obesity (in patients with chronic lung disease)	Decreased caloric needs resulting from decreasing metabolic rate with aging (metabolic rate declines by 2%/decade after age 30) or decreased activity to compensate for impaired respiratory function	Weight >120% of desirable or BMI >27	
Elevated respiratory quotient (RQ)*	Overfeeding usually with total parenteral nutrition or tube feeding	Tachypnea, shortness of breath	RQ ≥1 Elevated V_{O_2} and V_{CO_2} Elevated Pa_{CO_2} (not always present)
Fluid volume excess	Administration of more than 35-50 ml fluid/kg/day Increased antidiuretic hormone (ADH) release resulting from stress and ventilator dependency	Dependent edema Pulmonary rales Bounding pulse Shortness of breath	Serum sodium <135 mEq/L BUN, hematocrit, and serum albumin decreased from previous values Serum triglyceride >150 mg/dL
Excess lipid intake	Administration of intravenous (IV) lipids		Low $V_A Q$†

Modified from Moore MC: *Pocket guide to nutritional care,* ed 3, St Louis, 1996, Mosby.

BUN, blood urea nitrogen.

*RQ, or CO_2 produced ÷ O_2 consumed, is measured by indirect calorimetry, which is not available in all institutions.

†The defect is not usually sufficient to alter Pa_{O_2} or Pa_{CO_2}, except in patients with the most severe lung disease.

crease caloric intake without increasing volume. The nurse plays a valuable role in continually reassessing the patient's state of hydration and alerting other team members to changes that may dictate an increase or decrease in fluid intake.

NUTRITION AND NEUROLOGIC ALTERATIONS

Because neurologic disorders tend to be long-term problems, they necessitate good nutritional care to prevent nutritional deficits and promote well-being.

Nutrition Assessment

Nutrition-related assessment findings vary widely in the patient with neurologic alterations, depending on the type of disorder present. Some common findings are shown in Table 6-5.

Nutrition Intervention

Prevention or correction of nutritional deficits

Oral feedings. Patients with dysphagia or weakness of the swallowing musculature often experience the greatest difficulty in swallowing foods that are dry or thin liquids, such as water, that are difficult to control.

Tube feedings or TPN. Patients who are unconscious or unable to eat because of severe dysphagia, weakness, ileus, or other reasons will need tube feedings or TPN. Prompt initiation of nutrition support must be a priority in the patient with neurologic impairments. Needs for protein and calories are increased by infection and fever, as may occur in the patient with encephalitis or meningitis. Needs for protein, calories, zinc, and vitamin C are increased during wound healing, as occurs in the trauma patient and the patient with decubitus ulcers.

Patients with neurologic deficits have an increased risk of certain complications, particularly pulmonary aspiration, during tube feeding and thus they require especially careful nursing management. Patients of most concern are (1) those with an impaired gag reflex, such as some patients with cerebral vascular accident; (2) those with delayed gastric emptying, such as patients in the early period after spinal cord injury and patients with head injury treated with barbiturate coma; and (3) patients likely to experience seizures. To help prevent pulmonary aspiration, the patient's head is kept elevated, if not contraindicated. When elevation of the head is not possible, administering feedings with the patient in the prone or lateral position will allow free drainage of emesis from the mouth and decrease the risk of aspiration.

Although case reports in the literature suggest that formulas for enteral feeding can interfere with phenytoin absorption, one controlled investigation failed to find any effect on overall absorption of phenytoin.[11] Until this is-

sue has been resolved, phenytoin levels should be monitored carefully in patients receiving enteral feedings.

Hyperglycemia is a common complication in patients receiving corticosteroids. Patients treated with these drugs should have blood glucose levels monitored regularly; they may require insulin to prevent substantial loss of glucose in the urine as well as osmotic diuresis, loss of excessive amounts of potassium, and other fluid and electrolyte disturbances.

Prompt use of nutrition support is especially important for patients with head injuries, because head injury causes marked catabolism, even in patients who receive barbiturates, which should decrease metabolic demands.[11] Head-injured patients rapidly exhaust glycogen stores and begin to use body proteins to meet energy needs, a process that can quickly cause PCM. The catabolic response to head injury is partly a result of the corticosteroids often used in treatment. However, the hypermetabolism and hypercatabolism are also caused by dramatic hormonal responses to this type of injury.[11] Levels of cortisol, epinephrine, and norepinephrine increase, with levels of norepinephrine elevating as much as 7 times normal. These hormones increase the metabolic rate and caloric demands, causing mobilization of body fat and proteins to meet the increased energy needs. Furthermore, head-injured patients undergo an inflammatory response and may be febrile, creating increased needs for protein and calories. Improved survival has been observed in head-injured patients who receive adequate nutrition support early in the hospital course.[11]

NUTRITION AND RENAL ALTERATIONS

Providing adequate nutritional care for the patient with renal disease can be extremely challenging. Although renal disturbances and their treatments can markedly increase needs for nutrients, necessary restrictions in intake of fluid, protein, phosphorus, and potassium make delivery of adequate calories, vitamins, and minerals difficult. Thorough nutrition assessment provides the basis for successful nutritional management in patients with renal disease.

Nutrition Assessment

Assessment is summarized in Table 6-6.

Nutrition Intervention

The goal of nutritional intervention is to administer adequate nutrients, including calories, protein, vitamins, and minerals, while avoiding excesses of protein, fluid, electrolytes, and other nutrients with potential toxicity.

Protein

Evidence suggests that a low-protein diet retards the progression of renal damage in selected patients. It is postulated that a high-protein intake increases glomeru-

TABLE 6-5

NUTRITION ASSESSMENT OF THE PATIENT WITH NEUROLOGIC ALTERATIONS

Area of Concern	Significant Findings		
	History	Physical Assessment	Laboratory Data
DISORDERS OF PROTEIN AND CALORIE NUTRITURE			

Protein-calorie malnutrition	Decreased intake because of the following:
	  Coma or confusion
	  Feeding/swallowing difficulties such as dribbling of food and beverages from mouth, dysphagia, weakness of muscles involved in chewing and swallowing
	  Ileus resulting from spinal cord injury or use of pentobarbital
	  Anorexia resulting from depression
	Increased needs because of the following:
	  Hypermetabolism and catabolism after head injury
	  Catabolism resulting from corticosteroid use
	  Trauma and surgical wounds
	Loss of protein from decubitus ulcers
		Muscle wasting
		Loss of subcutaneous fat
		Weight <85% of desirable or BMI <19
		Change in hair texture, loss of hair
			Serum albumin <3.5 g/dL (or low transferrin or prealbumin value)
			Negative nitrogen balance
			Total lymphocyte count <1200/mm³
			Creatinine excretion <17 mg/kg/day (women) or <23 mg/kg/day (men)

Overweight/obesity	Decreased caloric needs resulting from inactivity Reliance on soft or pureed foods, which are often more dense in calories than higher fiber foods Increased food intake resulting from depression/boredom	Weight >120% of desirable or BMI >27	
VITAMIN AND MINERAL DEFICIENCIES			
Iron (Fe)	Poor intake of meats resulting from chewing difficulties (e.g., as occurs with myasthenia gravis) Loss of blood in trauma	Pallor, blue sclerae	Microcytic anemia (low Hct, Hgb, MCV, MCH, MCHC) Serum Fe <50µg/ml
Zinc (Zn)	Poor intake of meat resulting from chewing problems Increased needs for healing decubitus ulcers, trauma, or surgical wounds	Hypogeusia, dysgeusia Diarrhea Seborrheic dermatitis Alopecia	Serum Zn <60 µg/ml
FLUID ALTERATIONS			
Fluid volume deficit	Poor intake resulting from difficulty in swallowing (e.g., as occurs with cerebrovascular accident) Inability to express thirst Fluid restriction in an effort to reduce intracranial edema	Poor skin turgor Decreased urinary output Dry, sticky mucous membranes	Serum sodium >145 mEq/L Serum osmolality >300 mOsm/kg Increased BUN and Hct levels Urine specific gravity >1.030

Modified from Moore MC: *Pocket guide to nutritional care*, ed 3, St Louis, 1996, Mosby.

lar flow and pressures, as the kidney attempts to excrete the urea and other nitrogenous products derived from the protein. The increase in glomerular pressures may hasten the death of the glomeruli.[12] Consequently, decreased protein intake (0.6 to 0.8 g/kg/day compared with the 0.8 g/kg/day recommended for the healthy person and the 1.7 g/kg/day actually consumed by the average American) is recommended for some patients with renal insufficiency who do not yet need dialysis. Women and patients with renal failure from diabetes or hypertension appear to benefit less from protein restriction than do men and patients with glomerulonephritis and interstitial nephritis.[12] Nutritional status of patients on a low-protein diet must be carefully monitored because protein undernutrition is apt to occur.[13]

Although uremia necessitates control of protein intake, the patient with renal failure often has other physiologic stresses that actually increase protein/amino acid needs:

TABLE 6-6

NUTRITION ASSESSMENT OF THE RENAL PATIENT

Area of Concern	History	Physical Assessment	Laboratory Data

Protein-calorie malnutrition	Poor dietary intake because of the following:
	  Dietary restrictions on protein-containing foods
	  Anorexia caused by zinc deficiency (lost in dialysis or decreased in diet because of restrictions on meats, whole grains, legumes)
	Increased protein and amino acid losses from the following:
	  Dialysis (hemodialysis losses ≈ 10-13 g/session; CAPD losses ≈ 5-15 g/day)*
	  Tissue catabolism resulting from corticosteroid use
	  Proteinuria (e.g., as occurs with nephrotic syndrome)
	  Increased needs for protein and calories during peritonitis and other infections
		Muscle wasting
		Loss of subcutaneous tissue
		Weight <85% of desirable or BMI <19
		(Loss of weight and subcutaneous fat may be masked by edema)
		Loss of hair, change of hair texture
			Serum albumin <3.5 g/dL or low transferrin or prealbumin level
			Total lymphocyte count <1200/mm³
			Negative nitrogen balance

Altered lipid metabolism	Nephrotic syndrome, with elevated cholesterol levels
	Excess carbohydrate (CHO) consumption from the following:
	  Emphasis on CHO in the diet to replace some of the calories normally provided by protein
	  Use of glucose as an osmotic agent in dialysis
			Serum cholesterol >250 mg/dL
			Serum triglyceride >180 mg/dL

Potential fluid volume excess	Patient knowledge deficit about or noncompliance with fluid restriction Oliguria or anuria	Edema Hypertension Acute weight gain (≥1%-2% of body weight)	Hematocrit decreased from previous levels
DISORDERS OF MINERALS/ELECTROLYTES			
Phosphorus (P) excess	Oliguria or anuria	Tetany	Serum P >4.5 mg/dL Calcium × P product (Ca in mg/dL × P in mg/dL) >70

Modified from Moore, MC: *Pocket guide to nutritional care,* ed 3, St Louis, 1996, Mosby.
CAPD, continuous ambulatory peritoneal dialysis.
*Increased by 50%-100% in peritonitis.

losses because of dialysis, wounds, and fistulae; use of corticosteroid drugs that exert a catabolic effect; increased endogenous secretion of catecholamines, corticosteroids, glucagon, and parathyroid hormone, all of which can cause or aggravate catabolism; and catabolic conditions, such as trauma, surgery, and sepsis associated or coincident with the renal disturbances. During hemodialysis and arteriovenous (A-V) hemofiltration, amino acids are freely filtered and lost, but proteins such as albumin and immunoglobulin are not. Both proteins and amino acids are removed during peritoneal dialysis, creating a greater nutritional requirement for protein.[14] Protein needs are estimated at approximately 1.2 g/kg/day for patients receiving hemodialysis or hemofiltration,[15] and 1.2 to 1.5 g/kg/day for those receiving peritoneal dialysis.[14,16] Although these amounts are greater than the recommended daily level for healthy adults, they are lower than the amount found in the diet of most adults, and thus many patients will perceive them as restrictions.

It is commonly recommended that at least 50% of protein be in the form of "high biologic value" protein. Foods containing protein of high biologic value—such as eggs, milk, beef, poultry, and fish—are richer in essential amino acids than are foods with lower biologic value protein—such as grains, legumes, and vegetables. The philosophy is to reduce urea formation by providing a diet in which the protein consists primarily of essential amino acids, those which the body cannot make, with the idea that the patient will form adequate amounts of nonessential amino acids via the process of transamination (transfer of amine groups from one carbon backbone, or keto acid, to another). Specialized products, in which almost all of the amino acids are essential, have been developed for enteral tube feeding and TPN. However, use of these products

TABLE 6-6

NUTRITION ASSESSMENT OF THE RENAL PATIENT—cont'd

Area of Concern	History	Physical Assessment	Laboratory Data
DISORDERS OF MINERALS/ELECTROLYTES—cont'd			
Zinc (Zn) deficit	Poor intake because of restriction of protein-containing foods Loss in dialysis	Hypogeusia, dysgeusia Alopecia Seborrheic dermatitis Diarrhea	Serum Zn <60 µg/ml
Iron (Fe) deficit	Decreased intake because of restriction of protein-containing foods Loss of blood in dialysis tubing	Fatigue Pallor, blue sclerae	Hematocrit <37% (women) or <42% (men); hemoglobin <12 g/dL (women) or <14 g/dL (men); low MCV, MCH, MCHC levels
Sodium excess	Oliguria or anuria	Edema Hypertension	Serum sodium >145 mEq/L
Potassium (K⁺) excess	Oliguria or anuria	Weakness, flaccid muscles	Serum K⁺ >5 mEq/L Elevated T wave and depressed ST segment on ECG
Aluminum (Al) excess	Use of aluminum-containing phosphate binders Al contamination of TPN constituents	Ataxia, seizures Dementia Renal osteodystrophy with bone pain and deformities	Plasma Al >100 µg/L
DISORDERS OF VITAMIN NUTRITURE			
A excess	Oliguria or anuria Daily administration of tube feedings, TPN, or oral supplement with vitamin A	Anorexia Alopecia, dry skin Hepatomegaly Fatigue, irritability	Serum retinol level >80 µg/dL
C deficit	Loss in dialysis Decreased intake resulting from restriction of K⁺-containing fruits and vegetables	Gingivitis Petechiae, ecchymoses	Serum ascorbate <0.4 mg/dL
B₆	Failure of the diseased kidney to activate vitamin B₆ Loss in dialysis	Dermatitis Ataxia Irritability, seizures	Plasma pyridoxal phosphate <34 nmol (normal levels not well-established)
Folic acid	Loss in dialysis Decreased intake resulting from restriction of meats, fruits, and vegetables	Glossitis (inflamed tongue) Pallor	Hematocrit <37% (women) or <42% (men), elevated MCV level Serum folate <6 ng/ml

has not been found to improve patient outcome or nutritional status, in comparison with products with balanced amino acid mixtures.[17] During growth and severe stress or critical illness, a number of "nonessential" amino acids are needed in greater amounts than usual, and the need for these amino acids exceeds the body's ability to synthesize them. These amino acids are referred to as "conditionally essential," and they include arginine, glutamine, histidine, serine, taurine, cysteine, and tyrosine. Standard amino acid solutions, containing both essential and nonessential amino acids, are more effective at promoting healing, immune function, and optimal organ function than solutions of essential amino acids alone.[17]

Fluid

The patient with renal insufficiency usually does not require fluid restriction until urine output begins to diminish. Patients receiving hemodialysis are generally limited to a fluid intake resulting in a gain of no more than 0.45 kg (1 lb) per day on the days between dialysis.

This results in a daily intake of 500 to 750 ml plus the volume lost in urine.[14,16] With the use of continuous peritoneal dialysis, hemofiltration, or arteriovenous hemodialysis, the fluid intake can be liberalized. Most patients receiving peritoneal dialysis can tolerate 2000 ml per day.[14] This more liberal fluid allowance permits more adequate nutrient delivery, whether by oral, tube, or parenteral feedings. Enteral formulas containing 1.5 to 2 calories/ml or more provide a concentrated source of calories for tube-fed patients who require fluid restriction. Intravenous lipids, particularly 20% emulsions, can be used to supply concentrated calories for the TPN patient.

Calories

It is essential that the renal patient receive an adequate number of calories to prevent catabolism of body tissues to meet energy needs. Catabolism not only reduces the mass of muscle and other functional body tissues but also releases nitrogen that must be excreted by the kidney.

Adults with renal insufficiency need about 35 to 40 calories/kg/day, compared with the 25 to 30 calories/kg/day needed by healthy adults, to prevent catabolism and ensure that all protein consumed is used for anabolism rather than to meet energy needs. After renal transplantation, when the patient usually receives large doses of corticosteroids, it is especially important to ensure that caloric intake is adequate (usually 25 to 35 calories/kg/day) to prevent undue catabolism.

High-carbohydrate foods such as hard candies, sugar, honey, jelly, jellybeans, and gumdrops are often used as a means of supplying calories to the patient with renal failure because these foods are low in sodium and potassium, which are retained in renal failure. However, hypertriglyceridemia is found in a substantial number of patients with renal disorders. This condition is worsened by excessive intake of simple refined sugars, such as sucrose (table sugar) or glucose. Glucose in the peritoneal dialysate may be a significant calorie source[18] and a contributing factor in hypertriglyceridemia. Approximately 70% of the glucose instilled during peritoneal dialysis to serve as an osmotic agent may be absorbed, and this must be considered part of the patient's carbohydrate intake.[19] The glucose monohydrate used in intravenous and dialysate solutions supplies 3.4 calories/g. Thus if the patient receives 4.25% glucose (4.25 g glucose/100 ml solution) in the dialysate, he or she receives the following:

42.5 g/L $\times$ 70% $\times$ 3.4 calories/g = 101 calories/L of dialysate

To help control hypertriglyceridemia and to provide concentrated calories in minimal fluid, fat may need to supply as much as 40% of the patient's calories.[16] Hypercholesterolemia is commonly found in patients with renal failure, so unsaturated fats and oils (corn, soybean, sunflower, safflower, cottonseed, canola, and olive) are preferred over saturated fats (primarily from meats and dairy products), which tend to raise cholesterol levels. The necessary restriction of meat, milk, and other protein foods in the diet will help lower cholesterol and saturated fat intake. For patients who need a caloric supplement, Lipomul (Upjohn) is a palatable oral lipid supplement providing 6 calories/ml with minimal sodium and potassium. Intravenous lipids and the long-chain fats found in most enteral formulas are primarily polyunsaturated.

Other nutrients

Table 6-7 summarizes the recommended nutrient intake for patients with renal disorders. The recommendations for healthy adults are included to provide a basis for comparison.

NUTRITION AND GASTROINTESTINAL ALTERATIONS

Because the gastrointestinal (GI) tract is so inherently related to nutrition, it is not surprising that catastrophic occurrences in the GI tract—hemorrhage, perforation, infarct, or related organ failure—have acute and severe adverse effects on nutritional status.

Nutrition Assessment

Assessment is summarized in Table 6-8. The area and amount of the GI tract affected determine, to a large extent, the likelihood and degree of nutritional deficits because each portion of the bowel has a role to play in absorption. The ileum is among the most nutritionally important areas. Bile salt absorption, which is necessary for optimal fat digestion and absorption, occurs in this area as does absorption of vitamin B_{12}. Patients with ileal disease or resection are likely to become malnourished as a result of significant loss of calories (fat) in the feces, as well as loss of minerals and fat-soluble vitamins trapped in the fat. The ileocecal valve is especially critical in maintaining adequate nutrition. Not only does it slow entry of GI contents into the large bowel, allowing more time for absorption to take place in the small bowel, but it also helps prevent migration of the microorganisms from the large bowel into the small bowel. Proliferating microorganisms in the small bowel deconjugate the bile salts, further impairing fat absorption. Deconjugated bile salts also irritate the intestinal mucosa and raise the osmolality level within the bowel, promoting diarrhea.[20] The ileum can absorb most of the nutrients normally absorbed in the upper half of the small bowel, but it is impossible for the duodenum and jejunum to compensate for the loss of the ileum function.

Nutrition Intervention

The GI tract is the preferred route for delivery of nutrients in GI disease as it is in all other disease states. Because hepatic failure and bowel dysfunction, including failure resulting from inflammatory bowel disease or bowel resection, are two of the most nutritionally challenging GI alterations, most of the following discussion is devoted to them.

Hepatic failure

Hepatic failure is associated with a wide spectrum of metabolic alterations. Because the diseased liver has impaired ability to deactivate hormones, levels of circulating glucagon, epinephrine, and cortisol are elevated. These hormones promote catabolism of body tissues and cause glycogen stores to be exhausted. Release of lipids from their storage depots is accelerated, but the liver has decreased ability to metabolize them for energy. Furthermore, as many as half of the patients with hepatic failure may have malabsorption of fat because of inadequate production of bile salts by the liver.[21] Therefore body proteins are increasingly used for energy sources, producing tissue wasting. The branched-chain amino acids (BCAAs)—leucine, isoleucine, and valine—are especially well-used for energy, and their levels in the blood decline. Conversely, levels of the aromatic amino acids

TABLE 6-7

DAILY NUTRITIONAL RECOMMENDATIONS FOR ADULTS WITH RENAL FAILURE

	Recommended Daily Nutrient Intakes	
Nutrient	**Healthy Adults**	**Adults in Renal Failure**
Protein or amino acids (g/kg)	0.8	0.6-0.8 (renal insufficiency)* 1.2-1.4 (hemodialysis)* 1.2-1.5 (peritoneal dialysis)* 1.3-1.5 (immediately after transplant) 1.0 (stable after transplant)
Energy (calories/kg)	25-30	30-35 (renal insufficiency, dialysis—include calories from peritoneal dialy-sate)* 25-35 (after transplant; fat no more than 30% of calories)
Electrolytes and minerals†		
Sodium (mg; 1 mEq = 23 mg)	<2400 mg desirable	1000-3000 mg (renal insufficiency) 2000-3000 mg (hemodialysis) 2000-4000 mg (peritoneal dialysis, after transplant)
Potassium (mg/kg)	Not specified	Not restricted (renal insufficiency—unless glomerular filtration rate [GFR] <10 ml/min—peritoneal dialysis, after transplant) 40 (hemodialysis)*
Phosphorus (mg)	800-1200	8-12/kg (renal insufficiency)* <17/kg (dialysis)* Unrestricted, monitor (after transplant)
Calcium (mg)	800-1200	1200-1600 (renal insufficiency) Usually >1000, depends on serum level (dialysis)
Iron (mg)	10-15	15+, as needed to prevent anemia (all groups)
Zinc (mg)	12-15	15+, as needed to prevent deficiency (all groups)
Vitamins‡		
C (mg)	60	60-100
B₆ (mg)	1.6-2.0	5.0-10
Folic acid (mg)	0.18-0.2	0.8-1.0

Data modified from Beto JA: *J Am Dietet Assoc* 95:898, 1995; Kopple JD: *Am J Kidney Dis* 24:1002, 1994; Coats KG, et al: *J Am Dietet Assoc* 93:637, 1993; National Research Council: *Recommended dietary allowances,* ed 10, Washington, DC, 1989, National Academy of Sciences—National Research Council; and National Research Council: *Nutrition and your health: dietary guidelines for Americans,* ed 4, Washington, DC, 1995, USDA and USDHHS.
*Based on estimated dry weight or ideal body weight.
†Do not supplement with magnesium; monitor magnesium levels.
‡Daily supplement providing recommended daily allowance of B complex vitamins and vitamin C is appropriate but do not supplement vitamin A.

(AAAs)—phenylalanine, tyrosine, and tryptophan—rise as a result of tissue catabolism and impaired ability of the liver to clear them from the blood. Hyperammonemia is a feature of hepatic failure, but it may not be the causative agent in encephalopathy. The "false neurotransmitter" hypothesis suggests that AAAs cause encephalopathy. According to this hypothesis, AAAs are transported across the blood-brain barrier where they are converted to false neurotransmitters, which compete with the normal neurotransmitters for binding sites. The net result is to impede normal neurotransmission and produce hepatic encephalopathy.[21]

Fluid and electrolyte status. Ascites and edema result because the diseased liver produces less albumin and other plasma proteins; there is also decreased colloid osmotic pressure in the plasma, increased portal pressure caused by obstruction, and renal sodium retention from secondary hyperaldosteronism. To control fluid retention,

restriction of sodium (usually 500 to 1500 mg [or 20 to 65 mEq] daily) and fluid (1500 ml or less daily) is generally necessary, in conjunction with administration of diuretics.[21] Patients must be weighed daily to evaluate the success of treatment. In addition, laboratory data and physical status must be closely observed for potassium deficits caused by diuretic therapy and hyperaldosteronism.

Nutritious diet and response to dietary protein. Nutrition intervention in hepatic failure is based on the metabolic alterations. A diet with adequate protein helps to suppress catabolism and promote liver regeneration. Stable patients with cirrhosis usually tolerate 0.8 to 1 g protein/kg/day. Patients with severe stress or nutritional deficits have increased needs—as much as 1 to 1.5 g/kg/day.[21] However, if encephalopathy occurs or appears to be impending, tolerance of protein is impaired and protein intake is reduced to 0.5 g/kg/day or less.[17] A diet adequate in calories (at least 30 calories/kg daily) is

TABLE 6-8

NUTRITION ASSESSMENT OF THE PATIENT WITH A GASTROINTESTINAL DISORDER

Area of Concern	History	Physical Assessment	Laboratory Data

Protein-calorie malnutrition	Decreased oral intake caused by the following:
	  Fear of symptoms—pain, cramping, diarrhea—associated with eating (e.g., as occurs with peptic ulcer, dumping syndrome)
	  Alcohol abuse
	  Nausea, vomiting, anorexia
	Increased losses because of the following:
	  Maldigestion or malabsorption (e.g., as occurs with inadequate bile salt production, increased loss of bile salts in short bowel syndrome, diarrhea, inadequate absorptive area in short bowel syndrome)
	  GI bleeding
	  Fistula drainage
	Increased requirements caused by following: Needs for healing (e.g., surgical wounds, fistulae)
		Muscle wasting
		Loss of subcutaneous fat
		Weight <85% of desirable, recent weight loss or BMI <19
		Hair loss or change in hair texture
			Serum albumin <3.5 g/dL or low transferrin level
			Total lymphocyte count <1200/mm^3
			Creatinine excretion <17 mg/kg/day (women) or <23 mg/kg/day (men)
			Negative nitrogen balance
			Fecal fat >5 g/day or >5% of intake

Potential fluid volume deficit	Losses caused by severe vomiting or diarrhea (e.g., as occurs with GI obstruction, short bowel syndrome)	Poor skin turgor Dry, sticky mucous membranes Complaint of thirst Loss of ≥ 0.23 kg (0.5 pounds) in 24 hr	Hct >52% (men) or >47% (women) BUN >20 mg/dL Serum sodium >145 mEq/L Serum osmolality >300 mOsm/kg Urine specific gravity >1.030

DISORDERS OF MINERAL/ELECTROLYTE NUTRITURE

Area of Concern	History	Physical Assessment	Laboratory Data
Calcium (Ca)	Increased loss from steatorrhea (Ca forms soaps with fat in the stool and thus becomes unabsorbable)	Tingling of fingers Muscular tetany and cramps Carpopedal spasm Convulsions	Serum Ca level of <8.5 mg/dL (severe deficits only)

Magnesium (Mg)	Inadequate intake from poor diet in alcoholism
	Increased losses because of the following:
	  Diarrhea or steatorrhea
	  Loss of small bowel fluid (e.g., as occurs with short bowel syndrome, fistulae)
		Tremor
		Hyperactive deep reflexes
		Convulsions
			Serum Mg <1.5 mEq/L

Iron (Fe)	Blood loss Impaired absorption because of decreased upper GI acidity with gastrectomy or use of antacids and cimetidine Inadequate intake (e.g., restriction of protein foods in hepatic failure)	Pallor, blue sclerae Fatigue	Hct <42% (men) or <37% (women); Hgb <14 g/dL (men) or <12 g/dL (women); low MCV, MCH, MCHC Serum Fe <60 μg/dL

Zinc (Zn)	Increased losses caused by the following:
	  Diarrhea, steatorrhea
	  Loss of small bowel fluid
	  Diuretic use (in hepatic failure)
	  Increased urinary losses (in alcoholism)
	Inadequate intake caused by the following:
	  Protein restriction (in hepatic failure)
	  Poor diet (in alcoholism)
		Anorexia
		Hypogeusia, dysgeusia
		Seborrheic dermatitis
			Serum Zn <60 μg/dL

Potassium (K$^+$)	Increased loss caused by the following:
	  Diarrhea
	  Diuretic use
	  Hyperaldosteronism (in hepatic failure)
	  GI suction
		Muscle weakness, ileus
		Diminished reflexes
			Serum K$^+$ <3.5 mEq/L

DISORDERS OF VITAMIN NUTRITURE

Area of Concern	History	Physical Assessment	Laboratory Data
A	Increased loss in steatorrhea (vitamin A dissolves in fatty stools) Impaired release of vitamin A from storage in the liver because of inadequate production of retinol-binding protein, the transport protein, in malnutrition or liver failure	Drying of skin and cornea Poor wound healing Follicular hyperkeratosis (resembles gooseflesh)	Serum retinol <20 μg/dL
K	Impaired absorption in steatorrhea Decreased production because of destruction of intestinal bacteria by antibiotic usage	Petechiae, ecchymoses Prolonged bleeding	Prothrombin time >12.5 sec (not always accurate in liver failure)

Modified from Moore MC: *Pocket guide to nutritional care*, ed 3, St Louis, 1996, Mosby.

provided to help prevent catabolism and to prevent the use of dietary protein for energy needs.[21] Moderate amounts of fat are given, unless the patient has steatorrhea, in which case it is necessary to rely heavily on carbohydrates and medium-chain triglycerides (MCTs) to meet caloric needs. Soft foods are preferred because the patient may have esophageal varices that might be irritated by high-fiber foods. Because alcoholism is often the cause of hepatic failure and the diets of alcoholics are often low in zinc, vitamin B complex, folate, and magnesium, supplements of these nutrients are usually provided daily.[22] Anorexia, malaise, and confusion may interfere with oral intake, and the nurse may need to provide much encouragement to the patient to ensure intake of an adequate diet. Small frequent feedings are usually better accepted by the anorexic patient than are three large meals daily. The nurse must assess the patient's neurologic status daily to evaluate tolerance of dietary protein. Increasing lethargy, confusion, or asterixis may signal a need for decreased protein intake. Anorexia—coupled with the unpalatable nature of the very low-sodium, low-protein diet required in impending coma—may result in a need for tube feedings.

The patient who undergoes successful liver transplantation is usually able to tolerate a regular diet with few restrictions. Intake during the postoperative period must be adequate to support nutritional repletion and healing; 1.5 to 2 g protein/kg/day may be needed in the immediate postoperative period and during episodes of rejection when corticosteroid dosages are high.[23] In stable patients, 1 to 1.2 g protein/kg/day and approximately 30 calories/kg/day are often sufficient. Immunosuppressant therapy (corticosteroids and/or cyclosporine) frequently contributes to glucose intolerance.[24] Dietary measures to control glucose intolerance include (1) obtaining approximately 30% of dietary calories from fat, (2) emphasizing complex sources of carbohydrates, and (3) eating several small meals daily, with some of the day's carbohydrates in each meal. Moderate exercise often helps to improve glucose tolerance.

Short bowel syndrome

The major nutritional problems associated with bowel resection are loss of absorptive area, with increased fecal losses of fluids, electrolytes, fat, protein, and other nutrients; increased loss of bile salts, especially if the terminal ileum was resected, with further malabsorption of fat; and micronutrient deficiencies, which result from trapping of minerals and fat-soluble vitamins within the excreted fat.[20,25] After bowel resection, the remaining intestine undergoes marked hyperplasia, with increasing length of the remaining villi, which increases the available absorptive area. The result is improved absorption of water, electrolytes, and glucose.[25] The adaptive response may take up to 1 year to become complete, and it does not occur without the stimulus of nutrients within the gut.[25,26]

Administration of fluids and electrolytes. Extensive bowel resection is associated with marked gastric hypersecretion. The increase in gastric juices, coupled with the sudden loss of absorptive area, results in the loss of several liters of fluid daily, along with potassium, magnesium, and zinc. The nurse's role in management of these patients during the period immediately after extensive bowel resection includes (1) keeping strict intake and output records, including volume or weight of stools if they are frequent or loose; (2) continually assessing the patient's state of hydration; and (3) administering fluids and electrolytes and evaluating the patient's response—including daily weight measurements—to evaluate the adequacy of fluid replacement.

Administration of nutrition support. The extent of the resection is a determinant of the amount and type of nutrition support required. If more than 50% of the small bowel remains, few dietary changes may be needed.[20] With more extensive resection, leaving only 120 to 150 cm (4 to 5 feet) of small bowel, TPN is usually initiated during the early postoperative period. Small amounts of enteral feedings are begun as soon as possible to stimulate intestinal adaptation. Enteral feedings may consist of an elemental, or predigested, diet given by tube. Fat is the most difficult nutrient to absorb, and the formula will ordinarily be very low in fat or high in MCTs, which are more readily absorbed than are the long-chain triglycerides predominating in most foods. Alternatively, a low-fat, high-starch diet may be given by mouth.[20] Lactose, or milk sugar, is often tolerated poorly by patients with bowel resection, but low-fat cheese and yogurt, which are relatively low in lactose, may be tolerated.[25] MCTs can be served in juice or used in food preparation to increase caloric intake. Alcohol and caffeine stimulate intestinal motility and may have to be avoided for at least 1 year after surgery. Patients receiving oral feedings often require much encouragement to eat because they may associate eating with worsening of diarrhea. As more and more enteral intake is tolerated, TPN is gradually tapered. Some patients with 70% to 80% resection of the small bowel can eventually be maintained on enteral feedings only, especially if the terminal ileum and ileocecal valve are retained, but patients with jejunostomy and less than 100 cm of jejunum and those with an intact colon but less than 50 cm jejunum and ileum remaining usually require TPN indefinitely.[26] Many patients show an extraordinary degree of adaptation, even with very extensive resection, and thus gastrointestinal tolerance of enteral feedings is continually assessed. Careful records must be kept of all enteral and parenteral intake to determine when TPN can be decreased or discontinued. Some patients have difficulty maintaining fluid and electrolyte balance. Oral rehydration solutions can be used to meet their needs.[26]

Administration of medications. In some patients with short bowel syndrome, in whom diarrhea is prolonged or especially severe and causes anal excoriation or copious ostomy output, antidiarrheal agents, such as diphenoxylate with atropine or codeine, may be beneficial. Anticholinergic drugs, such as glycopyrrolate, can also be used to counteract gastric hypersecretion.

NUTRITION AND ENDOCRINE ALTERATIONS

Endocrine alterations have far-reaching effects on all body systems, and thus they affect nutritional status in a variety of ways.

Nutrition Assessment

The nutrition assessment process is summarized in Table 6-9. Because of the prevalence of non–insulin-dependent diabetes mellitus (NIDDM) patients among the hospitalized population, the nutritional problems most commonly noted in patients with endocrine alterations are overweight and obesity.

Nutrition Intervention

Underweight and malnourished patients

The most severely undernourished patients are usually those with pancreatitis, because of loss of pancreatic exocrine function. Pancreatic insufficiency—with inadequate release of trypsin, chymotrypsin, and pancreatic lipase and amylase—results in impaired digestion and subsequent loss of nutrients in the stool. Fat malabsorption is the most marked effect of pancreatic insufficiency. Fat lost in the stools is accompanied by calcium, zinc, and other minerals, along with the fat-soluble vitamins.

Patients with insulin-dependent diabetes mellitus (IDDM) or endocrine dysfunction caused by pancreatitis often have weight loss and malnutrition as a result of tis-

---

TABLE 6-9

NUTRITION ASSESSMENT OF THE PATIENT WITH AN ENDOCRINE DISORDER

Area of Concern	History	Physical Findings	Laboratory Data

Underweight or protein-calorie malnutrition	Increased losses of calories in urine or feces caused by the following:
	  Impaired glucose metabolism and glucosuria in type I diabetes mellitus
	  Steatorrhea (in pancreatitis)
	Decreased intake because of the following:
	  Discomfort with eating (in pancreatitis)
	  Alcoholism (often a cause of pancreatitis)
		Weight <85% of desirable or BMI <19
		Recent weight loss
		Wasting of muscle and subcutaneous tissue
			Urine glucose >0.5%
			Fecal fat >5 g/24 hr or <95% of intake
			Serum albumin <3.5 g/dL, or low transferrin or prealbumin level
			Total lymphocyte count <1200/mm³
			Creatinine excretion <17 mg/kg/day (women) or <23 mg/kg/day (men)

Overweight	NIDDM Sedentary life-style	Weight >120% of desirable or BMI >27	
Risk for fluid volume deficit	Diuresis (from diabetes insipidus or osmotic diuresis of HHNK or ketoacidosis)	Poor skin turgor Dry, sticky mucous membranes Thirst Loss of >0.25 kg (0.5 pound) in 24 hr Increased urine output	Serum glucose >250 mg/dL Urine glucose >0.5% Serum sodium >145 mEq/L Increasing Hct BUN >20 mg/dL
Risk for fluid volume excess	Fluid retention caused by SIADH	Edema (peripheral and/or pulmonary) Gain of >0.23 kg (0.5 pound) in 24 hr	Serum sodium <135 mEq/L Decreasing Hct
Potential zinc deficiency	Impaired absorption (in steatorrhea associated with pancreatitis) Increased urinary losses (in diuresis, diabetes mellitus, and alcoholism) Poor intake (in alcoholism)	Hypogeusia, dysgeusia Alopecia Seborrheic dermatitis Impaired wound healing	Serum zinc <60 μg/ml

Modified from Moore MC: *Pocket guide to nutritional care,* ed 3, St Louis, 1996, Mosby.
NIDDM, Non–insulin-dependent diabetes mellitus; *HHNK,* hyperglycemic hyperosmolar nonketotic (coma); *SIADH,* syndrome of inappropriate secretion of antidiuretic hormone.

sue catabolism because they cannot use dietary carbohydrates to meet energy needs. Although patients with NIDDM are more likely to be overweight than underweight, they too may become malnourished as a result of chronic or acute infections, trauma, major surgery, or other illnesses. Delivery of nutrition support to these patients, especially control of blood glucose, can be challenging. Blood glucose is monitored regularly, usually several times a day until the patient is stable. Regular insulin added to the solution is the most common method of managing hyperglycemia in the patient receiving TPN. The dosage required may be larger than the patient's usual subcutaneous dose because some of the insulin adheres to glass bottles and plastic bags or administration sets.

In patients receiving enteral tube feedings, the transpyloric route (via nasoduodenal, nasojejunal, or jejunostomy tube) may be the most effective because gastroparesis may make intragastric tube feedings impossible or inadequate. Transpyloric feedings are given continuously or by slow intermittent infusion, because dumping syndrome and poor absorption often occur if feedings are given rapidly into the small bowel. For the continuously tube-fed diabetic patient, control of blood glucose may be improved either with continuous insulin infusion or by use of a formula containing fiber, if such a formula is not contraindicated. Fiber slows the absorption of the carbohydrate in the formula, producing a more delayed and sustained glycemic response.

Overweight patients

Aggressive attempts at weight loss are rarely warranted among very ill patients, although weight loss in overweight patients with NIDDM improves glucose tolerance. Instead of suggesting a low-calorie diet, nurses must encourage patients to select foods providing fiber and starches. Diets rich in complex carbohydrates have been reported to lower insulin requirements, increase the sensitivity of the peripheral tissues to insulin, and decrease serum cholesterol levels.[27]

Nutrition support should not be neglected simply because a patient is obese; PCM develops even among such patients. When a patient is not expected to be able to eat for at least 5 to 7 days or inadequate intake persists for that period, the nurse needs to consult with the physician regarding initiation of tube feedings or TPN, if no steps have been taken to do so. No disease process benefits from starvation, and development or progression of nutritional deficits may contribute to complications (e.g., decubitus ulcers, pulmonary or urinary tract infections, and sepsis, all of which prolong hospitalization, increase the costs of care, and may even result in death).

Severe vomiting or diarrhea in the insulin-dependent diabetic patient

When insulin-dependent patients experience vomiting and diarrhea severe enough to interfere significantly with oral intake or result in excessive fluid and electrolyte losses, adequate carbohydrates and fluids must be supplied. If patients are receiving oral feedings, they may not be able to adhere to their usual diet, but they generally are to consume 10 to 20 g of carbohydrates every 1 to 2 hours[28]; the physician usually provides guidelines as to the amount. Small amounts of liquids taken every 15 to 20 minutes are generally tolerated best by the patient with nausea and vomiting. Blood glucose and urine ketone levels are monitored frequently, and the physician is notified of increasing hyperglycemia, ketonuria, difficulty retaining fluids, or signs of dehydration.

NUTRITION AND HEMATOIMMUNE ALTERATIONS

Malnutrition has well-known adverse effects on hematoimmune function. Generalized PCM, for example, depresses cell-mediated immunity, secretory immunity, complement levels, and phagocyte activity. Deficiencies of single nutrients—especially iron, zinc, selenium, folic acid, and vitamins B_{12}, B_6, C, and A—also impair immunologic function.[29,30] Therefore, in the patient with an existing hematoimmune disorder, maintenance of adequate nutrition is essential to prevent additional immunologic deficits.

Nutrition Assessment

Assessment of the patient with a hematoimmune disorder is summarized in Table 6-10. Acquired immunodeficiency syndrome (AIDS) is the hematoimmune disorder most likely to have profound nutritional consequences. Unfortunately, generalized PCM is a common sequela of AIDS. There are multiple etiologic factors for the malnutrition. AIDS itself may be associated with a poorly understood enteropathy that causes diarrhea and malabsorption. Furthermore, opportunistic GI infections caused by various fungi, viruses, bacteria, and protozoas may cause diarrhea.[31] *Cryptosporidium*, a particularly resistant protozoa, can cause intractable, profuse, watery diarrhea lasting for months. Calorie and protein needs are elevated in persons with AIDS because metabolic rate and catabolism increase as a result of infection, fever, and malignancies such as lymphoma and Kaposi's sarcoma. At the same time, oral intake is frequently suppressed by emotional reactions to the personal, family, and financial stresses imposed by AIDS; by oral and esophageal pain from lesions of Kaposi's sarcoma, herpes, candidiasis, and/or chemotherapy; by nausea, vomiting, and anorexia associated with antibiotic therapy, by chemotherapy for malignancies or antiviral agents used in the treatment of AIDS; and by impaired motor ability, confusion, and dementia caused by AIDS encephalitis or opportunistic central nervous system infections. AIDS patients often have marked weight loss, hypoalbuminemia, and low levels of zinc, selenium, and other minerals.[29,30]

TABLE 6-10

NUTRITION ASSESSMENT OF THE PATIENT WITH A HEMATOIMMUNE DISORDER

Area of Concern	History	Physical Findings	Laboratory Data

Protein-calorie malnutrition	Nutrient losses caused by malabsorption and diarrhea
	Increased needs caused by infection and fever
	Poor intake caused by the following:
	  Anorexia (related to respiratory or other infections, emotional stress, medication side effects)
	  Pain associated with eating (e.g., *Candida*, esophagitis, and endotracheal Kaposi's sarcoma)
	  Dementia or CNS infections
	  Dysphagia
		Weight <85% of desirable or BMI <19
		Recent weight loss
		Wasting of muscle and subcutaneous tissue
			Serum albumin <3.5 g/dL, or low transferrin or prealbumin level
			Negative nitrogen balance
			Creatinine excretion <17 mg/kg/day (women) or <23 mg/kg/day (men)

DISORDERS OF MINERAL AND VITAMIN NUTRITURE			

Iron (Fe)	Poor intake of meats, whole-grain or enriched breads and cereals, and legumes because of the following:
	  Anorexia
	  Pain associated with eating
		Pallor, blue sclerae
		Fatigue
		Tachycardia
			Hct <37% (women) or <42% (men); Hgb <12 g/dL (women) or <14 g/dL (men); low MCV, MCH, MCHC

Zinc (Zn)	Poor intake of meats, whole-grain or enriched breads and cereals, and legumes because of the following:
	  Anorexia
	  Pain associated with eating
		Hypogeusia, dysgeusia
		Alopecia
		Dermatitis
		Impaired wound healing
		Diarrhea
			Serum Zn <60 µg/dL

Vitamin B$_{12}$	Small intestinal disease with malabsorption Macrobiotic or other vegetarian diet that does not include vitamin B$_{12}$ sources	Pallor Glossitis Neuropathy Psychiatric symptoms	Hct <37% (women) or <42% (men); Hgb <12 g/dL (women) or <14 g/dL (men); increased MCV

Modified from Moore MC: *Pocket guide to nutritional care,* ed 3, St Louis, 1996, Mosby.

Nutrition Intervention

Nutritional needs may be quite high in some patients with AIDS, particularly those with sepsis. It is estimated that AIDS increases calorie needs 20% to 60%,[5] and patients may require 1.2 to 1.8 g amino acids/kg/day to maintain a zero or positive nitrogen balance.[32] Ideally, nutrition intervention in patients with AIDS can be achieved via the GI tract. Enteral feedings (oral or tube) maintain the integrity of the gut mucosa, are relatively inexpensive, and are the most physiologic acceptable means of nutritional support. As mentioned, a host of factors may interfere with adequate oral intake in the individual with AIDS. However, with thorough assessment and careful planning to meet the needs of the individual, it is often possible to increase oral intake significantly. If nutritional supplements must be given to improve intake, it is usually best to choose those that are lactose-free. Patients with disease of the small bowel often have lactose intolerance, which causes diarrhea when lactose is ingested. Awareness of the effects of drugs on nutrient intake helps the nurse to plan appropriate interventions and patient teaching to maximize oral intake. Megesterol acetate and dronabinol are appetite-stimulating drugs often used in AIDS therapy.[33] A daily vitamin-mineral supplement (100% of the recommended dietary intake) helps to ensure adequate micronutrient intake.[34]

Despite dietary modifications and encouragement, some patients may find consuming an adequate diet impossible. Temporary oral or esophageal disorders—such as candidiasis, which produces painful lesions—may temporarily impair oral intake. Other individuals may have such severe diarrhea and malabsorption that they are unable to maintain their nutritional state with oral feedings alone. Nasogastric, nasoduodenal, or nasojejunal feeding tubes can be used to administer tube feedings if the patient does not have severe oral or esophageal disease. Gastrostomy or jejunostomy tubes are used when long-term feedings are needed or when oral and/or esophageal complications prevent nasal intubation. Continuous feedings (given either 24 hours a day or only nocturnally) may improve absorption in individuals with small bowel disease. For patients with malabsorption, elemental formulas often are used. These contain no lactose and little fat or fat that is primarily in the form of MCTs, thereby maximizing absorption in the patient with impaired absorptive ability.

Parenteral nutrition is reserved for patients for whom enteral feeding is not feasible or beneficial. Strict asepsis is maintained to reduce the risk of catheter-related infection. Patients with sepsis often are glucose-intolerant, and therefore it is especially important to monitor their blood glucose levels frequently.

ADMINISTERING NUTRITION SUPPORT

Enteral Nutrition Support

The enteral route is the preferred method of feeding whenever possible because this route is generally safer, more physiologically acceptable, and much less expensive than is parenteral feeding. There are a variety of commercial enteral feeding products, some of which are designed to meet the specialized needs of very sick patients. Some products can be consumed orally, but it is difficult for the critically ill patient to consume enough orally to meet the increased needs associated with stress. Table 6-11 provides more information about the major categories of products.

Oral supplementation

For patients who can eat and have normal digestion and absorption but simply cannot consume enough regular foods to meet caloric and protein needs, oral supplementation may be necessary. Patients with mild-to-moderate anorexia, burns, or trauma sometimes fall into this category.

Enteral tube feedings

Tube feedings are used for patients who have at least some digestive and absorptive capability but are unwilling or unable to consume enough by mouth. Patients with profound anorexia and those experiencing severe stress that greatly increases their nutritional needs (e.g., those with major burns or trauma) often benefit from tube feedings.[26] Individuals who require elemental formulas because of impaired digestion or absorption or the specialized formulas for altered metabolic conditions (see Table 6-11) usually require tube feeding because the unpleasant flavors of the components used in these formulas are very difficult to mask.

Location and type of feeding tube. Nasal intubation is the simplest and most commonly used route for gaining access to the GI tract; this method allows access to the stomach, duodenum, or jejunum. Using a small-bore, soft (e.g., polyurethane or silicone rubber) feeding tube promotes comfort. Tube enterostomy—a gastrostomy or jejunostomy—is used primarily for long-term feedings (6 to 12 weeks or more) and when obstruction makes the nasoenteral route inaccessible. Tube enterostomies may also be used for the patient who is at risk

for tube dislodgement because of severe agitation or confusion. A conventional gastrostomy or jejunostomy is often performed at the time of other abdominal surgery. The percutaneous endoscopic gastrostomy (PEG) tube has become extremely popular because it can be inserted without the use of general anesthetics. A jejunostomy tube can be placed by inserting it through the PEG site and advancing it through the pylorus and duodenum.

Transpyloric feedings via nasoduodenal, nasojejunal, or jejunostomy tubes are commonly used when there is a risk of pulmonary aspiration, because theoretically the pyloric sphincter provides a barrier that lessens the risk of regurgitation and aspiration.

Because transpyloric feedings can be given without regard to the rate of gastric emptying, they often have an advantage over intragastric feedings for patients with gastric atony, such as those with head injury, gastroparesis associated with uremia or diabetes, or postoperative ileus. Small bowel motility returns more quickly than gastric motility after surgery, and thus it is often possible to deliver transpyloric feedings within 1 to 2 days of trauma or surgery.[35,36]

Nursing management. The nurse's role in delivery of tube feedings usually includes insertion of the tube if a temporary tube is used, maintenance of the tube, administration of the feedings, prevention and detection of complications associated with this form of therapy, and participation in assessment of the patient's response to tube feedings.

Tube placement. Critical care nurses are usually familiar with tube insertion, and therefore this topic is not discussed in depth here. However, transpyloric passage of tubes deserves special mention. Tubes with mercury, stainless steel, or tungsten weights on the proximal end are often used when transpyloric tube placement is desired, in the belief that the weight will encourage transpyloric passage of the tube or that the weight will help the tube maintain its position once it passes into the bowel. However, unweighted tubes are either just as likely or more likely to migrate through the pylorus than weighted tubes.[24,37] Because the weights sometimes cause discomfort while being inserted through the nares, unweighted tubes may be preferable. Administration of metoclopramide or erythromycin before tube insertion increases the likelihood of tube passage through the pylorus.[37,38]

Correct tube placement must be confirmed before initiation of feedings and regularly throughout the course of enteral feedings. Radiographs are the most accurate way of assessing tube placement, but repeated radiographs are costly and can expose the patient to excessive radiation. The pH of fluid removed from the feeding tube can be used to confirm tube placement; some tubes are equipped with pH monitoring systems. If the pH is less than 4 in patients not receiving gastric acid inhibitors, or less than 5.5 in patients who are receiving acid inhibitors, the tube tip is likely to be in the stomach.[39] Intestinal se-

TABLE 6-11

ENTERAL FORMULAS

Formula Type	Nutritional Uses	Clinical Examples
FORMULAS USED WHEN GI TRACT IS FULLY FUNCTIONAL		
Polymeric (standard): Contains whole proteins (10%-15% of calories), long-chain triglycerides (25%-40% of calories), and glucose polymers or oligosaccharides (50%-60% of calories); most provide 1 calorie/ml	Inability to ingest food Inability to consume enough to meet needs	Oral or esophageal cancer Coma, stroke Anorexia resulting from chronic illness Burns or trauma
High-nitrogen: Same as polymeric except protein provides >15% of calories	Same as polymeric, plus mild catabolism and protein deficits	Trauma or burns Sepsis
Concentrated: Same as polymeric except concentrated to 2 calorie/ml	Same as polymeric, but fluid restriction needed	Congestive heart failure Neurosurgery COPD Liver disease
FORMULAS USED WHEN GI FUNCTION IS IMPAIRED		
Modified fat: High MCT, intact protein	Impaired fat digestion and absorption	HIV infection Inflammatory bowel disease Cystic fibrosis Short bowel syndrome Pancreatitis
Elemental or predigested: Contains hydrolyzed (partially digested) protein, peptides (short chains of amino acids), and/or amino acids, little fat (<10% of calories) or high MCT, and glucose polymers or oligosaccharide	Impaired digestion and/or absorption (severe)	HIV infection Inflammatory bowel disease Cystic fibrosis Short bowel syndrome Pancreatitis
DIETS FOR SPECIFIC DISEASE STATES*		
Renal failure: Concentrated in calories; low sodium, potassium, magnesium, phosphorus, and vitamins A and D; low protein for renal insufficiency; higher protein formulas for dialyzed patients	Renal insufficiency Dialysis	Predialysis Hemodialysis or peritoneal dialysis
Hepatic failure: Enriched in BCAA; low sodium	Protein intolerance	Hepatic encephalopathy
Pulmonary dysfunction: Low carbohydrate, high fat	Respiratory insufficiency	Ventilator dependence COPD
Glucose intolerance: Moderately high fat, low carbohydrate; high in monosaturated fat, fortified with antioxidants; fiber-containing	Glucose intolerance	Individuals with diabetes mellitus whose blood sugar is poorly controlled with standard formulas
Critical care: High protein; most contain MCT to improve fat absorption; some have increased zinc and vitamin C for wound healing; some are high in antioxidants (vitamin E, β-carotene); some are enriched with arginine, glutamine, and/or omega-3 fatty acids	Critical illness	Severe trauma or burns Sepsis

*These diets may be beneficial for selected patients, but there is no evidence that they are needed by all patients with these disease states.

cretions usually have a pH greater than 6, and respiratory tract fluids usually have a pH greater than 5.5. The esophagus may have an acid pH, which may cause confusion between esophageal and gastric placement. However, other clues can help in identifying a tube with its distal tip in the esophagus—it may be especially difficult to aspirate fluid out of the tube, a large portion of the tube may extend out of the body (but a tube inserted to the proper length could be coiled in the esophagus), and belching often occurs immediately after air is injected into the tube.[39] Food coloring (usually blue, which is un-likely to be confused with any body secretion) can be added to the formula as an aid to detection of formula in the respiratory system.

Formula delivery. Careful attention to administration of tube feedings can prevent many complications. Very clean or aseptic technique in the handling and administration of the formula can help prevent bacterial contamination and a resultant infection.[35] The optimal schedule for delivery of feedings also is important. Tube feedings may be administered intermittently or continuously. Bolus feedings, which are intermittent feedings delivered rapidly into the stomach or small bowel, are likely to cause distention, vomiting, and dumping syndrome with diarrhea. Instead of using bolus feedings, nurses can gradually drip intermittent feedings, with each feeding lasting 20 to 30 minutes or longer, to promote optimal assimilation. The question of which feeding schedule—continuous or intermittent—is superior in critically ill patients remains unanswered.

Prevention and correction of complications. Some of the more common complications of tube feeding are pulmonary aspiration, diarrhea, constipation, tube occlusion, and delayed gastric emptying. Nursing management of these problems is detailed in Table 6-12.

Total Parenteral Nutrition

Total parenteral nutrition (TPN) refers to the delivery of all nutrients by the intravenous route. It is used when the GI tract is not functional or when nutritional needs cannot be met solely via the GI tract. Likely candidates for TPN include patients who have severely impaired absorption (as in short bowel syndrome, collagen-vascular diseases, or radiation enteritis), intestinal obstruction, peritonitis, or prolonged ileus. It may also be useful in selected patients who can benefit from a period of bowel rest to promote healing, including those with gastrointestinal fistulae.[26] In addition, some postoperative, trauma, or burn patients may need temporary TPN.

Routes for TPN

TPN may be delivered through either central or peripheral veins. Because it requires an indwelling catheter, central vein TPN carries an increased risk of sepsis, as well as potential insertion-related complications, such as pneumothorax and hemothorax.[26] Air embolism is also more likely with central vein TPN. However, a central venous catheter provides very secure IV access and allows delivery of a more hyperosmolar solution than does peripheral TPN. TPN solutions containing 25% to 35% dextrose are commonly used via central veins, and this provides an inexpensive source of calories. Patients requiring multiple IV therapies and frequent blood sampling usually have multilumen central venous catheters, and TPN is often infused via these catheters. Some clinical studies have reported that catheter-related sepsis is higher with multilumen catheters; others have found no difference in comparison to single lumen catheters.[40] Clearly, patients requiring multilumen catheters are likely to be very ill and immunocompromised, and scrupulous aseptic technique is essential in maintaining multilumen catheters. The manipulation involved in frequent changes of IV fluid and obtaining blood specimens through these catheters increases the risk of catheter contamination. Peripherally inserted catheters (PICs) allow central venous access through long catheters inserted in peripheral sites. This reduces the risk of complications associated with percutaneous cannulation of the subclavian vein (e.g., subclavian vein laceration, pneumothorax, and chylothorax).

Peripheral TPN rarely is associated with serious infectious or mechanical complications, but it does require good peripheral venous access. Therefore it may not be appropriate for long-term nutrition support or for patients receiving multiple IV therapies.

Nursing management

Nursing management of the patient receiving TPN includes catheter care, administration of solutions, prevention or correction of complications, and evaluation of patient responses to IV feedings.

The indwelling central venous catheter provides an excellent nidus for infection.[40] The nurse has a major role in preventing this complication of TPN therapy. Catheter care includes maintaining an intact dressing at the catheter insertion site and manipulating the catheter and administration tubing with aseptic technique. Dressings for TPN catheters may consist of transparent film, gauze and tape, or hydrocolloid.

TPN solutions usually consist of amino acids, dextrose, electrolytes, vitamins, minerals, and trace elements. Although dextrose-amino acid solutions are commonly thought of as good growth media for microorganisms, they actually suppress the growth of most organisms usually associated with catheter-related sepsis, except yeasts. However, because the many manipulations required to prepare solutions increase the possibility of contamination, TPN solutions are best used with caution. They need to be prepared under laminar flow conditions in the pharmacy, with avoidance of additions on the nursing unit. Solution containers need to be inspected for cracks or leaks before hanging, and solutions must be discarded within 24 hours of hanging. An in-line 0.22 μm filter, which eliminates all microorganisms but not endotoxins, may be used in administration of solutions. Use of the filter, however, cannot be substituted for scrupulous aseptic technique because there is no conclusive evidence that filters decrease sepsis rates.

In contrast to dextrose-amino acid solutions, IV lipid emulsions support the proliferation of many microorganisms. Furthermore, lipid emulsions cannot be filtered through an in-line 0.22 μm filter because some particles in the emulsions have larger diameters than this. Lipid emulsions are handled with strict asepsis, and they must be discarded within 12 to 24 hours of hanging. There is a trend toward mixing lipid emulsions with dextrose-amino acid TPN solutions. Although this saves nursing time, the nurse must be extremely careful in administering these solutions. TPN solutions containing lipids cannot be filtered through an in-line 0.22 μm filter, and they support the growth of most bacteria and *Candida albicans* better than do dextrose-amino acid TPN solutions.

Prevention or correction of complications

Some of the more common and serious complications of TPN include catheter-related sepsis, air embolism,

TABLE **6-12**

NURSING MANAGEMENT OF ENTERAL TUBE FEEDING COMPLICATIONS

Complication	Contributing Factor(s)	Prevention/Correction
Pulmonary aspiration	Feeding tube positioned in esophagus or respiratory tract	Check tube placement before intermittent feeding and every 4-6 hr during continuous feedings by checking the pH of fluid aspirated from the tube (usually gastric juice pH is <3.5); be aware that an in-rush of air can sometimes be auscultated over the right upper quadrant even when the distal tip of the tube is in the esophagus or respiratory tract; consider intermittent feedings for disoriented or combative patients
	Regurgitation of formula	Elevate head to 45° during feedings unless contraindicated; if head cannot be raised, position patient in lateral (especially right lateral, which facilitates gastric emptying) or prone position to improve drainage of vomitus from the mouth; if head must be in a dependent position, discontinue feedings 30-60 min earlier and restart them only when the head can be raised
		Keep cuff of endotracheal or tracheostomy tube inflated during feedings, if possible
		Cisapride or metoclopramide may improve gastric emptying and decrease the risk of regurgitation
		Add food coloring to formula to facilitate diagnosis of aspiration
		Evaluate feeding tolerance every 2 hr initially, then less frequently as condition becomes stable; intolerance may be manifested by bloating, abdominal distention and pain, lack of stool and flatus, diminished or absent bowel sounds, tense abdomen, increased tympany, nausea and vomiting; if intolerance is suspected, abdominal radiographs may be done to check for distended gastric bubble/loops of bowel
Diarrhea	Medications with GI side effects (antibiotics, digitalis, laxatives, magnesium-containing antacids, quinidine, caffeine, etc.)	Evaluate the patient's medications to determine their potential for causing diarrhea, consulting the pharmacist if necessary
	Hypertonic formula or medications (e.g., oral suspensions of antibiotics, potassium, or other electrolytes), which cause dumping syndrome	Evaluate formula administration procedures to be sure that feedings are not being given by bolus infusion; administer the formula continuously or by slow intermittent infusion
		Dilute enteral medications well
	Bacterial contamination of the formula	Use scrupulously clean technique in administering tube feedings; prepare formula with sterile water if there are any concerns about the safety of the water supply or if the patient is seriously immunocompromised; keep opened containers of formula refrigerated and discard them within 24 hr; hang formula no more than 4-8 hr unless it comes prepackaged in sterile administration sets; be especially careful with feedings given to patients being fed transpylorically or those receiving cimetidine or antacids because these patients lack the normal antibacterial barrier of the stomach's acid
	Fecal impaction with seepage of liquid stool around the impaction	Perform a digital rectal examination to rule out impaction; see guidelines for prevention of constipation that follow
Constipation	Low-residue formula, creating little fecal bulk	Consult with the physician regarding the possibility of using a fiber-containing formula
Tube occlusion	Medications administered via tube (which either physically plug the tube or coagulate the formula, causing it to clog the tube)	If medications must be given by tube, avoid use of crushed tablets; irrigate tube with water before and after administering any medication; *never* add any medication to the formula unless the two are known to be compatible
	Sedimentation of formula	Irrigate tube after every intermittent feeding and every 4-8 hr during continuous feedings; or use an enteral feeding pump with automatic flush
	Aspirating gastric contents to measure residual volumes (acidified protein from the formula clots in the tube)	It has been suggested that aspiration of gastric residuals be avoided with small-bore feeding tubes (8 French) and that patient tolerance be assessed by physical examination; if residuals are measured, flush the tube thoroughly after returning the formula to the stomach and use a tube as large as is compatible with patient comfort (usually 10 French)
Gastric retention	Delayed gastric emptying related to head trauma, sepsis, diabetic or uremic gastroparesis, electrolyte imbalance, or other illness	The cause must be corrected if possible; consult with the physician about use of transpyloric feedings or metoclopramide or cisapride to stimulate gastric emptying; encourage patient to lie in right lateral position frequently, unless contraindicated

Data adapted from McClave SA, et al: *J Parenter Enteral Nutr* 16:99, 1992; Powell KS, et al: *J Parenter Enteral Nutr* 17:243, 1993; and Spapen HD, et al: *Crit Care Med* 23:481, 1995.

TABLE 6-13

NURSING MANAGEMENT OF TPN COMPLICATIONS

Complication	Clinical Manifestations	Prevention/Correction
Catheter-related sepsis	Fever, chills, glucose intolerance, positive blood culture	Maintain an intact dressing, change if contaminated by vomitus, sputum, and so on; use aseptic technique when handling catheter, IV tubing, and TPN solutions; hang a bottle of TPN no longer than 24 hr, lipid emulsion no longer than 12-24 hr; use an in-line 0.22 µm filter with TPN to remove microorganisms; avoid drawing blood, infusing blood or blood products, piggybacking other IV solutions into TPN IV tubing, or attaching manometers or transducers via the TPN infusion line, if at all possible If catheter-related sepsis is suspected, remove catheter or assist in changing the catheter over a guidewire and administer antibiotics as ordered
Air embolism	Dyspnea, cyanosis, apnea, tachycardia, hypotension, "millwheel" heart murmur; mortality estimated at 50% (depends on quantity of air entering)	Use Luer-Lok syringe or secure all connections well; use an in-line 0.22 µm air-eliminating filter; have patient perform Valsalva maneuver during tubing changes; if the patient is on a ventilator, change tubing quickly at end expiration; maintain occlusive dressing over catheter site for at least 24 hr after removing catheter to prevent air entry through catheter tract If air embolism is suspected, place patient in left lateral decubitus and Trendelenburg positions (to trap air in the apex of the right ventricle, away from the outflow tract) and administer oxygen and CPR as needed; immediately notify physician, who may attempt to aspirate air from the heart
Pneumothorax	Chest pain, dyspnea, hypoxemia, hypotension, radiographic evidence, needle aspiration of air from pleural space	Thoroughly explain catheter insertion procedure to patient, because when a patient moves or breathes erratically he or she is more likely to sustain pleural damage; perform x-ray examination after insertion or insertion attempt If pneumothorax is suspected, assist with needle aspiration or chest tube insertion, if necessary; chest tubes are usually used for pneumothorax of >25%
Central venous thrombosis	Edema of neck, shoulder, and arm on same side as catheter; development of collateral circulation on chest; pain in insertion site; drainage of TPN from the insertion site; positive findings on venogram	Follow measures to prevent sepsis; repeated or traumatic catheterizations are most likely to result in thrombosis. If thrombosis is suspected, remove catheter and administer anticoagulants and antibiotics as ordered
Catheter occlusion or semi-occlusion	No flow or a sluggish flow through the catheter	If infusion is stopped temporarily, flush catheter with saline or heparinized saline If catheter appears to be occluded, attempt to aspirate the clot; if this is ineffective, physician may order a thrombolytic agent such as urokinase instilled in the catheter
Hypoglycemia	Diaphoresis, shakiness, confusion, loss of consciousness	Infuse TPN within 10% of ordered rate; observe patient carefully for signs of hypoglycemia after discontinuance of TPN If hypoglycemia is suspected, administer oral carbohydrate; if the patient is unconscious or oral intake is contraindicated, the physician may order a bolus of IV dextrose
Hyperglycemia	Thirst, headache, lethargy, increased urinary output	Administer TPN within 10% of ordered rate; monitor blood glucose level at least daily until stable; the patient may require insulin added to the TPN if hyperglycemia is persistent; sudden appearance of hyperglycemia in a patient who was previously tolerating the same glucose load may indicate onset of sepsis

pneumothorax, central venous thrombosis, catheter occlusion, and metabolic imbalances such as hypoglycemia and hyperglycemia. These complications, along with nursing approaches to their management, are described in Table 6-13.

References

1. Buckley S, Kudsk KA: Metabolic response to critical illness and injury, *AACN Clin Issues Crit Care Nurs* 5:443, 1994.
2. Coats KG, et al: Hospital-associated malnutrition: a reevaluation 12 years later, *J Am Dietet Assoc* 93:27, 1993.

3. Detsky AS, et al: Is this patient malnourished? *JAMA* 271:54, 1994.

4. McWhirter JP, Pennington CR: Incidence and recognition of malnutrition in hospital, *BMJ* 308:945, 1994.

5. Messner RL, et al: Effect of admission nutritional status on length of hospital stay, *Gastroenterol Nurs* 13:202, 1991.

6. Freeman LM, Roubenoff R: The nutritional implications of cardiac cachexia, *Nutr Rev* 52:340, 1994.

7. National Education Programs Working Group: Report on the management of patients with hypertension and high blood cholesterol, *Ann Intern Med* 114:224, 1991.

8. Malone AM: Is a pulmonary enteral formula warranted for patients with pulmonary dysfunction? *Nutr Clin Prac* 12:168, 1997.

9. Pezza M, et al: Nutritional support for the patient with chronic obstructive pulmonary disease, *Monaldi Arch Chest Dis* 49(3 suppl 1):33, 1994.

10. Pinard B, Geller E: Nutritional support during pulmonary failure, *Crit Care Clin* 11:705, 1995.

11. Ott L, Young B: Nutrition in the neurologically injured patient, *Nutr Clin Prac* 6:223, 1991.

12. Weltz CR, Morris JB, Mullen JL: Surgical jejunostomy in aspiration risk patients, *Ann Surg* 215:140, 1992.

13. Brodsky IG, et al: Effects of low protein diets on protein metabolism in insulin-dependent diabetes mellitus patients with early nephropathy, *J Clin Endocrinol Metab* 75:351, 1992.

14. Kopple JD: Effect of nutrition on morbidity and mortality in maintenance dialysis patients, *Am J Kidney Dis* 24:1002, 1994.

15. Hakim RM, Levin N: Malnutrition in hemodialysis patients, *Am J Kidney Dis* 21:125, 1993.

16. Beto JA: Which diet for renal failure: making sense of the options, *J Am Diet Assoc* 95:898, 1995.

17. Zaloga G, Ackerman MH: A review of disease-specific formulas, *AACN Clin Issues Crit Care Nurs* 5:421, 1994.

18. Kaiser BA, et al: Growth of children following the initiation of dialysis: a comparison of three dialysis modalities, *Pediatr Nephrol* 8:733, 1994.

19. Grodstein GP, et al: Glucose absorption during continuous ambulatory peritoneal dialysis, *Kidney Int* 19:564, 1981.

20. Grant JP, et al: Malabsorption associated with surgical procedures and its treatment, *Nutr Clin Prac* 11:43, 1996.

21. Nompleggi DJ, Bonkovsky HL: Nutritional supplementation in chronic liver disease: an analytical review, *Hepatology* 19:518, 1994.

22. Gecelter GR, Comer GM: Nutritional support during liver failure, *Crit Care Clin* 11:675, 1995.

23. Hasse JM: Diet therapy for organ transplantation: a problem-based approach, *Nurs Clin N Am* 32:863, 1997.

24. Plevak DJ, et al: Nutritional support for liver transplantation: identifying calorie and protein requirements, *Mayo Clin Proc* 69:225, 1994.

25. Purdum PP III, Kirby DF: Short-bowel syndrome: a review of the role of nutrition support, *J Parenter Enteral Nutr* 14:93, 1991.

26. Klein S, et al: Nutrition support in clinical practice: review of published data and recommendations for future research directions. Summary of a conference sponsored by the National Institutes of Health, American Society for Parenteral and Enteral Nutrition, and American Society for Clinical Nutrition, *J Parenter Enteral Nutr* 21:133, 1997.

27. American Diabetes Association: *Medical management of non-insulin-dependent (type II) diabetes,* ed 3, Alexandria, Va, 1994, The Association.

28. American Diabetes Association: *Medical management of insulin-dependent (type I) diabetes,* ed 2, Alexandria, Va, 1994, The Association.

29. Beal JA, Martin BM: The clinical management of wasting and malnutrition in HIV/AIDS, *AIDS Patient Care STDs* 9:66, 1995.

30. Berger DS: Combating malnutrition in HIV infection, *AIDS Patient Care STDs* 10:94, 1996.

31. Bowers JM, et al: Diarrhea in HIV-infected individuals: a review, *AIDS Patient Care STDs* 10:25, 1996.

32. Suttmann U, et al: Nitrogen balance in HIV-infected patients during total parenteral nutrition, *Int Conf AIDS* 9:77, 1993 (abstract WSB344).

33. Herrington AM, Herrington JD, Church CA: Pharmacologic options for the treatment of cachexia, *Nutr Clin Prac* 12:101, 1997.

34. Gerrior JL, Bell SJ, Wanke CA: Oral nutrition for the patient with HIV infection, *Nurs Clin N Am* 32:813, 1997.

35. Heyland DK, Cook DJ, Guyatt GH: Enteral nutrition in the critically ill patient: a critical review of the evidence, *Intens Care Med* 19:435, 1993.

36. Moore FA, et al: Early enteral feeding, compared with parenteral, reduces postoperative septic complications: the results of a meta-analysis, *Ann Surg* 216:172, 1992.

37. Lord LM, et al: Comparison of weighted vs unweighted enteral feeding tubes for efficacy of transpyloric intubation, *J Parenter Enteral Nutr* 17:271, 1993.

38. Clevenger F, Rodriguez DJ: Decision-making for enteral feeding administration: the why behind where and how, *Nutr Clin Prac* 10:104, 1995.

39. Metheny N, et al: pH testing of feeding-tube aspirates to determine placement, *Nutr Clin Prac* 9:185, 1994.

40. Collins E, et al: Care of central venous catheters for total parenteral nutrition, *Nutr Clin Prac* 11:109, 1996.

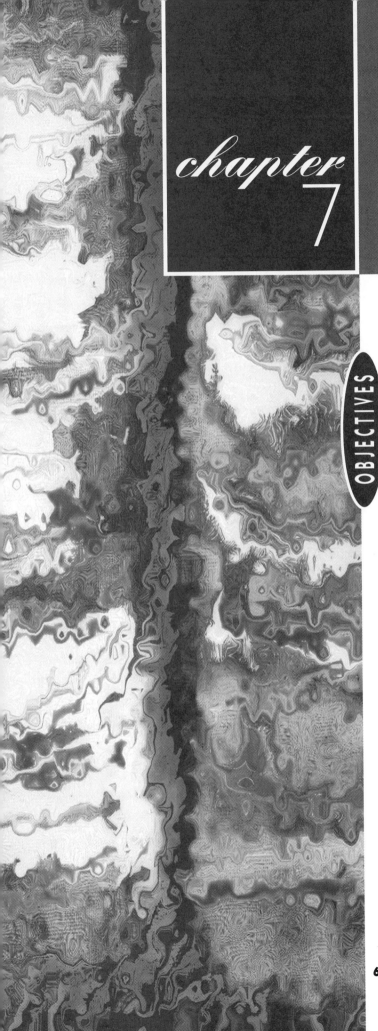

chapter 7

Gerontologic Alterations

Jeannine Forrest

OBJECTIVES

- Describe the age-associated physiologic changes that occur in the cardiovascular, respiratory, renal, gastrointestinal, hepatic, integumentary, and central nervous systems.

- State the clinical significance of age-related physiologic changes and the expected nursing considerations or interventions used in caring for older critical care patients.

- Relate the age-related changes in hepatic function and the accompanying pharmacokinetic changes to the administration of various cardiovascular medications.

Advancing age is accompanied by physiologic changes in the cardiovascular, respiratory, renal, gastrointestinal, hepatic, integumentary, immune, and central nervous systems. The incidence of disease increases with advancing age, with cardiovascular and neoplastic diseases being the most common causes of death.[1-2] However, although physiologic decline and disease processes influence each other, physiologic decline occurs independently of disease. The degree of physiologic decline is currently under investigation to differentiate true age-related changes from lifestyle, environmental, or genetic factors in later years.[3,4] The purpose of this chapter is to acquaint the critical care nurse with literature and research on the age-associated changes in physiologic function in healthy older adults and to describe implications for this population in critical care.

CARDIOVASCULAR SYSTEM

Advancing age has many effects on the cardiovascular system. With advancing age both the myocardium and the vascular system undergo a multitude of anatomic, cellular, and genetic changes that alter the function of both the myocardium and peripheral vascular system.[5]

Morphologic Changes in the Myocardium

Myocardial collagen content increases with age.[6,7] Collagen is the principal noncontractile protein occupying the cardiac interstitium.[8] Increased myocardial collagen content renders the myocardium less compliant. The decrease in myocardial compliance can adversely affect diastolic filling (through decreased distensibility and dilation) and myocardial relaxation. Consequently, the left ventricle must develop a higher filling pressure for a given increase in ventricular volume. The functional consequence could be an increase in myocardial oxygen consumption. Under normal physiologic conditions, an increase in myocardial oxygen demand is met with a corresponding increase in coronary artery blood flow. However, in the presence of coronary artery disease, coronary artery blood flow can be limited because of atherosclerotic-mediated narrowing of the coronary arteries. Hence the patient is at risk for developing myocardial ischemia and/or infarction. Clinical manifestations of myocardial ischemia include electrocardiographic (ECG) changes and chest pain. However, the sensation of chest pain is altered in the elderly person. Muller and others[9] found that complaints of chest pain were absent in 75% of elderly patients (older than 85 years) who sustained a myocardial infarction. Others[10] have also reported that chest pain in the elderly is less intense and of shorter duration and originates in other areas of the chest besides the substernal region.

The aging heart undergoes a modest degree of hypertrophy that is similar to pressure-overload–induced hypertrophy. Such hypertrophy entails a thickening of the left ventricular wall without appreciable changes in left ventricular cavity size.[11] The increase in left ventricular wall thickness is primarily a result of myocyte hypertrophy (increase in cell size). In elderly individuals, the myocardial hypertrophy may be caused by corresponding increases in aortic impedance and systemic vascular resistance.[12]

Myocardial Contraction and Relaxation

The prolonged duration of contraction (systole) is caused in part by a slowed or delayed rate of myocardial relaxation.[5,13,14] Myocardial relaxation depends on removal of calcium from the cell by uptake into the sarcoplasmic reticulum (SR) and extrusion of calcium across the plasma membrane (sarcolemma) by the action of the sarcolemmal sodium-calcium exchanger and sarcolemmal Ca^2-ATPase pump.[15] In heart cells, the decrease in intracellular calcium ion concentration at the start of diastole results primarily from uptake into the SR and, to a lesser extent, from efflux out of the cell via the sarcolemmal sodium-calcium exchanger and Ca^2-ATPase pump. The age-associated decrease in the rate of relaxation may be partly the result of a reduced rate of calcium uptake (sequestration) by the SR.[16,17] Calcium uptake by the SR occurs via a Ca^2-ATPase pump, which is embedded in the membrane of the SR.

Hemodynamics and the Electrocardiogram

Resting (supine) heart rate decreases with age.[18,19] Cinelli and others[18] reported a decrease in the resting heart rate from 78.8 beats/minute in young adults to 62.3 beats/minute in elderly adults. Heart rate is an important determinant of cardiac output (CO), and the normal resting heart beats approximately 70 times a minute. At rest or with minimal activity, the elderly person probably will not experience any untoward cardiovascular effect (i.e., a decrease in CO) with a heart rate of 62 beats/minute. However, if the heart rate response is attenuated during exercise, the elderly person's capacity for exercise may be limited.

Intrinsic heart rate decreases with aging.[20] The intrinsic heart rate is the heart rate in the absence of parasympathetic and sympathetic influences. In healthy resting individuals, parasympathetic (cholinergic) influences predominate, which cause a heart rate of approximately 70 beats/minute.[15] In the absence of both parasympathetic and sympathetic influences, the heart rate of young adults averages about 100 beats/minute (intrinsic heart rate).

Resting CO and stroke volume do not change with advancing age. At rest, left ventricular end-diastolic volume (preload), end-systolic volume (the volume of blood remaining in the ventricle after systole), and the ejection fraction are not affected by age.[21] In the elderly human myocardium, the early diastolic filling period and isovolumic phase of myocardial relaxation are prolonged.[22,23] However, these changes, although suggestive of diastolic dysfunction, do not translate into decreases in end-diastolic volume or stroke volume.[22,23] Finally, aging is associated with a moderate increase in pulmonary artery pressure.[24]

Advancing age produces changes in the ECG. R-wave and S-wave amplitude significantly decrease in persons older than 49 years, whereas Q-T duration increases (Table 7-1).[25] The increase in the duration of the Q-T interval is reflective of the prolonged rate of relaxation.[25]

The incidence of asymptomatic cardiac dysrhythmias increases in elderly patients.[26] The most common dysrhythmia occurring in elderly individuals is premature ventricular contraction (PVC). Other common types of dysrhythmias are sinus node dysfunction (atrial fibrillation, atrial flutter, or paroxysmal supraventricular tachycardia) and atrioventricular conduction disturbances.[25,26]

TABLE 7-1				
AGE-RELATED CHANGES IN ELECTROCARDIOGRAPHIC VARIABLES				
ECG Variable	<30 Years	30-39 Years	40-49 Years	>49 Years
R-wave amplitude (mm)	10.43	10.53	9.01	9.25
S-wave amplitude (mm)	15.21	14.21	12.22	12.42
Frontal plane axis (degrees)	48.93	48.13	36.50	38.83
P-R duration (ms)	15.89	16.23	16.04	16.25
QRS duration (ms)	7.64	7.51	7.36	8.00
Q-T duration (ms)	37.83	37.50	37.99	39.58
T-wave amplitude (ms)	5.21	4.57	4.31	4.42

Data from Bachman S, Sparrow D, Smith LK: *Am J Cardiol* 48:513, 1981.

Because the majority of patients are asymptomatic, the use of antidysrhythmics is generally not recommended. The side effects and toxic effects of antidysrhythmics impose more of a risk, as compared with the risk of mortality or morbidity related to the dysrhythmia.[26] In contrast, in patients who are symptomatic and have malignant ventricular dysrhythmias (sustained ventricular tachycardia and/or fibrillation), pharmacologic therapy is warranted.[26]

Baroreceptor Function

Baroreceptor-reflex function is altered with aging.[27] Baroreceptors are mechanoreceptors that respond to stretch and other changes in the blood vessel wall and are located at the bifurcation of the common carotid artery and aortic arch.[15] Abrupt changes in blood pressure caused by increases in peripheral resistance, CO, or blood volume are sensed by the baroreceptors, resulting in an increase in the impulse frequency to the vasomotor center within the medulla. This increase inhibits vasoconstrictor impulses arising from the vasoconstrictor region within the medulla.[15] The result is a decrease in heart rate and peripheral vasodilation; both of these effects return the blood pressure to within normal limits.

It was once thought that postural hypotension occurred more frequently in elderly subjects and was age-related. However, recent studies have shown that the prevalence of postural hypotension is quite low in elderly persons.[28,29] The prevalence of orthostatic hypotension is greater in institutionalized elderly patients who are receiving antihypertensive medications.[30]

Left Ventricular Function During Exercise

In most individuals, aging is associated with a decline in exercise performance. Exercise performance depends on a multitude of physiologic variables. With advancing age, the maximal heart rate achieved during exercise is attenuated; however, the decreased heart rate response is accompanied by an increase in left ventricular end diastolic volume (LVEDV) and stroke volume (SV). This augmentation in LVEDV and SV offsets the attenuated heart rate response and maintains cardiac output (CO) in exercise. In healthy older individuals there is no age-associated decline in CO during exercise; however, other factors such as neural functioning, skeletal and joint functioning, as well as pulmonary function, may limit an older individual's ability to exercise.

Peripheral Vascular System

The effects of aging on the peripheral vascular system are reflected in the gradual, but linear, rise in systolic blood pressure.[31,32] Diastolic blood pressure is less affected by age and generally remains the same or decreases.[32] Important determinants of systolic blood pressure include the compliance of the vasculature and the blood volume within the vascular system. Similar to the heart, the compliance of the vasculature is determined by its cell-type and tissue composition. With advancing age, the intimal layer thickens, principally because of an increase in smooth muscle cells, and the amount of connective tissue increases.[31] These changes occur in the intima of the large and distal arteries. This gradual decrease in arterial compliance or "stiffening of the arteries" is sometimes referred to as *arteriosclerosis*. The consequences of arteriosclerotic and atherosclerotic processes are that the arteries become progressively less distensible and the vascular pressure-volume relationship is altered. These changes are clinically significant, because small changes in intravascular volume are accompanied by disproportionate increases in systolic blood pressure.[13,33] The decrease in arterial compliance and disproportionate increase in systolic blood pressure may lead to an increase in afterload and the development of concentric (pressure-induced) ventricular hypertrophy in the elderly patient.[33]

Arterial pressure is also governed by the amount of blood volume, which in turn is regulated by plasma levels of sodium and water and the activity of the renin-angiotensin system (RAS).[34] Plasma renin activity declines with age, but aging per se has no appreciable effect on sodium and water homeostasis.[35] However, there are age-related changes in tubular function as well as a de-

---

TABLE 7-2

AGE-RELATED CHANGES IN COMMONLY PERFORMED PULMONARY FUNCTION TESTS

Pulmonary Function Test	Description	Standard Lung Volume and Capacity (ml)	Age-Related Change (ml)
Total lung capacity	Vital capacity plus residual volume	6000	No change
Vital capacity	Amount of air exhaled after a maximal inspiration	5000	↓3750
Tidal volume (V_T)	Amount of air inhaled or exhaled with each breath	500	No change
Residual volume (RV)	Amount of air left in lungs after forced exhalation	1200	↑1800
Inspiratory reserve volume (IRV)	Amount of air that can be forcefully inhaled after inspiring a normal V_T	3100	↓2800
Expiratory reserve volume (ERV)	Amount of air that can be forcefully exhaled after expiring a normal V_T	1200	↓1000
Forced expiratory volume in 1 sec (FEV_1)	Volume exhaled in the first second of a single forced expiratory volume; expressed as a percent of the forced vital capacity	80%	↓75%

crease in the glomerular filtration rate (GFR), both of which can affect overall sodium and water homeostasis. Circulating levels of sodium-regulating hormones—such as natriuretic hormone, aldosterone, and antidiuretic hormone (ADH)—are not appreciably altered by advancing age.[35,36] However, a delayed natriuretic response after sodium loading and plasma volume expansion and diminished renal response to ADH secretion have been reported in elderly persons.[36]

Lipoprotein levels increase with advancing age. In men, the serum total cholesterol level (all of the lipoproteins combined) increases progressively from 150 to 200 mg/dL between the ages of 20 and 50 years and remains relatively unchanged until the age of 70 years.[37] There are relatively few age-related changes in VLDL and HDL levels in men. In men, serum triglyceride levels peak at approximately age 40 and then decrease.[37,38]

In women, serum total cholesterol levels are low between the ages of 20 and 50 years.[37,38] However, between the ages 55 to 60 years, serum total cholesterol levels progressively increase, usually simultaneously with changes in the hormonal production of estrogen.[37] The increase in total serum cholesterol levels is primarily the result of an increase in the LDL fraction and, to a lesser extent, the VLDL and HDL fractions, which do not change appreciably with age in women. In women, serum triglyceride levels progressively increase with age.[37]

RESPIRATORY SYSTEM

Many of the changes in the pulmonary system that occur with aging are reflected in tests of pulmonary function and include changes in thoracic wall expansion and respiratory muscle strength, morphology of alveolar parenchyma, and decreases in arterial oxygen tension (PaO_2)[39] (Tables 7-2 and 7-3). These changes occur progressively as age advances and should not alter the elderly person's ability to breathe effortlessly.

TABLE 7-3

PROGRESSIVE CHANGES IN ARTERIAL OXYGEN TENSION (PaO_2) AND CARBON DIOXIDE TENSION ($PaCO_2$)

Age-Group	PaO_2 (mm Hg)	$PaCO_2$ (mm Hg)
<30 years	94	39
31-40	87	38
41-50	84	40
51-60	81	39
>60	74	40

Modified from Sorbini CA, et al: *Respiration* 25:3, 1968.

Thoracic Wall and Respiratory Muscles

With advancing age, the chest wall (thoracic skeleton) and vertebrae undergo a small degree of osteoporosis, and at the same time the costal cartilages that connect the rib cage together become calcified and stiff. These changes may produce kyphosis and reduce chest wall compliance, respectively[39-41] (Fig. 7-1). The functional effect is a decrease in thoracic wall excursion. Other factors, such as an increase in abdominal girth and change in posture, also decrease thoracic excursion. These anatomic structural changes are reflected by an increase in residual volume and decrease in vital capacity.

There is a gradual decrease in the strength of the respiratory muscles: the diaphragm and both the external and internal intercostal muscles. During aging, skeletal muscle progressively atrophies and its energy metabolism decreases, which may partially explain the declining strength of the respiratory muscles.[42,43] In addition, there is an age-associated decrease in the effectiveness of the cough reflex, which is possibly caused by a decrease in ciliary responsiveness and motion.[44]

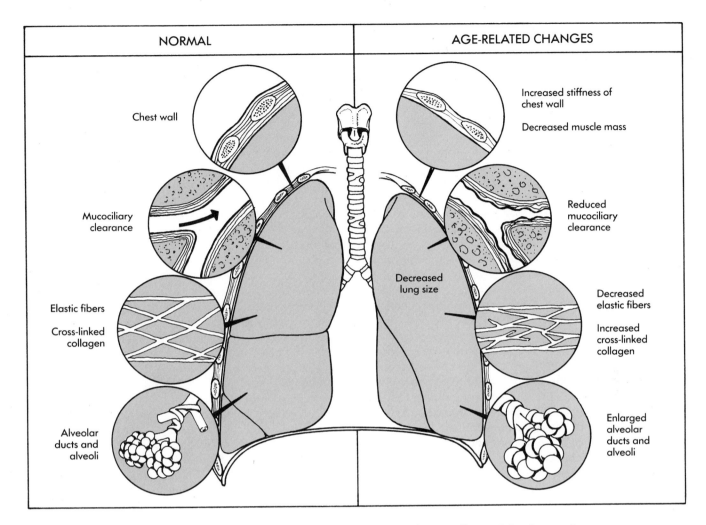

NORMAL	AGE-RELATED CHANGES

Chest wall

Mucociliary clearance

Elastic fibers

Cross-linked collagen

Alveolar ducts and alveoli

Increased stiffness of chest wall

Decreased muscle mass

Reduced mucociliary clearance

Decreased lung size

Decreased elastic fibers

Increased cross-linked collagen

Enlarged alveolar ducts and alveoli

Fig. **7-1** Age-related changes in the respiratory system. With advancing age, the compliance of the chest wall and lung tissue changes. There is also a reduced clearance of mucus by the cilia that line the pulmonary tree and an enlargement of the alveolar ducts and alveoli. More age-related changes in respiratory function are described in the text. (From Webster JR, Kadah H: *Geriatrics* 46:31, 1991.)

Alveolar Parenchyma

With advancing age a diminished recoil (or increased compliance) of the lung occurs.[45] The reduced recoil results from the increase in the ratio of elastin to collagen content that occurs with advancing age.[46] Whereas total lung collagen remains unaltered, the amount of elastin increases with age in the interlobular septa and pleura and possibly within the bronchi and their vessels.[47,48] These anatomic structural changes are reflected by an increase in residual volume and a decrease in forced expiratory volume. An additional anatomic structural change is the increase in the size of the alveolar ducts, which occurs after 40 years of age.[39] The bronchial enlargement displaces inhaled air volume away from the alveoli that line the alveolar ducts[39] (see Fig. 7-1). Ventilation and the process of oxygen and carbon dioxide exchange (diffusion) depend on numerous factors, one of which is the surface area available for diffusion. A displacement of inhaled air volume away from the alveoli limits the surface area avail-able for gas exchange. This may in part explain the progressive and linear decrease in the pulmonary diffusion capacity, which depends on both the surface area and capillary blood volume. There are reports that capillary blood volume and surface area decrease with advancing age.[49]

Pulmonary Gas Exchange

The arterial oxygen tension (PaO_2) decreases with age, such that the median PaO_2 for healthy persons older than 60 years is 74.3 mm Hg, as compared with 94 mm Hg for younger adults.[50] In contrast, arterial carbon dioxide ($PaCO_2$) does not change with advancing age[50,51] (see Table 7-3).

Lung Volumes and Capacities

With advancing age, total lung capacity and tidal volume do not change.[40] Residual volume (RV) increases with age, paralleling the decrease in chest wall compliance and reduced strength of the respiratory muscles.[39] The increase in RV may also add to the diminished strength of the inspiratory muscles by stretching the diaphragm and altering the tension-length relationship. Age-related changes in various pulmonary function tests are summarized in Table 7-2.

RENAL SYSTEM

Aging produces changes in renal structure and function, many of which begin at approximately 30 to 40 years of age.[52] One of the prominent changes is a decrease in the number and size of the nephrons, which begins in the cortical regions and progresses toward the medullary portions of the kidney.[53] The decrease in the number of nephrons corresponds to a 20% decrease in the weight of the kidney between 40 and 80 years of age.[53] Initially, this loss of nephrons does not appreciably alter renal function because of the large renal reserve. However, with time the geriatric patient also loses this "renal reserve."[53] Nephron loss is caused by a gradual reduction in blood flow to the glomerular capillary tuft.[54] Total renal blood flow declines after the fourth decade of life[52] because of hyaline arteriolosclerosis.[54,55] The etiology of this vascular lesion within the glomerular tuft is unknown. By the eighth decade of life, 50% of the glomeruli are lost as a result of this arteriolar hyalinization.[53]

The glomerular filtration rate (GFR), measured as creatine clearance, decreases with advancing age.[52,53,56] In elderly persons, the decrease in GFR is most likely caused by the decrease in nephron number as well as the decrease in renal blood flow.[52]

Even though the remaining nephrons adapt to the loss of nephrons by glomerular hyperfiltration and increased solute load per nephron, the reduced GFR predisposes the elderly patient to adverse drug reactions and drug-induced renal failure. In addition, the senescent kidney is more susceptible to injury by hypotensive episodes because of the age-related decrease in renal blood flow and reduced pressure gradient across the afferent arteriole.[56]

There are also age-related changes in tubular function. These changes in tubular function become apparent when there are extreme changes in the body fluid composition or acid-base balance. For example, with systemic acidosis the rate and amount of total acid excretion (bicarbonate, titratable acid, and ammonium) are reduced.[52,56] This predisposes the elderly patient to metabolic acidosis, volume depletion, and hyperchloremia. However, at a normal pH level, the kidney of an elderly person is able to maintain acid-base homeostasis.

There is a diminished ability of the senescent kidney to excrete a free water load, conserve water during periods of dehydration, and conserve sodium during periods of low salt intake.[52,56] There are also age-related changes in extrarenal mechanisms, such as the decreased activity and responsiveness of the senescent kidney to

the sympathetic nervous system and renin-angiotensin-aldosterone system, which are important in integrating overall fluid homeostasis and maintaining blood pressure in response to changes in body position.[57]

GASTROINTESTINAL SYSTEM

Age-related gastrointestinal changes occur in the processes of swallowing, motility, and absorption.[58,59] Swallowing may be difficult for the elderly person because of incomplete mastication of food.[59] Deteriorating dentition, diminished lubrication (secondary to salivary dysfunction), and ill-fitting dentures result in insufficient mastication of food within the oral cavity, thereby predisposing the elderly patient to aspiration.[58] In addition, the number and velocity of the peristaltic contractions of the elderly person's esophagus decrease and the number of nonperistaltic contractions increases.[59]

These changes in esophageal motility are referred to as *presbyesophagus*. These changes may predispose the patient to erosion of the esophageal wall (recurrent esophagitis) because food remains in the esophagus longer. In addition, bedrest and reclining in a supine position for a prolonged period can cause esophageal reflux, which also can lead to esophagitis.

The aging process produces thinning of the smooth muscle within the gastric mucosa.[60] The epithelial layer of the gastric mucosa, which contains the chief and parietal cells, undergoes a modest degree of atrophy, resulting in the hyposecretion of pepsin and acid, respectively.[61]

Mucin secretion from the mucus cells decreases, thereby altering the protective function of the gastric mucosal (bicarbonate) barrier. Because of this, the stomach wall is more susceptible to acid injury, thus increasing the incidence of gastric ulcerations.[62] Aging does not appreciably alter gastric emptying of solid foods.

Alterations within the small intestine include a decrease in intestinal weight after the age of 50 and a flattening and shortening of jejunal villi.[63] Age produces no change in the small intestine's absorption of fats and proteins; however, decreased carbohydrate absorption has been reported.[64,65] There is essentially no change in vitamin or mineral absorption, except for a decrease in calcium absorption from the aged duodenum.[59]

THE LIVER

With advancing age, both hepatocyte number and liver weight decrease.[66] There is also a significant decrease in total liver blood flow, such that between 25 and 65 years of age there is a 50% decrease in total liver blood flow.[66-68] Despite changes in hepatocyte number and blood flow, liver function is not appreciably altered.[68] Several tests of liver function—such as serum bilirubin, alkaline phosphatase, and glutamic oxaloacetic transaminase levels—are not altered with advancing age. However, because of the decrease in total liver blood flow, there is some reduction in first-pass clearance of drugs.

The most important age-related change in liver function is the decrease in the liver's capacity to metabolize drugs.[69,70] Although clinical tests of liver function do not reflect this change in metabolism, it is well-recognized that drug side effects and toxic effects occur more frequently in older adults than in young adults.[70]

Changes in Pharmacokinetics and Pharmacodynamics

There are many age-related changes in drug *pharmacokinetics,* which is the manner in which the body absorbs, distributes, metabolizes, and excretes a drug.[71,72] The aging process is associated with changes in gastric acid secretion, which can alter the ionization or solubility of a drug and hence its absorption[70,71] (Table 7-4).

Drug distribution depends on body composition as well as the physiochemical properties of the drug. With advancing age, fat content increases, lean body mass decreases, and total body water decreases, which can alter the drug disposition.[71] For example, because of the increase in the ratio of body fat content to body weight, lipophilic drugs have a greater volume of distribution per body weight in elderly persons, as compared with younger adults. Other age-related factors[73] affecting drug disposition are listed in Table 7-4.

As noted previously, the senescent liver has a decreased ability to metabolize drugs, which also affects the clearance of some drugs. For example, there is a reduced clearance of loop diuretics in elderly patients, which reduces the peak plasma concentration of the diuretic as well as decreases the magnitude of the diuretic response.[74] Other drugs—such as angiotensin II-converting enzyme (ACE) inhibitors—have delayed excretion, increased serum concentration, and more prolonged duration of action because their excretion parallels GFR (which decreases with age).[75] See Table 7-4 for age-related changes in drug pharmacokinetics and Table 7-5[56,73,75-80] for the potential side effects, nursing interventions, and/or special considerations for frequently used pharmacologic agents in the elderly patient in the critical care unit.

CENTRAL NERVOUS SYSTEM
Cognitive Functioning

Marked deterioration of any component of cognitive functioning is not a normal expectation of the aging process.[81] Cognitive impairment in older adults more commonly results from acute and chronic etiologies. Acute problems such as infection, electrolyte imbalance, or pharmacologic toxicity are generally reversible once identified. Uncontrolled pain is currently recognized as a strong contributor to cognitive impairment in the elderly.[82] On the other hand, chronic long-term cognitive impairment develops more from organic causes such as multiinfarct dementia or dementia of the Alzheimer's type.

Changes in Structure and Morphology

The brain decreases approximately 20% in size between 25 and 95 years of age[83] (Fig. 7-2). The reduced brain

---

TABLE 7-4

AGE-RELATED CHANGES IN PHARMACOKINETICS

Pharmacokinetic Parameters	Definition	Age-Related Changes
Absorption	Receptor-coupled or diffusional uptake of drug into tissue	Decreased absorptive surface area of small intestine Decrease in splanchnic blood flow Increase in gastric acid pH Decrease in gastrointestinal motility
Distribution	Theoretic space (tissue) or body compartment into which free form of drug distributes	Decreased lean body mass and total body water Increased total body fat Decreased serum albumin level Increased alpha$_1$ acid glycoprotein
Metabolism	Chemical change in drug that renders it active or inactive	Decreased liver mass Decrease in activity of microsomal drug-metabolizing enzyme system Decrease in total liver blood flow
Excretion	Removal of drug through an eliminating organ, which is often the kidney; some drugs are excreted in the bile or feces, in the saliva, or via the lungs	Decreased renal blood flow and GFR Decrease in distal renal tubular secretory function

Data from Gilman, et al, editors: *Goodman and Gilman's the pharmacological basis of therapeutics,* London, 1990, Pergamon Press; and Vestal RE, Cusack BJ: Pharmacology and aging. In Schneider EL, Rowe JW, editors: *Handbook of the biology of aging,* San Diego, 1990, Academic Press.

TABLE 7-5

PHARMACOLOGIC AGENTS USED IN THE CRITICAL CARE UNIT AND FREQUENT SIDE EFFECTS EXPERIENCED BY THE GERONTOLOGIC PATIENT

Pharmacologic Agent	Drug Actions	Adverse Drug Effects*	Nursing Interventions and/or Special Considerations
ACE INHIBITORS			
Enalapril	Inhibits the conversion of angiotensin I to angiotensin II	Hypotension, especially in patients taking diuretics Hypokalemia	Monitor HR and BP Monitor serum creatinine level Monitor serum K^+ level Excreted by the kidney so the dosage reduced if GFR reduced
DIURETICS			
Lasix	Inhibits Na^+ and Cl^- absorption from the proximal tubule and loop of Henle	Hypokalemia Volume depletion	Reduced rate of clearance and magnitude of the diuretic response
CARDIAC GLYCOSIDES			
Digoxin	Inhibits the sarcolermal Na^+ K^+-ATPase	Digitalis toxicity	Monitor HR and serum K^+ and serum digoxin levels Verapamil, quinidine, and amiodarone increase serum digoxin levels
ANTIDYSRHYTHMICS			
Procainamide	Decreases myocardial conduction velocity and excitability and prolongs myocardial refractoriness	Procainamide toxicity	Procainamide is converted to its active metabolite, N-acetyl-procainamide (NAPA), in the liver; NAPA may accumulate and cause side effects
Lidocaine	Decreases automaticity (especially in Purkinje fibers) and prolongs conduction and refractoriness	Dizziness, paresthesia, and drowsiness at lower plasma concentrations	Can be administered only parenterally
CALCIUM CHANNEL BLOCKERS			
Verapamil	Blocks the entry of Ca^{2+} through voltage-dependent Ca^{2+} channels and decreases SA automaticity and AV conduction	Constipation May alter liver function	Monitor liver function tests Contraindicated in heart failure, sick sinus syndrome, or first-degree AV block
Nifedipine	Same as verapamil	Headaches, tachycardia, palpitations, flushing, and ankle edema	Calcium channel blockers have a negative inotropic effect, but nifedipine produces less of a negative inotropic effect as compared with verapamil
Diltiazem	Same as verapamil	Constipation	Monitor liver function tests Contraindicated in heart failure, sick sinus syndrome, or first-degree AV block
NARCOTIC ANALGESICS			
Meperidine	Blocks the transmission of pain and inhibits the release of substance P; site of action is within the CNS	Respiratory depression and oversedation Tremors and muscle twitches related to effects of the metabolite normeperidine	Accumulation of normeperidine can produce CNS hyperexcitability, confusion
Morphine	Synthetic analgesic; mechanism similar to meperidine	Respiratory depression and oversedation	The volume of distribution for morphine is small; hence plasma and tissue levels are greater at a specific plasma concentration

Data modified from Creasy WA, et al: *J Clin Pharmacol* 26:264, 1986; Gilman AG, et al, editors: *Goodman and Gilman's the pharmacological basis of therapeutics*, London, 1990, Pergamon Press; Hockings N, Ajayi AA, Reid JL: *Br J Pharmacol* 21:341, 1986; Lynch RA, Horowitz LN: *Geriatrics* 46:41, 1991; Pederson KE: *Acta Med Scand* 697(suppl 1):1, 1985; Vidt GD, Borazanian RA: *Geriatrics* 46:28, 1991; Wall RT: *Clin Geriatr Med* 6:345, 1990; and Watters JM, McClaran JC: The elderly surgical patient. In Wilmore DW, et al, editors: *In care of the surgical patient*, vol III, *Special problems*, New York, 1990, Scientific American.
*Not all side effects are listed for each drug.

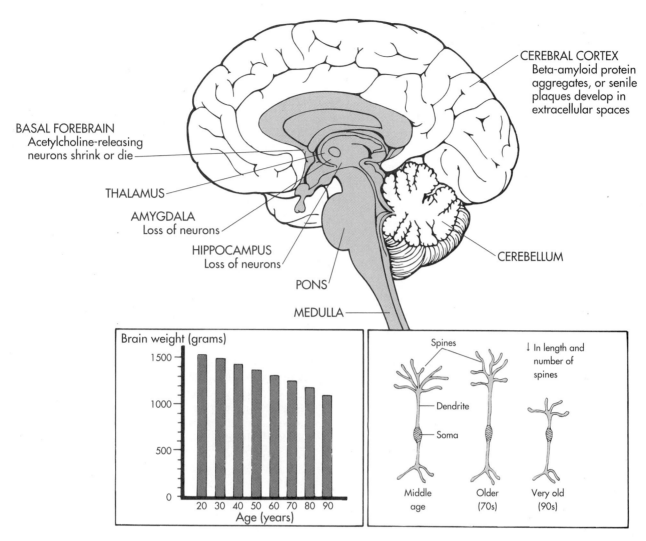

BASAL FOREBRAIN
Acetylcholine-releasing
neurons shrink or die

THALAMUS

AMYGDALA
Loss of neurons

HIPPOCAMPUS
Loss of neurons

PONS

MEDULLA

CEREBRAL CORTEX
Beta-amyloid protein
aggregates, or senile
plaques develop in
extracellular spaces

CEREBELLUM

Brain weight (grams)

Spines

↓ In length and
number of
spines

Dendrite

Soma

Middle
age

Older
(70s)

Very old
(90s)

Fig. **7-2** Summary of age-related changes in the brain. (From Soelkoe DJ: *Sci Am* 267:135, 1992.)

weight may be related in part to the overall decrease in the number of neurons that occurs with advancing age. Intracranial white matter decreases significantly more than gray matter.[84] In addition, portions of the cerebral cortex atrophy, principally the frontal and temporal cortical association areas.[85]

The cerebral ventricles enlarge and develop an asymmetric appearance.[86] Cerebrospinal fluid (CSF) also accumulates in the ventricles; however, total brain CSF is not increased.[86] Accompanying the loss of neurons are changes in the ultrastructure and intracellular structures of the neuron.[87] There are also reports of large neuron shrinking and degenerative changes occurring in the cell bodies and axons of certain acetylcholine-secreting neurons. These changes may explain alterations in processing and receiving information.[83]

In the senescent brain, synaptogenesis (synaptic regeneration) still occurs after partial nerve degeneration.[87] After a nerve fiber is damaged, neighboring undamaged neurons often sprout new fibers and form new connec-

tions. However, synaptogenesis occurs at a slower rate in the older brain.[87]

Cerebral Metabolism and Blood Flow

Cerebral blood flow (CBF) decreases with advancing age. This decrease parallels the decrease in brain weight and is most likely caused by the reduction in neuron number and metabolic needs of the cerebral tissue.[88]

Pain and Aging

Although animal studies indicate decreases in neurotransmitter function and diminished concentrations of opioid receptors in various regions of the cortex (Hiller, et al), there is little evidence to suggest that pain or its perception is altered in elderly people.[89,90] For the individual who is 60 years or older, pain often results from various chronic disease entities such as arthritis, osteoarthritis, cancer, and peripheral vascular disease.[91] In aging, pain is associated with a disease process, rather than being a product of aging in itself.[92-94]

IMMUNE SYSTEM

There are several changes in immune function that render the elderly person more susceptible to infections.[92,93,95-98] Infections in the elderly population are associated with higher rates of mortality.[98] Common infections in the elderly include bacterial pneumonia, urinary tract infection, intraabdominal infections, gram-negative bacteremia, and decubitus ulcers. The reasons for the increased susceptibility are multifactorial and include changes in cell-mediated and humoral-mediated immunity, breakdown in physical barriers such as the skin and oral mucosa, and changes in nutrition.

Cell-Mediated and Humoral-Mediated Immunity

Immune system function depends on many cell types with distinct functions. T cells are the primary effector of cell-mediated immunity whereas bone marrow-derived B cells produce antibodies that are the effector cells of humoral-mediated immunity.[95,97] With aging, there is a decline in cell-mediated immunity. Even though the total number of T cells remains unchanged with advancing age, there is a decrease in T cell function.[95,97] Similarly, the number of natural killer cells (NK) remains constant, but the function and activity of NK cells diminish with advancing age.[99]

Additional Risk Factors

Multiple concurrent chronic illnesses produce systemic stressors that ultimately diminish immune functioning. An exacerbation of preexisting illness such as diabetes or emphysema may present itself before infection is suspected. Introducing bacteria through invasive devices such as central lines or chest tubes may threaten an already suppressed immune system.

One must also consider how nutritional deficiencies, particularly protein malnutrition, are a common problem among the elderly. Inadequate protein intake can develop from prolonged anorexia and cognitive impairment. Protein malnutrition is associated with a shrinkage of lymphoid tissue, which then diminishes T cell functioning and cell-mediated immunity.[96]

INTEGUMENTARY AND MUSCULOSKELETAL SYSTEMS

The loss of elastic and connective tissue causes the skin to wrinkle; both skin wrinkles and sagging may be found over many areas of the body. The appearance and number of skin wrinkles also depends greatly on environmental agents and exposure to ultraviolet rays.[100] Underlying structures, such as the veins and muscles, are more visible because of the transparency of the skin. Table 7-6 outlines age-related changes in the skin and their corresponding nursing interventions.

There may be multiple ecchymotic areas because of decreased protective subcutaneous tissue layers, increased capillary fragility, and flattening of the capillary bed, all of which predispose elderly persons to developing ecchymosis.[101-104] In conjunction with frequent aspirin use, these physiologic factors result in increased bleeding tendencies and the appearance of ecchymotic areas. However, areas of unexplained ecchymosis may also indicate elder abuse.

Changes that occur in the musculoskeletal system are a decrease in lean body mass, a compression of the spinal column that results from the thinning of cartilage between vertebra, and a decrease in the mobility of skeletal

TABLE 7-6		
AGE-RELATED CHANGES IN THE INTEGUMENTARY SYSTEM		
Skin Problem	**Underlying Mechanisms**	**Nursing Interventions**
Delayed wound healing	↓ Vascular supply to dermis ↓ Connective tissue layer ↓ SQ tissue layer Impaired inflammatory response ↓ New connective tissue proliferation	Use nonrestrictive dressings Weigh patient daily Support nutritional needs
Thermoregulation	↓ SQ tissue layer ↓ Number of capillary arterioles supplying skin ↓ Number of eccrine (sweat) glands	Monitor room temperature
Pressure ulcers	↓ Flattening of capillary bed ↓ Thinning of epidermis	Reposition patient every 2 hr Use pressure-relieving devices
IV infiltrations	↓ Connective tissue layer Vascular fragility	Monitor peripheral IV site hourly Discontinue IV at first sign of infiltration
Diminished skin turgor	↓ Connective tissue layer ↓ Eccrine and sebaceous gland activity	Bathe with tepid water Avoid use of deodorant soap

↓, Decreased.

joints.[105] Despite the ubiquitous finding of reduced joint mobility, no exact physiologic process gives rise to the altered mobility. It is possible that the reduced synovial fluid production that occurs with aging causes changes in function. There is also an increase in muscle rigidity, especially in the neck, shoulders, hips, and knees.[106] This may produce some changes in range of motion.

Bone demineralization afflicts both men and women as they age; however, it occurs four times more often in women than in men. *Bone demineralization* refers to an increase in osteoplast and osteoclast activity, which decreases calcium absorption into the bone.[105] Mineral loss (calcium and phosphorous), along with a decrease in bone mass, is referred to as *osteoporosis*.[105] Osteoporosis produces bones that are more "porous" or fragile. With extensive bone demineralization, an elderly patient may sustain multiple fractures. There is an accelerated inci-

dence of osteoporosis in women that occurs after the onset of menopause. A decrease in estrogen is implicated in this process; estrogen replacement may arrest the osteoporosis process, but it will not reverse it.

SUMMARY

The elderly patient requires more intense observation and consideration in the critical care unit because his or her system has become less adaptable to stress and illness. Box 7-1 delineates the effects of aging on various laboratory values.[107-108] Table 7-7 summarizes the major changes in the various systems along with clinical considerations.[109] As shown in Fig. 7-3, many physiologic changes occur with advancing age, and each change may render a particular system less adaptable to stress. In addition, a change in one system may affect another system in the presence of disease.

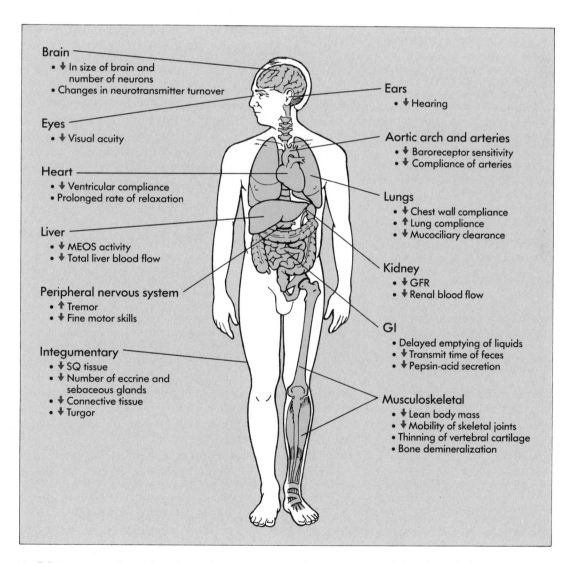

Fig. **7-3** Summary of the physiologic changes that occur in all systems and that the critical care nurse must consider in caring for the elderly patient in the critical care unit. *MEOS,* microsomal enzyme oxidative system; *GFR,* glomerular filtration rate; *GI,* gastrointestinal; *SQ,* subcutaneous.

TABLE 7-7

SUMMARY OF AGE-RELATED PHYSIOLOGIC CHANGES AND RELATED CLINICAL CONSIDERATIONS

Age-Related Effect	Clinical Considerations
CARDIOVASCULAR SYSTEM	
↓ Inotropic and chronotropic response of myocardium to catecholamine stimulation	The increase in CO achieved during stress or exercise is achieved by an increase in diastolic filling (increased dependence on Starling's law of the heart)
↑ Myocardial collagen content	Leads to a decrease in the compliance of the ventricle (higher filling pressures are needed to maintain stroke volume)
↓ Baroreceptor sensitivity	↑ Tendency for orthostatic hypotension after prolonged bedrest or if patient is taking antihypertensive medication or has systolic hypertension
Prolonged rate of relaxation	May predispose the elderly patient to hemodynamic derangements in the presence of tachydysrhythmias, hypertension, or ischemic heart disease
↓ Compliance of blood vessels	↑ Peripheral vascular resistance and blood pressure
RESPIRATORY SYSTEM	
↓ Strength of the respiratory muscles, recoil of lungs, chest wall compliance, and efficiency and number of cilia in airways	↑ Susceptibility to aspiration, atelectasis, and pulmonary infection Patient may require more frequent deep breathing, coughing, and position change
↓ Pa_{O_2} level	↓ Ventilatory response to hypoxia and hypercapnia ↑ Sensitivity to narcotics
RENAL SYSTEM	
↓ GFR	Careful observation of patient when administering aminoglycosides, antibiotics, and contrast dyes
↓ Ability to concentrate and conserve water	May predispose patient to development of dehydration and hypernatremia, especially if patient is fluid restricted and insensible losses are high (e.g., during mechanical ventilation or fever)
↓ Ability to excrete salt and water loads as well as urea, ammonia, and drugs	Observe for clinical manifestations of fluid overload and drug reactions
↓ Response to an acid load	After an acid load (i.e., metabolic acidosis), the elderly patient may be in a state of uncompensated metabolic acidosis for a longer period
LIVER	
↓ Total liver blood flow	Adverse drug reactions, especially with polypharmacy
GASTROINTESTINAL SYSTEM	
Diminished ability to swallow	May predispose elderly patient to aspiration pneumonia Assess for proper fit of dentures and ability to chew Flex head forward 45 degrees
Impaired esophageal motility	Develop awareness for complaints of food or medications "sticking in throat" Assess for complaints of heartburn or epigastric discomfort Avoid prolonged supine position
Delayed emptying of liquids	Examine abdomen for distention Investigate complaints of anorexia
↓ Stool weight and transit time	Obtain thorough bowel history and note routine use of laxatives Increase intake of dietary fiber and assess for fecal incontinence and impaction
NEUROLOGIC SYSTEM	
↑ Cranial dead space	Elderly persons may sustain a significant amount of hemorrhage before symptoms are apparent
↓ Number of neurons and dendrites and length of dendrite spines	Delayed or impaired processing of sensory and motor information
Delay in the rate of synaptogenesis	
Changes in neurotransmitter turnover	May cause desynchronization of neurotransmission

Modified from Rebenson-Piano M: *Crit Care Q* 12:1, 1989.

BOX **7-1**

EFFECTS OF AGING ON VARIOUS LABORATORY VALUES

VALUES THAT DO NOT CHANGE WITH AGE

Calcium
Hemoglobin/hematocrit or slight ↓
Platelet count
White blood cell count with differential
Serum electrolytes
Coagulation profile
Liver function tests
Thyroid function tests or slight ↓
Serum blood urea nitrogen or slight ↑
Serum creatinine

VALUES THAT CHANGE WITH AGE AND HAVE CLINICAL SIGNIFICANCE

↓ Erythrocyte sedimentation rate
↓ Arterial oxygen pressure
↑ Blood glucose
↓ or ↑ Serum lipid profile
↓ Albumin
↓ Creatinine clearance

↓, Decreased; ↑, increased.

References

1. Abrass IB: Biology of aging. In Wilson JD, et al, editors: *Harrison's principles of internal medicine,* ed 12, New York, 1991, McGraw-Hill.
2. Fried, et al: Heart health in older adults: importance of heart disease and opportunities for maintaining cardiac health, *West J Med* 167(4):240-246, 1997.
3. Rowe JW, Kahn R: Successful aging, *Gerontologist* 37(4):433-440, 1997.
4. Vijg J, Wei JY: Understanding the biology of aging: the key to prevention and therapy, *J Am Geriatr Soc* 43(4):426-434, 1995.
5. Weisfeldt ML, Lakatta EG, Gerstenblith G: Aging and the heart. In Braunwald E, editor: *Heart disease,* Philadelphia, 1992, WB Saunders.
6. Eghbali M, et al: Collagen accumulation in heart ventricles as a function of growth and aging, *Cardiovasc Res* 23:723, 1989.
7. Wegelius O, von Knorring J: The hydroxyproline and hexosamine content in human myocardium at different ages, *Acta Med Scand* (suppl)412:233, 1964.
8. Katz AM: Heart failure. In Fozzard HA, et al, editors: *The heart and cardiovascular system,* New York, 1991, Raven Press.
9. Muller RT, et al: Painless myocardial infarction in the elderly, *Am Heart J* 119:202, 1990.
10. Mukerji V, Holman AJ, Alpert MA: The clinical description of angina pectoris in the elderly, *Am Heart J* 117:705, 1989.
11. Gerstenblith G, et al: Echocardiographic assessment of normal adult aging population, *Circulation* 56:273, 1977.
12. Walsh RA: Cardiovascular effects of the aging process, *Am J Med* 82:34, 1987.
13. Weisfeldt M: Aging changes in the cardiovascular system and responses to stress, *Am J Hypertension* (3pt 2):41S-45S, March 11, 1998.
14. Lakatta EG, et al: Prolonged contraction duration in the aged myocardium, *J Clin Invest* 55:61, 1975.
15. Opie LH: *The physiology of the heart and metabolism,* New York, 1991, Raven Press.
16. Spurgeon HA, Steinbach MF, Lakatta EG: Prolonged contraction duration in senescent myocardium is prevented by exercise, *Am J Physiol* 244:H513, 1983.
17. Froehlich JP, et al: Studies of sarcoplasmic reticulum function and contraction in young and aged rat myocardium, *J Mol Cell Cardiol* 10:427, 1978.
18. Cinelli P, et al: Effects of age on mean heart rate variability, *Aging* 10:146, 1987.
19. Ribera JM, et al: Cardiac rate and hyperkinetic rhythm disorders in healthy elderly subjects: evaluation by ambulatory electrocardiographic monitoring, *Gerontology* 35:158, 1989.
20. Jose AD: Effect of combined sympathetic and parasympathetic blockage on heart rate and cardiac function in man, *Am J Cardiol* 18:476, 1966.
21. Lakatta EG: Heart and circulation. In Schneider EL, Rowe JW, editors: *Handbook of the biology of aging,* San Diego, 1990, Academic Press.
22. Bonow RO, et al: Effects of aging on asynchronous left ventricular regional function and global ventricular filling in normal human subjects, *J Am Coll Cardiol* 11:50, 1988.
23. Miller TR, et al: Left ventricular diastolic filling and its association with age, *Am J Cardiol* 58:531, 1986.
24. Davidson WR, Fee WC: Influence of aging on pulmonary hemodynamics in a population free of coronary artery disease, *Am J Cardiol* 65:1454-1458, 1990.
25. Bachman S, Sparrow D, Smith LK: Effect of aging on the electrocardiogram, *Am J Cardiol* 48:513, 1981.
26. Horwitz LN, Lynch RA: Managing geriatric arrhythmias, I. General considerations. *Geriatrics* 46:31, 1991.
27. Docherty JR: Cardiovascular responses in ageing: a review, *Pharmacol Rev* 42:103, 1990.
28. Smith JJ, et al: The effect of age on hemodynamic response to graded postural stress in normal men, *J Gerontol* 42:406, 1987.
29. Dambrink JHA, Wieling W: Circulatory response to postural change in healthy male subjects in relation to age, *Clin Sci* 72:335, 1987.
30. Applegate WB, et al: Prevalence of postural hypotension at baseline in the systolic hypertension in the elderly program (SHEP) cohort, *J Am Geriatr Soc* 39:1057, 1991.
31. Bierman EL: Arteriosclerosis and aging. In Finch CE, Schneider EL, editors: *Handbook of the biology of aging,* New York, 1985, Van Nostrand Reinhold.
32. Schoenberger JA: Epidemiology of systolic and diastolic systemic blood pressure elevation in the elderly, *Am J Cardiol* 57:45c, 1986.
33. Rowe JW: Clinical consequences of age-related impairments in vascular compliance, *Am J Cardiol* 60:68G, 1987.
34. Rose BD: *Clinical physiology of acid-base and electrolyte disorders,* New York, 1989, McGraw-Hill.
35. Crane MG, Harris JJ: Effect of aging on renin activity and aldosterone excretion, *J Lab Clin Med* 87:947, 1976.
36. Sica DA, Harford A: Sodium and water disorders in the elderly. In Zawada ET, Sica DA, editors: *Geriatric nephrology and urology,* Littleton, Mass, 1985, PSG Publishing.
37. Davis CE, et al: Lipoprotein-cholesterol distributions in selected North American populations: The Lipid Research Clinics Program Prevalence Study, *Circulation* 2:302, 1980.
38. Kreisberg RA, Kasim S: Cholesterol metabolism and aging, *Am J Med* 82:54, 1987.
39. Webster JR, Kadah H: Unique aspects of respiratory disease in the aged, *Geriatrics* 46:31, 1991.
40. Levitzky MG: Effects of aging on the respiratory system, *Physiologist* 27:102, 1984.
41. Mittman C, et al: Relationship between chest wall and pulmonary compliance and age, *J Appl Physiol* 20:1211, 1965.

42. Rizzato G, Marazzine L: Thoracoabdominal mechanisms in elderly men, *J Appl Physiol* 28:457, 1970.

43. Gutmann E, Hanzlikova V: Fast and slow motor units in aging, *Gerontology* 22:280, 1976.

44. Pontoppidan HH, Beecher HK: Progressive loss of protective reflexes in the airway with advance of age, *JAMA* 1974:2209, 1960.

45. Knudson RJ, et al: Changes in the normal maximal expiratory flow-volume curve with growth and aging, *Am Rev Respir Dis* 127:725, 1983.

46. Turner JM, Mead J, Wohl ME: Elasticity of human lungs in relation to age, *J Appl Physiol* 25:664, 1968.

47. Pierce JA, Hocott JB: Studies on the collagen and elastin content of the human lung, *J Clin Invest* 39:8, 1960.

48. Pierce JA, Ebert RV: Fibrous network of the lung and its change with age, *Thorax* 20:469, 1965.

49. Semmens M: The pulmonary artery in the normal aged lung, *Br J Dis Chest* 64:65, 1970.

50. Sorbini CA, et al: Arterial oxygen tension in relation to age in healthy subjects, *Respiration* 25:3, 1968.

51. Cardus J, et al: Increase in pulmonary ventilation-perfusion inequality with age in healthy individuals, *Am J Resp Crit Care Med* 156(2pt 1):648-653, 1997.

52. Weder AB: The renally compromised older hypertensive: therapeutic considerations, *Geriatrics* 46:36, 1991.

53. Gilbert BR, Vaughan ED: Pathophysiology of the aging kidney, *Clin Geriatr Med* 6(1):12, 1990.

54. Kasiske BL: Relationship between vascular disease and age-associated changes in the human kidney, *Kidney Int* 31:1153, 1987.

55. Anderson S, Brenner BM: Effects of aging on the renal glomerulus, *Am J Med* 80:435, 1986.

56. Watters JM, McClaran JC: The elderly surgical patient. In Wilmore DW, et al, editors: *In care of the surgical patient*, vol VII, *Special problems*, New York, 1990, Scientific American.

57. Hall JE, Coleman TG, Guyton AC: The renin-angiotensin system: normal physiology and changes in older hypertensives, *J Am Geriatr Soc* 37:801, 1989.

58. Brandt LJ: Gastrointestinal disorders in the elderly. In Rossman I, editor: *Clinical geriatrics*, ed 3, Philadelphia, 1986, JB Lippincott.

59. Williams SA, Fogel RP: Common gastrointestinal problems in the elderly, *JAMA* 87:29, 1989.

60. Altman DF: Changes in gastrointestinal, pancreatic, biliary and hepatic function in aging, *Gastroenterol Clin North Am* 19:227, 1990.

61. Thomson AB, Keelan M: The aging gut, *Can J Physiol Pharmacol* 64:30, 1986.

62. Bansal SK, et al: Upper gastrointestinal hemorrhage in the elderly: a record of 92 patients in a joint geriatric/surgical unit, *Age Ageing* 16:279, 1987.

63. Schuster MM: Disorders of the aging GI system, *Hosp Prac* 11:95, 1976.

64. Curran J: Overview of geriatric nutrition, *Dysphagia* 5:72, 1990.

65. Ausman LM, Russel RM: Nutrition and aging. In Schneider EL, Rowe JW, editors: *Handbook of the biology of aging*, San Diego, 1990, Academic Press.

66. Sato TG, Miwa T, Tauchi H: Age changes in the human liver of the different races, *Gerontology* 16:368, 1970.

67. Bach B, et al: Disposition of antipyrine and phenytoin correlated with age and liver volume in man, *Clin Pharmacokinet* 6:389, 1981.

68. Kampmann JP, Sinding J, Moller-Jorgensen I: Effect of age on liver function, *Geriatrics* 30:91, 1975.

69. Schmucker DL, Wang RK: Age-related changes in liver drug metabolism: structure versus function, *Proc Soc Exp Biol Med* 165:178, 1980.

70. Vestal RE, Cusack BJ: Pharmacology and aging. In Schneider EL, Rowe JW, editors: *Handbook of the biology of aging*, San Diego, 1990, Academic Press.

71. Yuen GJ: Altered pharmacokinetics in the elderly, *Clin Geriatric Med* 6:257, 1990.

72. Schwertz DW, Bushmann MT: Pharmacogeriatrics, *Crit Care Q* 12:26, 1989.

73. Gilman AG, et al, editors: *Goodman and Gilman's the pharmacological basis of therapeutics*, ed 8, London, 1990, Pergamon Press.

74. Mooradian AD: An update of the clinical pharmacokinetics, therapeutic monitoring techniques, and treatment recommendations, *Clin Pharmacokinet* 18:165, 1988.

75. Creasy WA, et al: Pharmacokinetics of captopril in elderly healthy male volunteers, *J Clin Pharmacol* 26:264, 1986.

76. Hockings N, Ajayi AA, Reid JL: Age and the pharmacodynamics of angiotensin-converting enzyme inhibitors, enalapril and enalaprilat, *Br J Pharmacol* 21:341, 1986.

77. Pederson KE: Digoxin interactions: the influence of quinidine and verapamil on the pharmacokinetics and receptor binding of digitalis glycosides, *Acta Med Scand* 697(suppl 1):1, 1985.

78. Lynch RA, Horowitz LN: Managing geriatric arrhythmias, II. Drug selection and use, *Geriatrics* 46:41, 1991.

79. Vidt GD, Borazanian RA: Calcium channel blockers in geriatric hypertension, *Geriatrics* 46:28, 1991.

80. Wall RT: Use of analgesics in the elderly, *Clin Geriatric Med* 6:345, 1990.

81. Foreman MD, Grabowski R: Diagnostic dilemma: cognitive impairment in the elderly, *J Gerontol Nurs* 18:5, 1992.

82. Lynch EP, et al: The impact of postoperative pain on the development of postoperative delirium, *Reg Anes Pain Manage* 86:781-785, 1998.

83. Selkoe DJ: Aging brain, aging mind, *Sci Am* 267:134, 1992.

84. Guttman DR, et al: White matter changes with normal aging, *Neurology* 50(4):972-978, 1998.

85. Morris JC, McManus DQ: The neurology of aging: normal versus pathologic change, *Geriatrics* 46:47, 1991.

86. Lytle LD, Altar A: Diet, central nervous system, and aging, *Fed Proc* 38:2017, 1979.

87. Cotman CW: Synaptic plasticity, neurotropic factors and transplantation in the aged brain. In Schneider EL, Rowe JW, editors: *Handbook of the biology of aging*, San Diego, 1990, Academic Press.

88. Gottstein U, Held K: Effects of aging on cerebral circulation and metabolism in man, *Acta Neurol Scand* (suppl)72:54-55, 1979.

89. Hiller JM, Fan L-Q, Simon EJ: Alterations in opioid receptor levels in discrete areas of the neocortex and in the globus pallidus of the aging guinea pig: a quantitative autoradiographic study, *Brain Res* 614:86, 1993.

90. Bonica JJ: *The management of pain*, Philadelphia, 1990, Lea & Febiger.

91. Egbert DA, et al: Help for the hurting elderly: pain relief, *Postgrad Med* 19:291, 1991.

92. Ferrell BR, Ferrell BA: Easing pain, *Geriatr Nurs* July/Aug:175, 1990.

93. Harkins SW, Kwentus J, Price DD: Pain and suffering in the elderly. In Bonica JJ, editor: *The management of pain*, Philadelphia, 1990, Lea & Febiger.

94. Schmitt-Luggen A: Chronic pain in older adults: a quality of life issue, *J Gerontol Nurs* 24(2):48-54, 1998.

95. Miller RA: Immune system. In Masoro EJ, editor: *Handbook of physiology: aging*, New York, 1995, Oxford University Press.

96. Terpenning MS, Bradley SF: Why aging leads to increased susceptibility to infection, *Geriatrics* 46:77, 1991.

97. Miller RA: The aging immune system: primer and prospectus, *Science* 273:70, 1996.

98. McClure CL: Common infections in the elderly, *Am Fam Phys* 45:2691, 1992.

99. Ogata K, et al: Natural killer cells in the late decades of human life, *Clin Immun Immunopath* 8(3):269-275, 1997.

100. Lapiere CM: The ageing dermis: the main cause for the appearance of "old skin," *Brit J Dermatol* 122(suppl 35):5, 1990.

101. Jones PL, Millman A: Wound healing and the aged patient, *Nurs Clin North Am* 25(1):263, 1990.

102. Kelly L, Mobily PR: Iatrogenesis in the elderly, *J Geron Nurs* 17(9):24, 1991.

103. Shenefelt PD, Fenske NA: Aging and the skin: recognizing and managing common orders, *Geriatrics* 45(10):57, 1990.

104. Wenger NK: Cardiovascular disease in the elderly, *Curr Probl Cardiol* October:611, 1992.

105. Kalu DN: Bone. In Masoro EJ, editor: *Handbook of physiology: aging*, New York, 1995, Oxford University Press.

106. Exton-Smith AN: Mineral metabolism. In Finch CE, Schneider EL, editors: *Handbook of the biology of aging*, New York, 1985, Van Nostrand Reinhold.

107. Cavalieri TA, et al: When outside the room is normal: interpreting lab data in the aged, *Geriatrics* 47(5):66-70, 1992.

108. Kane RL, et al: *Essentials of clinical geriatrics*, ed 3, New York, 1994, McGraw-Hill.

109. Piano MR: The physiologic changes that occur with aging, *Crit Care Q* 12:1, 1989.

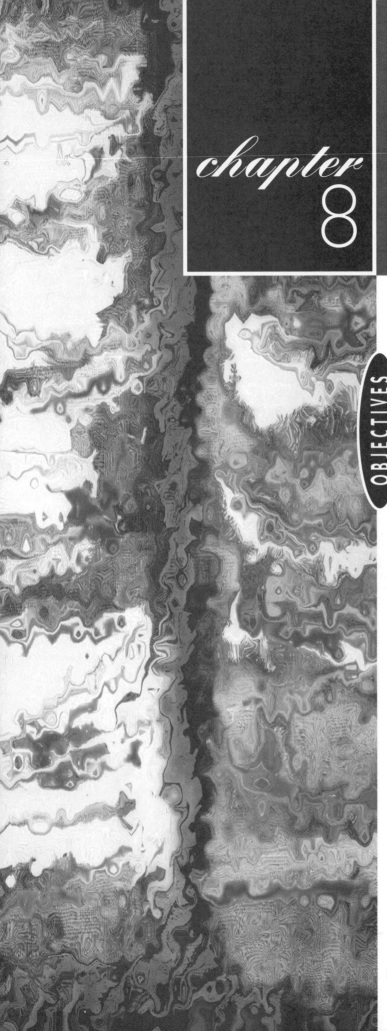

chapter 8

Pain Management

Lynne Jett

● **Explain the physiology of pain.**

● **Discuss how to perform a pain assessment in the critically ill patient.**

● **Identify patient and health care professional barriers to a pain assessment.**

● **Describe pharmacologic and nonpharmacologic interventions for pain management.**

● **Describe nursing interventions that are essential in the treatment of acute pain.**

OBJECTIVES

Pain is defined in a number of ways. Pain is a warning signal from the body that an injury has occurred. Unlike other sensations, pain is the protective signal for a threat to survival.[1] Pain is an unpleasant sensory experience that is associated with actual and potential tissue damage. Pain is not simply a pure physiologic response to an injury but is associated with an emotional response to the sensation.[2] Pain is an extremely complex set of responses to a physical stimulus. The definition with the most clinical significance is that pain is whatever the person experiencing it says it is, and it occurs when that person says it does.[3] Pain is a common thread that binds critical care patients together. Whether the pain is from an elective procedure or trauma, its presence is ubiquitous.[4] Studies examining the ability of the critically ill surgical patient to sleep identified pain and the inability to get comfortable as the most commonly cited barriers to sleep.[5]

With the frequency of the diagnosis of pain and the professional responsibility to manage pain, the critical care nurse must understand the mechanisms, the assessment technique, and the appropriate therapeutic measures to manage the pain state. Unfortunately, studies of pain management reflect that the critical care patient is commonly undermedicated. On average the nurse administered only 30% to 36% of the maximum opioid dose ordered.[6] One study of critically ill patients revealed that the second most commonly recalled memory of their illness was that of a painful, uncomfortable experience.[7,8]

PATHOPHYSIOLOGY OF PAIN

The pathophysiology of pain involves both the peripheral and central nervous systems.

Peripheral Nervous System

The peripheral nervous system contains a multitude of free nerve endings. The sensation of pain requires the activation of some of these free nerve endings. Other similar nerve endings are responsible for the transmission of sensations of touch, pressure, and warmth. The nerve endings responsible for pain, the nociceptors, are specialized. Because the role of pain in the body is protective, the nerve endings do not adapt to repeated painful stimuli. On the contrary, repeated stimulation heightens their sensitivity. The supersensitive state lowers the threshold for stimulation and increases the response to stimulation.[2] This phenomenon is responsible for the hypersensitive state of many critically ill patients. In this hypersensitive state, known as *hyperalgesia,* the slightest painful stimulus is interpreted as very painful.[9] Nociceptors are present in numerous organs in the body. They are primarily located in skin, joints, muscle, fascia, viscera, and the smooth muscle of the arterial walls. They are activated by thermal, mechanical, and chemical stimuli. There are two types of afferent nerve fibers that transmit painful stimuli from the site of injury through distinct neural pathways. Fig. 8-1 illustrates the dual pathways for pain transmission.

One type of fiber, Aδ, conducts the rapid acute pain sensation described as prickling, sharp, and fast. This type of fiber is activated by mechanical and thermal stimuli. The second type of nociceptor is the polymodal C fiber. C fibers are implicated in the transmission of pain

described as dull, diffuse, prolonged, and delayed. These fibers are activated by chemicals released when cell damage occurs. Some of these chemicals, or neurotransmitters, are potassium, histamine, bradykinin, serotonin, and acetylcholine.[1,2] These chemical transmitters are responsible for irritating the nerve endings and for activating the peripheral nerve system for transmission of other neurotransmitters that are active in the inhibition of the transmission of pain. These mediators are released when there is tissue damage of any type. Depending on which of the mediators is active, there are other associated reactions at the site of injury, including vasoconstriction, vasodilatation, or altered capillary permeability.

Both the Aδ fibers and the C fibers have roots in the dorsal horn of the spinal column. They are the afferent arm of the ascending spinal pathways of pain. In the dorsal horn at the laminae, the nociceptor neurons release substance P; substance P has as excitatory effect on the spinal cord and enhances the transmission of pain.[10] This is the point of integration of the peripheral and central nervous systems for the transmission of the pain impulse (Table 8-1).

Central Nervous System

The central nervous system has two components used in the pain response, the ascending, or conducting, pathways and the descending, or modulating, pathways.

Ascending pain pathways

The ascending tracts synapse with primary Aδ and C afferent nerve fibers that terminate in laminae I through V of the spinal cord. Aδ terminal fibers have been found in laminae I and V. Type C fibers are predominantly found in the laminae II, or the substantia gelatinosa. Most C fiber transmission immediately synapses with neurons to ascend to the thalamus. The sensations are transmitted via the spinothalamic tract (Fig. 8-2). Two other tracts are responsible for the transmission of nociceptor messages. The spinoreticular tract transmits to the brainstem reticular formation and terminates in the thalamus. The third nociceptor tract is the spinomesencephalic tract. This tract terminates in the midbrain reticular formation and the midbrain periaqueductal gray. This area of the

TABLE 8-1

NERVE FIBERS FOR PAIN TRANSMISSION

Nerve Fiber (Description)	General Location	Type of Pain Transmitted	Patient Descriptors	Rate of Transmission
Aδ fibers (thinly myelinated)	Skin, cutaneous tissue	Mechanical, thermal stimulus; easily localized	Sharp, pricking, electric, acute	Rapid, within 0.1 sec; velocity 6-30 m/sec
C fibers (primitive, unmyelinated)	Subcutaneous tissue, fascia, tendons, joints, ligaments, muscles	Mechanical, chemical, or thermal stimulus; difficult to localize	Throbbing, aching, burning, gnawing, chronic	Slow, 1+ sec, increases slowly; velocity 0.5-2 m/sec

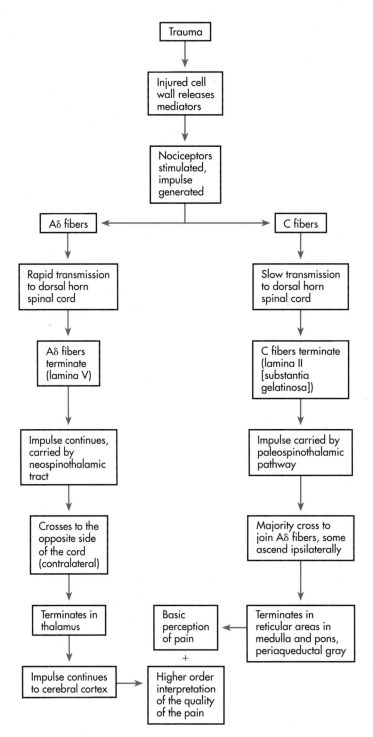

Fig. **8-1** Dual pathways of pain transmission using Aδ and C fibers for nociception.

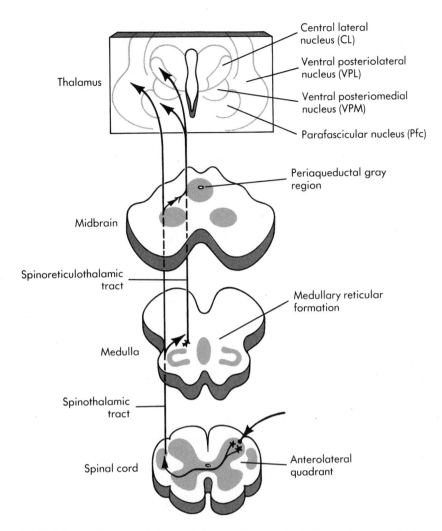

Fig. **8-2** Ascending somatosensory system. (From Barker E: *Neuroscience nursing*, St Louis, 1994, Mosby.)

brain is also responsible for strong inhibitory responses to pain transmission. Nociception continues to the somatosensory cortex of the brain. Cortical interpretation of the stimulus is necessary to finalize the perception of the pain; to discretely locate the pain, identify its intensity, and interpret its meaning; and to add the emotional component. This cortical process underlies the patient's individual, unique perception of the pain.

Descending pain pathways

The descending analgesia system is the endogenous pain modulation system, which is responsible for the body's attempt to intrinsically manage pain.[11] The system consists of a series of neurons in the brain and spinal cord that synapse with the ascending neurons. Fig. 8-3 illustrates the endogenous pain modification system. In the brain, the cortex and the hypothalamus activate the periaqueductal gray that influences fibers in the dorsal horns to release neurotransmitters that inhibit the action of the neurons transmitting pain impulses. These neurotransmitters that inhibit or modulate the transmission of pain

are produced in the body at sites along the neural synapses. The sites are located in both the brain and the descending pathways. These neurotransmitters are the endogenous opioid peptides known as *endogenous opioids* and are considered morphine-like. There are primarily three types of endogenous opioids: β-endorphins, enkephalins, and dynorphins, all three are from different chemical families.[9] Upon release, the endogenous opioids, or endorphins, bind to the nerve receptor sites located throughout the ascending pain transmission system and significantly modify the transmission of pain (Fig. 8-4). The binding sites, or receptors, are generally classified as the mu (μ) effect, kappa (κ) effect, and delta (δ) effect. Each receptor type acts differently when stimulated (Table 8-2). Different levels of these pain-modifying endorphins in individuals are responsible for the difference in response to the same painful stimulus among individuals.

β-endorphins are located primarily in the hypothalamus and the midbrain. They are the most morphine-like. Research indicates that the β-endorphins are released during accupuncture and transcutaneous stimulation.[2]

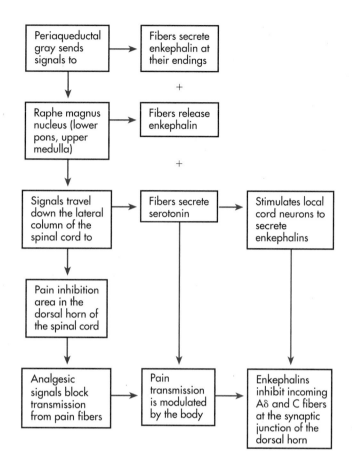

Fig. **8-3** The body's endogenous pain modification, or analgesia, system.

TABLE 8-2

OPIATE RECEPTOR CLASSIFICATION AND ACTIONS

Affected Area	μ Effect	δ Effect
Pupils	Miosis	Mydriasis
Respiratory system	Stimulates, then depresses	Stimulates
Heart	Bradycardia	Tachycardia
Temperature	Hypothermia	
Gastrointestinal (GI)	Constipation	Nausea

Modified from Willens J: Pain management in the trauma patient. In Cardona D, et al, editors: *Trauma nursing: from resuscitation through rehabilitation,* ed 2, Philadelphia, 1994, WB Saunders.

A second, less-discussed inhibitory pathway contributes to pain modification. This pathway is a nonopioid form of endogenous analgesia. It is the monoamine system. The primary neurotransmitters involved in this system are serotonin and norepinephrine. Serotonin is a major pain-inhibiting factor from the medulla to the spinal cord descending pathway.[2,10,11] At the dorsal horn, serotonin is responsible for the release of enkephalins.[10] Norepinephrine's role in pain modulation is in its attachment to α_2-adrenergic receptors and the resulting inhibition of nociception.[2]

TYPES OF ACUTE PAIN

Although all pain uses primarily the same nociception, pain experts describe the type of pain by differentiating the location of the fibers that are sensitized. The fibers are most commonly grouped as cutaneous, somatic, visceral, and deafferentation.

Cutaneous Pain

Cutaneous, or superficial pain, begins with injury at the skin, such as an incision or insertion of a needle. This trauma to the tissue activates the nociceptors on the skin. The mediators histamine, bradykinin, potassium, or hydrogen ions are released into the extracellular fluid around the wound. The cell wall injury causes the release of serotonin from platelets, prostaglandins, and substance P. All of the active mediators will sensitize and activate the cutaneous fibers to transmit the noxious stimuli to the central nervous system.[1,2] The cutaneous Aδ fibers are now sensitive to noxious stimuli that would not ordinarily be interpreted as painful, such as touch, pressure, or stretch. Normally, the patient is able to discretely locate this type of pain.

Somatic Pain

Somatic pain originates in the subcutaneous tissue, the joints, tendons, muscles, and fascia. It is also associated

They are also released in response to stress, fear, restraint, hypertension, and hypoglycemia. Endorphin release is well-documented during labor and delivery and exercise.[10] Endorphin release during stress accounts for a person's ability to perform normally or supranormally with an apparent unawareness of pain after an injury. This response is referred to as *stress analgesia.*

The enkephalins are located primarily in the limbic system and the hypothalamus as well as the midbrain. The endings of many of the nerves in these areas secrete enkephalins. In an associated response, fibers originating in the same area but with their endings in the dorsal horn secrete serotonin. The serotonin, in turn, acts on yet another set of neurons to incite the release of additional enkephalins.[10] The enkephalins block the presynaptic transmission of both Aδ and C fibers.[10] This inhibition can last from minutes to hours, providing analgesia for that period.

The dynorphins are found in minute quantities in the nervous system, primarily in the midbrain and the spinal cord. They are extremely powerful opiates; they appear to have as much as 200 times the pain-killing effect of morphine.

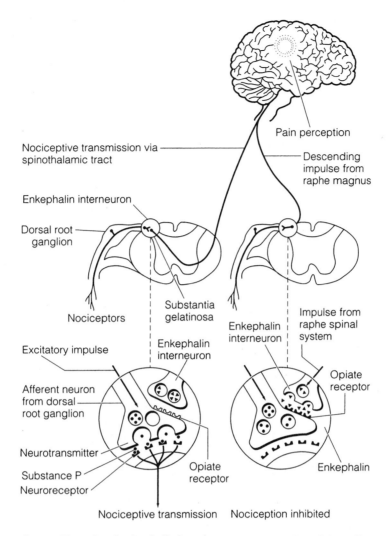

Fig. **8-4** The role of enkephalin in pain management. (From Salerno E, Willens J: *Pain management: an interdisciplinary approach,* St Louis, 1996, Mosby).

with muscle ischemia and spasm.[2] Bradykinin and histamine release are associated with somatic pain. C fibers are responsible for the transmission of this type of pain. Somatic pain is difficult for the patient to locate. It can be either dull, aching, or diffuse.[1,2,8] In addition, deep somatic pain is associated with an autonomic nervous system response that may cause nausea, vomiting, and cold, clammy skin.

Visceral Pain

In general, the viscera has only sensory receptors for pain. The unique characteristic of visceral pain is that highly localized stimulation of pain receptors in the viscera can cause minimal discomfort. However, diffuse stimulation of multiple receptors can cause extreme pain.[10] Visceral pain results from compression, distention, or stretching of the viscera in the thoracic or abdominal cavity. The pain of myocardial ischemia or infarction is considered visceral. Visceral pain is described

as pressure, deep, and squeezing. It is sometimes difficult to localize and is associated with referred pain. The visceral pain fibers are unique in that they travel to the spinal cord with the fibers of the sympathetic nervous system. This may account for the intense sympathetic nervous system response often seen with this type of pain.[2]

Deafferentation Pain

Deafferentation pain is seen most commonly in the cancer patient. The mechanism of this pain is an injury to either a central or peripheral nerve component from either the disease or its treatment. The injury is normally a consequence of tumor invasion, thermal damage from radiation, or chemical injuries from radiation.[1] This is also considered to be the type of pain stemming from a number of chronic pain syndromes. In this regard the origin of the pain may be peripheral or central. Neuralgia and phantom pain are peripheral deafferentation pains, in which

thalamic lesions related to cerebrovascular accidents (CVAs) cause central deafferentation pain.[11]

PAIN ASSESSMENT

Adequate assessment of pain in the critically ill patient is made more difficult by the complexity of the critical care experience. For instance, there may be the complicating factor of altered communication, or the patient may be unconscious and unable to communicate pain. Pain assessment in the critically ill population has three major components: assessment technique, patient barriers to assessment, and nurse and/or physician barriers to complete or accurate assessment. The complexity of assessment requires the use of multiple strategies by critical care practitioners.

Multidimensional Assessment

Because pain is a multidimensional phenomenon, it requires a multidimensional assessment. Complete assessment involves the collection of subjective and objective data about the patient's physiologic, cognitive, and emotional response to the pain.[12] Because of the life/death immediacy of most actions in the critical care environment, assessment is normally one-dimensional.[13] The evaluation of pain includes type, location, intensity, aggravating factors, and alleviating factors. The most important consideration in assessment is that pain is an entirely subjective experience. Pain is whatever the patient says it is and however the patient describes it.[3,14] In the assessment of pain type, the verbal patient can give de-

scriptive terms. The patient may describe the pain as dull, aching, or sharp and stabbing. This provides the nurse with data regarding the type of pain the patient is experiencing (i.e., visceral or cutaneous). The differentiation between types of pain may contribute to the determination of cause and management. A patient who has had defibrillation and cardiopulmonary resuscitation (CPR) after a heart attack may complain of chest pain that is prickling or stinging. This information would lead the nurse to investigate for cutaneous injuries, such as defibrillation burns. The same patient may describe a dull, aching pain with radiation that might lead the nurse to consider a visceral anginal pain from myocardial ischemia. Furthermore, a verbal description of pain is important because it provides a baseline description, allowing the critical care nurse to monitor changes in the type of pain, which could indicate a change in the underlying pathology.

Pain Assessment Tools

Intensity or severity of pain is a measurement that has undergone a great deal of recent investigation. Studies have shown that the consistent use of a visual tool aids both the patient and the practitioner in correctly identifying the intensity of the patient's pain.[3,7,14,15] Multiple visual analog scales are available (Fig. 8-5). Many critical care units have identified a specific tool to be used. The use of a single tool provides consistency of assessment and documentation. The employment of a pain grading scale is also useful in the critical care environment.[13] Asking the patient to grade his or her pain on a scale of 1 to

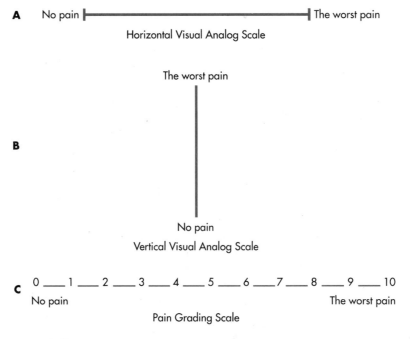

Fig. **8-5** Visual analog scales. **A,** Horizontal Visual Analog Scale; **B,** Vertical Visual Analog Scale; **C,** Pain Grading Scale.

10 is a consistent method and aids the nurse in objectifying the subjective nature of the patient's pain. The pain grading scale is also useful in establishing a baseline for comparison of future episodes of pain. A unique part of the assessment of pain is the need to have the patient identify exactly what amount or level of pain allows functionality and is acceptable to the patient. This level of acceptable pain is the target for subsequent pain management techniques.[3,14]

Pain Location

The next area of evaluation is the location of the patient's pain. Location is normally easy for the patient to identify, although visceral pain is more difficult for the patient to localize.[1,2] If the patient has difficulty naming the location, ask that he or she point to the location on himself or herself or on a simple anatomic drawing. This technique is also helpful in identifying multisites of pain.[16]

Asking the patient to identify factors that moderate pain is an important evaluation component for the critical care nurse. Position or movement as a component of pain may contribute significantly to the final evaluation of the pain occurrence; the example of deep breathing intensifying the chest pain because of pericarditis is an illustration of this. Moderating factors that reduce the pain or discomfort are also important findings. The moderation of pain continues after the patient leaves the critical care environment. A knowledge of any alleviation activities contributes to the patient's plan of care throughout the continuum of care.

The subjective data of intensity, type, location, and moderating factors form a single component of pain assessment. The critical care nurse also completes a physiologic assessment on any patient who reports pain. It is important to note that lack of a physiologic response to pain does not mean that the patient is reporting pain that does not exist.[3,7,9,16] A number of things may explain the lack of a physiologic response. Many of the therapies employed in the critical care area are designed to block the sympathetic nervous system response to stress, successfully blocking the same response to pain. If there is a response to pain, the nurse assesses for the following findings: tachycardia, hypertension, tachypnea, increased muscle tone in the area of pain, sweating, pallor, and hypervigilence. Any of the body's responses to sympathetic nervous system stimulation might be expected. Complicating this finding in the critical care patient is the possibility that the original illness or injury is the cause of the sympathetic response.[2,7]

Some critical care patients respond to pain or painful stimuli by simply withdrawing from the painful stimuli. This patient is able to perceive the pain, but the higher somatosensory cortical contribution of interpretation of the pain is absent. There are also patients who do not respond at all to painful stimuli. These patients lack integrity in the nociceptive system and are unable to perceive the pain. These phenomena are usually associated with pathologies in the brain or spinal cord that interrupt the system.

Behavioral Assessment

Certain behaviors may be manifested in the patient with pain. It is important to remember that not all patients have an observable behavioral response. Diligent observation of the patient experiencing pain may uncover behavioral cues (Table 8-3). These behaviors may indicate pain, or they may indicate an attempt to control pain with types of distraction.[9,13,16]

Patient Barriers to Pain Assessment
Communication

The most obvious patient barrier to the assessment of pain in the critical care population is an alteration in the ability to communicate. The patient who is intubated is unable to verbalize a description of the pain. If the patient is able to communicate in any way, then he or she may report the pain in that manner. If the patient is able to write a description, he or she may be able to thoroughly describe the pain in writing. It is the nonverbal patients whom the nurse relies on most intensely for nonverbal clues or behaviors to assess the presence and intensity of pain. Because the nurse cannot be assured of predictable pain behaviors, other sources of assessment need to be addressed. The patient's family can contribute significantly in the assessment of behavioral clues to pain. The

TABLE 8-3
BEHAVIORS ASSOCIATED WITH PAIN

Type	Examples
Expression	Grimacing, frowning, eyes squeezed close, withdrawn expression, staring, crying, teeth clenched, wrinkled brow
Noises	Groaning, moaning, sighing, sobbing, grunting
Speech	Cussing, shouting, praying, calling for help, chanting
Body movements	Rocking, thrashing, tossing/turning
Behaviors	Guarding, protective posturing, massaging or applying pressure, reading, watching TV, wandering

Modified from Salerno E, Willens J: *Pain management handbook,* St Louis, 1996, Mosby.

family is intimately familiar with the patient's normal responses to pain and can assist the nurse in identifying such clues. If there is absolutely no observable evidence to support a diagnosis of pain, the practitioner needs to use the concept that if the trauma, disease, injury, or procedure is a painful one for most patients, it is painful for this patient.[3]

Altered level of consciousness

The presence of delirium, dementia, or altered mentation related to psychoactive therapies or disease states presents a unique pain assessment barrier. It has been erroneously thought that the confused patient is unable to perceive pain. Research now supports that the patient with altered cognitive abilities is able to accurately report pain when questioned or upon the actual painful event. The limitation for this population is in pain recall and the ability to integrate the pain experience over time.[14] The critical care nurse needs to assess for pain frequently in cognitively impaired patients and not anticipate that these patients will initiate a pain discussion.

The patient in a coma presents a dilemma for the critical care nurse. Because pain relies on cortical response to provide recognition, there is the belief that the patient without higher cortical functioning has no perception of pain.[1,17] Conversely, the inability to interpret the nociceptive transmission does not negate the transmission. The critical care nurse can initiate a discussion with the other members of the health care team to formulate a plan of care for the coma patient's comfort.

Cultural influences

Another barrier to accurate pain assessment is the cultural influences on pain and pain reporting.[12,15,17,18] The cultural influences may be compounded by the patient who speaks another language than that of the health team members. Although this chapter does not address specific cultural groups and their typical responses to pain, a few generalizations can be made. The first consideration in assessing a patient from a different cultural group is to avoid the assumption that the patient will have a specific response to pain or exhibit a particular behavior because of culture. Patients are uniquely individual in their response to pain, and the health care practitioner might unjustly assign or expect behaviors that a patient will not exhibit. A second consideration that is commonly overlooked is the role of pain in the life of the patient. The nurse must communicate with the patient or the family to ascertain this role. Some cultures believe that God's test or punishment takes the form of pain. Persons of such cultures would not necessarily believe that the pain should be relieved. Other cultures perceive pain as being associated with an imbalance in life, hot and cold, for instance. Persons of these cultures believe they need to manipulate the environment to restore balance to accomplish pain control.[18] The complexities and intricacies of cultural beliefs require much greater discussion. Many critical care units have established references or re-

sources for dealing with cultural diversity in the critically ill patient. It is important for the nurse to support, whenever possible, the special beliefs and needs of the patient and his or her family to provide the most therapeutic environment for healing to occur.

Knowledge deficit

A relatively overlooked patient barrier to accurate pain assessment is the public knowledge deficit regarding pain and pain management. Many patients and their families are scared by the risk of addiction to pain medication. They fear that addiction will occur if the patient is medicated frequently or with sufficient amounts of opiates necessary to relieve the pain. This belief is compounded by programs such as the "Just Say No to Drugs" campaign that increase the public's concern regarding drugs.[19] The concern is powerful enough for some that they will deny or deliberately underreport the frequency or intensity of pain. Another inaccurate belief on the part of some patients is the expectation that unrelieved pain is part of a critical illness or procedure.[20] As part of the patient plan for pain management, the critical care nurse must teach both the family and patient the importance of pain control and the use of opioids in treating the critically ill patient.

Health Professional Barriers to Pain Assessment

The health professional's beliefs and attitudes about pain and pain management are commonly a barrier to accurate and adequate assessment of pain that can lead to poor management practices.[3,6,7,9,14] It is well-documented that the study of pain assessment and management is lacking in most schools of nursing.[7,20] Multiple studies have documented nurses' misconceptions or lack of knowledge regarding addiction, physiologic dependence, drug tolerance, and respiratory depression. The most problematic misconception on the part of nurses is the belief that the patient must have a physiologic and behavioral response to pain that matches the nurses' picture of what a patient in pain looks like (i.e., the patient must have a marked change in vital signs and be moaning, writhing, and crying to truly be in pain). This misbelief hampers appropriate management of the patient's pain. The critical care nurse must remember that pain is what the patient states it is and that no additional finding is necessary to treat the patient's pain.[3] When a patient is denied pain management based on the misconception that there is a certain behavior that always accompanies pain, an ethical conflict arises.[20,21]

Nursing concerns with addiction can contribute to misinterpretation of signs during the pain assessment process. Addiction rates for patients in acute pain who receive opioid analgesics are less than 1%.[3,22] Some of the misbeliefs that surround addiction result from lack of knowledge about the terms *addiction* and *tolerance*. Addiction is defined "as a pattern of compulsive drug use that is characterized by an incessant longing for a drug and the need to use the drug for effects other than pain control." Tolerance is defined as a decreasing duration of opioid action.[3,23-25] Physical dependence and tolerance to opioids may develop if the drugs are given over a long period. If this is an anticipated problem, withdrawal may be avoided by simply weaning the patient from the opioid slowly to allow the brain to reestablish neurochemical balance in the absence of the opioid.[2] Tolerance to an opioid is a rare phenomenon in the critical care patient.

Another concern on the behalf of the health care professional is the fear that aggressive management of pain with opiates will cause critical respiratory depression.[10,14,26,27] Opioids can cause respiratory depression, but in the critically ill this is a rare phenomenon. Like addiction, the incidence is less than 1%.[22]

PAIN MANAGEMENT

The management of pain in the critically ill patient is as multidimensional as the assessment and is a multidisciplinary task. The control of pain can be pharmacologic, nonpharmacologic, or a combination of both. The most commonly used course for pain control in critical care is in the pharmacologic domain.

Pharmacologic Methods

The pharmacologic management of pain has infinite variety in the critical care unit. Although this is not an indepth discussion of pharmacology, some commonly administered agents are discussed. Pain pharmacology is divided into four categories of action:

- Opioid agonists (morphine, hydromorphone, fentanyl, and meperidine)
- Partial agonists and agonist-antagonists (buprenorphine, pentazocine)
- Nonopioids (acetaminophen, nonsteroidal antiinflammatory drugs [NSAIDs])
- Adjuvants (anticonvulsants, antidepressants).

How the pain is approached and managed is a progression or combination of the available agents, the type of pain, and the patient response to the therapy. See Table 8-4 for more information on pharmacologic management of pain.[28-31]

Delivery Methods

The most common route for drug administration is the intravenous route, via continuous infusion, bolus administration, or patient-controlled analgesia (PCA). Traditionally, the choice has been IV bolus administration. The benefits of this method are rapid onset of action and ease of titration. The major disadvantage is the rise and fall of the serum level of the opioid, leading to periods of pain control with periods of breakthrough pain.[32]

Continuous infusion of the opioids via an infusion pump provides constant blood levels of the ordered opioid; this promotes a consistent level of comfort. It is a particularly helpful method of administration during sleep because the patient awakens with an adequate level of pain relief.[33] It is important that the patient be given the loading dose that relieves the pain and raises the circulating dose of the drug. After the basal rate is established, the patient maintains a steady state of pain control, unless there is additional pain from a procedure, an activity, or a change in the patient's condition. Orders for additional boluses of opioid need to be available.

Patient-controlled analgesia

Patient-controlled analgesia is a method of delivery, via an infusion pump, that allows the patient to self-administer small doses of analgesics. This method of medication delivery allows the patient to control the level of pain and sedation and to avoid the peaks and valleys of intermittent dosing by the health care professional. The patient can self-administer a bolus of medication the moment the pain begins, thus acting preemptively.

Although a variety of routes can be used with PCA, it is traditionally administered via an IV route.[34] Certain patients are not candidates for PCA. Alterations in the level of consciousness or mentation preclude understanding the use of the equipment. The very elderly or patients with renal or hepatic insufficiency may require careful screening for PCA.

Allowing the patient to self-administer opioid doses does not diminish the role of the critical care nurse in pain management. The nurse advises for necessary changes to the prescription and continues to monitor the effects of the medication and doses. The patient is closely monitored during the first 2 hours of therapy and after every change in the prescription. If the patient's pain does not respond within the first 2 hours of therapy, a total reassessment of the pain state is essential. The nurse monitors the number of boluses the patient delivers. If he or she is bolusing more often than the prescription, the dose may be insufficient to maintain pain control. Naloxone must be readily available to reverse adverse opiate respiratory effects. Ideally, the patient undergoing an elective procedure requiring opioid analgesia postoperatively is instructed in the use of PCA during preoperative teaching. This allows the patient to become comfortable with the concept of self-medication before use.

Intraspinal pain control

Intraspinal anesthesia uses the concept that the spinal cord is the primary link in nociceptive transmission. The goal is to mimic the body's endogenous opioid pain modification system by interfering with the transmission of pain by providing an opiate receptor binding agent directly into the spinal cord. The benefits of the intraspinal route include good-to-excellent pain control with typically lower doses of opioids, increased patient mobility, minimal sedation, and, typically, increased patient satisfaction.[34] There is also very little change in the hemodynamic status of the patient. Intraspinal anesthesia is par-

TABLE 8-4

SELECTED PHARMACOLOGIC AGENTS USED FOR PAIN MANAGEMENT

Drug	Dosage	Action	Special Considerations
Amitriptyline (Elavil)	PO 10 mg/day	Blocks reuptake of serotonins	Can be sedating
Bupivacaine (Marcaine)	Epidural 1-5 mg/hr	Local hydrophilic anesthetic; blocks C and Aδ fiber transmission	May be given alone or in combination with an opioid; monitor carefully for hypotension, respiratory depression
Butorphanol (Stadol)	1-2 mg q 3-4 hr IM or slow IV	Agonist-antagonist	Psychometric effects, anxiety, hallucinations, nightmares
Capsaicin	Topical 3-4 times/day	Causes release and depletion of substance P	Effective for peripheral neuropathies, neuralgias
Codeine	15-30 mg q 4 hr	Weak μ agonist	Effective for minor pain; constipating
Diazepam (Valium)	IV 2-5 mg PO 2.5-10 mg	Adjuvant agent for pain; antilytic	Must not be given directly with an opioid, which can increase side effects, sedation
Fentanyl	IV 0.1 mg Epidural 25-250 μg or 10-25 μg/hr	Moderate-dose analgesia High-dose anesthesia opioid agonist	80 times as potent as morphine Transdermal onset 72 hr
Hydromorphone (Dilaudid)	PO 2 mg q 4 hr IM 1.5 mg	μ agonist	Shorter duration of action than morphine
Ibuprofen (Advil, Motrin)	200-600 mg q 6 hr	NSAID	GI upset, prolonged bleeding time
Ketorolac (Toradol)	15-30 mg IM qid	Parenteral NSAID; prevents production of prostaglandins	Platelet aggregation interrupted; inhibits maintenance of gastric mucosa
Meperidine (Demerol)	IM 75-150 mg q 4 hr	μ agonist	Short half-life, very neurotoxic, limited use advised
Methadone (Dolophine)	PO 20 mg q 4 hr IV 5-10 mg	μ agonist	Very efficient orally; accumulates with multiple dosing, causing serious sedation (2-5 days)
Oxycodone (Percocet with Tylenol; Percodan with aspirin)	PO 2 tabs (10 mg total) q 4 hr	Moderately strong μ agonist	Combination with aspirin and Tylenol to block both peripheral and central pathways
Pentazocine (Talwin)	PO 50-100 mg q 3-4 hr SQ/IM 30-60 mg q 3-4 hr IV 30 mg	Mixed agonist-antagonist, blocks μ and activates κ receptors, considered a weak agent	Has ceiling effect, increases cardiac workload
Propoxyphene (Darvocet-N)	PO 1-2 tabs q 4 hr	Weak μ agonist	CNS toxic metabolite, not for long-term use, for minor pain
Morphine	IV 2-15 mg/hr bolus IV 1-10 mg/hr continuous infusion IM 5-15 mg q 3-4 hr SQ 5-15 mg q 3-4 hr Epidural 1-5 mg/hr bolus Epidural 0.5-2.0 mg/hr continuous infusion PO 8-20 mg q 4 hr	Analgesia, antianxiety, opioid agonist	Respiratory depression, hypotension, nausea, vomiting, sedation, pruritus; titrate to effect

ticularly appropriate for pain in the thorax, the upper abdomen, and the lower extremities. There are two intraspinal routes: intrathecal and epidural. Regardless of the route, the effects of the opioid agonist used will be the same so assessment parameters will mimic those used for other routes.

Intrathecal analgesia

Intrathecal (subarachnoid) opioids are placed directly into the cerebral spinal fluid and attach to spinal cord re-

ceptor sites. Opioids introduced at this site act quickly at the dorsal horn. However, the dural sheath is punctured, eliminating any barrier for pathogens between the environment and the cerebral spinal fluid. This creates the risk for serious infections. The intrathecal route is usually reserved for intraoperative use. Single-bolus dosing provides short-term relief for pain that is short lived (e.g., the pain of labor and delivery is well managed using this regimen).[33] Side effects of intrathecal pain control include postdural puncture headache and infection.

TABLE 8-5

EQUIANALGESIA CHART

This chart is designed to assist the practitioner in identifying approximate doses of medication that will provide similar pain relief. All dosing of drugs should be based on the patient's response to the medication. This chart is based on the recommendations of the American Pain Society. *Single IV doses are equivalent to ½ the IM dose.* All IM and PO doses in this chart are considered equivalent to 10 mg of morphine in clinical effect

Analgesic	IM Route (mg)	PO Route (mg)	Comments
Morphine	10	30-60	PO 3-6 × IM dose; morphine is the gold standard to which the effect of other opiates is compared
Fentanyl	1.0		
Meperidine (Demerol)	75	300	PO 4 × IM dose; neurotoxic metabolite; use with extreme caution
Hydromorphone (Dilaudid)	1.5	7.5	PO 5 × IM dose; shorter duration than MS
Oxycodone		15-30	Effect may last up to 6 hr
Codeine	130	200	PO 1.3-1.5 × IM dose; very constipating; high doses may cause nausea and vomiting
Nalbuphine (Nubain)	10		May precipitate withdrawal in opiate-dependent patients
Butorphanol (Stadol)	2		Same as above

From Jacox A, et al: *Acute pain management: operative or medical procedures and trauma. Clinical practice guidelines,* Publication 92-0032, Rockville, Md, 1992, Agency for Health Care Policy and Research, US Department of Health and Human Services.
×, Times.

Epidural analgesia

Epidural analgesia is commonly used in the critical care unit after major abdominal surgery, nephrectomy, thoracotomy, and major orthopedic procedures.[22] Certain conditions preclude the use of this pain control method: systemic infection, anticoagulation, and increased intracranial pressure. Epidural delivery of opiates provides longer-lasting pain relief with less dosing of opiates. When delivered into the epidural space, 5 mg of morphine may be effective for 6 to 24 hours, compared with 3 to 4 hours when delivered intravenously. Opioids infused in the epidural space are more unpredictable than those administered intrathecally. The epidural space is filled with fatty tissue and is external to the dura mater. The fatty tissue interferes with uptake and the dura acts as a barrier to diffusion, making the diffusion rate difficult to predict. The rapidity of the diffusion of the drug is determined by the type of drug used. The drugs are either hydrophilic or lipophilic. Hydrophilic drugs are water-soluble and penetrate the dura slowly, giving them a longer onset and duration of action. Morphine is hydrophilic. Lipophilic drugs are lipid-soluble; they penetrate the dura rapidly and therefore have a rapid onset and a shorter duration of action.[22] Fentanyl is lipophilic. The dura itself acts as a physical barrier and causes delay in diffusion, which in comparison to the intrathecal route allows more drug to be absorbed in the systemic circulation, requiring greater doses for pain relief.[34] Drugs delivered epidurally may be bolused or continuously infused. Epidural analgesia is experiencing increased usage in the critical care environment and requires careful monitoring. The nurse must assess the patient for respiratory depression using the unit protocol. This phenomenon may occur early in the therapy or as late as 24 hours after initiation. The epidural catheter also puts the patient at risk for infection.

Equianalgesia

At some point in the patient's recovery, strong opioids are replaced by more moderate agents. In doing any conversion, the goal is to provide equal analgesic effects with the new agents. This concept is referred to as *equianalgesia.* The critical care nurse is the practitioner most likely to convert the patient from parenteral medication to oral medication in preparation for a change in the level of care or in preparation for discharge. Studies have identified that nurses lack knowledge regarding equal doses between IV and oral administration. There is the misconception that when a patient is able to take oral medication the pain is less severe. The change to oral medications does not indicate a need for less medication. The nurse needs to practice equianalgesia when converting the patient. Because of the variety of agents and routes, the professional pain organizations have developed equianalgesia charts for use by the health care professional. All critical care units need to have a chart posted for easy referral. Table 8-5 is an equianalgesia chart used in clinical practice.[35]

Non-Pharmacologic Methods

There are numerous methods of pain management other than drugs that appear in the critical care literature.[23] In most instances, these therapies augment and enhance the pharmacologic management of the patient's pain. Stimulating other non-pain sensory fibers present in the periphery modifies pain transmission. These fibers are stimulated by thermal changes, as occurs in the application of heat or cold, simple massage, or action of the transcutaneous electrical nerve stimulator (TENS). The use of massage has been a mainstay in the nursing management of the patient in pain. It is an appropriate pain management technique for most critically ill patients.

The use of TENS has contraindications in the critical care unit. Because the device is controlled by the patient, mentation must be intact. TENS is also contraindicated in patients with pacemakers or automatic implantable defibrillators because these devices may recognize and erroneously interpret the TENS electrical signal. TENS therapy is efficient, patient-controlled pain management for orthopedic, obstetric, and some postoperative pain states.

Using the cortical interpretation of pain as the foundation, there are a number of interventions known to reduce the patient's pain report. These modalities include cognitive techniques: patient teaching, relaxation, distraction, guided imagery, music therapy, and hypnosis.[23,36]

Relaxation is a well-documented method for reducing the distress associated with pain.[37] While not a substitute for pharmacology, relaxation is an excellent adjunct to control pain. Relaxation decreases oxygen consumption and muscle tone and can decrease heart rate and blood pressure. Relaxation gives the patient a sense of control over the pain and reduces muscle tension and anxiety. Not all patients are interested in relaxation therapy. For such patients, deep-breathing exercises may be helpful and frequently lead to relaxation. Excellent references for thorough techniques in relaxation therapy are available.[3]

Guided imagery is a technique that uses the imagination to provide control over pain. It can be used to distract or relax. Guiding a patient to a place that is pain-free and relaxing takes a considerable time commitment on the part of the nurse. Although this may be difficult in the critical care environment, guiding a patient to a place in his or her imagination that is free from pain can be done rapidly and may be very beneficial.[23]

Music therapy is a commonly used intervention for relaxation. Music that is pleasing to the patient may have very soothing effects.[38] Ideally, the music should be supplied by a small set of very light headphones. This method also serves to minimize the distracting and anxiety-producing noises of a critical care unit.[39] It is important to educate the patient and family regarding the role of music in relaxation and pain control and also to provide music of the patient's choice.

The patient and family may provide information about other sources of distraction for the patient. Determining what distraction therapies the patient normally uses may provide a clue to which might work during the illness. Some persons are distracted by television; however, for others, television is a source of increased anxiety. Do not assume that the patient does or does not want to watch television until you determine whether it will be beneficial or harmful to the patient.

The key to success with any of these therapies is to understand their mechanism of action so that the therapy matches the needs of the patient. All of the previously mentioned interventions require the patient's cooperation. There must be some commitment on the part of the patient to the treatment. When handled efficiently, non-pharmacologic tools can assist in pain management.

Today's health care environment mandates that patients experience positive outcomes as rapidly as possible. Because pain is a major barrier to early mobility and rapid return to a pre-illness state, pain management is of paramount importance to the critical care nurse. The critically ill patient is the most difficult to assess and manage; therefore, it is imperative that the critical care nurse develop the skill and intervention techniques necessary to manage the most difficult of the pain states. **As patient advocate, the nurse assumes the responsibility for establishing pain control as a priority for the health care team.**[40]

References

1. Caillet R: *Pain: mechanisms and management,* Philadelphia, 1993, FA Davis.
2. Puntillo K: Physiology of pain and its consequences in critically ill patients. In Puntillo K, editor: *Pain in the critically ill: assessment and management,* Gaithersburg, Md, 1991, Aspen.
3. McCaffery M, Beebe A: *Pain: clinical manual for nursing practice,* St Louis, 1989, Mosby.
4. Carson M, Barton D, Morrison C: Managing pain during mediastinal chest tube removal, *Heart Lung* 23(6):500, 1994.
5. Simpson T, Lee E, Cameron C: Patients' perceptions of environmental factors that disturb sleep after cardiac surgery, *Am J Crit Care* 5:173, 1996.
6. Sun X, Weissman C: The use of analgesics and sedatives in the critically ill patient: physicians order versus medication administered, *Heart Lung* 23:169, 1994.
7. Alpen M, Titler M: Pain management in the critically ill: what do we know and how can we improve? *AACN Clin Issues Crit Care Nurs* 5:159, 1994.
8. Maxam-Moore V, Wilkie D, Woods S: Analgesics for cardiac surgery patients in critical care: describing current practice, *Am J Crit Care* 3:31, 1994.
9. Willens J: Introduction to pain management. In Salerno E, Willens J, editors: *Pain management handbook: an interdisciplinary approach,* St Louis, 1996, Mosby.
10. Guyton A: *Textbook of medical physiology,* ed 8, Philadelphia, 1991, WB Saunders.
11. Barker E: *Neuroscience nursing,* St Louis, 1994, Mosby.
12. Jurf J, Nirschl A: Acute postoperative pain review and update, *Crit Care Nurs Q* 16:8, 1993.
13. McGuire D: Comprehensive and multidimensional assessment and measurement of pain, *J Pain Symptom Manage* 7:312, 1992.
14. Jacox A, et al: *Acute pain management: operative or medical procedures and trauma. Clinical practice guidelines,* Publication 92-0032, Rockville, Md, 1992, Agency for Health Care Policy and Research, US Department of Health and Human Services.
15. Villaire M: An interview with Kathleen Puntillo. Pain: assessment, treatment and the coming thunder, *Crit Care Nurs* 15:159, 1995.
16. Voight L, Paice J, Pouilot J: Standardized pain flowsheet: impact on patient reported experiences after cardiovascular surgery, *Am J Crit Care* 4:308, 1995.

17. Halloran T, Pohlman A: Managing sedation in the critically ill patient, *Crit Care Nurs* suppl 1, 1995.

18. Bozeman M: Cultural aspects of pain management. In Salerno E, Willens J, editors: *Pain management handbook: an interdisciplinary approach,* St Louis, 1996, Mosby.

19. Douglas M: Cultural diversity in response to pain. In Puntillo K, editor: *Pain in the critically ill: assessment and management,* Gaithersburg, Md, 1991, Aspen.

20. Ulmer J: Identifying and preventing pain mismanagement. In Salerno E, Willens J, editors: *Pain management handbook: an interdisciplinary approach,* St Louis, 1996, Mosby.

21. Faucett J: Care of the critically ill patient. In Puntillo K, editor: *Pain in the critically ill: assessment and management,* Gaithersburg, Md, 1991, Aspen.

22. Puntillo K: Dimensions of procedural pain and its analgesic management in critically ill surgical patients, *Am J Crit Care* 3:116, 1994.

23. Gujol M: A survey of pain assessment and management practices among critical care nurses, *Am J Crit Care* 3:123, 1994.

24. Henknleman W: Inadequate pain management: ethical considerations, *Nurs Manage* 25(1):48a, 1994.

25. Salerno E: Pharmacologic approaches to pain. In Salerno E, Willens J, editors: *Pain management handbook: an interdisciplinary approach,* St Louis, 1996, Mosby.

26. Watt-Watson J: Misbeliefs about pain. In Watt-Watson J, Donovan M, editors: *Pain management: nursing perspective,* St Louis, 1992, Mosby.

27. Spross J, Singer M: Patients with cancer. In Watt-Watson J, Donovan M, editors: *Pain management: nursing perspective,* St Louis, 1992, Mosby.

28. Paice J: Pharmacologic management. In Watt-Watson J, Donovan M, editors: *Pain management: nursing perspective,* St Louis, 1992, Mosby.

29. Wild L: Intravenous methods of analgesia for pain in the critically ill. In Puntillo K, editor: *Pain in the critically ill: assessment and management,* Gaithersburg, Md, 1991, Aspen.

30. Mather I, Denson D: Pharmacokinetics of systemic opioids for the management of pain. In Sinatra R, et al, editors: *Acute pain: mechanisms and management,* St Louis, 1992, Mosby.

31. American Society of Hospital Pharmacists: *American hospital formulary service drug information '98,* Bethesda, Md, 1998, The Association.

32. McKenry L, Salerno E, editors: *Mosby's pharmacology in nursing,* ed 19, St Louis, 1995, Mosby.

33. Collins P, Spunt A, Huml M: Symptom management. In Salerno E, Willens J, editors: *Pain management handbook: an interdisciplinary approach,* St Louis, 1996, Mosby.

34. Dyble K: Epidural and intrathecal methods of analgesia in the critically ill. In Puntillo K, editor: *Pain in the critically ill: assessment and management,* Gaithersburg, Md, 1991, Aspen.

35. Kaiser K: Assessment and management of pain in the critically ill trauma patient, *Crit Care Nurs Q* 15(2):14, 1992.

36. McCaffery M, Ferrell B: Opioid analgesics: nurses' knowledge of doses and psychological dependence, *J Nurs Staff Dev* 8:72, 1994.

37. Herr K, Mobily P: Interventions related to pain, *Nurs Clin North Am* 27(2):347, 1992.

38. Courts N: Non-pharmacologic approaches to pain. In Salerno E, Willens J, editors: *Pain management handbook: an interdisciplinary approach,* St Louis, 1996, Mosby.

39. Edgar L, Smith-Hanrahan C: Non-pharmacologic pain management. In Watt-Watson J, Donovan M, editors: *Pain management: nursing perspective,* St Louis, 1992, Mosby.

40. Meehan D, et al: Analgesic administration, pain intensity, and patient satisfaction in cardiac surgical patients, *Am J Crit Care* 4:435, 1995.

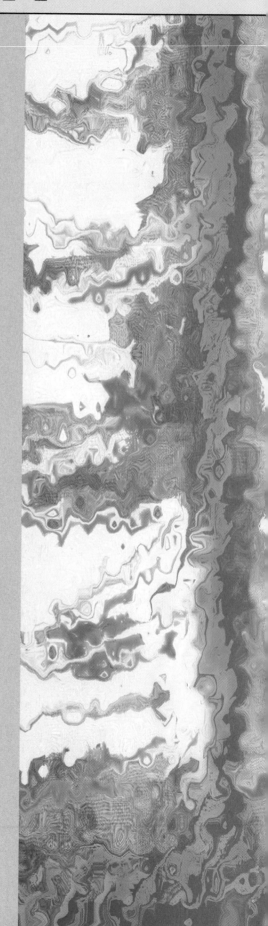

CARDIOVASCULAR ALTERATIONS

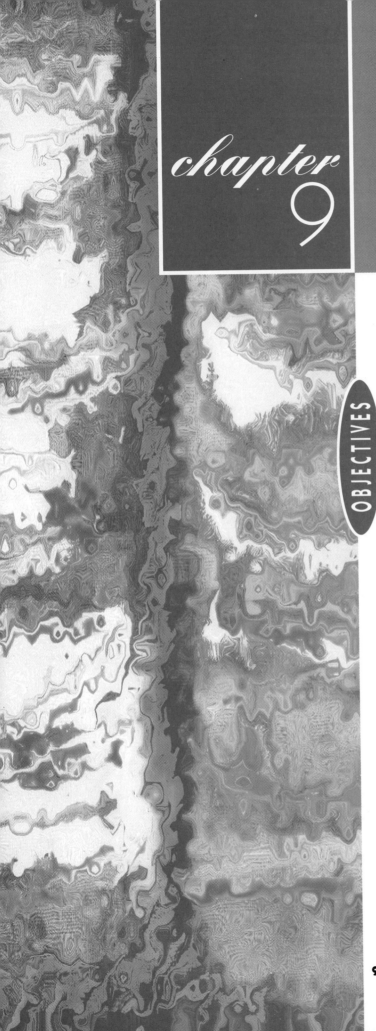

chapter 9

Cardiovascular Assessment and Diagnostic Procedures

Jennifer Bloomquist
and Martha M. Love

OBJECTIVES

- Identify the components of a cardiovascular history.

- Describe inspection, palpation, percussion, and auscultation of the patient with cardiovascular dysfunction.

- Delineate the clinical significance of selected laboratory tests used in the assessment of cardiovascular disorders.

- Describe key diagnostic procedures used in assessment of the patient with cardiovascular dysfunction.

- Discuss the nursing management of a patient undergoing a cardiovascular diagnostic procedure.

- Illustrate the proper placement of the electrodes for monitoring MCL_1 or V_1, MCL_6 or V_6, and Lead II.

- Outline the steps in analyzing an electrocardiographic rhythm strip.

- Explain the electrocardiographic findings and nursing actions for a variety of atrial, ventricular, and junctional dysrhythmias.

- Delineate the use of intraarterial and pulmonary artery catheters for bedside monitoring.

Assessment of the patient with cardiovascular dysfunction is a systematic process that incorporates both a history and a physical examination. The purpose of the assessment is twofold: (1) to recognize changes in the patient's cardiovascular status that would necessitate nursing or medical intervention and (2) to determine the ways in which the patient's cardiovascular dysfunction is interfering with self-care activities.[1] To complete the assessment, the patient's laboratory studies and diagnostic tests must be reviewed. This chapter focuses on priority clinical assessments, laboratory studies, and diagnostic tests for the critically ill patient with cardiac dysfunction.

HISTORY

The patient history is important for providing data that contribute to the cardiovascular diagnosis and treatment plan. The patient's presenting symptoms or complaints direct the history-taking part of the assessment. For a patient in acute distress, the history is curtailed to just a few questions about the patient's chief complaint, precipitating events, and current medications. For a patient in no obvious distress, the history focuses on four different areas: (1) review of the patient's present illness, (2) overview of the patient's general cardiovascular status including previous cardiac diagnostic studies or interventional procedures, (3) examination of the patient's general health status including family history of coronary artery disease, hypertension, diabetes, and stroke, and (4) survey of the patient's lifestyle including risk factors for coronary artery disease.[2]

A thorough description of the patient's current symptoms is also obtained. Symptoms that are common in the cardiovascular patient include dyspnea, chest pain, palpitations, cough, fatigue, edema, leg pain or cramps, nocturia, syncope, and cyanosis. Information is elicited regarding the location, character, onset, duration, precipitating and aggravating factors, associated symptoms, setting in which symptoms occur, and efforts to treat the symptoms.[2]

PHYSICAL EXAMINATION

Inspection

The four priorities for inspection of the patient with cardiovascular dysfunction are (1) assessment of general appearance, (2) examination of the nailbeds and extremities, (3) evaluation of jugular veins, and (4) observation of the apical impulse.

Assessment of general appearance and face

The weight in proportion to the height is assessed to determine whether the patient is obese (a cardiac risk factor) or cachectic (which can indicate chronic heart failure). The face is observed for the color of the skin (cyanotic, pale, or jaundiced) and expressions of apprehension or pain. Body posture can indicate the amount of effort it takes to breathe or the position of comfort the patient chooses (e.g., sitting upright to breathe may be necessary with acute heart failure or leaning forward may be the least painful position for the patient with pericarditis).[3] The patient is also observed for diaphoresis, confusion, or lethargy, each of which could indicate hypotension or low cardiac output. It is important to systematically inspect the skin, lips, tongue, mucous membranes, and conjunctiva for hydration, pallor, or cyanosis. Central cyanosis is a bluish discoloration of the tongue and sublingual area, indicating the presence of reduced arterial hemoglobin either from cardiac or pulmonary causes, which is considered life-threatening.[4]

TABLE 9-1

INSPECTION AND PALPATION OF EXTREMITIES: COMPARISON OF ARTERIAL AND VENOUS DISEASE

CHARACTERISTICS	ARTERIAL DISEASE	VENOUS DISEASE
Hair loss	Present	Absent
Skin texture	Thin, shiny, dry	Flaking, stasis, dermatitis, mottled
Ulceration	Located at pressure points; painful, pale, dry with little drainage; well-demarcated with eschar or dried; surrounded by fibrous tissue; granulation tissue scant and pale	Usually at the ankle; painless, pinkish, moist with large drainage; irregular, dry and scaly; surrounded by dermatitis; granulation tissue healthy
Skin color	Elevational pallor, dependent rubor	Brawny, brown, cyanotic when down
Nails	Thick, brittle	Normal
Varicose veins	Absent	Present
Temperature	Cool	Warm
Capillary refill	>3 seconds	<3 seconds
Edema	None or mild, usually unilateral	Usually present foot to calf, unilateral or bilateral
Pulses	Weak or absent (0 to 1+)	Normal, strong and symmetric

Modified from Krenzer ME: *AACN Clin Issues* 6(4):631, 1995.

Examination of the nailbeds and extremities

The nailbeds are inspected for signs of discoloration or peripheral cyanosis. Peripheral cyanosis indicates reduction of peripheral blood flow as a result of vascular disease or decreased cardiac output.[4] The extremities yield multiple signs of vascular disease. The parameters to be assessed are hair loss (sparse or lacking), skin texture (shiny, dry, cracked, or ulcerated), temperature (cool or warm), color (pale, dusky, or hyperpigmented), and the presence of edema. With arterial insufficiency, pallor is present when the legs are elevated. With venous thrombosis, the color of the extremity may be dusky and the circumference of the affected calf or thigh may be slightly larger compared with the other extremity.[5] The lower extremities are specifically inspected for varicosities that may predispose a patient to thrombophlebitis. Table 9-1 lists the specific information to be obtained through inspection of the extremities and separates the abnormal findings into arterial or venous disease etiologies.

Evaluation of jugular veins

The jugular veins of the neck are inspected for a noninvasive estimate of intravascular volume and/or pressure. The external jugular veins are observed for jugular vein distention (Box 9-1 and Fig. 9-1), and the right internal jugular vein pulsation is observed to estimate central venous pressure (Box 9-2 and Fig. 9-2). This data provides an information on right ventricular function. Jugular venous distention occurs when central venous pressure is elevated, as it is with right ventricular dysfunction.[6-7]

Observation of the apical impulse

The anterior thorax must also be inspected for the apical impulse, sometimes referred to as the point of maximal impulse (PMI). The apical impulse occurs as the left ventricle contracts during systole and rotates forward, causing the left ventricular apex to hit the chest wall. The impulse is a quick, localized, outward movement normally located just lateral to the left midclavicular line at the 5th intercostal space in the adult patient (Fig. 9-3). The apical impulse is the only normal pulsation visualized on the chest wall, and its location, size, and character are noted if apparent.

Palpation

The five priorities for palpation of the patient with cardiovascular dysfunction are (1) assessment of arterial pulses, (2) evaluation of capillary refill, (3) estimation of edema, (4) observation for signs of thrombophlebitis, and (5) evaluation of thoracic and abdominal pulsations.

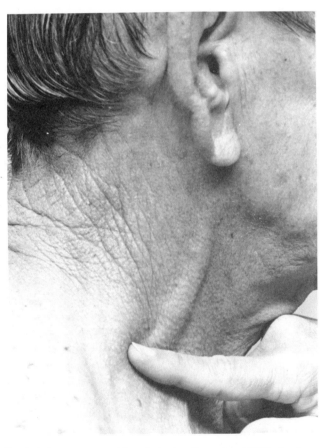

Fig. **9-1** Assessment of jugular vein distention (JVD). Applying light finger pressure over the sternocleidomastoid muscle, parallel to the clavicle, helps identify the external jugular vein by occluding flow and distending it. Release the finger pressure and observe for true distention. If the patient's trunk is elevated to 30 degrees or more, JVD should not be present.

BOX 9-1

PROCEDURE FOR ASSESSING JUGULAR VEIN DISTENTION

1. Patient reclines at a 30- to 45-degree angle.
2. The examiner stands on the patient's right side and turns the patient's head slightly toward the left.
3. If the jugular vein is not visible, light finger pressure is applied across the sternocleidomastoid muscle just above and parallel to the clavicle. This pressure will fill the external jugular vein by obstructing flow (see Fig. 9-1).
4. Once the location of the vein has been identified, the pressure is released and the presence of JVD is assessed.
5. Because inhalation decreases venous pressure, JVD should be assessed at the end of exhalation.
6. Any fullness in the vein extending more than 3 cm above the sternal angle is evidence of increased venous pressure. Generally the higher the sitting angle of the patient when JVD is discovered, the higher the central venous pressure.
7. *Documentation:* JVD is reported by including the angle of the head of the bed at the time JVD was evaluated (e.g., "presence of JVD with head of bed elevated to 45 degrees").

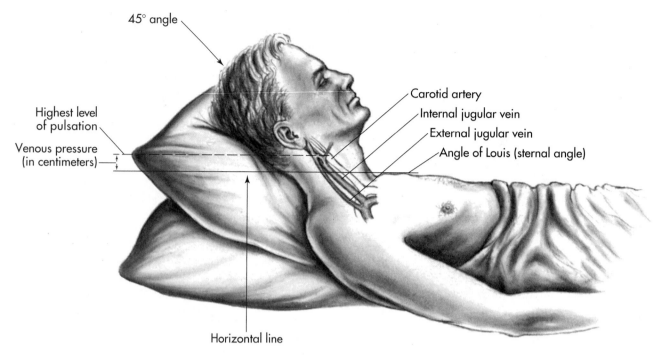

Fig. **9-2** Position of internal and external jugular veins. Pulsation in the internal jugular vein can be used to estimate central venous pressure. (Modified from Thompson JM, et al: *Mosby's clinical nursing*, ed 4, St Louis, 1997, Mosby.)

BOX **9-2**

PROCEDURE FOR ASSESSING CENTRAL VENOUS PRESSURE

1. The patient reclines in bed. The highest point of pulsation in the internal jugular vein is observed during exhalation.
2. The vertical distance between this pulsation, which is at the top of the fluid level, and the sternal angle is estimated or measured in centimeters (cm).
3. This number is then added to 5 cm for an estimation of CVP. The 5 cm is the approximate distance of the sternal angle above the level of the right atrium (see Fig. 9-2).
4. *Documentation:* The degree of elevation of the patient is included in reporting this finding (e.g. "central venous pressure estimated at 13 cm, using the internal jugular vein pulsation, with the head of the bed elevated 45 degrees").

BOX **9-3**

PULSE PALPATION SCALE

SCALE	DESCRIPTION
0	Not palpable
1+	Faintly palpable (weak and thready)
2+	Palpable (normal pulse)
3+	Bounding (hyperdynamic pulse)

Assessment of arterial pulses

Seven major areas are palpated for arterial pulses. The examination incorporates bilateral assessment of the carotid, brachial, radial, ulnar, popliteal, dorsalis pedis, and posterior tibial arteries. The pulses are palpated separately and compared bilaterally to check for consistency. Pulse volume is graded on a scale of 0 to +3 (Box 9-3). A diminished or absent pulse may indicate the presence of arterial stenosis or occlusion proximal to the site of the examination. An abnormally strong or bounding pulse

suggests the presence of an aneurysm or an occlusion distal to the examination site.[5]

Evaluation of capillary refill

Capillary refill assessment is a maneuver done on the nailbeds to evaluate arterial circulation to the extremity. The nailbed is compressed to produce blanching, and release of the pressure should result in a return of blood flow and nail color in less than 3 seconds. The severity of arterial insufficiency is directly proportional to the amount of time necessary to reestablish flow and color.

Estimation of edema

Edema is fluid accumulated in the extravascular spaces of the body, such as the abdomen and the dependent tissues of the legs and sacrum. One must note whether the edema is dependent, unilateral or bilateral, and pitting or nonpitting. The amount of edema is quantified by measuring the circumference of the limb or by pressing the skin of the feet, ankles, and shins against the

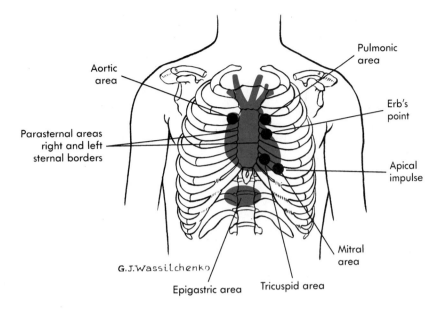

Fig. **9-3** Thoracic palpation and auscultation points.

BOX **9-4**

PITTING EDEMA SCALE

SCALE	DESCRIP-TION	DEPTH OF INDENTATION	TIME TO RETURN TO BASELINE
0	None present	0	—
1+	Trace	0-¼" (<6.4 mm)	Rapid
2+	Mild	¼-½" (6.4-12.8 mm)	10-15 sec
3+	Moderate	½-1" (12.8 mm-2.5 cm)	1-2 min
4+	Severe	>1" (>2.5 cm)	2-5 min

underlying bone. If an impression is left in the tissue when the thumb is removed, it is called pitting edema (Box 9-4).

Observation for signs of thrombophlebitis

The veins of the lower extremities are assessed with palpation, specifically for thrombophlebitis, which is an inflammation of the vein with thrombus formation. Squeezing or pressing the calves against the tibia may elicit pain, tenderness, increased firmness, or tension in the muscle. These signs suggest phlebitis and should alert the examiner to check other parameters that may aid in diagnosis, such as comparing leg circumferences and checking for increased heat in the extremity, unexplained fever, or tachycardia. Also, Homan's sign, in the presence of the other signs, can assist in the diagnosis of phlebitis.[6] To elicit Homan's sign, the examiner flexes the patient's knee and forcefully and abruptly dorsiflexes the patient's foot. The sign is positive when pain is reported in the popliteal region and the calf.

Evaluation of thoracic and abdominal pulsations

The chest wall is palpated for the apical impulse described previously. Its location, size, amplitude, and duration are recorded. An enlarged left ventricle (left ventricular hypertrophy secondary to ventricular failure or hypertension) is suspected when the apical impulse is enlarged (greater than 2 cm) and is displaced laterally. When the apical impulse is difficult to locate, the patient can be turned to the left lateral decubitus position. This facilitates palpation of the impulse because the left ventricle is against the chest wall in the left lateral position. Although this makes palpation of the apical impulse easier, it may also distort the placement and size of the impulse.[8] Once the apical impulse has been examined, the entire precordium must be assessed for pulsations, vibrations, heaves, or thrills (see Fig. 9-3). The abdomen is palpated for pulsations of the femoral arteries and the descending aortic artery. The femoral arteries are palpated by pressing deeply into the groin beneath the inguinal ligament, approximately midway between the anterior superior iliac spine and the symphysis pubis on both the right and left sides. The aortic pulsation is normally located in the epigastric area (see Fig. 9-3) and can be felt as a forward movement by using firm fingertip pressure above the umbilicus. If the pulsation is prominent or diffuse, it may indicate an abdominal aneurysm. The normal width of the aorta is approximately the width of the patient's own thumb. To estimate aortic width, lay two to three fingers on one side of the aorta and the thumb, of the same hand, on the other side. Compare that width to the patient's thumb. A widened aorta also may indicate an aortic aneurysm.[5]

Auscultation

The four priorities for auscultation of the patient with cardiovascular dysfunction are (1) measurement of blood pressure, (2) detection of bruits, (3) assessment of normal heart sounds, and (4) identification of abnormal heart sounds, murmurs, and pericardial friction rubs.

Measurement of blood pressure

Blood pressure is measured in both arms to rule out aortic or subclavian stenosis. Normally the blood pressure between both arms varies only 5 to 10 mm Hg. A difference of 20 mm Hg or more suggests arterial compression or obstruction on the side with the lower pressure. Clearly document asymmetry, so that all subsequent measurements are made on the arm with the higher pressure.[5] Evaluation of pulse pressure, pulsus alternans, pulsus paradoxus, and orthostatic blood pressure changes may be necessary (Table 9-2).

Detection of bruits

The carotid and femoral arteries are auscultated for bruits. A bruit is a high-pitched "sh-sh" extracardiac vascular sound, that vacillates in volume with systole and diastole, resulting from either blood flow through a tortuous or a partially occluded vessel or increased blood flow through a normal vessel. The auscultation of a bruit can expedite the diagnosis of arterial obstruction suspected with inspection and palpation of the lower extremities.

Assessment of normal heart sounds

Normal heart sounds are referred to as sound one (S_1) and sound two (S_2). S_1 is produced by the rapid deceleration of blood flow when the atrioventricular (mitral and tricuspid) valves close at the beginning of systole. S_2 is heard at the end of systole when the semilunar (aortic and pulmonic) valves reach closure. The actual sounds are caused not by the valve leaflets touching each other when they close, but by the vibrations created by the abrupt interruption of retrograde blood flow against the closed, tensed valve leaflets.[3,8] Both sounds are high-pitched and heard best with the diaphragm of the stethoscope. Each sound is loudest in an auscultation area located "downstream" from the actual valvular component of the sound. For example, S_2 (associated with aortic and pulmonary valve closure) can be heard best at the base of the heart, at the second intercostal space to the right and left of the sternum, and in the areas labeled aortic and pulmonic (see Fig. 9-3). S_1 (associated with mitral and tricuspid valve closure) is heard best in the mitral and tricuspid areas. Technically both S_1 and S_2 are split sounds because the left side of the heart contracts milliseconds before the right (Fig. 9-4). However, in the healthy heart, the left-sided heart valves, mitral and aortic, are the first heard components of each sound and are usually the

loudest, and S_1 and S_2 are heard as a single sound in their respective areas.[2]

Identification of abnormal heart sounds, murmurs, and pericardial friction rubs

The abnormal heart sounds are labeled sound three (S_3) and sound four (S_4) and are referred to as gallops when auscultated during tachycardia. Low pitched, they occur during diastole and are best heard with the bell of stethoscope positioned lightly over the apical impulse when the patient in the left lateral decubitus position. S_3 is related to diastolic motion and rapid filling of the ventricles in early diastole and is sometimes referred to as a ventricular gallop. The presence of S_3 is normal in persons younger than age 40 years because of rapid filling of the ventricle and the motion it causes in the young, healthy heart.[3,6,9] An S_3 may be heard in the presence of ventricular dysfunction with an increase in end-systolic volume (e.g., myocardial infarction, heart failure, or valvular disease) or hyperdynamic states. S_4 is related to diastolic motion and ventricular dilation with atrial contraction in late diastole and is sometimes referred to as an atrial gallop. It may occur with or without cardiac decompensation. An S_4 may be heard in the presence of ventricular hypertrophy with a decrease in ventricular compliance (e.g., systemic hypertension, aortic stenosis or cardiomyopathy), hyperkinetic states, and acute valvular regurgitation.[3,6,9]

Heart murmurs are prolonged extra sounds that occur during systole or diastole. The sounds are vibrations caused by turbulent blood flow through the cardiac chambers as a result of an increased rate of flow through cardiac structures (e.g., fever or exercise), blood flow across a partial obstruction or irregularity (e.g., valvular stenosis), shunting of blood through an abnormal passage from high to low pressure (e.g., patent foramen ovale), and backflow across an incompetent valve (e.g., valvular insufficiency).[10] Murmurs are characterized by their timing (systolic/diastolic), location and radiation, quality (blowing, grating, harsh), pitch (high or low), and intensity (loudness graded on a scale of I to VI [Box 9-5]). Table 9-3 describes the most common murmurs and usual characteristics heard on auscultation. When auscultating mur-

---

BOX 9-5

GRADING OF CARDIAC MURMURS

GRADE	DESCRIPTION
I/VI	Very faint, may be heard only in a quiet environment
II/VI	Quiet, but clearly audible
III/VI	Moderately loud
IV/VI	Loud: may be associated with a thrill
V/VI	Very loud; thrill easily palpable
VI/VI	Very loud; may be heard with stethoscope off the chest; thrill palpable and visible

TABLE 9-2

BEYOND SYSTOLIC AND DIASTOLIC BLOOD PRESSURE

LOOK FOR	TECHNIQUE	FINDINGS/SIGNIFICANCE
Pulse pressure	The difference between systolic and diastolic blood pressure (SBP and DBP)	Normal pulse pressure 30 to 40 mm Hg Reflects both stroke volume and vascular resistance A narrow pulse pressure signals a fall in cardiac output. Common in all shock states except neurogenic or early septic shock where vascular resistance is decreased. A narrow pulse pressure may also be seen in severe aortic stenosis, constrictive pericarditis, and pericardial effusions which compromise forward blood flow. A wide pulse pressure may be seen in situations of high cardiac output and low vascular resistance. For this reason, it is seen in early phase septic shock and in neurogenic shock. A wide pulse pressure is common in aortic insufficiency and may also be seen in disease states with a hyperdynamic circulation such as anemia and thyrotoxicosis.
Pulsus alternans	When auscultating the BP, look for a sudden increase in Korotkoff or (k) sounds that is not related to a pulse rate or rhythm change and that is not affected by the timing of inspiration or expiration.	Reflects inconsistent stroke volume. Pulses from a higher stroke volume are heard first. When k sounds suddenly increase, pulses from a lower stroke volume are being appreciated. In the absence of atrial fibrillation or repetitive ectopy, pulsus alternans suggest LV dysfunction with stroke volume changing in relation to abnormal contractility.
Pulsus paradoxus	Inflate cuff 30 mm Hg above point where radial pulse is lost. Deflate cuff. Note point at which k sounds are heard. K sounds normally first occur on expiration. Begin deflating the cuff in 2- to 3-mm Hg increments encompassing full inspiratory/expiratory cycle. Note point at which k sounds are heard on both inspiration and expiration. Difference between where k sounds are first heard on expiration only and where they are heard on both inspiration and expiration is normally 10 mm Hg.	Pulsus paradoxus is present when the value between where k sounds are first heard on expiration to where k sounds are heard on both inspiration and expiration is >10 mm Hg. Most often occurs as a result of pericardial effusions. With pericardial effusion, pulsus paradoxus occurs as a result of inspiratory descent of the diaphragm of the creating traction on an already taut pericardium impeding left ventricular outflow causing a fall in cardiac output. Once an effusion produces a paradox, as little as 50 to 100 ml additional fluid may cause cardiac tamponade and circulatory collapse. An important note is that a *pulsus paradoxus* cannot be appreciated in patients on controlled mechanical ventilation since the normal intrathoracic pressure changes on inspiration do not occur. A *pulsus paradoxus* associated with acute asthma signals severe airway obstruction. Orthostatic changes may take several forms.
Orthostatic blood pressure changes	The nature of an orthostatic episode can only be assessed if both BP and heart rate (HR) changes are evaluated. First check the patient's BP and pulse in supine position. Then position patient sitting with feet dangling over side of bed or stand the patient. Ask about orthostatic symptoms such as dizziness. After 2 minutes at the new position, repeat patient's BP and pulse.	*Orthostatic tachycardia* is defined as an HR increase >10 beats per minute (BPM) without a systolic blood pressure (SBP) drop. This may be seen in mild intravascular volume depletion in a person with good vascular tone. *Orthostatic hypotension* is defined as an HR increase >10 BPM, an SBP fall >15 mm Hg, and a DBP fall > 5 mm Hg. Orthostatic hypotension may precipitated by (1) volume depletion, (2) vasodilation, (3) autonomic dysfunction. Volume depletion and peripheral vasodilation present with appropriate HR increase and SBP and/or DPB fall. The clinical picture determines origin of the event. Autonomic dysfunction is suggested by a blood pressure decrease without a pulse rate increase. Beta-blockers and calcium channel blockers block normal HR increases to volume shifts causing hypotension when position changes are made. Autonomic dysfunction may also accompany diabetic neuropathy and is seen with spinal cord injuries with spinal cord transection T6 or above also leading to positional blood pressure changes.

From Kinney MR, et al: *AACN's clinical reference for critical care nursing,* ed 4, St Louis, 1998, Mosby.

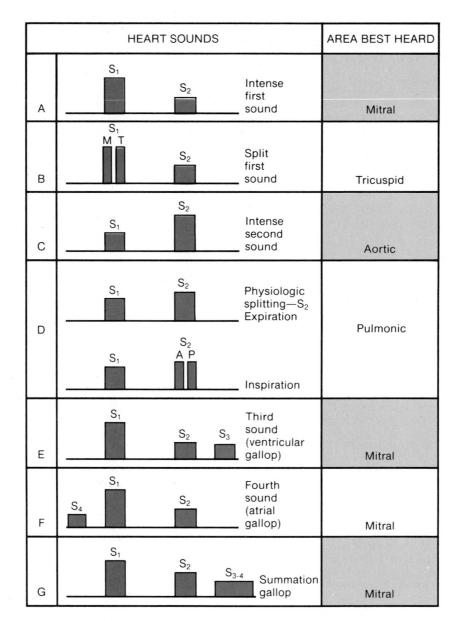

HEART SOUNDS		AREA BEST HEARD
A	S_1 S_2 Intense first sound	Mitral
B	S_1 M T S_2 Split first sound	Tricuspid
C	S_1 S_2 Intense second sound	Aortic
D	S_1 S_2 Physiologic splitting—S_2 Expiration / S_1 S_2 A P Inspiration	Pulmonic
E	S_1 S_2 S_3 Third sound (ventricular gallop)	Mitral
F	S_4 S_1 S_2 Fourth sound (atrial gallop)	Mitral
G	S_1 S_2 S_{3-4} Summation gallop	Mitral

Fig. **9-4** Characteristics of normal and abnormal heart sounds and the auscultatory area where each is best heard.

murs, the examiner visualizes the cardiac anatomy, specifically the location of the heart valves and the direction of sound transmission with valve closure and murmur. Generally the systolic valvular murmurs radiate downstream from the valve that is narrowed (stenotic), and the diastolic valvular murmurs (indicating a backflow of blood through an incompetent valve) are auscultated best directly over the area of the valve (see Fig. 9-3).

A pericardial friction rub is a sound that can occur within 2 to 7 days of a myocardial infarction and/or cardiac surgery and is secondary to pericardial inflammation or pericarditis. Classically, it is a three-phase grating or scratching sound that is both systolic and diastolic, corresponding with cardiac motion within the pericardial sac. It is high-pitched, often transient, and best auscultated at Erb's point during inhalation (see Fig. 9-3). It is often associated with chest pain, which can be aggravated by deep inspiration, coughing, swallowing, and changing position. It is important to differentiate pericarditis from myocardial ischemia, and the detection of the pericardial friction rub through auscultation can assist in this differentiation, leading to the proper diagnosis and treatment.

LABORATORY ASSESSMENT

Potassium

During depolarization and repolarization of nerve and muscle fiber, potassium and sodium exchange occurs intracellularly and extracellularly. Thus either an excess or a deficiency of potassium can alter cardiac muscle function. The normal serum level is 3.5 to 5.5 mEq/L.

TABLE 9-3

CHARACTERISTICS OF SOME MURMURS

DEFECT	TIMING IN THE CARDIAC CYCLE	PITCH, INTENSITY, QUALITY	LOCATION, RADIATION
SYSTOLIC MURMURS			
Mitral regurgitation	S₁ — S₂	High Harsh Blowing	Mitral area May radiate to axilla
Tricuspid regurgitation	S₁ — S₂	High Often faint, but varies Blowing	Tricuspid RLSB, apex, LLSB, epigastric areas Little radiation
Ventricular septal defect	S₁ — S₂	High Loud Blowing	Left sternal border
Aortic stenosis	S₁ ◇ S₂	Chhhh hh Medium Rough, harsh	Aortic area to suprasternal notch, right side of neck, apex
Pulmonary stenosis	S₁ ◇ S₂	Low to medium Loud Harsh, grinding	Pulmonic area No radiation
DIASTOLIC MURMURS			
Mitral stenosis	S₂ — S₁ (Atrial kick)	Low Quiet to loud with thrill Rough rumble	Mitral area Usually no radiation
Tricuspid stenosis	S₂ — S₁ (Atrial kick)	Medium Quiet; louder with inspiration Rumble	Tricuspid area or epigastrium Little radiation
Aortic regurgitation	S₂ — S₁	High Faint to medium Blowing	Aortic area to LLSB and aorta Erb's point
Pulmonic regurgitation	S₂ — S₁	Medium Faint Blowing	Pulmonic area No radiation

RLSB, Right lower sternal border; *LLSB,* left lower sternal border.

Hyperkalemia

High serum potassium (hyperkalemia) decreases the rate of ventricular depolarization, shortens repolarization, and also depresses atrioventricular (AV) conduction. As serum potassium rises above the normal range, changes are seen on the electrocardiogram (ECG) (Fig. 9-5, *A*). Tall, peaked T waves are usually, although not uniquely, associated with early hyperkalemia and are followed by widening of the QRS complex and prolongation of the P wave and PR interval. With severe hyperkalemia (greater than 8 mEq/L), depressed AV conduction leads to cardiac standstill or ventricular fibrillation. Co-existing low serum sodium, calcium, or pH levels potentiate the cardiac effects of hyperkalemia.

Hypokalemia

Low serum potassium (hypokalemia) is commonly caused by gastrointestinal losses, diuretic therapy with insufficient replacement, and chronic steroid therapy. Hypokalemia is also reflected by the ECG (Fig. 9-5, *B*). Myocardial conduction is impaired, and ventricular repolarization is prolonged, as evidenced by a prominent U

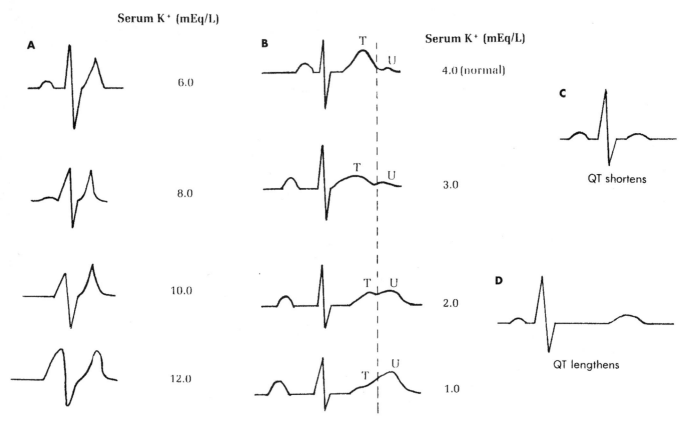

Fig. **9-5** Effects electrolyte imbalances on ECG tracing. **A,** Hyperkalemia: the earliest electrocardiogram (ECG) change with hyperkalemia is peaking (tenting) of the T wave. With progressive increases in the serum potassium level, the QRS complexes widen, P waves disappear, and finally ventricular fibrillation occurs. **B,** Hypokalemia: variable ECG patterns, ranging from slight T wave flattening to the appearance of U waves, sometimes with ST segment depressions or T wave inversions, may be seen. **C,** Hypercalcemia. **D,** Hypocalcemia.

wave. The U wave is not totally unique to hypokalemia, but its presence is a signal for the nurse to check the serum potassium level. The occurrence of or increase in numbers of premature ventricular contractions (PVCs) can also be a result of decreased potassium levels. Other ECG indicators of hypokalemia are the occurrence of bradycardia, AV block, atrial flutter, and an exaggeration of toxic effects of digitalis.[11] All of these dysrhythmias are usually reversible with potassium replacement.

Calcium

Calcium is an important mediator of many cardiovascular functions because of its effect on vascular tone, myocardial contractility, and cardiac excitability. Although the most commonly performed blood test for calcium levels is total serum calcium (8.5 to 10.5 mg/dL), the portion of the total calcium called ionized or "free" calcium is what is biologically active. The inactive forms of plasma calcium are bound to protein (primarily albumin) and complexed to anions such as chloride and phosphate. Ionized calcium is primarily responsible for the pathophysiologic effects of hypercalcemia and hypocalcemia. The serum concentration of ionized calcium is maintained within

very narrow limits (4 to 5 mg/dL), and direct measurement is considered to be the most accurate method for assessing calcium status.[12] Calcium levels are disrupted by tumors of the bone and lung, endocrine disorders, hypomagnesemia or hypermagnesemia, excessive intake or deficiency of vitamin D, intestinal malabsorption, kidney failure, and pancreatitis.

Hypercalcemia

High serum calcium (hypercalcemia) is an increased amount of ionized calcium (greater than 4.8 mg/dL) or total serum calcium (greater than 10.5 mg/dL). This condition has a cardiovascular effect of strengthening contractility and shortening ventricular repolarization. The ECG demonstrates the shortened repolarization with a shortened QT interval (Fig. 9-5, C). Rhythm disturbances may include bradycardia; first-, second-, and third-degree heart block; and bundle branch block. Hypercalcemia can potentiate the effects of digitalis, precipitate digitalis toxicity, and cause hypertension.[12]

Hypocalcemia

Low serum calcium (hypocalcemia) is a decreased amount of ionized calcium (less than 4.0 mg/dL) or total

TABLE 9-4

SUMMARY OF INCREASED SERUM MARKERS AFTER ACUTE MI

SERUM MARKER	EARLIEST INCREASE (HOURS)*	PEAK (HOURS)*	RETURN TO NORMAL (DAYS)*	AMPLITUDE OF INCREASE
Total CK	3-6	24-36	3	6-12
CK-MB	4-8	15-24	3-4	16
CK-MB$_2$/MB$_1$	2	4-6	2	
Total LD	10-12	48-72	11	3
LD$_1$	8-12	72-144	8-14	
LD$_1$/LD$_2$	>6		>3	
Myoglobin	2-3	6-9	Often 12 hours	10
Troponin T	4-6	10-24	10-15	
Troponin I	4-6	10-24	10-15	

Modified from Wallach J: *Interpretation of diagnostic tests*, ed 6, Boston, 1996, Little, Brown.
*Time periods represent average reported values.
NOTE: There is a range of reported values because different studies used different time periods after onset of symptoms, different benchmarks for establishing the diagnosis, and different patient populations, etc.
CK, Creatine phosphokinase; *LD,* lactate dehydrogenase.

serum calcium (less than 8.5 mg/dL). Hypocalcemia is common in critically ill and postsurgical patients because of blood transfusions, magnesium imbalances, shock, or alkalosis.[12] The cardiovascular effects of hypocalcemia include decreased myocardial contractility, reduced cardiac output, decreased cardiac responsiveness to digitalis, and hypotension. Rhythm disturbances range from bradycardia to ventricular tachycardia and asystole. When the ionized calcium is less than 3.2 mg/dL, the ECG commonly demonstrates a prolonged QT interval, which predisposes a patient to the life-threatening ventricular dysrhythmia torsades de pointes (Fig. 9-5, *D*). An ionized calcium level this low is considered a medical emergency and requires immediate reversal with an intravenous infusion of calcium.[11]

Magnesium

Magnesium is essential for many enzyme, protein, lipid, and carbohydrate functions in the body and is critical for the production and use of energy.[13] In the blood stream, it is found predominantly within the cells, although an adequate serum level (extracellular) is essential to normal cardiac and skeletal muscle function. The normal serum level is 1.5 to 2.0 mEq/L or 1.8 to 2.4 mg/dL.

Hypomagnesemia

A serum magnesium concentration less than 1.5 mEq/L is called hypomagnesemia. It is commonly associated with other electrolyte imbalances, most notably alterations in potassium, sodium, calcium, and phosphorous. Both hypokalemia and hypocalcemia are likely to be unresponsive to replacement therapy until the hypomagnesemia is corrected.[13] Cardiac-related changes with hypomagnesemia are hypertension and vasospasm, including coronary artery spasm. The ECG changes are similar to those seen with hypokalemia and hypocalcemia. Car-

diac dysrhythmias may be supraventricular or ventricular and include torsades de pointes. Dysrhythmias associated with hypomagnesemia may not respond to usual antidysrhythmic treatment, but they often respond well to magnesium infusions. The American Heart Association is currently recommending intravenous magnesium as the treatment of choice for torsades de pointes.[11] It is important to evaluate renal function when administering magnesium to avoid hypermagnesium states.

Cardiac Enzymes

Cardiac enzymes are proteins that are released from irreversibly damaged myocardial tissue cells. The traditional "gold standard" for diagnosing myocardial infarction (MI) is the rise and fall of the serum MB fraction of the enzyme creatine phosphokinase (CK) within 24 hours after the onset of symptoms.[14] The CK-MB serum levels elevate 4 to 8 hours after MI, peak at 15 to 24 hours, and remain elevated for 2 to 3 days. Serial samples are drawn routinely every 6 to 12 hours, and three samples are usually sufficient to support or rule out the diagnosis of MI. Newer methods of detection include evaluating myoglobin, troponin T, and troponin I levels (Table 9-4).

Lactate dehydrogenase (LDH, or LD) is another cardiac enzyme that is almost always elevated after MI. Its levels are useful for late diagnosis of MI, when CK-MB levels have returned to normal. LDH levels begin to increase 10 to 12 hours after injury, peak at 48 to 72 hours, and remain elevated for 10 to 14 days. LDH isoenzymes, LDH$_1$ and LDH$_2$, delineate the tissue source (increase the cardiac specificity) of the elevated LDH. Normally, serum levels of LDH$_1$ are less than those of LDH$_2$ (LDH$_1$/LDH$_2$ less than or equal to 1.0), and with MI, both levels rise, but LDH$_1$ levels become greater than LDH$_2$ levels. This is called a "flipped" LDH$_1$-to-LDH$_2$ ratio (LDH$_1$/LDH$_2$ greater than 1.0). The flipped ratio usually appears in 12 to 24 hours after injury and never appears before CK-MB elevation. It may flip back and forth, making it important to collect serial specimens, and it may remain flipped for longer than the total LDH stays elevated[15] (Table 9-4).

Coagulation Studies

Coagulation studies are ordered to determine serum clotting effectiveness. Anticoagulants, most notably heparin, warfarin, and platelet inhibitory agents (e.g., aspirin) are administered to reduce the incidence of reocclusion after successful reperfusion and to decrease myocardial infarct extension.[14] Patients who have stasis of blood (e.g., with atrial fibrillation or prolonged bed rest), valvular heart disease, or a history of thrombosis are at risk for developing a thrombus and usually require anticoagulation. Coagulation studies are ordered to guide dosage of these anticoagulating drugs.

Most coagulation study results are reported as the length of time in seconds it takes for blood to form a clot in the laboratory test tube. The prothrombin time (PT) is used to determine the therapeutic dosage of warfarin necessary to achieve anticoagulation. The PT is also reported as an international normalized ratio (INR). The INR was developed by the World Health Organization (WHO) in an attempt to standardize PT results between clinical laboratories worldwide. The partial thromboplastin time (PTT) and activated partial thromboplastin time (APTT) are used to measure the effectiveness of intravenous or subcutaneous heparin administration. An additional test of heparin effect is the activated coagulation time (ACT). The ACT can be performed outside of the laboratory setting in areas such as the cardiac catheterization laboratory, the operating room, or the critical care unit.[16]

Serum Lipid Studies

Four primary blood lipid levels are important in evaluating an individual's risk of developing and/or progressing coronary artery disease: total cholesterol; low density lipoprotein–cholesterol (LDL-C); triglycerides; and high density lipoprotein-cholesterol (HDL-C). When levels of cholesterol, LDLs, and triglycerides are elevated or the level of HDLs is low, the patient is considered "at risk" for developing or progressing coronary heart disease (CHD) and is offered intensive interventions in diet therapy, exercise prescription, and/or drug therapy.

Total cholesterol

Cholesterol is a fatlike substance (lipid) that is present in cell membranes and is a precursor of bile acids and steroid hormones. It is produced by the liver. The cholesterol level in the blood is determined partly by genetics and partly by acquired factors such as diet, calorie balance, and level of physical activity. Cholesterol in excess amounts (more than 200 mg/dL) in the serum forces the progression of atherosclerosis (athrogenesis).

Low density lipoproteins

About 60% to 70% of the total serum cholesterol is found in low density lipoproteins-cholesterol (LDL-C). Both the LDL-C and total serum cholesterol levels are directly correlated with risk for CHD, and high levels of each are significant predictors of future myocardial infarctions in patients with established coronary artery atherosclerosis.[17] LDL-C is the major atherogenic lipoprotein and thus is the primary target for cholesterol-lowering efforts. In the patient with coronary artery disease, the desired level of LDL-C is less than 100 mg/dL.

Very low density lipoproteins and triglycerides

The very low density lipoproteins (VLDL) contain 10% to 15% of the total serum cholesterol along with most of the triglycerides in fasting serum; VLDLs are precursors of LDL-C, and some forms of VLDL (phenotype B) appear to be atherogenic.[17] Elevated triglyceride levels (greater than 200 mg/dL) are often associated with reduced HDL-C levels and directly correlate with the phenotype B of LDL-C.

High density lipoproteins

High density lipoproteins-cholesterol (HDL-C) are particles that carry 20% to 30% of the total serum cholesterol. A low HDL-C level (less than 35 mg/dL) is another independent, significant risk factor for CHD. Several studies, however, also support a protective role of HDL-C against atherogenesis, and a level greater than 60 mg/dL may act as a "shield" against the risk of CHD.[17]

DIAGNOSTIC PROCEDURES

Table 9-5 presents an overview of the various diagnostic procedures used to evaluate the patient with cardiovascular dysfunction.

Nursing Management

The nursing management of a patient undergoing a diagnostic procedure involves a variety of interventions. **Priorities are directed toward preparing the patient psychologically and physically for the procedure, monitoring the patient's responses to the procedure, and assessing the patient after the procedure.** Preparing the patient includes teaching the patient about the procedure, answering any questions, and transporting and/or positioning the patient for the procedure. Monitoring the patient's responses to the procedure includes observing the patient for signs of pain, anxiety or hemorrhage and monitoring vital signs. Assessing the patient after the procedure includes observing for complications of the procedure and medicating the patient for any postprocedure discomfort. **Any evidence of bleeding or chest pain should be immediately reported to the physician, and emergency measures to maintain circulation and increase myocardial oxygen supply must be initiated.**

TABLE 9-5

CARDIOVASCULAR DIAGNOSTIC PROCEDURES

PROCEDURES	EVALUATES	COMMENTS
Aortography	• Aortic valve insufficiency • Aneurysms or dissection of ascending aorta • Coarctation of the aorta • Injuries to the aorta and major branches	• Contrast medium used: check for allergy to iodine, shellfish, dye; ensure hydration post procedure
Cardiac biopsy	• Effect of cardiotoxic drugs • Evidence of cardiac transplant rejection • Inflammatory heart disease • Tumors • Cardiomyopathy	• Observe closely for signs of cardiac perforation and/or cardiac tamponade
Cardiac catheterization and coronary arteriography	• Severity of coronary artery stenosis • Cardiac muscle function • Pressures within the heart • Cardiac output and ejection fraction • Blood gas analysis with chambers • Allows angioplasty, atherectomy, intracoronary stents, or lasers to reduce coronary artery obstruction	Before the test • Contrast medium used: check for allergy to iodine, shellfish, dye After the test • Contrast medium used: ensure hydration postprocedure • Keep extremity in which catheter was placed immobilized in a straight position for 6-12 hours • Monitor arterial puncture point for hemorrhage or hematoma • Monitor neurovascular status of affected limb • Monitor for indications of systemic emboli
Chest x-ray	• Cardiac size • Presence of pulmonary congestion or pleural effusions • Presence of thoracic aneurysm or calcification of the aorta	• Inquire about possibility of pregnancy
Computed tomography (CT)	• Left ventricular wall motion • Cardiac tumors • Myocardial infarction • Pericardial effusion • Aortic aneurysm • Aortic dissection	• May be done with or without contrast medium • If contrast medium used, check for allergy to iodine, shellfish, dye; ensure hydration post-procedure
Digital subtraction angiography	• Vascular disease (excluding coronary arteries) and degree of occlusion	• Contrast medium used: check for allergy to iodine, shellfish, dye; ensure hydration post procedure

Echocardiography
• M-mode: single ultrasound beam
• 2-D: planar ultrasound beam; wider view of heart and structures
• Doppler: addition of Doppler to demonstrate flow of blood through the heart
	• Chamber size and wall thickness
	• Valve functioning
	  • Papillary muscle functioning
	  • Prosthetic valve functioning
	• Ventricular wall motion abnormalities
	• Intracardiac masses
	• Presence of pericardial fluid
	• Intracardiac pressures (Doppler)
	• Ejection fraction and cardiac output (Doppler)
	• Valve gradients (Doppler)
	• Intracardiac shunts (Doppler)
		• Transesophageal echocardiography is better if patient is obese, has COPD, chest wall deformity, chest trauma, or thick chest dressings

Electrocardiography (ECG)	• Dysrhythmias • Conduction defects including intraventricular blocks • Electrolyte imbalance • Drug toxicity • Myocardial ischemia, injury, infarction • Chamber hypertrophy	• List what drugs the patient is receiving on ECG request • Be alert to electrical safety hazards
Electrophysiologic studies (EPS)	• Dysrhythmias under controlled circumstances • Best therapy for control of dysrhythmia: drug, required dosage of therapy, pacemaker, catheter ablation	• Patient may have near-death experience during EPS; encourage expression of fears, concerns, and anxieties

From Dennison RD: *Pass CCRN!* St Louis, 1996, Mosby.   *Continued*

TABLE **9-5**

CARDIOVASCULAR DIAGNOSTIC PROCEDURES—cont'd

PROCEDURES	EVALUATES	COMMENTS
Holter monitor	• Suspected dysrhythmias over 24-hour period • Pacemaker function • Silent ischemia	• Instruct patient on importance of diary-keeping
Magnetic resonance imaging (MRI)	• Three-dimensional view of the heart • Changes in chemistry of tissues before structural changes occur	• Do not use in patients with any implanted metallic device, including pacemakers
Multiple-gated acquisition (MUGA) scan (radionuclide angiography)	• Ventricular size and ventricular wall motion • Cardiac output, cardiac index, end-systolic volume, end-diastolic volume, and ejection fraction • Intracardiac shunts	• Assure patient that amount of radioactive material is minimal
Myocardial infarction indicators: technetium pyrophosphate-99	• Presence of MI: infarcted areas showing increased uptake of radioactivity ("hot spots") 1 to 7 days after MI	• Assure patient that amount of radioactive material is minimal • Peak accuracy at 48 hours after initial symptoms
Myocardial perfusion imaging: thallium-201	• Myocardial ischemia; ischemic or infarcted areas showing decreased uptake of radioactivity ("cold spots")	• Assure patient that amount of radioactive material is minimal
Pericardiocentesis	• Presence of blood, pus, pathogens, or malignancy • Emergency relief of cardiac tamponade	• Observe closely for signs of cardiac tamponade
Peripheral arteriography and venography	• Atherosclerotic plaques, occlusion, aneurysms, or traumatic injury	Before the test • Contrast medium used: check for allergy to iodine, shellfish, dye After the test • Contrast medium used, ensure hydration post procedure • Keep extremity in which catheter was placed immobilized in a straight position for 6 to 12 hours • Monitor arterial puncture point for hemorrhage or hematoma • Monitor neurovascular status of affected limb • Monitor for indications of systemic emboli
Phonocardiography	• Extra heart sounds and murmurs in relation to the cardiac cycle and ECG	• It is rarely used today
Positron emission tomography (cardiac PET scan)	• Severity of coronary artery stenosis • Collateral circulation • Patency of bypass grafts • Size and location of infarcted tissue	• Assure patient that amount of radioactive material is minimal
Stress electrocardiography	• High-risk patients, patients with known CAD, or postsurgical patients for ischemia with exercise or pharmacologic agents (e.g., adenosine, dipyridamole, dobutamine) • Exercise-induced dysrhythmias	• One millimeter or greater transient ST segment depression 80 msec after the J point suggests CAD • Patients may also have exercise-induced hypotension or ventricular dysrhythmias
Thallium stress electrocardiography	• Myocardial ischemia: ischemic areas showing decreased uptake of radioactivity ("cold spots")	• Assure patient that amount of radioactive material is minimal
Vectorcardiography	• Chamber hypertrophy • Bundle branch blocks and hemiblocks • Myocardial ischemia or infarction	
Ventriculography	• Ventricular wall motion • Wall thickness • Ventricular aneurysm • Mitral valve motion • LV end-diastolic volume, end-systolic volume, stroke volume, ejection fraction • Shunt	• Contrast medium used: check for allergy to iodine, shellfish, dye: ensure hydration post-procedure

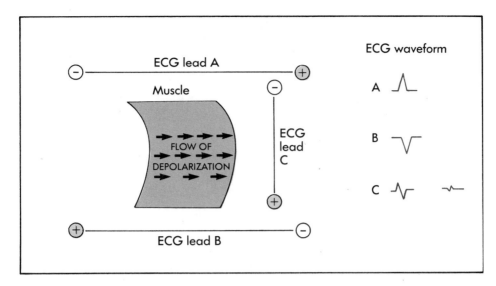

Fig. **9-6** Effect of lead position on the ECG tracing *A,* Flow of depolarization toward the positive electrode results in a positive deflection on the ECG. *B,* Flow of depolarization away from the positive electrode results in a negative deflection on the ECG. *C,* Flow of depolarization perpendicular to the positive electrode results in a biphasic or nearly isoelectric deflection on the ECG. This basic principle applies to both the P wave and the QRS complex.

BEDSIDE MONITORING

Electrocardiography

This section provides a general discussion of bedside electrocardiography (ECG) and dysrhythmias interpretation. The ECG records electrical changes in heart muscle. It does not record mechanical contraction, which usually immediately follows electrical depolarization.

ECG leads

All ECGs use a system of one or more leads designed to record electrical activity. A lead consists of three electrodes: a positive electrode, a negative electrode, and a ground electrode that prevents the display of background electrical interference on the ECG tracing. Leads do not transmit any electricity to the patient—they just sense and record it.

The positive electrode on the skin functions like the lens of a camera. If the wave of depolarization travels toward the positive electrode, an upward stroke, or positive deflection, is written on the ECG paper (Fig. 9-6, *A*). If the wave of depolarization travels away from the positive electrode, a downward line, or negative deflection, is recorded on the ECG (Fig. 9-6, *B*). When depolarization moves perpendicularly to the positive electrode, a biphasic complex occurs. Sometimes the complex may even appear almost flat or isoelectric if the electrical forces traveling in opposite directions are equal and have the effect of canceling out each other (Fig. 9-6, *C*). The size of the muscle mass being depolarized also has an effect, with the larger muscle mass having the greatest influence on the direction of the complex.

The portion of the tracing between the various wave-forms, referred to as the baseline, must be flat. Two forms of artifact can distort the baseline: 60-cycle interference and muscular movement. Sixty-cycle interference (Fig. 9-7, *A*) results from leakage of electrical current somewhere within the system and appears as a generalized thickening of the baseline. It can usually be resolved by ensuring that all electrical equipment at the bedside is well-grounded. Occasionally, it may be necessary to unplug one piece of equipment at a time until the offending device is found. Muscular movement (Fig. 9-7, *B*) is displayed as a coarse, erratic disturbance of the baseline.

During continuous cardiac monitoring, adhesive, pregelled electrodes are used to obtain the ECG tracing. At a minimum, this requires three electrodes: one positive, one negative, and one ground. In many clinical areas, five electrodes are used, either to monitor two leads simultaneously or to allow selection of several different leads at any time through a lead selector switch on the monitor. Though lead II is probably the most widely selected lead for monitoring, MCL_1 (three electrode system) or V_1 (five electrode system) are considered the best leads for bedside dysrhythmia monitoring while MCL_6 (three electrode system) or V_6 (five electrode system) are considered the second-best leads.[18] Fig. 9-8 describes the proper placement of the electrodes for the different leads.

ECG paper

ECG paper records the speed and magnitude of electrical impulses on a grid composed of small and large boxes (Fig. 9-9). There are five small boxes in every large box. At a standard paper speed of 25 mm/second, one small box (1 mm) is equivalent to 0.04 second, and one large box (5 mm) represents 0.20 second. Distances

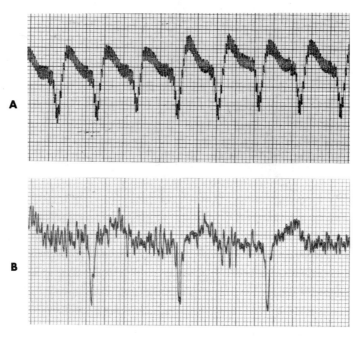

Fig. **9-7** Artifact. **A,** 60-cycle interference. **B,** Muscular movement.

along the horizontal axis represent speed and are stated in seconds rather than in millimeters or number of boxes. The vertical axis represents magnitude or strength of force. At standard calibration, one small box equals 0.1 mV, and one large box equals 0.5 mV. It is important to look for the standardization mark, which is usually located at the beginning of the tracing. The mark indicates 1 mV and at standard calibration goes up two large boxes (Fig. 9-10).

ECG waveforms

The analysis of waveforms and intervals provide the basis for ECG interpretation (Figure 9-9). The P wave represents atrial depolarization. The QRS complex represents ventricular depolarization. It is referred to as a complex because it can actually consist of several different waves, depending on the placement of the positive electrode and the direction of the spread of electrical activity in the heart. Basically, the letter *Q* is used to describe an initial negative deflection; in other words, only if the first deflection from the baseline is negative will it be labeled a Q wave. The letter *R* applies to any positive deflection. If there are two positive deflections in one QRS complex, the second is labeled *R'* (read "R prime"). The letter *S* refers to any subsequent negative deflections. Any combination of these deflections can occur and is collectively called the QRS complex. The QRS duration is normally 0.10 second (2½ small boxes) or less. The T wave represents ventricular repolarization. The PR interval is measured from the beginning of the P wave to the beginning of the QRS complex. Normally, the PR interval is 0.12 to 0.20 second in length and represents the time between sinus node discharge and the beginning of ventricular depolarization. Because most of this time period results

from delay of the impulse in the AV node, the PR interval is an indicator of AV nodal function. The portion of the wave that extends from the end of the QRS to the beginning of the T wave is labeled the ST segment. Its duration is not measured. Instead, its shape and location are evaluated. The ST segment is normally flat and at the same level as the isoelectric baseline. Elevation or depression is expressed in millimeters and may indicate ischemia. The QT interval is measured from the beginning of the QRS complex to the end of the T wave and indicates the total time interval from the onset of depolarization to the completion of repolarization. At normal heart rates, the QT interval is less than half of the RR interval (measured from one QRS complex to the next). However, the normal value of a QT interval depends on heart rate and must be adjusted according to the heart rate to be evaluated in a meaningful way. The corrected QT interval (QTc) can be calculated by dividing the measured QT interval, in seconds, by the square root of the R to R interval.[19]

Dysrhythmia interpretation

In clinical practice the terms *dysrhythmia* and *arrhythmia* often are used interchangeably. There may be discussion over which word is the most accurate. Both are correct, and either may be used in practice. In this textbook, *dysrhythmia* is the more commonly used term. A dysrhythmia is any disturbance in the normal cardiac conduction pathway. Dysrhythmias can be detected on a 12-lead ECG, but very often they occur only sporadically. For this reason patients in a critical care unit are monitored continuously, using a single or dual lead system, and rhythm strips are recorded routinely, as well as any time there is a change in the patient's rhythm. A systematic approach to evaluation of a rhythm strip is intro-

A

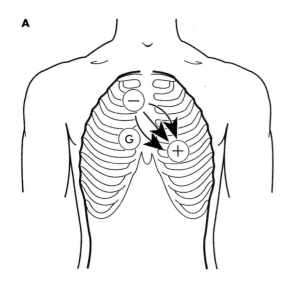

B

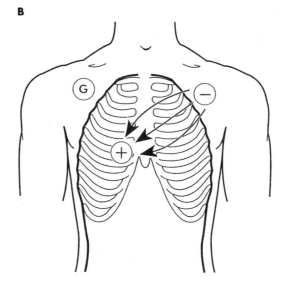

C

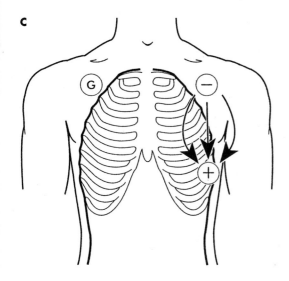

D

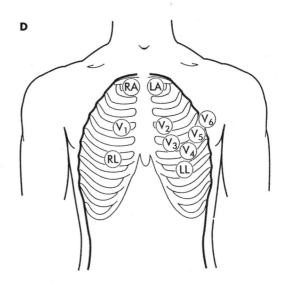

Three-lead system:
(A) Lead II
  (1) Apply negative electrode to first intercostal space, right sternal border.
  (2) Apply positive electrode to fourth intercostal space, left midclavicular line.
  (3) Apply ground electrode at fourth intercostal space, right sternal border.

(B) MCL₁ (modified chest lead V₁)
  (1) Apply negative electrode just inferior to left clavicle, midclavicular line.
  (2) Apply positive electrode to fourth intercostal space, right sternal border.
  (3) Apply ground electrode just inferior to right clavicle, midclavicular line.

(C) MCL₆ (modified chest lead V₆)
  (1) Apply negative electrode inferior to left clavicle, midclavicular line.
  (2) Apply positive electrode to fifth intercostal space, midclavicular line.
  (3) Apply ground electrode inferior to right clavicle, midclavicular line.

(D) Five-lead system
  (1) Apply RA electrode inferior to right clavicle, midclavicular line.
  (2) Apply LA electrode inferior to left clavicle, midclavicular line.
  (3) Apply RL electrode on sixth intercostal space, right midclavicular line.
  (4) Apply LL electrode on sixth intercostal space, left midclavicular line.
  (5) Apply chest lead electrode on selected chest sites V₁, V₂, V₃, V₄, V₅, or V₆ position.

Fig. **9-8** Electrode placement for continuous bedside cardiac monitoring. **A,** Lead II provides clear P wave and tall, distinct R wave. **B,** MCL₁ (modified chest lead V₁) identifies bundle branch blocks, atrial and ventricular dysrhythmias, and ventricular conduction. **C,** MCL₆ (modified chest lead V₆) is used for patients with median sternotomy incisions and for telemetry monitoring; it provides a good R wave and identifies ventricular dysrhythmias and bundle branch blocks. **D,** Five-lead system. The fifth (V) lead electrode can be applied to a selected chest site; obtains a precise, multiplaned view of the heart's activity; detects hemiblocks. (Modified from Millar S, et al: *AACN procedure manual for critical care,* ed 2, Philadelphia, 1985, WB Saunders.)

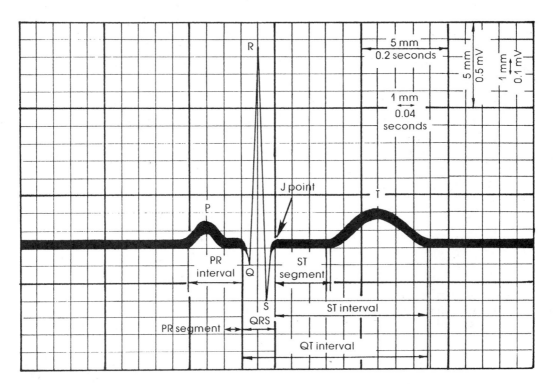

Fig. **9-9** ECG graph paper and normal ECG waveforms. The horizontal axis represents time, and the vertical axis represents magnitude of voltage. Horizontally, each small box is 0.04 second and each large box is 0.2 second. Vertically, each large box is 5 mm. Markings are present every 3 seconds at the top of the paper for ease in calculating heart rate. The **P wave** represents atrial depolarization, followed immediately by atrial systole. The **QRS complex** represents ventricular depolarization, followed immediately by ventricular systole. The **ST segment** corresponds to time the heart muscle is completely depolarized and contraction normally occurs. The **T wave** represents ventricular repolarization. The **PR interval** corresponds to atrial depolarization and impulse delay in the AV node. The **QT interval** represents the time from initial depolarization of the ventricles to the end of ventricular repolarization. (From The Methodist Hospital: *Basic electrocardiography: a modular approach,* St Louis, 1986, Mosby.)

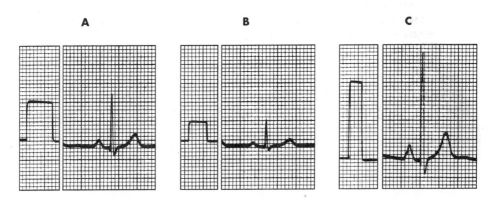

Fig. **9-10** Standardization mark. **A,** Normal standardization mark, in which the machine is calibrated so that the standardization mark is 10 mm tall. **B,** Half standardization, used whenever QRS complexes are too tall to fit on the paper. **C,** Twice normal standardization, used whenever QRS complexes are too small to be adequately analyzed. (From Goldberger AL, Goldberger E: *Clinical electrocardiography: a simplified approach,* ed 5, St Louis, 1994, Mosby.)

duced first in this section, followed by specific criteria for common dysrhythmias encountered in clinical practice.

Heart rate determination. The first element to assess when evaluating a rhythm strip is the ventricular rate. Regardless of the dysrhythmia involved, the ventricular rate holds the key to whether the patient is able to tolerate the dysrhythmia (i.e., maintain adequate blood pressure, cardiac output, and mentation). If the ventricular rate is consistently greater than 200 or less than 30, emergency measures must be started to correct the rate. A

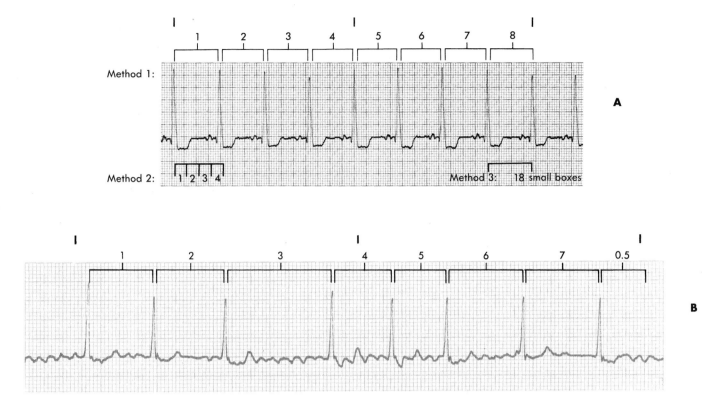

Fig. **9-11** Calculation of heart rate. **A,** Regular rhythm. *Method 1:* number of RR intervals in 6 seconds multiplied by 10 (e.g., 8 × 10 = 80/min). *Method 2:* number of large boxes between QRS complexes divided into 300 (e.g., 300 ÷ 4 = 75/min). *Method 3:* number of small boxes between QRS complexes divided into 1500 (e.g., 1500 ÷ 18 = 84/min). **B,** Rate calculation if the rhythm is irregular. Only Method 1 can be used (e.g., 7.5 intervals × 10 = 75/min).

detailed analysis of the underlying rhythm disturbance can proceed later when the immediate crisis is over. The three methods for calculating rate are described in Fig. 9-11. In the healthy heart, the atrial rate and the ventricular rate are the same. However, in many dysrhythmias the atrial and ventricular rates are different; thus both must be calculated. To find the atrial rate, the P wave to P wave interval, instead of the R to R interval, is used as outlined in method 1 (see Fig. 9-11).

Rhythm determination. The term *rhythm* refers to the regularity with which the P waves or R waves occur. Calipers assist in determining rhythm. One point of the calipers is placed on the beginning of one R wave, while the other point is placed on the very next R wave. Leaving the calipers "set" at this interval, each succeeding R to R interval is checked to be sure it is the same width. In describing the rhythm, three terms are used. If the rhythm is *regular,* the R to R intervals are the same, ±10%. If the rhythm is *regularly irregular,* the R to R intervals are not the same, but some sort of pattern is involved, which could be grouping, rhythmic speeding up and slowing down, or any other consistent pattern. If the rhythm is *irregularly irregular,* the RR intervals are not the same, and no pattern can be found.

P wave evaluation. The P wave is analyzed by answering the following questions. First, is the P wave present or absent? Second, is it related to the QRS? It is hoped that one P wave will be in front of every QRS. Sometimes there may be two, three, or four P waves in front of every QRS. If this pattern is consistent, the P wave and QRS are still related, although not on a 1:1 basis.

PR interval evaluation. The duration of the PR interval, which normally is 0.12 to 0.20 second, is measured first. This is done by measuring from the start of a P wave to the beginning of the following QRS (see Fig. 9-9). Next, all PR intervals on the strip are checked to be sure they are the same duration as the original interval.

QRS evaluation. The entire ECG strip must be evaluated to ascertain that the QRS complexes are consistently the same shape and width. The normal QRS duration is 0.06 to 0.10 second. If more than one QRS shape is on the strip, each QRS must be measured. The QRS is measured from where it leaves the baseline to where it returns to the baseline (see Fig. 9-9).

Dysrhythmias. The most common atrial, junctional, and ventricular dysrhythmias are outlined in Figs. 9-12 through 9-30.

Nursing management

Nursing priorities for the patient with bedside cardiac monitoring include positioning electrodes prop-

Text continued on p. 130

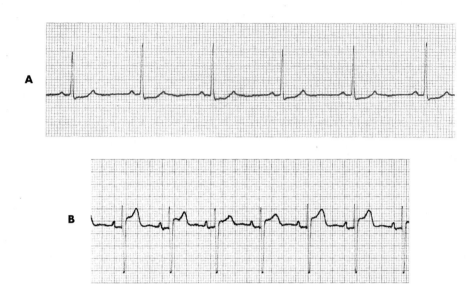

Fig. **9-12** Normal sinus rhythm (NSR).

RATE: 60 to 100 beats per minute.
RHYTHM: Regular, plus or minus 10%.

P WAVE: Present, all the same shape, with only one preceding each QRS complex.
PR INTERVAL: 0.12 to 0.20 of a second.
QRS DURATION: 0.06 to 0.10 of a second.

QRS COMPLEX: The shape and whether the deflection is positive or negative will vary depending on lead placement. For example, in lead II the normal complex is positive (Strip **A**) and in MCL$_1$ or V$_1$ the normal complex is negative (Strip **B**).
ETIOLOGY: Normal conduction.
TREATMENT: None required.

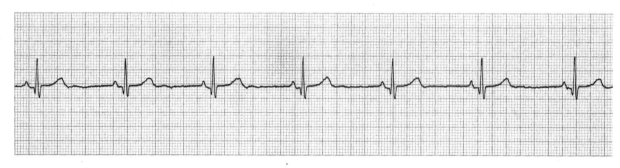

Fig. **9-13** Sinus bradycardia (SB).

RATE: Less than 60 beats per minute.
RHYTHM: Regular.

P WAVE: Present, all the same shape, with only one preceding each QRS complex.
PR INTERVAL: 0.12 to 0.20 of a second.
QRS DURATION: 0.06 to 0.10 of a second.

QRS COMPLEX: Same as NSR. Narrow complex QRS.
ETIOLOGY: Vagal stimulation, increased intracranial pressure, ischemia of the sinus node caused by an acute inferior wall myocardial infarction or as a side effect of cardiac drugs such as beta blockers or digoxin. SB is also normal in well-conditioned, healthy athletes at rest.
TREATMENT: Only treated if it is accompanied by symptoms of hypoperfusion such as hypotension, dizziness, chest pain, or changes in level of consciousness. If the patient becomes symptomatic, Advanced Cardiac Life Support (ACLS) measures, such as atropine and transcutaneous pacing, will be required (see Appendix A).

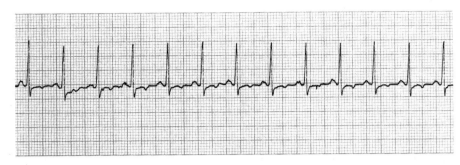

Fig. **9-14** Sinus tachycardia (ST).

RATE: Greater than 100 beats per minute. Rates may be as high as 180 bpm in young healthy adults during strenuous exercise. However, in the critically ill patient a heart rate above 150 is usually caused by other dysrhythmias.

RHYTHM: Regular.

QRS COMPLEX: Same as NSR. Narrow complex QRS.

P WAVE: Present, all the same shape, with only one preceding each QRS complex.

PR INTERVAL: 0.12 to 0.20 of a second.

QRS DURATION: 0.06 to 0.10 of a second.

ETIOLOGY: Pain, fever, hemorrhage, shock, and acute heart failure. Many medications used in the critical care unit cause sinus tachycardia. A few of these include aminophylline, dopamine, hydralazine, nitroglycerin, epinephrine, and atropine.

PHYSIOLOGY: Tachycardia is detrimental to anyone with ischemic heart disease. The rapid heart rate shortens the time for ventricular filling, decreasing both stroke volume and cardiac output. This occurrence increases myocardial oxygen demand while decreasing oxygen supply because of decreased coronary artery filling time.

TREATMENT: Treatment varies according to the cause. If the cause of the tachycardia is evident (fever or pain), the cause should be treated rather than treating the heart rate directly. If the problem is cardiac-related, both calcium channel blockers and beta blockers are widely used to decrease rapid heart rates. However, clinical assessment is required before these drugs are administered. Cardiac output (CO) is determined by heart rate and stroke volume. If an injured heart can no longer maintain an adequate stroke volume, the body increases heart rate to maintain CO and supply an adequate blood flow to vital body tissues. If a drug is administered to force the sinus node to slow down and the heart cannot increase stroke volume, severe sudden heart failure can result.

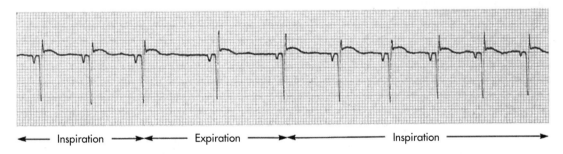

← Inspiration → ← Expiration → ← Inspiration →

Fig. **9-15** Sinus dysrhythmia. Note the increase in heart rate during inspiration and decrease in heart rate during expiration.

RATE: 60 to 100 beats per minute.

RHYTHM: Irregular, rate varying with the respiratory cycle. It increases with inhalation and decreases with exhalation.

QRS COMPLEX: Same as with NSR. Narrow complex QRS.

ETIOLOGY: Normal variant. Also frequently called sinus arrhythmia.

TREATMENT: None required.

P WAVE: Present, all the same shape, with only one preceding each QRS complex.

PR INTERVAL: 0.12 to 0.20 of a second.

QRS DURATION: 0.06 to 0.10 of a second.

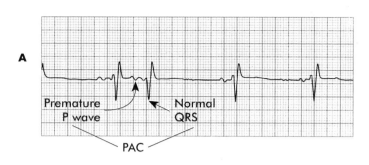

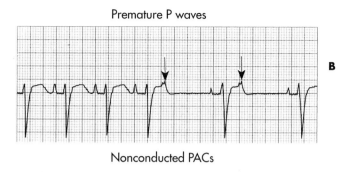

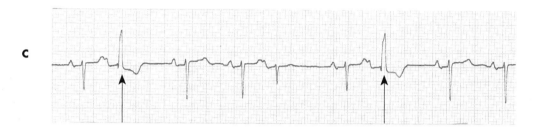

Fig. **9-16** Premature atrial contraction (PAC).

RATE: Determined by underlying rhythm, which is usually sinus related.

RHYTHM: Variable. Underlying rhythm may be regular, but PACs create irregularity.

P WAVE: Present, different shape from other P waves, may be inverted. The early P wave may be buried in the preceding T wave.

PR INTERVAL: 0.12 to 0.20 of a second. The PR interval may be longer, shorter, or the same as the PR interval of a sinus beat.

QRS DURATION: 0.06 to 0.10 of a second.

QRS COMPLEX: The QRS usually has a normal appearance because conduction through the AV node and ventricular conduction system is normal (Strip **A**). However, there are exceptions, as shown in Strip **C**.

ETIOLOGY: Can occur normally. Often accentuated by emotional disturbances, caffeine, nicotine, digitalis, mitral valve prolapse, and heart failure.

PHYSIOLOGY: The PAC originates from an ectopic focus in the atria, somewhere other than the sinus node. The ectopic impulse occurs prematurely before the normal sinus impulse is due to occur.

   a. Usually the premature P wave initiates a normal QRS complex (Strip **A**).
   b. If the beat is so early that the AV node remains refractory to stimuli, a pause as a result of a nonconducted PAC is seen (Strip **B**).
   c. Occasionally the early ectopic P wave can be conducted through the AV node, but part of this conduction pathway through the ventricles is blocked. On the ECG, this will appear as an early, abnormal P wave, followed by an abnormally wide QRS (Strip **C**). This is termed *aberrant conduction*.

TREATMENT: None if infrequent. If frequent and the patient is symptomatic, treat the cause. For example, reduce stress, eliminate caffeine and nicotine, modify digitalis dosage, and treat symptoms of heart failure.

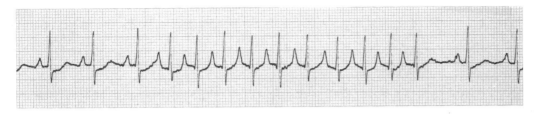

Fig. **9-17** Paroxysmal supraventricular tachycardia (PSVT). Note that the atrial rate during the tachycardia is 158 beats per minute. The run starts and stops abruptly.

RATE: Atrial rate 150 to 250 beats per minute.
RHYTHM: Regular.

P WAVE: Present, may have an abnormal shape. Not all P waves may be conducted to the ventricle.
PR INTERVAL: 0.12 to 0.20 of a second.
QRS DURATION: 0.06 to 0.10 of a second.

QRS COMPLEX: The QRS is usually narrow and normal in appearance.
ETIOLOGY: PSVT has causal factors similar to those of PACs, but it has greater clinical significance. *PSVT* refers to the sudden interruption of sinus rhythm by an atrial ectopic focus that fires repetitively and rapidly and is sustained by a reentry or circular movement. It eventually stops as suddenly as it began. *Paroxysmal* means starting and stopping abruptly.
TREATMENT: PSVT usually responds rapidly to medical treatment. IV adenosine is the drug of choice to slow conduction through the AV node and unmask the ectopic P waves; often it will also restore normal sinus rhythm. Other options include vagal maneuvers, calcium channel blockers, digitalis, or cardioversion.

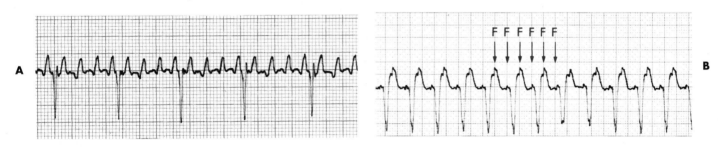

Fig. **9-18** Atrial flutter (AF). **A,** Atrial flutter with 4:1 conduction through the AV node. **B,** Atrial flutter with flutter waves hidden in T waves.

RATE: An atrial rate of 250 to 350 beats per minute. When evaluating the rate of atrial flutter, both the atrial and ventricular rates must be calculated. Usually the atrial rate is faster.
RHYTHM: Regular flutter waves. The ventricular response (QRS complexes) may be regular or irregular.
QRS COMPLEX: QRS shape is usually narrow and normal.
PHYSIOLOGY: Atrial flutter (AF) is believed to be caused by a circular reentry pathway through which the wave of depolarization is continually moving. At this rapid rate, individual P waves form the classic saw-tooth pattern shown in Strip **A.**

P WAVE: Flutter (F) waves.
PR INTERVAL: No longer applies; instead a conduction ratio of P waves to QRS complexes (e.g., 2:1, 3:1, or 4:1) is used. The conduction ratio is clearly visible in Strip **A.** However sometimes the flutter waves are hidden by the QRS complex or T wave as shown in Strip **B.**

TREATMENT: Sometimes it is difficult to identify the flutter waves, especially if the conduction ratio is 2:1. Intravenous adenosine or vagal maneuvers can be useful diagnostic tools to increase briefly the refractory period of the AV node and allow better visualization of the F waves. Vagal maneuvers or IV adenosine terminate atrial flutter. Electrical or pharmacologic cardioversion is usually required to restore sinus rhythm. Type I antidysrhythmic drugs, such as quinidine, procainamide, or disopyramide, cause the flutter waves to become slower but may result in an increase in the ventricular response rate, which may not be well-tolerated.[20] A new class III IV antidysrhythmic agent, Ibutilide, has also shown promise in pharmacologic cardioversion of atrial flutter and atrial fibrillation.[21] If cardioversion is unsuccessful, ventricular rate control can be achieved using digoxin, calcium channel blockers, or beta-adrenergic blockers.

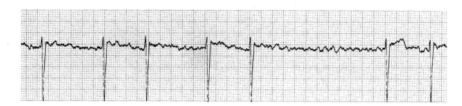

Fig. **9-19** Atrial fibrillation (AF). Note the irregularly irregular ventricular rhythm.

RATE: Atrial: 350-600 fibrillatory waves per minute.
    Ventricular: 60-100 (controlled by medication).
    Greater than 100 (uncontrolled by medication).
RHYTHM: Irregularly irregular ventricular rhythm.

P WAVE: Replaced by fibrillating baseline or waves.
PR INTERVAL: Absent. Replaced by fibrillating baseline.
QRS DURATION: 0.06 to 0.10 of a second.

QRS COMPLEX: The QRS complex is usually normal because the pathway through the ventricles is unchanged once the impulse leaves the AV node.

ETIOLOGY: Small sections of atrial muscle are activated individually, resulting in quivering of the atrial muscle without effective contraction.

PHYSIOLOGY: When numerous sites in the atria fire spontaneously and rapidly, an organized spread of depolarization can no longer take place and atrial fibrillation results. Atrial fibrillation can be either acute or chronic.

TREATMENT: There are two approaches: (1) convert the atrial fibrillation back to sinus rhythm using electrical cardioversion or chemical cardioversion with pharmacologic agents or (2) allow the atrial fibrillation to exist and use pharmacologic measures to control the ventricular response rate. Electrical cardioversion may be successful in converting the rhythm to sinus if attempted within a few days or weeks of the onset of atrial fibrillation. Cardioversion also carries with it the threat of precipitating emboli. During atrial fibrillation the atria do not contract; hence blood may pool in areas of the atrial walls. This pooling can promote thrombus formation (mural thrombi) within the atria. If cardioversion is successful and normal sinus rhythm is restored, the atria again contracts forcibly and, if thrombus formation has occurred, clots may be sent traveling through the pulmonary or systemic circulation. To prevent this, it is recommended that patients who have been in atrial fibrillation for 3 or more days be anticoagulated for 3 weeks before elective cardioversion.[22] Transesophageal echocardiography (TEE) may be helpful in identifying the presence of thrombi in the atria and is sometimes used as a screening tool before elective cardioversion. However, thrombi may be missed or may be transient. Inability to visualize thrombi on the echocardiogram does not negate the need for anticoagulation. Calcium channel blockers, beta-blockers, and digoxin are the most commonly used drugs to control ventricular response rate in atrial fibrillation.

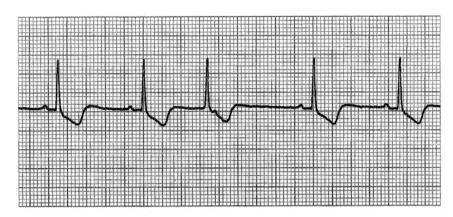

Fig. **9-20** Premature junctional contraction (PJC).

RATE: Depends on the underlying rhythm, usually a NSR.

RHYTHM: On the ECG, the rhythm is regular from the sinus node except for the early QRS complex (PJC) of normal shape and duration.

P WAVE: a. P wave may be entirely absent.
b. P wave may be seen in the T wave.
c. P wave may be inverted with PR interval < 0.12 sec.

PR INTERVAL: Usually absent. The lack of a normal PR interval is a defining characteristic of junctional rhythms.

QRS DURATION: 0.06 to 0.10 of a second.

QRS COMPLEX: The QRS complex is usually narrow and normal.

ETIOLOGY: A PJC is a single ectopic impulse that originates in the AV junctional area.

PHYSIOLOGY: Only certain areas of the AV node have the property of automaticity. The entire area around the AV node is collectively called the *junction;* hence impulses generated there are called *junctional.* After an ectopic impulse arises in the junction, it spreads in two directions at once. One wave of depolarization spreads upward into the atria, depolarizes the atria, and causes a P wave that is usually seen following the QRS. At the same time another wave of depolarization spreads downward into the ventricles through the normal conduction pathway and results in a normal QRS complex.

TREATMENT: Usually none required. PJCs have virtually the same clinical significance as do PACs. However, if the patient is receiving digoxin, digitalis toxicity should at least be suspected. Although digoxin slows conduction through the AV node, it also increases automaticity in the junction.

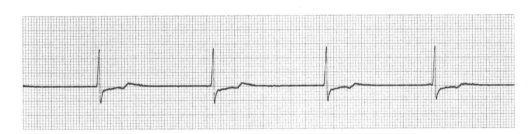

Fig. **9-21** Junctional escape rhythm. The ventricular rate is 38 beats per minute. P waves are absent, and the QRS is normal width.

RATE: Sometimes the junction becomes the dominant pacemaker of the heart. The intrinsic rate of the junction is 40 to 60 beats per minute.

RHYTHM: Regular.

P WAVE: Same as for PJC.
PR INTERVAL: Usually absent.
QRS DURATION: 0.06 to 0.10 of a second.

QRS COMPLEX: QRS complex is usually narrow and normal because the impulse originates above the ventricles.

ETIOLOGY: A junctional escape rhythm originates in the junction following failure of the sinus node.

PHYSIOLOGY: Under normal conditions the junction never has a chance to "escape" and depolarize the heart because it is overridden by the faster sinus node. However, if the sinus node fails, the junction of impulses can depolarize completely and pace the heart. This junctional escape rhythm is a protective mechanism to prevent asystole in the event of sinus node failure.

TREATMENT: Generally a junctional escape rhythm is well tolerated hemodynamically, although efforts should be directed toward restoring sinus rhythm. Sometimes a pacemaker is inserted as a protective measure because of concern that the junction may fail.

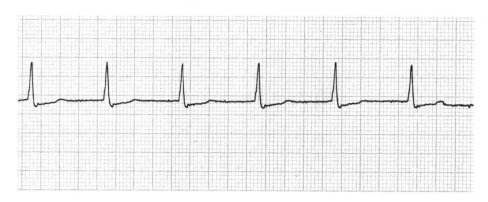

Fig. **9-22** Accelerated junctional rhythm.

RATE: Accelerated junctional rhythm: 60 to 100 bpm.
   Junctional tachycardia: greater than 100 bpm.
RHYTHM: Regular.
QRS COMPLEX: The QRS is usually narrow and normal.

P WAVE: Same as PJC.
PR INTERVAL: Usually absent.
QRS DURATION: 0.06 to 0.10 of a second.

ETIOLOGY: Rapid junctional rhythms originate in the junction. This may indicate irritability in the junctional area caused by AV node ischemia or digitalis toxicity.

PHYSIOLOGY: Accelerated junctional rhythms are usually well tolerated hemodynamically by patients, mainly because the heart rate is within the normal range.

   Junctional tachycardia may not be so well tolerated, depending on patients' tolerance of the rapid rate.

TREATMENT: No treatment if patients have a good blood pressure and no unusual symptoms. If this is a recent rhythm change and patients are on digoxin, digitalis toxicity should be suspected. This is because digoxin enhances automaticity of the AV node. If digitalis toxicity is present, the only treatment is to withhold digoxin until the dysrhythmia resolves.

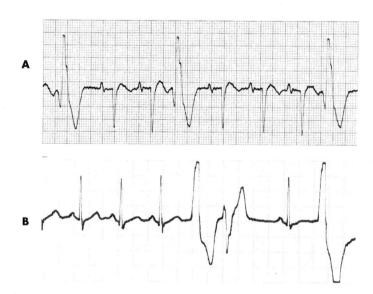

Fig. **9-23** Premature ventricular contraction (PVC). **A,** Unifocal PVCs. **B,** Multifocal PVCs.

RATE: Depends on the underlying heart rate, usually NSR.
RHYTHM: Early QRS complexes interrupt the underlying rhythm.
QRS COMPLEX: The QRS complex is wide, with a bizarre shape.

P WAVE: Absent or following the early QRS complex.
PR INTERVAL: Absent.
QRS DURATION: >0.12 of a second. The prolonged width of the QRS is diagnostic for ventricular ectopy.

UNIFOCAL PVCs: If all of the ventricular ectopic beats look the same in a particular lead, they are called *unifocal PVCs*, which means that they probably all result from the same irritable focus (Strip **A**).

MULTIFOCAL PVCs: If the ventricular ectopics are of various shapes in the same lead, they are called *multifocal PVCs* (Strip **B**). Multifocal PVCs are more serious than unifocal ventricular ectopics because they indicate that a greater area of irritable myocardium is involved, and they are more likely to deteriorate into ventricular tachycardia or fibrillation.

FUSION BEATS: If a ventricular ectopic impulse and the sinus beat meet in the middle of the ventricles, a fusion beat results. Fusion beats are narrower than are the ventricular beats and look like a cross between patient's sinus QRS and the ventricular ectopic QRS.

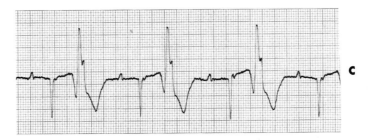

Fig. **9-23—cont'd C,** Ventricular bigemeny.

VENTRICULAR BIGEMENY: When a PVC follows each normal beat, it is called *ventricular bigemeny* (Strip **C**).
COUPLET: Two consecutive PVCs.
TRIPLET: Three consecutive PVCs.

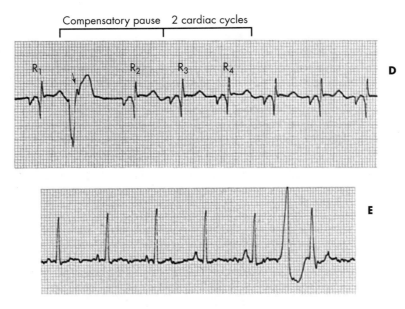

Fig. **9-23—cont'd D,** PVC with a full compensatory pause. **E,** Interpolated PVC.

COMPENSATORY PAUSE: If the interval from the last normal QRS preceding the PVC to the one following the PVC is exactly equal to two complete cardiac cycles, it is called a *compensatory pause* (Strip **D**).
INTERPOLATED PVC: The PVC falls between two normal QRS complexes without disturbing the rhythm. Note that the RR interval between sinus beats remains the same (Strip **E**).
R ON T: If a PVC occurs on the T wave during the relative refractory period (latter half of T wave) when only a part of the muscle is repolarized, individual segments of muscle can depolarize separately from each other, resulting in ventricular fibrillation.
ETIOLOGY: The many causes of PVCs include myocardial ischemia; electrolyte imbalances; hypoxia; acidosis; heart diseases such as cardiomyopathy, ventricular aneurysm, and previous MI; and medications that are prodysrhythmic.
PHYSIOLOGY: Ventricular dysrhythmias result from an ectopic focus in any portion of the ventricular myocardium. The usual conduction pathway through the ventricles is not used, and the wave of depolarization spreads from cell to cell.
DOCUMENTATION: The underlying rhythm must always be described first: for example, "sinus bradycardia with frequent unifocal PVCs" or "atrial fibrillation with occasional multifocal PVCs."
TREATMENT: Not all ventricular ectopy requires treatment. In individuals without significant underlying heart disease, PVCs do not represent an increased risk for sudden death and are considered benign.[23] If possible, the cause of the PVCs should be treated: for example, PVCs caused by hypokalemia and hypomagnesemia are treated by administration of potassium and magnesium. Hypoxia is treated by administration of oxygen, ventilation if required, and correction of acidosis.

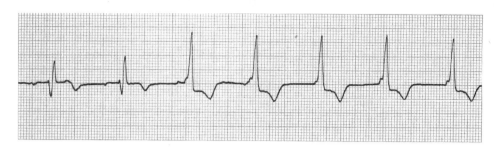

Fig. **9-24** Idioventricular rhythm (IVR) and accelerated idioventricular rhythm (AIVR). The QRS duration is 0.14 second, and the ventricular rate is 65.

RATE: Idioventricular rhythm: 20-40 beats per minute
Accelerated idioventricular rhythm: 40-100 beats per minute
RHYTHM: Regular
QRS COMPLEX: Wide and bizarre because the complexes originate in the ventricles.

P WAVE: Present, but not associated with the QRS complex.
PR INTERVAL: Absent.
QRS DURATION: Greater than 0.12 of a second.

ETIOLOGY: The SA and AV nodes may be damaged by degenerative heart disease or an acute MI or depressed by drug toxicity.

PHYSIOLOGY: At times an ectopic focus in ventricle can be the dominant pacemaker of the heart. If both the SA node and AV junction fail, the ventricles will depolarize at their own intrinsic rate of 20 to 40 times per minute (idioventricular rhythm). When a ventricular focus assumes control of the heart at a rate greater than 100 per minute an accelerated idioventricular rhythm occurs.

TREATMENT: Rather than trying to abolish the ventricular beats, the aim of treatment is to increase the effective heart rate and to reestablish a higher pacing site, such as the SA node or AV junction. The heart rate may be increased pharmacologically with an infusion of isoproteronal (Isuprel). More commonly a transvenous temporary pacemaker is inserted and the heart is paced at a faster rate until the underlying problems that caused failure of faster pacing sites can be resolved. Drugs such as lidocaine are contraindicated in treatment of idioventricular rhythms because if the ventricular ectopic focus is abolished, patients could become asystolic.

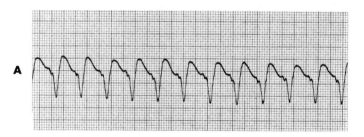

Fig. **9-25 A,** Ventricular tachycardia (VT).

RATE: Greater than 100 beats per minute.
RHYTHM: Mostly regular. May have some irregularities.

P WAVE: P wave is not related to the QRS. In most cases the sinus node is unaffected and will continue to depolarize the atria on schedule. Therefore P waves can sometimes be seen on the ECG tracing. They are not related to the QRS and may even conduct a normal impulse to the ventricles if the timing is just right.
PR INTERVAL: Absent.
QRS DURATION: Greater than 0.12 of a second.

QRS COMPLEX: Wide, with a bizarre shape compared to the sinus QRS (Strip **A**).
NONSUSTAINED VT: Three or more consecutive PVCs, rate greater than 110 beats per minute, lasts less than 30 seconds without hemodynamic collapse, and self-terminates.[24]

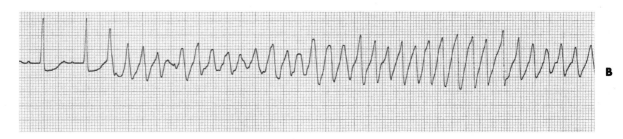

Fig. **9-25, cont'd B,** Torsades de pointes.

TORSADES DE POINTES (twisting of the points): This is a specific form of ventricular tachycardia. Its name refers to the twisting appearance of the VT on the ECG strip (Strip **B**). It may be precipitated by antidysrhythmic drugs that prolong the QT interval and ventricular refractory period. Quinidine is an example of a drug that prolongs the QT interval.
ETIOLOGY: VT may be caused by all of the same factors that cause PVCs, as described in that section; myocardial ischemia, digitalis toxicity, electrolyte disturbances, and as an adverse side effect of certain antidysrhythmic drugs. Some antidysrhythmic drugs can actually cause more serious dysrhythmias than those they were intended to treat.[23]
PHYSIOLOGY: VT results from a repeating ectopic focus in the ventricular myocardium. The usual conduction pathway through the ventricles is bypassed, and the wave of depolarization spreads from cell to cell.
TREATMENT: VT may be treated pharmacologically or with electrical cardioversion or defibrillation.

Acute Sustained VT: If the patient is pulseless, Advanced Cardiac Life Support (ACLS) measures, such as immediate defibrillation, epinephrine, and cardiopulmonary resuscitation (CPR), will be required (see Appendix A). If the patient has a pulse but is unstable (e.g., chest pain, shortness of breath, decreased level of consciousness, or hypotensive). Advanced Cardiac Life Support (ACLS) measures, such as immediate synchronized cardioversion and lidocaine, will be required (see Appendix A). If the patient has a pulse and is stable, Advanced Cardiac Life Support (ACLS) measures, such as lidocaine, procainamide, and bretylium will be required (see Appendix A). If hypoxia, acidosis, electrolyte imbalances, or drug toxicity is the cause, these must also be corrected to prevent the recurrence of the VT.

Chronic VT: Many patients with underlying heart disease from cardiomyopathy or an old myocardial infarction (MI) have frequent PVCs and episodes of VT. Traditionally these dysrhythmias have been treated aggressively with oral antidysrhythmic drugs. However, a landmark clinical study known as the *Cardiac Arrhythmia Suppression Trial (CAST)* suggests that treatment of this ventricular ectopic activity may increase the risk of sudden cardiac death.[23] Another option for treatment of chronic VT is an implantable cardioverter defibrillator (ICD).

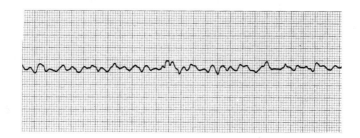

Fig. **9-26** Ventricular fibrillation (VF).

RATE: Indeterminable.
RHYTHM: Irregular, wavy baseline without recognizable QRS complexes.

P WAVE: Absent. Cannot be distinguished from the fibrillating ventricular baseline.
PR INTERVAL: Absent.
QRS DURATION: Absent. No QRS complexes are present.

QRS COMPLEX: The normal QRS is missing. In VF the ECG appears as a wavy baseline. Sometimes VF is described as "coarse" or "fine." Coarse VF is seen on the ECG as large, erratic undulations of the baseline, whereas in fine VF the ECG baseline exhibits only a mild tremor. In either case, patients have no pulse, no blood pressure, and are unconscious.
ETIOLOGY: VT is the most common precursor of VF. Therefore all of the factors that predispose patients to VT apply.
PHYSIOLOGY: Ventricular fibrillation is the result of electrical impulses from single or multiple foci in the ventricles that prevent the ventricles from contracting. The ventricles merely quiver, and there is no forward flow of blood.
TREATMENT: Defibrillation is the emergency treatment of choice. See Appendix A for Advanced Cardiac Life Support (ACLS) guidelines. Epinephrine may be used to try to change fine VF to coarse VF and facilitate defibrillation attempts. Antidysrhythmic drugs such as intravenous lidocaine and bretylium are also given if initial attempts at defibrillation fail. As with any cardiac arrest situation, supportive measures such as CPR, intubation, and correction of metabolic abnormalities are performed concurrently with definitive therapy.

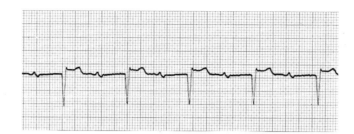

Fig. **9-27** First-degree AV block. The PR interval is prolonged to 0.44 second.

RATE: Depends on the underlying rhythm, usually normal sinus rhythm.

RHYTHM: Regular if NSR.

QRS COMPLEX: Unaffected by first-degree AV block.

P WAVE: Present, normal shape.

PR INTERVAL: Greater than 0.20 of a second.

QRS DURATION: 0.06 to 0.10 of a second.

ETIOLOGY: All atrial impulses that should be conducted to the ventricles are conducted, but the PR interval is prolonged.

TREATMENT: None required. Many older patients have first-degree AV block as a chronic condition associated with aging of the AV junction.

Acute MI: Patients with an acute MI should be monitored for degeneration into more serious forms of AV block.

Drug side effect: If the development of first-degree AV block is new and related to recent antidysrhythmic drug administration, the medication regimen must be evaluated.

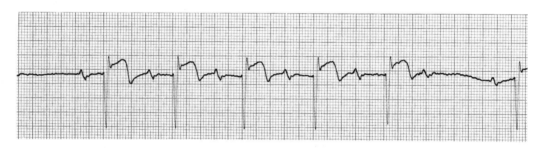

Fig. **9-28** Second-degree AV block, type I (Mobitz I or Wenckebach). Note that PR intervals gradually increase from 0.36 to 0.46 second until finally a P wave is not conducted to the ventricles.

RATE: *Atrial:* Depends on the underlying sinus rate.

Ventricular: Depends on the P wave to QRS ratio.

RHYTHM: Regular, irregular pattern. P waves will be regular. As part of the Mobitz I pattern the R to R intervals become progressively shorter until the sinus P wave is not conducted. This causes a pause. After the pause the cycle repeats itself.

QRS COMPLEX: The conducted QRS complexes are normal.

P WAVE: Normal shape.

PR INTERVAL: The PR intervals progressively lengthen until a P wave is not conducted to the ventricles and is therefore not followed by a QRS.

QRS DURATION: 0.06 to 0.10 of a second.

ETIOLOGY: In Mobitz I block the anatomic site of the block is at the level of the AV node. If it is associated with an acute inferior wall MI, the block is caused by ischemia and is usually transient.

PHYSIOLOGY: In Mobitz I block the AV conduction time progressively lengthens until a P wave is not conducted to the ventricles.

DOCUMENTATION: The P wave to QRS complex ratio is documented. For example, if four P waves are conducted to the ventricles and the fifth one is not, a 5:4 conduction ratio is present (five P waves to four QRS complexes).

TREATMENT: No treatment is required if the ventricular rate is sufficient to sustain hemodynamic stability. In certain clinical conditions, such as an acute MI, the possibility of progression to a more serious conduction disturbance exists, and patients are closely monitored. If hemodynamic compromise is present or deemed likely, a temporary transvenous pacemaker may be inserted.

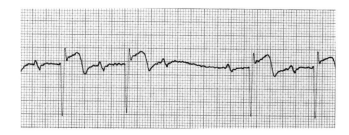

Fig. **9-29** Second-degree AV block, type II (Mobitz II). PR intervals of the conducted beats remain constant.

RATE: *Atrial:* Usually 60-100 range.
    Ventricular: The ventricular rate is slower and depends upon the number of conducted P waves.
RHYTHM: *Regular:* If the AV node conducts every second or third P wave in a consistent pattern.
    Irregular: If the P waves are conducted irregularly.
QRS COMPLEX: May be narrow and normal or widened due to a coexisting BBB.
ETIOLOGY: Usually Mobitz II indicates block below the AV node, either in the His bundle or in both bundle branches. It most frequently occurs when one bundle branch is blocked and the other is ischemic. Mobitz II block is more ominous clinically than Mobitz I and often progresses to complete AV block.
PHYSIOLOGY: Mobitz II block occurs in the presence of a long absolute refractory period with virtually no relative refractory period. This results in an "all or nothing" situation. Sinus P waves may be conducted. When conduction does occur, all PR intervals are the same.
TREATMENT: Mobitz II can be serious and often precedes complete AV block. Use of a temporary transvenous pacemaker is usually necessary, but its insertion can be elective if patients remain hemodynamically stable.

P WAVE: Normal in shape. There are more P waves than QRS complexes.
PR INTERVAL: 0.12 to 0.20 of a second. The PR interval is constant for the P waves that conduct to the ventricles.
QRS DURATION: 0.06 to 0.10 of a second. Will be wider if a bundle branch block (BBB) is present.

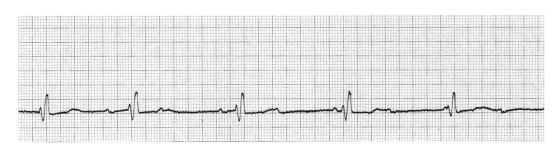

Fig. **9-30** Third-degree AV block with ventricular escape pacemaker (QRS >0.10)

RATE: Depends on underlying rhythm.
RHYTHM: Usually regular.

QRS COMPLEX: *Junctional focus:* If a junctional focus is pacing the heart, the QRS complex looks normal but is not related to the P waves.
    Ventricular focus: If a ventricular focus is pacing the heart, the QRS complex is wide and unrelated to the P waves.
ETIOLOGY: Degeneration of the AV node caused by underlying heart disease or an acute MI Blockage of the AV node is a side effect of some antidysrhythmic drugs.
PHYSIOLOGY: In third-degree, or complete, AV block, no atrial impulses can conduct through the AV node to cause ventricular depolarization. The opportunity for conduction is optimal but does not occur. Ideally a junctional or ventricular focus depolarizes spontaneously at its intrinsic rate of 20 to 60 beats per minute and ventricular contraction continues. If not, asystole occurs, the pulse stops, and death results if intervention is not immediate.
TREATMENT: Complete heart block almost always requires use of a pacemaker. If patients are hemodynamically unstable, an external pacemaker can be used to maintain an adequate ventricular rate until a temporary transvenous pacemaker can be inserted.

P WAVE: Normal shape.
PR INTERVAL: P waves are not related to the QRS complexes, so the PR intervals will vary widely.
QRS DURATION: Greater than 0.10 of a second.

erly for obtaining specific leads, selecting the optimal lead for monitoring based on the patient's clinical situation, and documenting significant changes in the patient's rhythm.[18]

Hemodynamic Monitoring

The range of medical diagnoses for which hemodynamic monitoring can be used is enormous. Arterial pressure monitoring is recommended for patients who require continuous blood pressure monitoring because of hemodynamic instability or titration of vasoactive drugs and for patients in whom noninvasive blood pressure monitoring is inadvisable because of extensive burns or in low cardiac output states. Patients who require frequent arterial blood gases are also candidates for arterial pressure monitoring.[25] Pulmonary artery (PA) pressure monitoring is recommended for patients who may experience complications after an acute myocardial infarction or cardiac surgery, for differentiating shock states, and for assessing hemodynamic instability. Patients in chronic heart failure may also require PA pressure monitoring to evaluate the effectiveness of their medical therapy.[26] Table 9-6 describe the different data points that can obtained using hemodynamic monitoring.

Equipment

A hemodynamic monitoring system has four component (Fig. 9-31): (1) the invasive catheter in the patient and the high pressure tubing connecting the patient and the transducer; (2) the transducer, which receives the physiologic signal from the catheter and tubing and converts it into electrical energy; (3) the flush system, which maintains catheter patency of the fluid-filled system; and (4) the bedside monitor containing the amplifier/recorder, which increases the volume of the electrical signal and displays it on an oscilloscope and on a digital scale in millimeters of mercury (mm Hg). Although many different invasive catheters are inserted to monitor hemodynamic pressures, all catheters are connected to similar equipment. This consists of a bag of 0.9% normal saline solution, which may contain 1 unit of heparin (range 0.25 to 2 units per milliliter of saline depending on the institutional protocol). A 300 mm Hg pressure infusion cuff, IV tubing, three-way stopcocks, and an in-line flow device for both continuous fluid infusion and manual flush are also attached. The high pressure tubing connects the invasive catheter to the transducer to prevent damping (flattening) of the waveform. The most commonly used transducers are disposable, use a silicon chip, and are highly accurate.[25]

Accuracy

The accuracy of hemodynamic pressure readings depends on several factors: (1) ensuring the air-fluid interface of the pressure monitoring system is level with the patient's phlebostatic axis; (2) zeroing the transducer to atmospheric pressure; (3) evaluating the dynamic response of the pressure system via the fast flush square wave test; and (4) positioning the patient.[26]

Leveling. Leveling aligns the transducer with the tip of catheter, thus eliminating the effect of hydrostatic pressure on the pressure monitoring system. This is accomplished by leveling the air-fluid interface of the pressure monitoring (the stopcock that is opened to air when zeroing the system) to the patient's phlebostatic axis. The phlebostatic axis is a physical reference point on the chest located at the fourth intercostal space midpoint between the anterior and posterior chest[26] (see Fig. 9-31). Error in measurement can occur if the transducer is placed below the phlebostatic axis because the fluid in the system will weigh on the transducer (hydrostatic pressure) and produce a false high reading. For every inch the transducer is below the tip of the catheter, the fluid pressure in the system increases the measurement by 1.87 mm Hg.[27] For example, if the transducer is positioned 6 inches below the tip of the catheter, this falsely elevates the displayed pressure by 11 mm Hg. If the transducer is placed above this atrial level, gravity and lack of fluid pressure will give an erroneously low reading. Once again, for every inch the transducer is positioned above the catheter tip, the measurement is 1.87 mm Hg less than the true value.[27]

Zeroing. Zeroing equilibrates the pressure monitoring system to atmospheric pressure. This is accomplished by turning the three-way stopcock nearest to the transducer (air-fluid interface) to open the transducer to air (atmospheric pressure) and to close it to the patient and the flush system.[26] The monitor is adjusted so that "0" is displayed, which equals atmospheric pressure. Atmospheric pressure is not actually "0"—it is 760 mm Hg at sea level. Using "0" to represent current atmospheric pressure provides a convenient baseline for hemodynamic measurement purposes.[28] Disposable transducers are now so accurate that once they are calibrated to atmospheric pressure, drift from the zero baseline is minimal.[28] While in theory this means that repeated calibration is unnecessary, clinical protocols in most units require the nurse to calibrate the transducer at the beginning of each shift.

Fast-flush square wave test. The monitoring system dynamic response can be checked at the bedside by performing the fast-flush square wave, or frequency response, test. This test involves use of the manual flush system on the transducer. Normally the flush device allows only 3 ml of fluid/hour. With the normal waveform displayed, the manual fast-flush is used to generate a rapid increase in pressure, which is displayed on the monitor oscilloscope. As shown in Fig. 9-32, the normal dynamic response waveform shows a square pattern with one or two oscillations before the return of the waveform. If the system is overdamped, a sloped—rather than square—pattern is seen. If the system is underdamped, there are additional oscillations—or vibrations—seen on the fast-flush square wave test. This test can be performed for any hemodynamic monitoring system.[29]

TABLE 9-6

HEMODYNAMIC PRESSURES AND CALCULATED HEMODYNAMIC VALUES

HEMODYNAMIC PRESSURE	DEFINITION AND EXPLANATION	NORMAL RANGE*
Mean arterial pressure (MAP)	Average perfusion pressure created by arterial blood pressure during the cardiac cycle. The normal cardiac cycle is one third systole and two thirds diastole. These three components are divided by 3 to obtain the average perfusion pressure for the whole cardiac cycle.	70-100 mm Hg
Central venous pressure (CVP)	Pressure created by volume in the right side of the heart. When the tricuspid valve is open, the CVP reflects filling pressures in the right ventricle. Clinically, the CVP is often used as a guide to overall fluid balance.	2-5 mm Hg 3-8 cm water (H_2O)
Pulmonary artery pressure (PAP) (PA systolic [PAS], PA diastolic [PAD], PA mean [PAM])	Pulsatile pressure in the pulmonary artery, measured by an indwelling catheter.	PAS 20-30 mm Hg PAD 5-10 mm Hg PAM 10-15 mm Hg
Pulmonary artery wedge pressure (PAWP)	Pressure created by volume in the left side of the heart. When the mitral valve is open, the PAWP reflects filling pressures in the pulmonary vasculature, and pressures in the left side of the heart are transmitted back to the catheter "wedged" into a small pulmonary arteriole.	5-12 mm Hg
Cardiac output (CO)	The amount of blood pumped out by a ventricle. Clinically, it can be measured using the thermodilution CO method, which calculates CO in liters per minute (L/min).	4-6 L/min (at rest)
Cardiac index (CI)	CO divided by body surface area (BSA), tailoring the CO to individual body size. A BSA conversion chart is necessary to calculate CI, which is considered more accurate than CO because it is individualized to height and weight. CI is measured in liters per minute per square meter BSA ($L/min/m^2$).	2.2-4.0 $L/min/m^2$
Stroke volume (SV)	Amount of blood ejected by the ventricle with each heartbeat. Hemodynamic monitoring systems calculate SV by dividing cardiac output (CO in L/min) by the heart rate (HR) then multiplying the answer by 1000 to change liters to milliliters (ml).	60-130 mL/beat
Stroke volume index (SI)	SV indexed to BSA.	40-50 ml/m^2
Systemic vascular resistance (SVR)	Mean pressure difference across the systemic vascular bed, divided by blood flow. Clinically, SVR represents the resistance against which the left ventricle must pump to eject its volume. This resistance is created by the systemic arteries and arterioles. As SVR increases, CO falls. SVR is measured in either units or $dynes/sec/cm^{-5}$. If the number of units is multiplied by 80, the value is converted to $dynes/sec/cm^{-5}$.	10-18 units or 800-1400 $dynes/sec/cm^{-5}$
Pulmonary vascular resistance (PVR)	Mean pressure difference across pulmonary vascular bed, divided by blood flow. Clinically, PVR represents the resistance against which the right ventricle must pump to eject its volume. This resistance is created by the pulmonary arteries and arterioles. As PVR increases, the output from the right ventricle decreases. PVR is measured in either units or $dynes/sec/cm^{-5}$. PVR is normally one sixth of SVR.	1.2-3.0 units or 100-250 $dynes/sec/cm^{-5}$
Left ventricular stroke work index (LVSWI)	Amount of work the left ventricle performs with *each heartbeat*. The hemodynamic formula represents pressure generated (MAP) multiplied by volume pumped (SV). A conversion factor is used to change ml/mm Hg to gram-meter (g-m). LVSWI is always represented as an indexed volume. LVSWI increases or decreases because of changes in either pressure (MAP) or volume pumped (SV).	50-62 $g\text{-}m/m^2$
Right ventricular stroke work index (RVSWI)	Amount of work the right ventricle does *each heartbeat*. The hemodynamic formula represents pressure generated (PAP mean) multiplied by volume pumped (SV). A conversion factor is used to change mm Hg to gram-meter (g-m). RVSWI is always represented as an indexed value (BSA chart). Similar to LVSWI, the RVSWI increases or decreases because of changes in either pressure (PAP mean) or volume pumped (SV).	7.9-9.7 $g\text{-}m/m^2$

*The formulas for these hemodynamic values are listed in Appendix B.

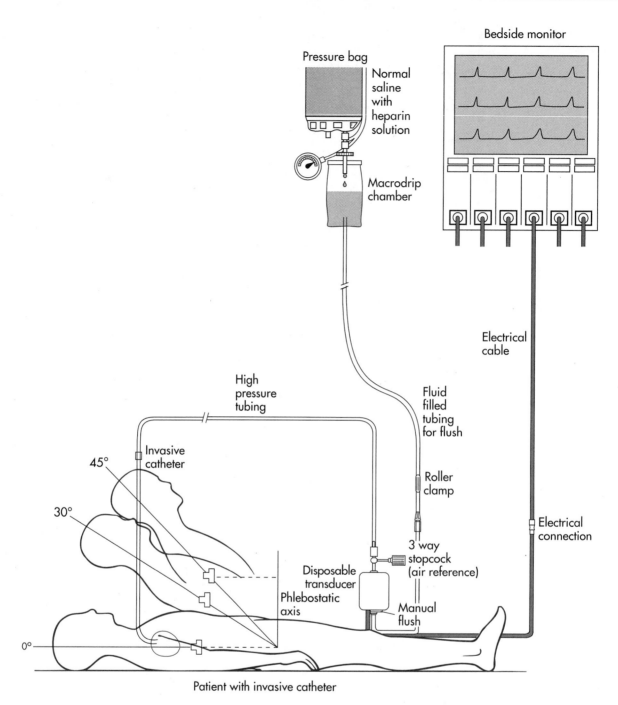

Fig. **9-31** The four parts of a hemodynamic monitoring are invasive catheter attached to high pressure tubing to connect to the transducer, transducer, flush system including a manual flush, and bedside monitor.

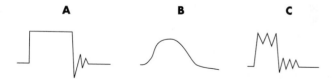

Fig. **9-32** Fast-flush square wave test. **A,** Normal system dynamic response. **B,** System overdamped. **C,** System underdamped.

Patient position. Checking patient position in hemodynamic monitoring would not be an issue if critical care patients always laid flat and supine in bed. However, this is not a comfortable position, especially if the patient is alert, or if the head of the bed needs to be elevated to decrease the work of breathing. Nurse researchers have determined that the central venous pressure (CVP), PA pressures, and pulmonary artery wedge pressure (PAWP) can be reliably measured at head-of-bed positions from 0 (flat) to 60 degrees if the patient is lying on his or her back.[30-33]

In general, if the patient is normovolemic and hemodynamically stable, raising the head of the bed does not affect hemodynamic pressure measurements. If the patient is so hemodynamically unstable or hypovolemic that raising the head of the bed negatively affects intravascular volume distribution, correcting the hemodynamic instability and leaving the patient in a supine position is the first priority. In summary, the majority of patients do not need the head of the bed to be lowered to "0" to obtain accurate CVP, PAP, or PAWP readings. However, there is no such agreement if patients are turned to the side in the lateral position. This is mainly because it is difficult to identify the true phlebostatic axis in this position and also because of the position of the heart in the left chest. Currently, measurements taken in the lateral position are not considered as accurate as measurements taken when the patient is lying on his or her back.[30,33]

Troubleshooting

Table 9-7 outlines common problems with hemodynamic monitoring systems and how to troubleshoot them.

Intraarterial blood pressure monitoring

Intraarterial blood pressure monitoring is indicated for any major medical or surgical condition that compromises cardiac output, tissue perfusion, or fluid volume status. The system is designed for continuous measurement of three blood pressure parameters—systole, diastole, and mean arterial blood pressure (MAP). In addition, the direct arterial access is helpful in the management of patients with acute respiratory failure who require frequent arterial blood gas (ABG) measurements.

Catheters. The size of the catheter used is proportionate to the diameter of the cannulated artery. In small arteries—such as the radial and dorsalis pedis—a 20-gauge, 3.8 to 5.1 cm, nontapered Teflon catheter is most often used. For larger femoral or axillary arteries, a 19- or 20-gauge, 16 cm, Teflon catheter is used. Teflon catheters are preferred because of their lower risk of causing thrombosis. The catheter insertion is usually percutaneous, although the technique varies with vessel size. Cannulas are most often inserted in the smaller arteries, using a "catheter-over-needle" unit in which the needle is used as a temporary guide for catheter placement. With this method, once the unit has been inserted into the artery, the needle is withdrawn, leaving the supple plastic cannula in place. Insertion of a cannula into a larger artery usually necessitates use of the Seldinger technique. This procedure involves (1) entry into the artery using a needle, (2) passage of a supple guidewire through the needle into the artery, (3) removal of the needle, (4) passage of the catheter over the guidewire, and (5) removal of the guidewire, leaving the cannula in the artery. If a cannula cannot be inserted into the artery using percutaneous methods, an arterial cutdown may be performed. This procedure is avoided if possible because it involves a skin incision to expose the artery directly and is associated with a higher risk of infection.

Monitoring sites. Several major peripheral arteries are suitable for receiving a cannula and for long-term hemodynamic monitoring. The most frequently used site is the radial artery. If this artery is not available, the femoral, dorsalis pedis, axillary, or brachial arteries may be used. The major advantage of the radial artery is that collateral circulation to the hand is provided by the ulnar artery and palmar arch in most of the population; thus there are other avenues of circulation if the radial artery becomes blocked after catheter placement. Before radial artery cannulation, collateral circulation must be assessed, either by using the Doppler flowmeter or by the Allen test. In the Allen test the radial and ulnar arteries are compressed simultaneously. The patient is asked to clench and unclench the hand until it blanches. One of the arteries is then released, and the hand should immediately flush from that side. The same procedure is repeated for the remaining artery.[25]

Clinical physiology. Intraarterial blood pressure monitoring is designed for continuous assessment of arterial perfusion to the major organ systems of the body. Mean arterial pressure (MAP) is the clinical parameter most frequently used to assess perfusion because MAP represents perfusion pressure throughout the cardiac cycle. Because one third of the cardiac cycle is spent in systole and two thirds in diastole, the MAP calculation must reflect the greater amount of time spent in diastole. The formula for calculating MAP is [(Diastole × 2) + Systole] ÷ 3 (thus a blood pressure of 120/60 mm Hg produces a MAP of 80 mm Hg). However, the bedside hemodynamic monitor may show a slightly different digital number because most computers calculate the area under the curve of the arterial line tracing. A MAP greater than 60 mm Hg is necessary to perfuse the coronary arteries, brain, and kidneys. Systolic and diastolic pressures are monitored in conjunction with the MAP as a further guide to the accuracy of perfusion. Should cardiac output decrease, the body compensates by constricting peripheral vessels to maintain the blood pressure. In this situation, the MAP may remain constant, but the pulse pressure (difference between systolic and diastolic pressures) narrows.

Arterial pressure waveform interpretation. As the aortic valve opens, blood is ejected from the left ventricle and is recorded as an increase of pressure in the arterial system (Fig. 9-33). The highest point recorded is called *systole*. After peak ejection (systole), force is decreased and pressure drops. A notch (the dicrotic notch) may be visible on the downstroke of this arterial waveform, representing closure of the aortic valve. The dicrotic notch signifies the beginning of diastole. The remainder of the downstroke represents diastolic runoff of blood flow into the arterial tree. The lowest point recorded is called *diastole*.[25] Note that electrical stimulation (QRS) is always first and that the arterial pressure tracing follows the initiating QRS.

TABLE 9-7

TROUBLESHOOTING PROBLEMS WITH HEMODYNAMIC MONITORING EQUIPMENT

PROBLEM	PREVENTION	RATIONALE	TROUBLESHOOTING
Overdamping of waveform	Provide continuous infusion of solution containing heparin through an in-line flush device (1 unit of heparin for each millimeter of flush solution).	To ensure that recorded pressures and waveform are accurate because a damped waveform gives inaccurate readings.	Before insertion, completely flush the line and/or catheter. In a line attached to a patient, back flush through the system to clear bubbles from tubing or transducer.
Underdamping, ("overshoot" or "fling")	Use short lengths of noncompliant tubing. Use fast-flush square wave test to demonstrate optimal system damping. Verify arterial waveform accuracy with the cuff blood pressure.	If the monitoring system is underdamped, both the systolic and diastolic values will be overestimated by both the waveform and the digital values. False high systolic values may lead to clinical decisions based on erroneous data.	Perform the fast-flush square wave test to verify optimal damping of the monitoring system.
Clot formation at end of catheter	Provide continuous infusion of solution containing heparin through an in-line flush device (1 unit of heparin for each millimeter of flush solution).	Any foreign object placed in the body can cause local activation of the patient's coagulation system as a normal defense mechanism. The clots that are formed may be dangerous if they break off and travel to other parts of the body.	If a clot in the catheter is suspected because of a damped waveform or resistance to forward flush of the system, gently aspirate the line using a small syringe inserted into the proximal stopcock. Then flush the line again once the clot is removed and inspect the waveform. It should return to a normal pattern.
Hemorrhage	Use Luer-Lok (screw) connections in line setup. Close and cap stopcocks when not in use.	A loose connection or open stopcock creates a low-pressure sump effect, causing blood to back into the line and into the open air.	Once a blood leak is recognized, tighten all connections, flush the line, and estimate blood loss.
	Ensure that the catheter is either sutured or securely taped in position.	If a catheter is accidentally removed, the vessel can bleed profusely, especially with an arterial line or if the patient has abnormal coagulation factors (resulting from heparin in the line) or has hypertension.	If the catheter has been inadvertently removed, put pressure on the cannulation site. When bleeding has stopped, apply a sterile dressing, estimate blood loss, and inform the physician. If the patient is restless, an armboard may protect lines inserted in the arm.
Air emboli	Ensure that all air bubbles are purged from a new line setup before attachment to an indwelling catheter.	Air can be introduced at several times, including when central venous pressure (CVP) tubing comes apart, when a new line setup is attached, or when a new CVP or pulmonary artery (PA) line is inserted. During insertion of a CVP or PA line, the patient may be asked to hold his or her breath at specific times to prevent drawing air into the chest during inhalation.	Because it is impossible to get the air back once it has been introduced into the blood stream, prevention is the best cure.

Central venous pressure monitoring

Central venous pressure (CVP) monitoring is indicated whenever a patient has significant alteration in fluid volume. The CVP can be used as a guide in fluid volume replacement in hypovolemia and to assess the impact of diuresis after diuretic administration in the case of fluid overload. In addition, when a major IV line is required for volume replacement, a central venous line is a good choice because large volumes of fluid can easily be delivered. To take CVP measurements the clinician can choose from two methods: either a mercury (mm Hg) system, using a transducer

TABLE **9-7**

TROUBLESHOOTING PROBLEMS WITH HEMODYNAMIC MONITORING EQUIPMENT—cont'd

PROBLEM	PREVENTION	RATIONALE	TROUBLESHOOTING
Air emboli—cont'd	Ensure that the drip chamber from the bag of flush solution is more than half full before using the in-line, fast-flush system. Some sources recommend removing all air from the bag of flush solution before assembling the system.	The in-line, fast-flush devices are designed to permit clearing of blood from the line after withdrawal of blood samples. If the chamber of the IV tubing is too low or empty, the rapid flow of fluid will create turbulence and cause flushing of air bubbles into the system and into the bloodstream.	If any air bubbles are noted, they must be vented through the in-line stopcocks and the drip chamber must be filled. The left atrial pressure (LAP) line setup is the only system that includes an air filter specifically designed to prevent air emboli.
Normal waveform with *low* digital pressure	Ensure that the system is calibrated to atmospheric pressure. Ensure that the transducer is placed at the level of the phlebostatic axis.	To provide a 0 baseline relative to atmospheric pressure. If the transducer has been placed *higher* than the phlebostatic level, gravity and the lack of hydrostatic pressure will produce a false *low* reading.	Recalibrate the equipment if transducer drift has occurred. Reposition the transducer at the level of the phlebostatic axis. Misplacement can occur if the patient moves from the bed to the chair or if the bed is placed in a Trendelenburg position.
Normal waveform with *high* digital pressure	Ensure that the system is calibrated to atmospheric pressure. Ensure that the transducer is placed at the level of the phlebostatic axis.	To provide a 0 baseline relative to atmospheric pressure. If the transducer has been placed *lower* than the phlebostatic level, the weight of hydrostatic pressure on the transducer will produce a false *high* reading.	Recalibrate the equipment if transducer drift has occurred. Reposition the transducer at the level of the phlebostatic axis. Misplacement can occur if the head of the bed was raised and the transducer was not repositioned. Some centers require attachment of the transducer to the patient's chest to avoid this problem.
Loss of waveform	Always have the hemodynamic waveform monitored so that changes or loss can be quickly noted.	The catheter may be kinked, or a stopcock may be turned off.	Check the line setup to ensure that all stopcocks are turned to the correct position and that the tubing is not kinked. Sometimes the catheter migrates against a vessel wall, and having the patient change position restores the waveform.

and a hemodynamic monitor, or a water (cm H_2O) manometer system. If a patient changes from one system to the other, the CVP value will also change because mercury is heavier than water and 1 mm Hg is equal to 1.36 cm H_2O. To convert water to mercury, the water value is divided by 1.36 ($H_2O \div 1.36$). To convert mercury to water, the mercury value is multiplied by 1.36 (mm Hg × 1.36).[34]

Catheters. CVP catheters are available as single-, double-, or triple-lumen infusion catheters, depending on the specific needs of the patient. They are made from polyvinyl chloride and are very soft and flexible.

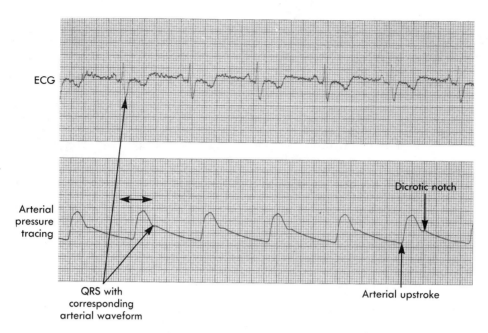

Fig. **9-33** Simultaneous ECG and normal arterial pressure tracing.

Insertion. The large veins of the upper thorax (subclavian [SC] or internal jugular [IJ]) are most commonly used for percutaneous CVP line insertion. During insertion using the SC or IJ veins, the patient may be placed in a Trendelenburg position. Placing the head in a dependent position causes the internal jugular veins in the neck to become more prominent, facilitating line placement. To minimize the risk of air embolus during the procedure, the patient may be asked to "take a deep breath and hold it" any time the needle or catheter is open to air. The tip of the catheter is designed to remain in the vena cava and should not migrate into the right atrium. If the IJ or SC veins are not available, the femoral veins can be used for CVP access. The femoral veins are further away from the heart, so for accurate measurement the tip of the catheter must be advanced into the inferior vena cava near the right atrium.[35] Because many patients are awake and alert when a CVP catheter is inserted, a brief explanation about the procedure will minimize patient anxiety and result in cooperation during the insertion. This cooperation is important because insertion is a sterile procedure and because the supine or Trendelenburg position may not be comfortable for many patients. After CVP catheter placement, a chest radiograph is obtained to verify placement and the absence of an iatrogenic hemothorax or pneumothorax. Other suitable insertion sites include the femoral and antecubital fossae veins. In the rare case that it is not possible to insert a CVP catheter percutaneously, a surgical cutdown may be performed.

Clinical physiology. The CVP catheter is used to measure the filling pressures of the right side of the heart. During diastole, when the tricuspid valve is open and blood is flowing from the right atrium to the right ventricle, the CVP accurately reflects right ventricular end-diastolic pressure (RVEDP). The normal CVP is 2 to 5 mm Hg (3 to 8 cm H_2O).[34]

A low CVP often occurs in the hypovolemic patient and suggests there is insufficient blood volume in the ventricle at end-diastole to produce an adequate stroke volume. Thus to maintain normal cardiac output, the heart rate must increase. This increase produces the tachycardia often observed in hypovolemic states and increases myocardial oxygen demand.

The CVP is used in combination with the MAP and other clinical parameters to assess hemodynamic stability. In the hypovolemic patient, the CVP falls before there is a significant fall in MAP because peripheral vasoconstriction keeps the MAP normal. Thus the CVP is an excellent early warning system for the patient who is bleeding, vasodilating, receiving diuretics, or rewarming after cardiac surgery.

An elevated CVP occurs in cases of fluid overload. To circulate the excess blood volume, the heart must greatly increase its contractile force to move the large volume of blood. This increases the cardiac workload and increases myocardial oxygen consumption. The critical care nurse follows the trend of the CVP measurements to determine subsequent interventions for optimal fluid volume management.

The CVP is not a reliable indicator of left ventricular dysfunction. Left ventricular dysfunction, which can occur after an acute myocardial infarction, increases filling pressures on the left side of the heart. The CVP, because it measures RVEDP, remains normal until the increase in pressure from the left side of the heart is reflected back through the pulmonary vasculature to the right ventricle. In this situation a pulmonary artery catheter that mea-

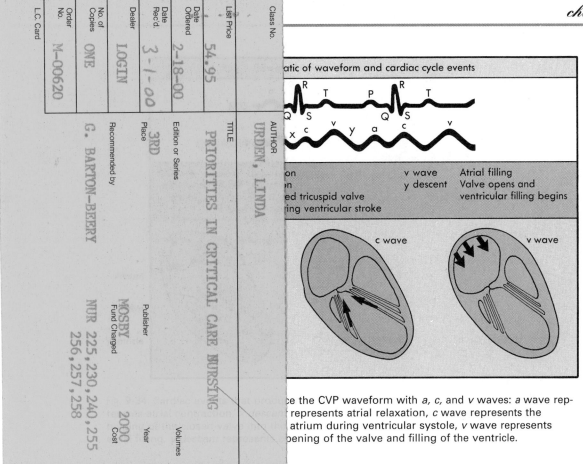

atic of waveform and cardiac cycle events

...ce the CVP waveform with *a*, *c*, and *v* waves: *a* wave represents atrial relaxation, *c* wave represents the ...atrium during ventricular systole, *v* wave represents ...pening of the valve and filling of the ventricle.

sures pressures on the left side of the heart is the monitoring method of choice.

CVP waveform interpretation. The normal CVP waveform has three positive deflections—called *a*, *c*, and *v* waves—that correspond to specific atrial events in the cardiac cycle[36] (Fig. 9-34). The *a* wave reflects atrial contraction and follows the P wave seen on the ECG. The downslope of the *a* wave is called the *x descent* and represents atrial relaxation. The *c* wave reflects the bulging of the closed tricuspid valve into the right atrium during ventricular contraction. The *c* wave is small and not always visible but corresponds to the QRS-T interval on the ECG. The *v* wave represents atrial filling and increased pressure against the closed tricuspid valve in early diastole. The downslope of the *v* wave is named the *y descent* and represents the fall in pressure as the tricuspid valve opens and blood flows from the right atrium to the right ventricle.

Pulmonary artery pressure monitoring

When specific hemodynamic and intracardiac data are required for diagnostic and treatment purposes, a thermodilution PA catheter may be inserted. A significant advantage of the PA catheter over the previously described methods of monitoring is that it simultaneously assesses several hemodynamic parameters, including right atrial pressure (RAP); PA systolic (S), diastolic (D), and mean (M) pressures; and the PAWP; and includes the capability of measuring cardiac output and of calculating additional hemodynamic parameters.[37]

Catheters. The traditional pulmonary artery (PA) catheter has four lumens for measurement of RAP, PA pressures, PAWP, and CO (Fig. 9-35, *A*). Multifunction catheters may have additional lumens, which can be used for IV infusion (Fig. 9-35, *B*), to measure continuous mixed venous oxygen saturation (SvO$_2$), right ventricular volume, continuous cardiac output, or to pace the heart using transvenous pacing electrodes.[38]

The PA catheter is 110 cm in length and is made of polyvinyl chloride. This supple material is ideal for flow-directional catheters. The most commonly used size is 7.5 or 8.0 Fr, although 5.0 and 7.0 Fr sizes are available. Each of the four lumens exits into the heart at a different point along the catheter length (see Figure 9-35, *A*). The proximal lumen is situated in the right atrium and is used for IV infusion, CVP measurement, withdrawal of venous blood samples, and injection of fluid for CO determinations. This port is often described as the RA or CVP port. The distal lumen is located at the tip of the catheter and is situated in the pulmonary artery; thus, it is referred to as the PA port. It is used to record PA pressures and can be used for withdrawal of blood samples to measure SvO$_2$. The third lumen opens into a latex balloon at the end of the catheter that can be inflated with 0.8 (7 Fr) to 1.5 (7.5 Fr) ml of air. The balloon is inflated during catheter insertion once the catheter reaches the right atrium to assist in forward flow of the catheter and to minimize right ventricular ectopy from the catheter tip. It is also inflated to obtain PAWP measurements when the PA catheter is correctly positioned in the pulmonary artery. The fourth lu-

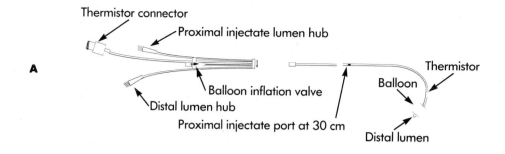

A

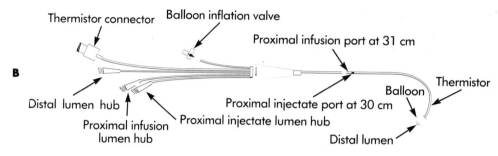

B

Fig. **9-35** Types of pulmonary artery catheters available for clinical use. **A,** Four-lumen catheter. **B,** Five-lumen catheter that includes an additional infusion lumen in the right atrium. (Courtesy Baxter Healthcare Corporation, Edwards Critical Care Division.)

men is a thermistor used to measure changes in blood temperature. It is located 4 cm from the catheter tip and is used to measure thermodilution CO. The connector end of the lumen is attached directly to the CO computer.

Insertion. If a PA catheter is to be inserted into a patient who is awake, a brief explanation about the procedure is helpful to ensure that the patient understands what is going to happen. The initial insertion techniques used for placement of a PA catheter are similar to those described in the section on CVP line insertion. In addition, because the PA catheter is positioned within the heart chambers and the pulmonary artery on the right side of the heart, catheter passage is monitored, using either fluoroscopy or waveform analysis on the bedside monitor. Before inserting the catheter into the vein, the physician—using sterile technique—tests the balloon for inflation and flushes the catheter with normal saline solution to remove any air. The PA catheter is then attached to the bedside hemodynamic line setup and monitor, so that the waveforms can be visualized while the catheter is advanced through the right side of the heart (Fig. 9-36). A larger introducer sheath (8.5 Fr)—which has the tip positioned in the vena cava and an additional IV side-port lumen—is often used to cannulate the vein first. This remains in place, and the supple PA catheter is threaded through the introducer. A sterile plastic sleeve is placed over the outside of the catheter when it is inserted to maintain sterility to the length of catheter that exits from the patient. If the catheter is not in the desired position or if it migrates out of position, the PA catheter can be repositioned.[26]

As the PA catheter is advanced into the right atrium during insertion, a right atrial waveform must be visible

on the monitor (see Figure 9-36). The normal range for RAP is 2 to 5 mm Hg. Before passage through the tricuspid valve, the balloon at the tip of the catheter is inflated for two reasons. First, it cushions the pointed tip of the PA catheter so that if the tip comes into contact with the right ventricular wall, it will cause less myocardial irritability and, consequently, fewer ventricular dysrhythmias. Second, inflation of the balloon assists the catheter to float with the flow of blood from the right ventricle into the pulmonary artery. It is because of these features and the balloon that PA catheters are described as flow-directional catheters.

The catheter is then advanced into the right ventricle (RV). The RV waveform is pulsatile, with distinct systolic and diastolic pressures (see Fig. 9-36). Normal RV pressures are 20 to 30 mm Hg systolic and 0 to 5 mm Hg diastolic. Even with the balloon inflated, it is not uncommon for some ventricular ectopy to occur during passage through the RV. All patients who have a PA catheter inserted must have simultaneous electrocardiographic monitoring, with defibrillator and emergency resuscitation equipment nearby.

As the catheter enters the pulmonary artery, the waveform again changes (see Fig. 9-36). The diastolic pressure rises. Normal PA pressures range from 20 to 30 mm Hg systolic (PAS) over 10 mm Hg diastolic (PAD). A dicrotic notch, visible on the downslope of the waveform, represents closure of the pulmonic valve.

While the balloon remains inflated, the catheter is advanced into the wedge position (see Fig. 9-36). Here, the waveform decreases in size and is pulsatile—reflective of a normal left atrial tracing with *a* and *v* wave de-

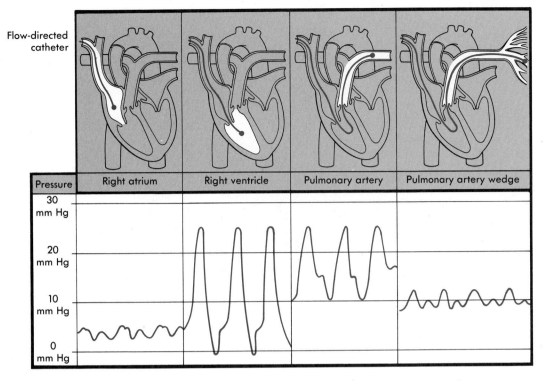

Fig. **9-36** PA insertion with corresponding waveforms.

flections (see Figure 9-34). This is described as a wedge tracing, because the balloon is "wedged" into a small pulmonary vessel. The balloon occludes the pulmonary vessel so that the PA lumen is exposed only to left atrial pressure and is protected from the pulsatile influence of the PA. When the balloon is deflated, the catheter should spontaneously float back into the PA. When the balloon is reinflated, the wedge tracing should be visible. Do not inflate the balloon with more air than specified on the catheter and for more than 8 to 15 seconds.[26] The normal PAWP ranges from 5 to 12 mm Hg.

After insertion, the catheter is sutured to the skin, and a chest radiograph is taken to verify the catheter's position and to make sure that it is not looped or knotted in the RV. In addition the radiograph is used to rule out a pneumothorax or other hemorrhage complication. If the catheter is advanced too far into the pulmonary bed, the patient is at risk for pulmonary infarction. If the catheter is not sufficiently advanced into the PA, it will not be useful for PAWP readings. However, in many critical care units, if the patient's PAD pressure and PAWP values approximate (within 0 to 4 mm Hg), the PAD can be used as reliable indirect measure of PAWP. This prevents possible trauma from frequent balloon inflation; in such a situation the PA catheter would be consciously pulled back into a nonwedging position in the pulmonary artery. If the pulmonary vascular resistance is increased or heart rate is greater than 130 beats per minute, the PAD cannot be used as a indirect measure of PAWP.[26]

Respiratory variation. All PAD and PAWP tracings are subject to respiratory interference, especially if the patient is on a positive-pressure, volume-cycled ventilator. During inhalation, the ventilator "pushes up" the PA tracing, which produces an artificially high reading (Fig. 9-37, *A*). During spontaneous respiration, negative intrathoracic pressure "pulls down" the waveform and can produce an erroneously low measurement (Fig. 9-37, *B*). To minimize the impact of respiratory variation, the PAD is read at end-expiration, which is the most stable point in the respiratory cycle. If the digital number fluctuates with respiration, a paper readout can be obtained to verify true PAD. In some clinical settings, airway pressure and flow are recorded simultaneously with the PAD/PAWP tracing to identify end-expiration.[26,39]

Positive end-expiratory pressure. Some forms of acute respiratory failure require the use of high levels of positive end-expiratory pressure (PEEP) to treat refractory hypoxemia. If greater than 10 cm H_2O is used, PAWP and PA pressures will be artificially elevated. Because of this impact of PEEP, in the past, patients in some critical care units were taken off the ventilator to record PA pressure measurements. It has since been shown that this practice decreases the patient's oxygenation and may result in persistent hypoxemia. Because patients remain on PEEP for treatment, they remain on it during measurement of PA pressures. In this situation the trend of PA readings is more important than one individual measurement.[26]

Thermodilution cardiac output. The PA catheter measures cardiac output (CO) using the bolus thermodilution method. This technique can be performed at the bedside and results in CO calculated in liters per minute. Generally, three cardiac outputs that are within a 10%

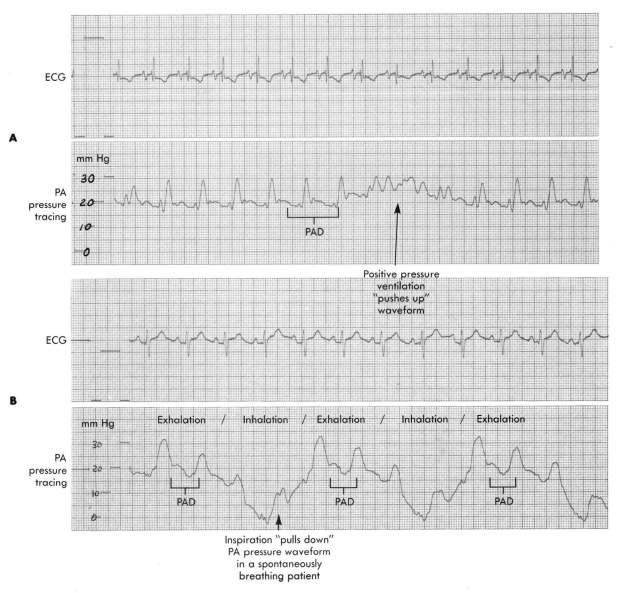

ECG

A

PA pressure tracing

mm Hg
30
20
10
0

PAD

Positive pressure ventilation "pushes up" waveform

ECG

B

PA pressure tracing

mm Hg
30
20
10
0

Exhalation / Inhalation / Exhalation / Inhalation / Exhalation

PAD   PAD   PAD

Inspiration "pulls down" PA pressure waveform in a spontaneously breathing patient

Fig. **9-37** The effects of ventilation on PA pressure readings. For accuracy, PA pressures are read at end-exhalation. **A,** Positive pressure ventilation: the increase in intrathoracic pressure during inhalation "pushes up" the PA pressure waveform, creating a false high reading. **B,** Spontaneous breathing: the decrease in intrathoracic pressure during normal inhalation "pulls down" the PA waveform, creating a false low reading.

mean range are obtained at one time and are averaged to calculate CO.[40] The normal range for CO is 4 to 6 L/min. The cardiac output should be indexed (divided by the patient's body surface area) to adjust it for the patient's body size.[40] The normal range for cardiac index (CI) is 2.2 to 4.0 L/min/m^2.

To obtain a thermodilution cardiac output a known amount (5 ml or 10 ml bolus) of iced or room temperature 5% dextrose in water (D_5W) is injected into the proximal lumen (RA port) of the catheter over 4 seconds or less at the end-expiratory phase of the patient's respiratory cycle.[40] The injectate exits into the right atrium (RA) and travels with the flow of blood past the thermistor (temperature sensor) at the distal end of the catheter in the

pulmonary artery. The injectate can be delivered by hand injection via individual syringes or, as done more commonly, by a closed in-line system attached to a 500 ml bag of D_5W.

Three clinical conditions produce errors in the thermodilution CO measurement: tricuspid valve regurgitation, intracardiac shunts, and cardiac dysrhythmias that affect beat-to-beat ejection.[40] If the patient has tricuspid valve regurgitation, the expected flow of blood from the right atrium to the pulmonary artery is disrupted by backflow from the right ventricle to the right atrium. This creates a lower CO measurement than the patient's actual output. If the person has an intracardiac left-to-right shunt, such as occurs with a ventricular septal defect

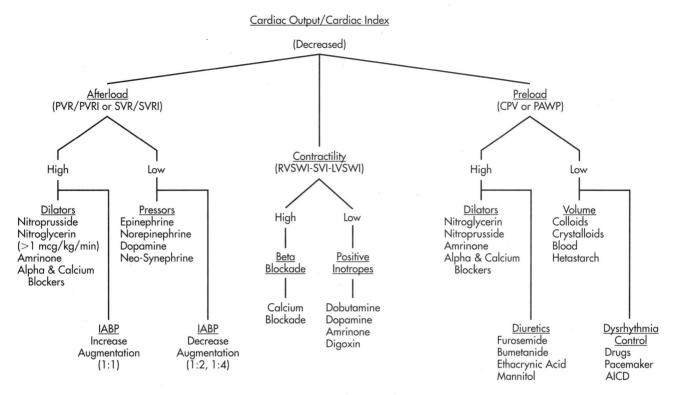

Fig. **9-38** Hemodynamic algorithm. (From Urban N: Hemodynamic clinical profiles, *AACN Clin Issues Crit Care Nurs* 1:119, 1990.)

(VSD), the thermodilution CO measures the large pulmonary volume and records a higher CO than the patient's true systemic output.

Clinical physiology. The function and viability of all body tissues depends on adequate tissue perfusion. The adequacy of the supply is primarily determined by the effectiveness of the pumping action of the heart and hemoglobin and arterial saturation. CO is a measure of the effectiveness of the heart as a pump. CO is the product of heart rate multiplied by stroke volume:

$$CO = HR \times SV$$

Stroke volume (SV) is the volume of blood ejected by the heart each beat in milliliters. The normal range for SV is 60 to 130 ml/beat. The clinical factors that contribute to the heart's stroke volume are preload, afterload, and contractility (Fig. 9-38). All three of these can be measured by the PA catheter. The other determinant of CO, heart rate, is measured via bedside cardiac monitoring.[41]

Preload. Preload is the filling pressure in the ventricles at the end of diastole (EDP). It is determined by the volume of blood stretching the ventricles at end-diastole, which is influenced by venous return and atrial kick. Because diastole is the filling stage of the cardiac cycle, the volume in the ventricle at end-diastole represents the presystolic volume available for ejection for that cardiac cycle. Preload influences myocardial fiber length and stretch (Starling's mechanism), and thus the amount of stretch determines in part the strength of contraction

(contractility). The more the muscle fiber is stretched, the more it will shorten in systole and the more force (contractility) will be used. Beyond a certain volume, however, the fibers become overstretched and the force (contractility) is decreased.[41]

The preload of the right side of the heart is measured by the RAP or CVP. The preload of the left side of the heart is measured by the PAWP. It is not possible to measure left ventricular volume directly in the critical care unit. However, the presence of blood within the ventricle creates pressures that can be measured by the PA catheter and transducer and that can be displayed on the bedside monitor. When the PA catheter is correctly positioned, with the tip in one of the large branches of the pulmonary artery, the only valve between the PA catheter tip and the left ventricle is the mitral valve. During diastole, when the mitral valve is open, there is no obstruction between the tip of the PA catheter and the left ventricle (Fig. 9-39).

Causes of decreased preload include volume loss (e.g., hemorrhage or third spacing), venous dilatation (e.g., hyperthermia or drugs), tachydysrhythmias or atrial fibrillation, increased intrathoracic pressure (e.g., positive pressure ventilation), and elevated intracardiac pressure (e.g., cardiac tamponade). Causes of increased preload include volume overload (e.g., excess intravenous fluid administration), venous constriction (e.g., hypothermia and drugs), and ventricular failure.[41]

Afterload. Afterload is defined as the pressure the ventricle has to generate (wall tension) to overcome the

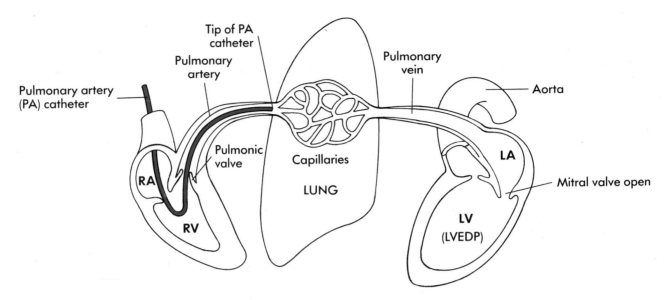

Fig. **9-39** Relationship of PAWP to LVEDP/preload. This diagram illustrates why, in the majority of clinical situations, the PAWP accurately reflects LVEDP, or preload. During diastole, when the mitral valve is open, there are no other valves or other obstructions between the tip of the catheter and the left ventricle. Thus the pressure exerted by the volume in the LV is reflected back through the left atrium through the pulmonary veins and to the pulmonary capillaries.

resistance to ejection created by the arteries and arterioles. It is a calculated measurement derived from information obtained from the PA catheter. As a response to increased afterload, ventricular wall tension rises. After a decrease in afterload, wall tension is lowered. The technical term for afterload is systemic vascular resistance. The afterload of the left side of the heart is measured by the systemic vascular resistance (SVR). The normal range is 800 to 1200 dynes/sec/cm^{-5}. The afterload of the right side of the heart is measured by the pulmonary vascular resistance (PVR). The normal range is 50 to 250 dynes/sec/cm^{-5}. Causes of decreased afterload include arterial dilatation (e.g., shock and hyperthermia) and of increased afterload include arterial constriction (e.g., shock and hypothermia).[41]

Pharmacologic manipulation of afterload to improve cardiac performance is commonly used with the critically ill patient. Many drugs, with different modes of action, are available. Drugs that vasodilate the arterial system and reduce SVR when given as a continuous infusion include sodium nitroprusside (Nipride) and high-dose nitroglycerin (NTG). Other vasodilators commonly used include IV hydralazine and oral ACE inhibitor drugs. If the SVR is extremely low (less than 500 dynes/sec/cm^{-5}) the cardiac output will be elevated and can induce cardiac failure because of the extreme work requirements. In this situation, medications may be used to "tighten up" the SVR. If the patient is refractory to dopamine or dobutamine, norepinephrine (Levophed) is used as a vasopressor to vasoconstrict the peripheral vasculature. The critical care nurse evaluates the effectiveness of the medication by the increase in SVR into the therapeutic range. Frequent assessment of the peripheral circulation is re-

quired when drugs that increase SVR are used because excessive vasoconstriction can negatively affect tissue perfusion.

Contractility. Contractility is described as the force of myocardial contraction. It is related to degree of myocardial fiber stretch (preload) and wall tension (afterload), and it influences myocardial oxygen consumption. Increased contractility increases myocardial workload and thus increases consumption and vice versa. The contractility of the right side of the heart is measured by the right ventricular stroke work index (RVSWI) and the contractility of the left side of the heart is measured by the left ventricular stroke work index (LVSWI). The normal range for the RVSWI is 7.9-9.7 g-m/m^2 and for LVSWI is 50-62 g-m/m^2. Causes of decreased contractility include excessive preload or afterload, drugs (negative inotropes), myocardial damage, and changes in the ionic environment (e.g., hypoxia, acidosis, or electrolyte imbalances). Causes of increased contractility include drugs (positive inotropes) and hyperthyroidism.[41]

PA waveform interpretation. The normal RAP and PAWP waveforms have three positive deflections—called *a, c,* and *v* waves—that correspond to specific atrial events in the cardiac cycle[36] (see Figure 9-34). The *a* wave reflects atrial contraction and follows the P wave seen on the ECG. The downslope of the *a* wave is called the *x descent* and represents atrial relaxation. The *c* wave reflects the bulging of the closed valve into the atrium during ventricular contraction. The *c* wave is small and not always visible but corresponds to the QRS-T interval on the ECG. The *v* wave represents atrial filling and increased pressure against the closed valve in early diastole. The downslope of the *v* wave is named the *y descent* and rep-

TABLE 9-8

COMPLICATIONS OF HEMODYNAMIC MONITORING

COMPLICATIONS	PREVENTION/DETECTION/TREATMENT
Air emboli	• Trendelenburg position is used for insertion of deep vein catheters • The physician usually puts gloved finger over needle hub with any disconnection during insertion to prevent air emboli • Aspirate air from flush solution bag to avoid air embolus with inadvertent emptying of flush solution bag • All lumens must be flushed with saline before insertion of catheters • Look for air bubbles in the pressure monitoring system • Use only Luer-Lok connections • Have patients hold their breath during catheter-tubing disconnects (e.g., tubing changes or removal of deep vein catheters) • If air embolus is suspected, turn patient to left side with head down
Arterial puncture (during venous cannulation)	• Hold pressure for at least 5-10 minutes; a longer time may be required for patients on anticoagulants or patients who have received thrombolytics
Balloon rupture	• Limit the length of time that catheter is left in place • Limit the number of times balloon is inflated (balloons are expected to last about 72 inflations); PAWP measurements are usually done every 4 hours unless clinical condition necessitates more frequent measurement • Do not overinflate balloon • Do not aspirate air from the balloon; allow passive deflation • Balloon rupture is particularly dangerous in right-to-left shunt (e.g., neonates; remember: adults shunt left-to-right) • Indications that the balloon has ruptured include inability to obtain PAWP waveform and absence of resistance during inflation • If balloon rupture has occurred, label balloon lumen accordingly so that others do not continue to try to inflate balloon
Clotting	• Maintain heparinized normal saline drip with intermittent flush device • Monitor for any change in waveform (e.g., dampening)

Dysrhythmias: usually ventricular dysrhythmias or RBBB	• Have emergency equipment (including transcutaneous pacemaker) available during insertion
	• Assess PAP waveform for indication that catheter is flipping back into RV
	  • Request catheter repositioning for catheter fling or RV waveform
	  • Turn patient to left side to encourage migration of catheter back into pulmonary artery

Emboli	• If you suspect a small clot, aspirate rather than flush
Exsanguination	• Use only Luer-Lok connections • Maintain alarms in ON position; pressure alarms are usually set 10-20 mm Hg above and below the patient's normal pressure
Fluid overload	• Limit the number of fast flushes • Use 5 ml instead of 10 ml for cardiac outputs when needed (if using 5 ml, injectate may need to be iced to provide adequate signal) • Limit frequency of cardiac outputs to every 4 hours
Hematoma	• Maintain pressure for 5-10 minutes with single-thickness pressure dressing after catheter removal; a longer time may be required for patients on anticoagulants or patients who have received thrombolytics

From Dennison RD: *Pass CCRN!* St Louis, 1996, Mosby.   *Continued*

resents the fall in pressure as the valve opens and blood flows from the atrium to the ventricle.

The normal PA waveform is similar to the arterial pressure waveform. As the pulmonic valve opens, blood is ejected from the right ventricle and is recorded as an increase of pressure in the pulmonary vascular system (see Figure 9-36). The highest point recorded is called *systole*. After peak ejection (systole), force is decreased and pressure drops. A notch (the dicrotic notch) may be visible on the downstroke of this waveform, representing closure of the pulmonic valve. The dicrotic notch signifies the beginning of diastole. The remainder of the downstroke represents diastolic runoff of blood flow into the pulmonary vasculature. The lowest point recorded is called *diastole*.

Nursing management

Nursing priorities for the patient with a hemodynamic pressure monitoring system are directed toward maintaining the system, ensuring the accuracy of the pressures, assessing the pressure waveforms, troubleshooting the system, and preventing complications.

Complications. Frequent patient and site assessment is essential for early identification of complications. Complications of hemodynamic monitoring are outlined on Table 9-8.

TABLE 9-8	

COMPLICATIONS OF HEMODYNAMIC MONITORING—cont'd

COMPLICATIONS	PREVENTION/DETECTION/TREATMENT
Hypothermia	• Use room temperature injectate • Apply blankets, radiant heaters as needed
Infection	• Percutaneous catheter insertion results in a much lower incidence of infection than does cutdown • Change flush solution bag every 24 hours • Change tubing every 48-72 hours or according to hospital protocol • Dress and inspect site using sterile technique every 24-48 hours or according to hospital protocol • Use normal saline for the heparinized flush • Do not allow dried blood to stay in stopcock ports or tubing • Limit the number of stopcocks in the pressure monitoring system • Replace all vented stopcock covers with nonvented "deadend" caps • Use strict sterile technique with blood sampling and cardiac outputs • Encourage use of catheter sleeve over PA catheter to ensure sterility and allow for sterile catheter manipulation • Limit the length of time that catheter is left in place (ideally <72 to 96 hours) • Monitor for signs/symptoms of catheter sepsis: fever, chills, leukocytosis, positive blood culture and/or catheter culture, redness, swelling, induration, and purulent drainage from catheter insertion site
Microshock	• Risk occurs because of elimination of the skin as a protection from microshock in patients with intracardiac catheters • Ensure that all electrical equipment is properly functioning and grounded • Do not touch the patient and a piece of electrical equipment at the same time
Nerve palsy	• Maintain limbs in functional position (i.e., do not keep the wrist hyperextended)
Pneumothorax, hemothorax, chylothorax during insertion	• Chest x-ray is taken after deep vein catheter cannulation • Treatment includes chest tube insertion
Pulmonary artery rupture	• Inflate balloon with only enough air to cause PAWP waveform; do not overwedge • If pulmonary artery rupture occurs, the primary clinical manifestation is hemoptysis; frank hemorrhage is possible
Pulmonary infarction	• Inflate balloon only long enough to record pressure value and waveform • Continuously monitor PAP so that if catheter advances into PAWP position, it will be noted and catheter repositioned • Request proximal repositioning if less than 1.25 ml is required to achieve wedge position because this indicates that the catheter's position is too distal and it may spontaneously wedge • If pulmonary infarction occurs, clinical manifestations include chest pain, dyspnea, decreased PaO_2 and SaO_2

Thrombosis	• Maintain heparinized normal saline drip with intermittent flush device (IFD); keep pressure bag at 300 mm Hg
	• Limit length of time that catheter is left in place (ideally less than 72 hours)
	• Use skillful catheter insertion technique to reduce trauma to intima
	• To prevent/detect arterial thrombosis with arterial catheters
	  • Ideally, select site with collateral flow (e.g., radial artery for arterial cannulation)
	  • Use smallest catheter feasible (e.g., 20 gauge for radial artery cannulation)
	  • Perform neurovascular assessment hourly
	• Arterial occlusion may be treated with local thrombolytic infusion or embolectomy

References

1. Lobert S: Cardiovascular assessment. In Kinny MR, Packa DR, editors: *Andreoli's comprehensive cardiac care*, ed 8, St Louis, 1996, Mosby.
2. Barkauskas VH, et al: *Health and physical assessment*, ed 2, St Louis, 1998, Mosby.
3. Perloff JK, Braunwald E: The physical examination of the heart and circulation. In Braunwald E, editor: *Heart disease: a textbook of cardiovascular medicine*, ed 5, Philadelphia, 1997, WB Saunders.
4. Carpenter KD: A comprehensive review of cyanosis, *Crit Care Nurs* 13(4):66, 1993.
5. Krenzer ME: Peripheral vascular assessment: finding your way through arteries and veins, *AACN Clin Issues Crit Care Nurs* 6(4):631, 1995.
6. Hurst JW: *Cardiovascular diagnosis: the initial examination*, St Louis, 1993, Mosby.
7. Cook DJ, Simel DL: Does this patient have abnormal central venous pressure? *JAMA* 275(8):630, 1996.
8. O'Rourke RA, et al: The history, physical examination, and cardiac auscultation. In Alexander RW, et al, editors: *Hurst's the heart, arteries, and veins*, ed 9, New York, 1998, McGraw-Hill.

9. Adolph RJ: The value of bedside examination in an era of high technology, III, *Heart Dis Stroke* 3:236, 1994.
10. Adolph RJ: The value of bedside examination in an era of high technology, IV, *Heart Dis Stroke* 3:312, 1994.
11. Conover MB: *Understanding electrocardiography,* ed 7, St Louis, 1996, Mosby.
12. Yucha CB, Toto KH: Calcium and phosphorus derangements, *Crit Care Clin North Am* 6:747, 1994.
13. Toto KH, Yucha CB: Magnesium homostasis, intolerances, and therapeutic uses, *Crit Care Clin North Am* 6:767, 1994.
14. Williams K, Morton PG: Diagnosis and treatment of acute myocardial infarction, *AACN Clin Issues Crit Care Nurs* 6:375, 1995.
15. Wallach JW: *Interpretation of diagnostic tests,* ed 6, Boston, 1996, Little, Brown.
16. Popma JJ, et al: Antithrombic therapy in patients undergoing coronary angioplasty, *Chest,* 108(Suppl):486S, 1995.
17. National Cholesterol Education Program: *Second report of the expert panel on detection, evaluation, and treatment of high blood cholesterol in adults (adult treatment panel II),* NIH Pub. No. 93-3095, 1993, U.S. Department of Health and Human Services.
18. Jacobson C: *Bedside cardiac monitoring,* Aliso Viejo, CA, 1996, American Association of Critical Care Nurses.
19. Futterman LG, Lemberg L: The long QT syndrome: when syncope is common to the young and the elderly, *Am J Crit Care* 4:405, 1995.
20. Chun HM, Sung RJ: Supraventricular tachyarrhythmias: pharmacologic versus nonpharmacologic approaches, *Med Clin North Am* 79:1121, 1995.
21. Stambler BS: Efficacy and safety of repeated intravenous doses of Ibutilide for rapid conversion of atrial flutter on fibrillation, *Circulation* 94:1613, 1996.
22. Ukani ZA, Ezekowitz MD: Contemporary management of atrial fibrillation, *Med Clin North Am* 79:1135, 1995.
23. Kellen JC, et al: The cardiac arrhythmia suppression trial: implications for nursing practice, *Am J Crit Care* 5(1):19, 1996.
24. Nicolai C: Ventricular dysrhythmias in ischemic heart disease, *AACN Clin Issues Crit Care Nurs* 6:452, 1995.
25. Imperial-Perez F, McRae M: *Arterial pressure monitoring,* Aliso Viejo, CA, 1998, American Association of Critical Care Nurses.
26. Keckeisen M: *Pulmonary artery pressure monitoring,* Aliso Viejo, CA, 1998, American Association of Critical Care Nurses.
27. Gardner RM: Accuracy and reliability of disposable pressure transducers coupled with modern pressure monitors, *Crit Care Med* 24:879, 1996.
28. Ahrens T, Penick JC, Tucker MK: Frequency requirements for zeroing transducers in hemodynamic monitoring, *Am J Crit Care* 4:466, 1995.
29. Quaal SJ: Quality assurance in hemodynamic monitoring, *AACN Clin Issues Crit Care Nurs* 4:197, 1993.
30. Doering LV: The effect of position change on hemodynamics and gas exchange in the critically ill: a review, *Am J Crit Care* 2:208, 1993.
31. Dobbin K, et al: Pulmonary artery mean pressure measurement in patients with elevated pressures: effect of backrest elevation and methods of measurement, *Am J Crit Care* 1(2)61, 1992.
32. Potger KC, Elliott D: Reproducibility of central venous pressures in supine and lateral positions: a pilot evaluation of the phlebostatic axis in critically ill patients, *Heart Lung* 23:285, 1994.
33. Emerson RJ, Banasik JL: Effect of position on selected hemodynamic parameters in postoperative cardiac surgery patients, *Am J Crit Care* 3:289, 1994.
34. Darovic GO: *Hemodynamic monitoring: invasive and noninvasive clinical application,* Philadelphia, 1995, WB Saunders.
35. Joynt GM, et al: Comparison of intrathoracic and intraabdominal measurements of central venous pressure, *Lancet* 347:1155, 1996.
36. Cook DJ, Simel DL: Does this patient have abnormal central venous pressure? *JAMA* 275:630, 1996.
37. Ginosak Y, Sprung CL: The Swan-Ganz catheter: twenty-five years of monitoring, *Crit Care Clin* 12:771, 1996.
38. Nelson LD: The new pulmonary arterial catheters, *Crit Care Clin* 12:795, 1996.
39. Booker KJ, Arnold JS: Respiratory-induced changes on the pulmonary capillary wedge pressure tracing, *Crit Care Nurs* 13(3):80, 1993.
40. Gawlinski A: *Cardiac output monitoring,* Aliso Viejo, CA, 1998, American Association of Critical Care Nurses.
41. Urban N: Integrating the hemodynamic profile with clinical assessment, *AACN Clin Issues Crit Care Nurs* 4:161, 1993.

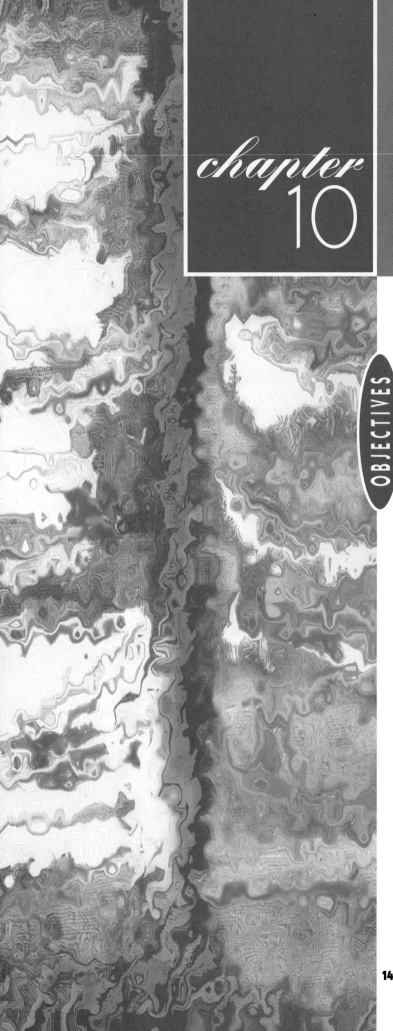

chapter 10

Cardiovascular Disorders

Mimi O'Donnell and Joni Dirks

OBJECTIVES

- Describe the etiology and pathophysiology of selected cardiovascular disorders.
- Identify the clinical manifestations of selected cardiovascular disorders.
- Explain the treatment of selected cardiovascular disorders.
- Discuss the nursing priorities for managing a patient with selected cardiovascular disorders.

Cardiovascular disease remains the leading cause of mortality in the United States. It claims more than 950,000 lives annually and places a heavy emotional and financial burden on society.[1] An understanding of the pathology of cardiovascular disease processes, the areas of assessment on which to focus, and current medical and nursing management allow the critical care nurse to accurately anticipate and plan interventions. This chapter focuses on cardiac disorders commonly seen in the critical care environment.

CORONARY ARTERY DISEASE

Description and Etiology

Coronary artery disease (CAD) is an insidious, progressive disease of the coronary arteries that results in their narrowing or complete occlusion. There are multiple causes of coronary artery narrowing, including thrombosis, spasm, dissection and aneurysm formation, but atherosclerosis is the most prevalent. Atherosclerosis affects not only the coronary arteries but also arterial vessels in the brain, kidneys, and peripheral arteries.

Any number of Diagnosis Related Groups (DRGs) may apply to the patient with CAD, depending on the underlying cause and whether the patient develops complications or comorbid conditions (CC). These include DRG 132 (Atherosclerosis with CC), DRG 133 (Atherosclerosis without CC), and DRG 140 (Angina Pectoris) with average lengths of stay of 3.3 days, 2.7 days, and 3.2 days respectively.[2]

CAD has a long latent period.[3] Fatty streaks can appear within the aorta during childhood, but symptoms occur only when the atherosclerotic plaque occludes 75% of the vessel lumen, usually in late middle age.[4]

Epidemiologic data collected during the past 40 years has demonstrated an association between specific risk factors and the development of CAD. One of the most important epidemiologic studies is the Framingham Heart Study, which began in 1948 and continues today with third and fourth generations of subjects. Blood cholesterol, smoking, activity level, blood pressure, and electrocardiographic results are checked on a regular basis for participants in this study. As a result, specific CAD risk factors that are associated with an increased probability of CAD development have been identified. These life-style habits are referred to as CAD risk factors.[5]

Factors that increase risk for development of CAD include age, gender, race, genetic inheritance (family history), elevated serum cholesterol, hypertension, cigarette smoking, glucose intolerance, sedentary life-style, stress, and a type A behavior pattern. These factors are further delineated into nonmodifiable and modifiable CAD risk factors (Box 10-1).

Nonmodifiable

The symptoms of CAD occur as a person ages. In general CAD is a disease of middle and old age.[3-5] CAD occurs approximately 10 years later in women than it does in men. After menopause, rates are the same for both genders.[5,6] A positive family history is one in which a close blood relative had a myocardial infarction or stroke before the age of 60 years. This family history suggests a genetic predisposition to the development of CAD.[5] Nonwhite populations of both genders have higher CAD mortality rates than do white populations.

Modifiable

Hyperlipidemia is a leading factor responsible for severe atherosclerosis and the development of CAD.[7] Total serum cholesterol levels more than 200 mg/dL are associated with a higher risk of CAD, and levels greater than 270 mg/dL carry a fourfold increase in risk.[7] In addition, elevated LDL-C, VLDL-C, and triglyceride levels are associated with an increased incidence of CAD as are low HDL-C levels.[7,8] Homocystinuria is a rare inborn error of metabolism. It has received attention recently because patients with high levels of plasma homocystine have a very high incidence of atherosclerotic coronary artery and vascular disease.[9,10] Hypertension is the elevation of either systolic blood pressure (SBP) or diastolic blood pressure (DBP). The higher the BP, the greater is the risk of coronary artery disease. Hypertension is a risk factor because of the damage it causes to the endothelium of the vessel. The risk of developing CAD is reduced when the SBP and DBP are less than 140/90 mm Hg.[11] Management of hypertension is initially directed toward life-style modifications such as weight loss, decrease of dietary sodium chloride, increase in physical activity, reduced alcohol consumption, stress management, and, if these are not successful, by pharmacologic therapy.[11,12] The greater the number of cigarettes smoked per day, the greater the CAD risk. Cigarette smoking unfavorably alters serum lipid levels, decreasing HDL-C levels and increasing LDL-C and triglyceride levels. Smoking results in cardiac electrical instability within cell membranes and impairs oxygen transport and use while increasing myocardial oxygen demand. Smoking also is thought to alter intimal endothelial permeability and to foster platelet agglutination. Fortunately, the damage from smoking is not unalterable, and after cessation the coronary risk falls rapidly, with a decrease of approximately 50% within 1 year.[6] Individuals with diabetes mellitus have a higher incidence of CAD than does the general population. In fact, diabetes triples or quadruples the risk of developing CAD.[13] Premenopausal women with diabetes are at increased risk of developing CAD, compared with nondiabetic women of the same age, because diabetes negates the protective effect of estrogen. CAD risk from diabetes also rises in the presence of increased serum cholesterol, hypertension, and cigarette smoking.[13] Oral contraceptives increase a woman's risk of developing CAD, especially after age 35 years, because they alter blood coagulation, platelet function, and fibrinolytic activity, and may inversely affect the integrity of vascular endothelium. The risk is increased more if the woman also smokes cigarettes. Obesity is often associated with a sedentary life-style. It also increases susceptibility to the develop-

---

BOX 10-1

CORONARY ARTERY DISEASE RISK FACTORS

NONMODIFIABLE
Age
Gender
Family history
Race

MODIFIABLE
Major
Elevated serum lipids
Hypertension
Cigarette smoking
Impaired glucose tolerance
Diet high in saturated fat, cholesterol, and calories
Physical inactivity

Minor
Psychologic stress
Personality type

ment of other risk factors, such as hypertension, impaired glucose tolerance, and hyperlipidemia, with increased LDL-C and decreased HDL-C levels. Evidence continues to accumulate that a sedentary life-style increases the risk for CAD. Physical inactivity is also associated with lower HDL-C levels, higher LDL-C levels, hypertension, obesity, increased glucose intolerance, and hyperlipidemia.[5] Type A behavior patterns that include time-urgency, hostility, anger, and anxiety have also been associated with the development of CAD.[14,15] How stress and behavior influences the development of CAD is not well-understood, but stress is associated with increased circulating catecholamines, which may precipitate hypertension, alteration in platelet function, increased fatty acid mobilization, and a resultant elevation of free fatty acids.

At present, researchers are uncertain why a risk factor in one individual may result in serious consequences but may not cause problems for another individual. Studies show that CAD is a multifactorial disease and as the number of known risk factors increases, the risk of developing the disease increases in an exponential, rather than additive, manner.

Pathophysiology

CAD is a progressive disorder of the coronary arteries that results in narrowing or complete occlusion. There are multiple causes for coronary artery narrowing, but atherosclerosis is the most prevalent. Atherosclerosis affects the medium-sized arteries perfusing the heart, brain, and kidneys and the large arteries branching off the aorta. Atherosclerotic lesions may take different forms, depending on their anatomic location; the individual's age, ge-

netic makeup, physiologic status; and the number of risk factors present. Normal arterial walls are composed of three cellular layers: the intima, or innermost endothelial layer; the media, or middle muscular layer; and the adventitia, or outermost connective tissue layer.

Three major elements are associated with atherosclerotic plaque development and luminal narrowing: (1) smooth muscle proliferation; (2) formation of a connective tissue matrix composed of collagen, elastic fibers, and proteoglycans; and (3) accumulation of lipids[16-18] (Fig. 10-1).

Stages of plaque development

Specific stages of atherosclerotic plaque development have been identified.[3,16-18] The first stage is the development of fatty streaks. These are broad-based lesions composed of lipid-laden macrophages and smooth muscle cells. During the second stage, streaks develop into fatty plaques. Subsequently, collagen and dense connective tissue create atherosclerotic fibrous plaques. Finally, the third stage—the advanced or complicated lesion phase—is when the fibrous plaque becomes vascularized, the core calcifies, and the surface ulcerates, resulting in hemorrhage and thromboembolic episodes. Furthermore, the media may develop aneurysmal changes resulting from the decrease in smooth muscle cells (see Fig. 10-1).

CAD hemodynamic effects

The major hemodynamic effect of CAD is the disturbance of the delicate balance between myocardial oxygen supply and demand. Atherosclerosis alters the normal coronary artery's response to increased demand in two

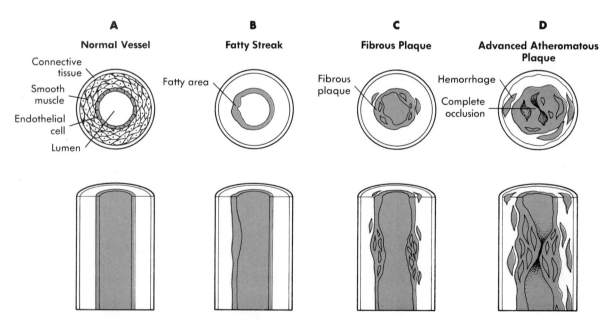

Fig. **10-1** The progression of atherosclerosis shown in both longitudinal and cross-sectional views. **A,** Normal vessel. **B,** First stage, fatty streaks. **C,** Second stage, fibrous plaque development. **D,** Third stage, advanced (complicated) lesions.

ways: (1) lesions that result in a 75% or more vessel-lumen occlusion restrict flow under resting conditions and (2) vessels become stiff and lose the ability to dilate. The result is decreased driving pressure beyond the site of the lesion and less oxygenated blood available to the myocardial cells perfused by that vessel. During periods of ischemia the myocardium is forced to shift from aerobic metabolism to anaerobic metabolism, the consequences of which are (1) less efficient energy production, (2) lactic acid build-up, (3) intracellular hypokalemia, (4) intracellular acidosis, (5) intracellular hypernatremia, and (6) interference with the release of calcium from its storage sites in the sarcoplasmic reticulum. Tissue hypoxia or ischemia is the end result of this process.

Plaque rupture

Superficial tears in vessel wall atherosclerotic plaque are found on autopsy in about 17% of patients who die from noncardiac causes.[19] This suggests that damage to atherosclerotic plaque is a routine event. In individuals who die from a known coronary event, the vessel luminal diameter is more than 75% occluded by plaque.[18,19] In individuals with more lumen than not occluded by plaque, there is a greater risk of plaque rupture from the damaged plaque surface. It is believed that unstable angina, acute myocardial infarction, and ischemic sudden cardiac death are the result of ruptured plaque and a rapidly evolving thrombus.[20] Deep fissures in the fibrous cap expose procoagulant factors within the plaque core to the blood plasma. When platelets in the blood are exposed to collagen, necrotic debris, von Willebrand factor, and thromboxane, a clot is formed that can occlude the coronary artery.[20] Highly fibrotic plaques do not rupture. The type of atherosclerotic plaque that is prone to rupture has a weak fibrous cap and a large amount of cholesterol within the core.[20] For this reason it is thought that reducing the plasma cholesterol, and ultimately the cholesterol within the plaque, will decrease the risk of an acute coronary event.[21,22]

Plaque regression

Reduction of blood cholesterol decreases the plaque size by decreasing the amount of cholesterol within the plaque core. It will not change the dimensions of the fibrous or calcified portions of the plaque. If diet is not effective in lowering blood cholesterol levels, lipid-lowering drugs are used to lower the LDL-C level to less than 100 mg/dL, the HDL-C level to less than 50 mg/dL, and triglycerides to less than 140 mg/dL.[7,21]

Assessment and Diagnosis

Angina pectoris, or chest pain caused by myocardial ischemia, is not a separate disease, but rather a symptom of CAD. It is caused by a blockage or spasm of a coronary artery, leading to diminished blood supply to the myocardium. The lack of oxygen causes ischemia, which is felt as pain. Angina may occur anywhere in the chest, neck, arms, or back, but the most commonly described location is behind the sternum. The pain often radiates to the left arm but can also radiate to both arms, the mandible, and/or the neck. Angina has other characteristics in addition to pain (Box 10-2). It is classified as stable, unstable, and variant.[23,24]

Stable angina

Stable angina is predictable and caused by similar precipitating factors each time, such as exercise, emotional upset, and tachycardia. Patients become used to the pattern of this type of angina and may describe it as "my usual chest pain." Control of pain is achieved by rest and administration of a coronary artery vasodilator such as sublingual nitroglycerin. Stable angina is the result of fixed lesions (blockages) of more than 75%. Ischemia and

---

BOX 10-2

CHARACTERISTICS OF ANGINA PECTORIS

LOCATION

Beneath sternum, radiating to neck and jaw
Upper chest
Beneath sternum, radiating down left arm
Epigastric
Epigastric, radiating to neck, jaw, and arms
Neck and jaw
Left shoulder, inner aspect of both arms
Intrascapular

DURATION

0.5 to 30 minutes (stable)
Duration of longer than 30 minutes, without relief from rest or medication, indicates unstable or preinfarction symptoms

QUALITY

Sensation of pressure or heavy weight on the chest
Feeling of tightness, like a vise
Visceral quality (deep, heavy, squeezing, aching)
Burning sensation
Shortness of breath, with feeling of suffocation
Most severe pain ever experienced

RADIATION

Medial aspect of left arm
Jaw
Left shoulder
Right arm

PRECIPITATING FACTORS

Exertion/exercise
Cold weather
Exercising after a large, heavy meal
Walking against the wind
Emotional upset
Fright, anger
Coitus

MEDICATION RELIEF

Usually within 45 seconds to 5 minutes of sublingual nitroglycerin administration

chest pain occur when myocardial demand exceeds blood oxygen supply. It can be managed medically for long periods.

Unstable angina

Unstable angina is defined as a change in a previously established stable pattern of angina or a new onset of severe angina. It usually is more intense than stable angina, may awaken the person from sleep, or may necessitate more than nitrates for pain relief. A change in the level or frequency of symptoms requires immediate medical evaluation.[24] Severe angina that persists for more than 20 minutes and is not relieved by three nitroglycerin tablets is called preinfarction, or crescendo, angina. This is a medical emergency, and the person must be taken to a hospital emergency room immediately.[25] The pathology underlying the change from stable to unstable angina may be plaque hemorrhage or fissure that causes an increase in localized platelet agglutination and acute thrombosis.[20]

Variant angina

Variant, or Prinzmetal's, angina is caused by coronary artery spasm. It is believed to result from spasm, with or without atherosclerotic lesions. Variant angina commonly occurs when the individual is at rest and also can be cyclic, occurring at the same time every day. It usually is associated with ST-segment elevation and occasionally with transient abnormal Q waves. Smoking tobacco and ingesting alcohol and cocaine also may precipitate spasm. Drugs of choice for the treatment of spasm are agents that vasodilate the coronary arteries, such as nitroglycerin or calcium channel blockers (e.g., nifedipine and diltiazem).

Silent ischemia

Silent ischemia is defined as objective ECG evidence of myocardial ischemia (ST-segment changes) without the patient experiencing any symptoms of angina.[26] It is classified into three clinical types (Box 10-3). Patients with type I ischemia are asymptomatic, without manifesta-

tions of cardiovascular disease, yet continuous monitoring or stress testing demonstrates myocardial ischemia. Often, these patients are found to have multivessel CAD when tested later using coronary arteriography. Type II patients are those who have had an acute myocardial infarction and demonstrate active ischemia but have no anginal symptoms. Patients with type III ischemia have some ischemic episodes that are accompanied by chest pain and other episodes without chest discomfort. Type III patients may or may not have had a prior infarction. Once identified, silent ischemia usually is treated in the same manner as classic angina—with nitrates, beta-blockers, calcium channel blockers, and lifestyle changes.[26,27]

Medical Management

The major goals of medical therapy for CAD and angina are to (1) increase coronary artery perfusion, (2) decrease myocardial workload, (3) prevent myocardial infarction (MI) disability or death, and (4) intervene in cases of unstable angina. Specific medical management depends on the frequency, severity, duration, and hemodynamic consequences of the angina.

Myocardial supply/demand balance

Pharmacologic therapy such as oxygen, nitrates, and vasodilators[23] are used to increase coronary artery perfusion and myocardial oxygen supply. Lytic therapy may be used to restore blood flow to the coronary artery if the patient arrives in the emergency department within 6 hours of the onset of chest pain. Bedrest, beta-blockers, ACE (angiotensin-converting enzyme) inhibitors, and calcium channel blockers are used to decrease myocardial oxygen demand. Analgesics such as morphine are used to relieve anginal pain.[23,28,29]

MI prevention

CAD risk factors, such as hypertension or hyperlipidemia, are treated aggressively. A low-sodium, low-cholesterol diet may be recommended. Activity is restricted until episodes of angina are controlled.

Angina management

The change from stable to unstable angina represents a serious problem. The patient is admitted to a hospital, and bedrest is prescribed. It is important that any identified precipitating problems be treated. If the anginal pain continues, cardiac catheterization, intraaortic balloon support, thrombolytic therapy, interventional cardiology procedure, or coronary artery bypass graft (CABG) surgery may be indicated.[28,29]

Nursing Management

Nursing management of the patient with CAD and angina incorporates a variety of nursing diagnoses (Box 10-4). **Nursing priorities are directed toward identifying**

BOX 10-3

SILENT ISCHEMIA

TYPE	CLINICAL CHARACTERISTICS
I	Objective evidence of myocardial ischemia without chest pain/symptoms
II	No anginal symptoms after a previous MI, but objective evidence of myocardial ischemia continues
III	Symptoms of angina with some episodes of ischemia, and asymptomatic with other ischemic events; may or may not have had a previous MI

Objective evidence of myocardial ischemia: ST-segment changes seen on ECG monitoring.

chest pain early, relieving chest pain, providing comfort and emotional support, and maintaining surveillance for complications.

Identifying chest pain

Complaints of chest discomfort are evaluated quickly. Factors to consider when assessing chest pain are listed in Box 10-5. Chest pain in the patient with known or suspected coronary disease may represent myocardial ischemia, which must be treated while it is still reversible. The patient is asked to rate the intensity of the chest discomfort on a scale of 1 to 10. The term *chest pain* is not to be used exclusively because some patients describe their

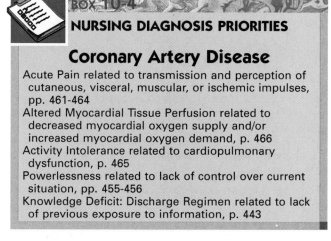

Box 10-4

NURSING DIAGNOSIS PRIORITIES

Coronary Artery Disease

Acute Pain related to transmission and perception of cutaneous, visceral, muscular, or ischemic impulses, pp. 461-464
Altered Myocardial Tissue Perfusion related to decreased myocardial oxygen supply and/or increased myocardial oxygen demand, p. 466
Activity Intolerance related to cardiopulmonary dysfunction, p. 465
Powerlessness related to lack of control over current situation, pp. 455-456
Knowledge Deficit: Discharge Regimen related to lack of previous exposure to information, p. 443

BOX 10-5

FACTORS TO CONSIDER WHEN ASSESSING CHEST PAIN

Onset (either sudden or gradual)
Precipitating factors (did visitors come or leave; was the patient up moving around?)
Location (was it substernal; was it located in same area as previous pain?)
Radiation (did it radiate to the jaw, neck, arm, or shoulder?)
Quality (was it similar to previous anginal pain; was it less or worse?)
Intensity (on a scale of 1 to 10, where would the patient rate it?)
Duration (did it last seconds or minutes; how soon after onset did the patient call for help?)
Relieving factors (what made it better—changing position, nitroglycerin, oxygen, the presence of the nurse?)
Aggravating factors (did the environment, telephone calls, waiting for help worsen the pain?)
Associated symptoms (was the pain accompanied by nausea, vomiting, diaphoresis, or dyspnea?)
Emotional response (how did the patient feel about the pain; anxious, fearful, angry?)

angina as *pressure* or *heaviness*. It is also important to document the characteristics of the pain, the patient's heart rate and rhythm, the presence of ectopic beats or conduction defects, the patient's mentation, and overall tissue perfusion. This includes skin color, temperature, peripheral pulses, and urine output. A 12-lead electrocardiogram (ECG) is used to identify the area of ischemic myocardium.[30] The major concern is that the chest pain may represent preinfarction angina, and early identification is essential so that the patient can be immediately transported to the cardiac catheterization laboratory for diagnosis and possibly treatment. If the hospital does not have a cardiac catheterization laboratory, thrombolytics may be prescribed to prevent the development of an acute myocardial infarction.

Relieving chest pain

In the critical care unit, control of angina is achieved by a combination of supplemental oxygen, nitrates, and analgesia. All patients with acute ischemic pain are administered supplemental oxygen to increase myocardial oxygenation. Those patients who develop symptoms of acute heart failure may require emergency intubation and mechanical ventilation to correct significant hypoxemia.[23,29] A combination of intravenous and sublingual nitroglycerin is used to vasodilate the coronary arteries and control pain. After nitrate administration, the nurse closely observes the patient for relief of chest pain, return of the ST segment to baseline, and for the development of unwanted side effects such as hypotension and headache.[23,29] Morphine is the analgesic of choice for preinfarction angina; it both relieves pain and decreases fear and anxiety. After administration, the critical care nurse assesses the patient for pain relief and the development of unwanted side effects such as hypotension and respiratory depression.[23,29]

Providing comfort and emotional support

Patients admitted to a critical care unit with acute angina experience extreme anxiety and fear of death. The critical care nurse is met with the challenge of combining the elements of a calm environment that can alleviate fear and anxiety, while at the same time always being ready to respond to an acute patient emergency such as a cardiac arrest or to assist with emergency intubation or insertion of hemodynamic monitoring catheters.

Patient education

Once the ischemic pain is controlled, patient and family education can begin. Points to cover include risk factor modification, signs and symptoms of angina, when to call the physician, medications to use, and dealing with emotions and stress.[31] However, since the acute hospital length of stay for uncomplicated angina is usually less than 4 days, referral to a cardiac rehabilitation program for a controlled exercise program and risk factor modification after discharge is perhaps the most helpful teaching intervention a critical care nurse can provide.

MYOCARDIAL INFARCTION

Description and Etiology

Myocardial infarction is the term used to describe irreversible myocardial necrosis (cell death) that results from an abrupt decrease or total cessation of coronary blood flow to a specific area of the myocardium.[29]

Myocardial infarction falls under three different DRGs depending on whether the patient develops complications or comorbid conditions (CC). These include DRG 121 (Circulatory Disorders with Acute Myocardial Infarction and Major Complications, Discharged Alive), DRG 122 (Circulatory Disorders with Acute Myocardial Infarction without Major Complications, Discharged Alive), and DRG 123 (Circulatory Disorders with Acute Myocardial Infarction, Expired) with average lengths of stay of 7.3 days, 4.7 days, and 4.6 days respectively.[2]

Pathophysiology

Atherosclerosis is responsible for most myocardial infarctions because it causes luminal narrowing and reduced blood flow, resulting in decreased oxygen delivery to the myocardium. The three mechanisms that are primarily responsible for the acute reduction in oxygen delivery to the myocardium are (1) coronary artery thrombosis, (2) plaque fissure or hemorrhage, and (3) coronary artery spasm. Infarction is more prevalent in the left ventricle, with multivessel occlusions, and in myocardium distal to vessels that have not developed collateral flow.

Coronary artery thrombi

Thrombi are now known to be present in almost all acute coronary artery occlusions. These thrombi, usually composed of platelets, fibrin, erythrocytes, and leukocytes, may be superimposed on a plaque or may be aligned adjacent to a plaque. They release thromboxane A_2, serotonin, and thrombin—all vasoconstricting substances that compound vessel narrowing and set up a vicious cycle of recurrent occlusion. Scientists have not determined the cause of thrombus formation, but plaque fissure or hemorrhage, or both, are thought to be predisposing events.[16-19]

Atherosclerotic plaques

Plaques are classified according to their composition. Hard plaques are heavily calcified and fibrotic, whereas soft plaques are composed of cholesterol esters and lipids. Coronary artery thrombosis has been associated with rupture, or cracks, of the plaques and release of the plaque material into the vascular lumen. Plaque rupture can induce thrombosis by (1) forming a platelet plug, (2) releasing tissue thromboplastin from the plaque material that activates the clotting cascade, and (3) obstructing the vessel lumen with plaque components. Coronary artery spasm is often present in acute occlusions. However, it is not known whether this results from hyperactive smooth muscle or whether it is a secondary response related to a plaque rupture and the release of vasoactive substances.[16-19]

Infarction

The area of cellular death and muscle necrosis in the myocardium is known as the zone of infarction (Fig. 10-2). On the ECG, evidence of this zone is seen by pathologic Q waves, which reflect a lack of depolarization from the cardiac surface involved in the myocardial infarction (Fig. 10-3, *D*). As healing takes place, the cells in this area are replaced by scar tissue.

Injury

The infarcted zone is surrounded by injured but still potentially viable tissue in an area known as the *zone of injury* (see Fig. 10-2). Cells in this area do not fully repolarize because of the deficient blood supply. This is recorded as elevation of the ST segment (Fig. 10-3, *C*).

Ischemia

The outer region of the myocardium is the zone of ischemia (see Fig. 10-2) and is composed of viable cells. Repolarization in this zone is impaired but eventually is restored to normal. Repolarization of the cells in this area manifests as T wave inversion (Fig. 10-3, *B*).

MI evolution

During the first 6 weeks after an infarction, the damaged myocardium undergoes many changes. Approximately 6 hours after the infarction, the muscle becomes distended, pale, and cyanotic. Over the next 2 days the myocardium becomes reddish purple, and an exudate may form on the epicardium. Leukocyte scavenger cells begin to infiltrate the muscle and carry away the necrotic debris, thereby thinning the necrotic wall. Approximately 3 to 4 weeks after the infarction, scar tissue begins to form and the affected wall becomes whiter and thicker.

Classification

Myocardial infarctions are classified according to their location on the myocardial surface and the muscle layers affected. A transmural MI involves all three muscle layers—the endocardium, the myocardium, and the epicardium—and involves significant ECG changes. Nontransmural infarctions are classified as either subendocardial, involving the endocardium, or subepicardial, involving the epicardium. Some myocardium may be involved in a nontransmural MI, but it is not a full thickness infarction. Generally, abnormal Q waves are not seen, so a nontransmural MI is commonly called a non-Q wave MI.

Assessment and Diagnosis

The definitive diagnosis of myocardial infarction is based on a combination of the patient's clinical symptoms, 12-lead ECG changes, and cardiac enzyme levels.[29] MI location can help predict risk of mortality. Anterior and an-

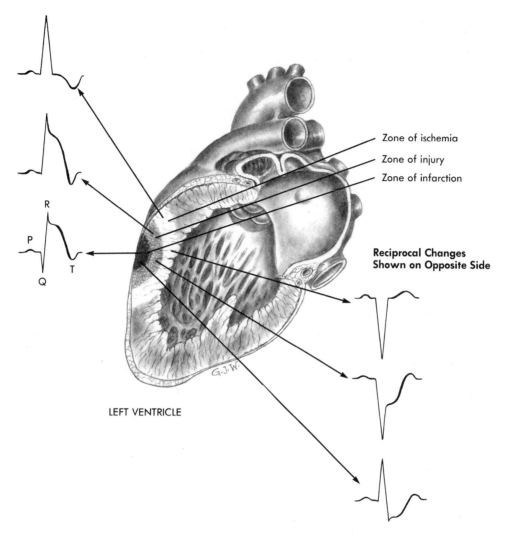

Fig. **10-2** Zone of ischemia, zone of injury, and zone of infarction, shown through ECG wave-forms and reciprocal waveforms corresponding to each zone.

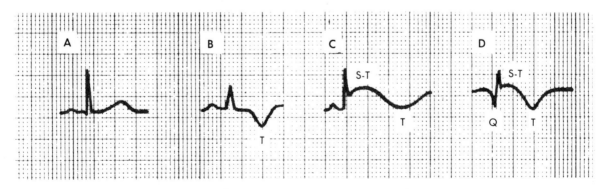

Fig. **10-3** ECG changes indicative of ischemia, injury, and infarction (necrosis) of the myocardium. **A,** Normal ECG. **B,** Ischemia indicated by inversion of the T wave. **C,** Ischemia and current injury indicated by T wave inversion and ST-segment elevation. The ST segment may be elevated above or depressed below the baseline, depending on whether the tracing is from a lead facing toward or away from the infarcted area and depending on whether epicardial or endocardial injury occurs. Epicardial injury causes ST elevation in leads facing the epicardium. **D,** Ischemia, injury, and myocardial necrosis. The Q wave indicates necrosis of the myocardium. (From Kinney M, et al: *Comprehensive cardiac care,* ed 8, St Louis, 1996, Mosby.)

CLINICAL MANIFESTATIONS OF ACUTE MYOCARDIAL INFARCTION

Tachycardia *with* or *without* ectopy
Bradycardia
Normotension or hypotension
Tachypnea
Diminished heart sounds, especially S_1
If left ventricular dysfunction present, may have S_3 and/or S_4
Systolic murmur
Pulmonary crackles
Pulmonary edema
Air hunger
Orthopnea
Frothy sputum
Decreased cardiac output
  Decreased urine output
  Decreased peripheral pulses
  Slow capillary refill
Restlessness
Confusion
Anxiety
Agitation
Denial
Anger

CORRELATION BETWEEN VENTRICULAR SURFACES, ECG LEADS, AND CORONARY ARTERIES

SURFACE OF LEFT VENTRICLE	ECG LEADS	CORONARY ARTERY USUALLY INVOLVED
Inferior	II, III, aV_F	Right coronary
Lateral	V_5-V_6, I, aV_L	Left circumflex
Anterior	V_2-V_4	Left anterior descending
Septal	V_1-V_2	Left anterior descending
Posterior	V_1-V_2 (reciprocal changes)	Left circumflex

teroseptal infarctions are associated with twice the mortality of inferior wall infarctions.

Clinical symptoms

The most common clinical manifestation of infarction is prolonged severe chest pain, which often is associated with nausea, vomiting, and diaphoresis. This pain generally lasts 30 or more minutes and usually is located in the substernal or left precordial area. Unlike angina, which often is described as discomfort, the pain of infarction may be described as the most severe pain the individual has ever experienced. Descriptions used are "like an elephant sitting on my chest" or a viselike tightness. The pain may radiate to the back, neck, jaw, or left arm, particularly down the ulnar aspect. Neither rest nor nitrates relieves the pain. Additional clinical manifestations are shown in Box 10-6.

Twelve-lead ECG changes

The ECG changes produced by a transmural infarction demonstrate alteration in both myocardial depolarization (QRS complex) and repolarization (ST segment). The changes in repolarization are seen by the presence of new Q waves. These Q waves are deeper (more than one third the height of the corresponding R wave) and wider than normal (more than 0.04 seconds).[30]

The location of infarction is determined by correlating the ECG leads with Q waves and the ST segment T wave abnormalities (Table 10-1). Infarction most commonly occurs in the left ventricle and the interventricular septum; however, almost 25% of patients who sustain an inferior

myocardial infarction have some right ventricular damage.[29] The ECG manifestations that are used to diagnose an MI and pinpoint the area of damaged ventricle include inverted T waves, ST-segment elevation, and pathologic Q waves.[30]

Anterior wall infarction. Anterior wall infarction results from occlusion of the proximal left anterior descending (LAD) artery and may involve the left main artery. ST-segment elevation is expected in leads V_1 through V_4, and T wave inversion may occur in leads I, aV_1, and V_2 through V_5 (Fig. 10-4). There is a loss of positive R wave progression in leads V_1 through V_6. A large anterior wall MI may be associated with left ventricular (LV) pump failure, cardiogenic shock, or death. Because the anterior wall is so large, it is commonly described in sections, as in the following discussion.

Anteroseptal infarction. Anteroseptal infarction results from an occlusion of the LAD artery. Leads V_1 through V_4 on the 12-lead ECG reflect the electrical activity of the anterior wall. There is a loss of R wave progression in V_1 and V_2, leaving a QS complex. Q waves are seen in leads V_2 through V_4. If the infarct involves only the septum, this will appear only in the V_1 lead. Reciprocal changes usually are not seen with an anteroseptal myocardial infarction.

Anterolateral infarction. Anterolateral infarction occurs as a result of occlusion of the circumflex coronary artery. On a 12-lead ECG, Q waves and ST-T wave changes are seen in leads I, aV_L, V_4, V_5, and V_6. Reciprocal changes occur in the inferior leads II, III, and aV_F.

Inferior wall infarction. Inferior wall infarction occurs with occlusion of the right coronary artery (RCA). This infarction is manifested by ECG changes in leads II, III, and aV_F. Reciprocal changes occur in leads I and aV_L (Fig. 10-5). Because the RCA perfuses the sinoatrial (SA) node, the proximal bundle of His, and the atrioventricular (AV) node, conduction disturbances may be seen with an inferior wall MI.

Right ventricular infarction. Infarction of the right ventricle occurs when there is a blockage in a proximal

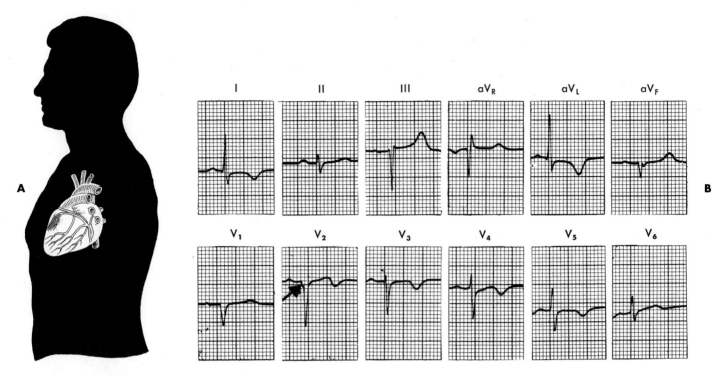

Fig. **10-4 A,** Position of an anterior wall infarction. **B,** ECG evidence of anterior wall infarction. Note the QS complexes in leads V$_1$ and V$_2$, indicating anteroseptal infarction. There is also a characteristic notching (*arrow,* V$_2$) of the QS complex, often seen in infarctions. In addition, note the diffuse ischemic T wave inversions in leads I, aV$_L$, and V$_2$ through V$_5$, indicating generalized anterior wall ischemia. (From Goldberger AL, Goldberger E: *Clinical electrocardiography: a simplified approach,* ed 5, St Louis, 1994, Mosby.)

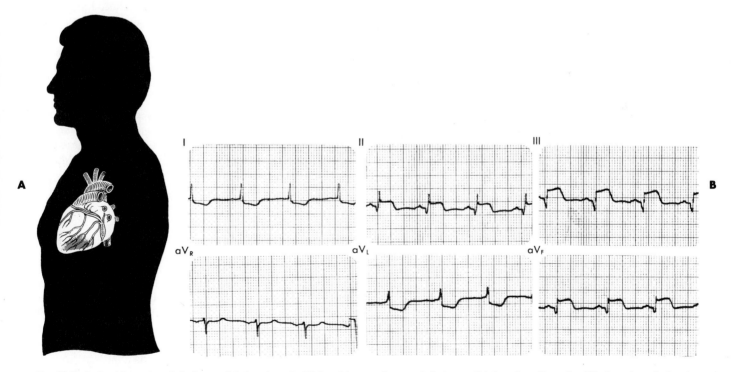

Fig. **10-5 A,** Position of an inferior wall infarction. **B,** ECG evidence of acute inferior wall infarction. Note the ST elevations in leads II, III, and aV$_L$, with reciprocal ST depressions in leads I and aV$_L$. Abnormal Q waves also are seen in leads II, III, and aV$_f$. Changes are not seen in leads V$_4$ to V$_6$, so these leads are not shown. (From Goldberger AL, Goldberger E: *Clinical electrocardiography: a simplified approach,* ed 5, St Louis, 1994, Mosby.)

section of the right coronary artery. This places all of the right ventricle and the inferior wall at risk.[29]

Posterior wall infarction. Posterior wall infarction occurs with occlusion of the circumflex branch of the left coronary artery. Because the standard 12-lead ECG does not directly record activity on the posterior surface of the myocardium, a posterior wall myocardial infarction is documented by reciprocal changes, seen as tall R waves and ST-segment depression in leads V_1 and V_2.[30]

Cardiac enzymes

Specific cardiac enzymes and isoenzymes are released in the presence of damaged or infarcted myocardial cells. To confirm the diagnosis of MI, serum CK-MB isoenzymes are measured at 6-hour intervals for the first 24 hours and then daily.[30] With a large anterior MI, the CK-MB level can rise to more than 150 U/L with a total CK level of more than 1000 U/L. Troponin levels also can be used for early detection of acute MI.

Medical Management

The goals of medical management during myocardial infarction include preservation of myocardium, pain control, pharmacologic therapy, and management of complications.

Preservation of myocardium

The first 6 hours after the onset of chest pain constitute the crucial period for salvaging the myocardium. During this period it may be possible to achieve reperfusion of the infarcting myocardium with either one or a combination of the following interventions: (1) intravenous or intracoronary thrombolysis, (2) emergency percutaneous transluminal coronary angioplasty (PTCA) or coronary atherectomy, or (3) emergency coronary artery bypass surgery.[29] Myocardial tissue can be salvaged for at least 4 hours after the onset of anginal symptoms, but in some patients this period may extend to 6 hours. Unfortunately, many persons do not seek treatment until this phase has passed.

Pain control

Pain control is a priority because continued pain is a symptom of ongoing ischemia, which places additional risk on noninfarcted myocardial tissue. Morphine remains the analgesic agent of choice; it decreases anxiety, restlessness, autonomic nervous system activity, and preload, thereby decreasing myocardial oxygen demands. Oxygen is used for a minimum of 24 to 48 hours after infarction to prevent tissue hypoxia.

Pharmacologic therapy

The major goals of drug therapy are anticoagulation, reduction in myocardial workload, and analgesia.

Anticoagulation may involve the use of three different types of agents—antiplatelet agents, anticoagulants, and thrombolytic agents. Antiplatelet agents act against the

---

> ### BOX 10-7
>
> ## COMPLICATIONS OF MYOCARDIAL INFARCTION
>
> Dysrhythmias
> Ventricular aneurysm
> Ventricular septal defect
> Papillary muscle rupture
> Pericarditis
> Cardiac rupture
> Sudden death
> Heart failure
> Pulmonary edema
> Cardiogenic shock

---

initial "white clot" that forms the platelet plug. Low-dose aspirin is used for many patients. Aspirin decreases platelet release of thromboxane A_2, which reduces vasoconstriction and further platelet aggregation.[32] This therapy may be continued for an indefinite period, and studies have documented the beneficial antiplatelet effect of low-dose prophylactic aspirin.[32] If a patient cannot tolerate aspirin, the antiplatelet agent ticlopidine (Ticlid) may be prescribed.[33] Anticoagulants are used to decrease the incidence of embolic complications (e.g., deep vein thrombosis and left ventricular thrombi), especially while bedrest is prescribed. Anticoagulants include heparin, as an IV infusion or by subcutaneous injection, or oral warfarin (Coumadin). The effectiveness of these agents is determined by measurement of blood coagulation times.[29,34,35] If an acute MI is diagnosed within 6 hours, lytic agents may be used to dissolve the clot and restore blood flow in the occluded artery.[29]

Beta-blocking agents are used to reduce infarct size by decreasing myocardial oxygen demand during the first few hours of infarction. However, beta-blockers are contraindicated if there is LV failure because they depress cardiac contractility.[29] Beta blockade is also used after the completed infarction to lower the risks of reinfarction or death. Calcium channel blockers are a diverse group of drugs that are used in conjunction with the other agents previously described to decrease coronary artery spasm and as antihypertensives.[29]

Complications

Many patients experience complications, occurring either early or late in the postinfarction course (Box 10-7). These complications may result from a pump problem or an electrical dysfunction. Pumping complications cause heart failure (HF), pulmonary edema, and cardiogenic shock. Electrical dysfunctions include bradycardia, bundle branch blocks, and varying degrees of heart block.[29] Almost 95% of patients who experience a MI will have dysrhythmias. There are many potential causes (Box 10-8). The major goal of treatment of any dysrhythmia is preservation, or return, of adequate cardiac output.

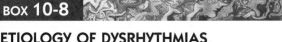

BOX 10-8

ETIOLOGY OF DYSRHYTHMIAS IN MYOCARDIAL INFARCTION

Tissue ischemia
Hypoxemia
Autonomic nervous system influences
Metabolic derangements
   Acid-base imbalances
Hemodynamic abnormalities
Drugs (especially digoxin toxicity)
Electrolyte imbalances (e.g., hypokalemia,
   hypomagnesemia)
Fiber stretch
   Chamber dilation
   Cardiomyopathy

Sinus bradycardia and sinus tachycardia. Sinus bradycardia (heart rate less than 60 beats/minute) occurs in approximately 40% of patients who sustain an acute myocardial infarction and is more prevalent with an inferior wall infarction. It is seen most frequently in the immediate postinfarction period. Symptomatic bradycardia with hypotension and low cardiac output is treated with atropine 0.5 mg IV push, repeated every 5 minutes to a maximum dose of 2 mg.[29] Sinus tachycardia (heart rate more than 100 beats/minute) most often occurs with anterior wall myocardial infarctions. Anterior infarctions impair left ventricular pumping ability, thereby reducing the ejection fraction and stroke volume. In an attempt to maintain cardiac output, the heart rate increases. Sinus tachycardia must be corrected, not only because it greatly increases myocardial oxygen consumption, but because it shortens diastolic filling time, thereby decreasing stroke volume, systemic perfusion, and coronary artery filling.

Atrial dysrhythmias. Premature atrial contractions (PAC) occur frequently in patients who sustain an acute infarction. PACs most commonly are caused by cell irritability, resulting from distention of the left atrium secondary to increased left ventricular end-diastolic pressure and volume. Atrial fibrillation is a common atrial dysrhythmia associated with acute MI and is more prevalent with an anterior wall infarction. It may occur spontaneously or be preceded by PACs or atrial flutter. With atrial fibrillation, there is loss of atrial contraction and hence a loss of atrial kick and the extra stroke volume it carries. It is estimated that cardiac output can decrease by 30% when atrial kick is lost.

Ventricular dysrhythmias. Premature ventricular contractions (PVCs) are seen in almost all patients within the first few hours after a myocardial infarction. They are controlled by administering oxygen to reduce myocardial hypoxia, by correcting acid-base or electrolyte imbalances, and by administering an IV lidocaine bolus and infusion. In the setting of an acute MI, PVCs are treated if they are (1) frequent (more than 6/minute), (2) closely coupled (R-on-T phenomenon), (3) multiform in shape,

and (4) occur in bursts of 3 or more.[29] PVCs and ventricular tachycardia (VT) occurring within the first few hours postinfarction usually are transient. When, however, these same dysrhythmias occur late in the course, they tend to be associated with high in-hospital mortality because they usually are related to the cumulative loss of myocardium. Ventricular fibrillation (VF) is a life-threatening dysrhythmia associated with high mortality in acute MI.

AV heart blocks. AV heart block during MI most frequently follows an inferior wall MI. Because the right coronary artery perfuses the AV node in 90% of the population, RCA occlusion leads to ischemia and infarction of the AV node cells. Symptomatic AV block with hemodynamic compromise is treated with IV atropine or by insertion of a temporary pacemaker.[29]

Ventricular aneurysm. A ventricular aneurysm (Fig. 10-6) is a noncontractile, thinned left ventricular wall, which results in a reduction of the stroke volume. It occurs in approximately 12% to 15% of patients who survive acute transmural infarction. The most common complications of a ventricular aneurysm are acute heart failure, systemic emboli, and VT. Treatment is directed toward management of these complications and surgical repair by left ventricular aneurysmectomy. The prognosis depends on the size of the aneurysm, overall left ventricular function, and the severity of co-existing CAD. Rupture of the aneurysm is rare, but nonetheless life-threatening, and usually occurs only if there is reinfarction of the border of the aneurysm.

Ventricular septal defect. Rupture of the ventricular septal wall (Fig. 10-7) affects approximately 1% to 2% of patients who sustain acute transmural MI and usually occurs in the first week after MI.[36] However, acute ventricular septal defect (VSD) patients make up 5% to 20% of acute MI associated deaths. The rupture often is followed by acute heart failure, shock, and death. Ventricular septal defect manifests as severe chest pain, syncope, hypotension, and sudden hemodynamic deterioration caused by shunting of blood from the high-pressure left ventricle into the low-pressure right ventricle through the new septal opening. A holosystolic murmur (accompanied by a thrill) can be auscultated and is best heard along the left sternal border. A diagnosis of postinfarction VSD can be made at the bedside with use of a pulmonary artery catheter or by transesophageal echocardiography (TEE). Rupture of the septum is a medical and surgical emergency. The patient's condition is stabilized with vasodilators and an intraaortic balloon pump (IABP) to decrease afterload. The goal of afterload reduction in these patients is to decrease the amount of blood being shunted to the right side of the heart and to increase the forward flow of blood to the systemic circulation. Mortality is very high with medical therapy alone; therefore most patients need emergency surgery to close the ventricular septum.[36]

Papillary muscle rupture. Papillary muscle rupture can occur when the infarct involves the area around the

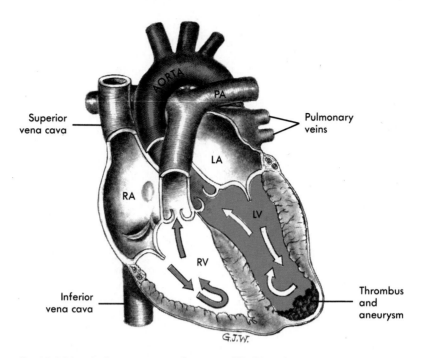

Fig. **10-6** Ventricular aneurysm after acute MI. *PA,* pulmonary artery. *LA,* left atrium. *RA,* right atrium. *LV,* left ventricle. *RV,* right ventricle.

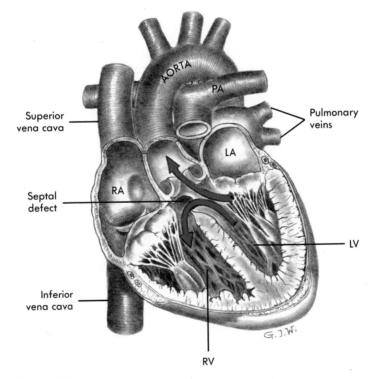

Fig. **10-7** Ventricular septal defect after acute MI. *PA,* pulmonary artery. *LA,* left atrium. *RA,* right atrium. *LV,* left ventricle. *RV,* right ventricle.

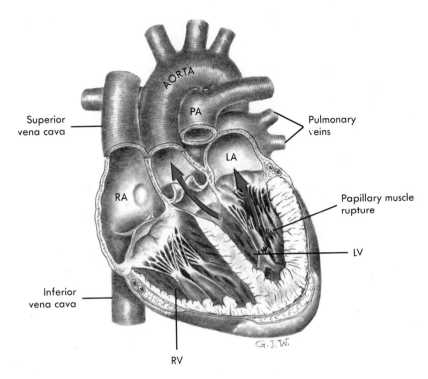

Fig. **10-8** Papillary muscle rupture after acute MI. *PA,* pulmonary artery. *LA,* left atrium. *RA,* right atrium. *LV,* left ventricle. *RV,* right ventricle.

mitral valve. It is rare but accounts for 1% to 5% of acute MI-related deaths.[11] Infarction of the papillary muscles results in ineffective mitral valve closure, and blood is forced back into the low-pressure left atrium during ventricular systole.[37] The rupture may be partial or complete. Complete rupture is catastrophic and precipitates severe acute mitral regurgitation, shock, and death. Partial rupture (Fig. 10-8) also results in mitral regurgitation, but usually the condition can be stabilized with aggressive medical management using the intraaortic balloon pump and vasodilators. Urgent surgical intervention is required to replace the mitral valve.[36]

Cardiac wall rupture. Of the deaths that occur after myocardial infarction, 3% to 4% can be attributed to cardiac rupture, which often occurs in older patients who have systemic hypertension during the acute phase of their infarction.[36,38] Rupture commonly occurs around the fifth postinfarction day when leukocyte scavenger cells are removing necrotic debris, thus thinning the myocardial wall. The onset is sudden and usually catastrophic. Bleeding into the pericardial sac results in cardiac tamponade, cardiogenic shock, electromechanical dissociation, and death. Survival is rare. If rupture occurs in the hospital, emergency pericardiocentesis is required to relieve the tamponade until a surgical repair can be attempted.[36,38]

Pericarditis

Pericarditis is inflammation of the pericardial sac. It can occur during a transmural MI after an acute MI when the damage extends into the epicardial surface of the heart. The damaged epicardium then becomes rough and tends to irritate and inflame the pericardium lying adjacent to it, precipitating pericarditis.[39] Pain is the most common symptom of pericarditis, and a pericardial friction rub is the most common sign. The friction rub is best heard at the sternal border and is described as a grating, scraping, or leathery scratching. Pericarditis may result in a pericardial effusion. Once the effusion (fluid) occurs, the friction rub may disappear. Pericarditis is treated with either aspirin or nonsteroidal antiinflammatory drugs.[39]

Nursing Management

Nursing management of the patient with an acute myocardial infarction incorporates a variety of nursing diagnoses (Box 10-9). **Nursing priorities are directed toward balancing myocardial oxygen supply/demand balance, providing comfort and emotional support, and maintaining surveillance for complications.**

Balancing myocardial oxygen supply and demand

Measures to limit myocardial oxygen consumption include administering analgesics and sedatives, positioning the patient for comfort, limiting activities, offering support to reduce anxiety, providing a calm and quiet environment, and teaching the patient about the condition. Measures to enhance oxygen myocardial supply include

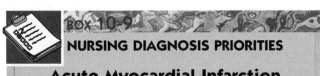

NURSING DIAGNOSIS PRIORITIES

Acute Myocardial Infarction

Acute Pain related to transmission and perception of cutaneous, visceral, muscular, or ischemic impulses, pp. 461-464

Altered Myocardial Tissue Perfusion related to decreased myocardial oxygen supply and/or increased myocardial oxygen demand, p. 466

Decreased Cardiac Output related to alterations in contractility, p. 464

Decreased Cardiac Output related to alterations in heart rate or rhythm, p. 470

Activity Intolerance related to cardiopulmonary dysfunction, p. 465

Anxiety related to threat to biologic, psychologic, and/or social integrity, pp. 448-450

Knowledge Deficit: Discharge Regimen related to lack of previous exposure to information, p. 443

administering supplemental oxygen, monitoring the patient's respiratory status, and administering prescribed medications.

Nursing research studies have shown that many of the "coronary precautions" previously practiced to decrease energy expenditure by the patient do not have a scientific basis.[40] These precautions included withholding iced oral fluids and caffeine, feeding patients, avoiding rectal temperatures, providing full bed baths, having patients use bedpans rather than bedside commodes, and avoiding vigorous backrubs.[40] One precaution that has proved valid is teaching patients to avoid the Valsalva maneuver.[40]

Acute MI patients who are stable and pain free can feed themselves and do not need to be fed by the nurse, although most acute MI patients do not have a large appetite. If patients are accustomed to drinking coffee at home, withholding it in the hospital can cause symptoms of acute caffeine withdrawal. Therefore coffee drinkers may have one to four cups of coffee a day during hospitalization.[40] There is no reason to withhold iced fluids because they do not have any clinical effect on dysrhythmias. Vigorous backrubs are not contraindicated and do not increase angina. In addition, full bed baths are no longer considered necessary for the stable patient who can assist with the bath. In the past many MI patients were given full bed baths to conserve their energy, even when the patients were pain free and stable. Most stable patients are also able, and prefer, to use the bedside commode, rather than a bedpan. Finally, the issue of obtaining rectal temperatures (not contraindicated) has largely been resolved by the increasing use of less invasive tympanic membrane thermometers that use the ear canal as the route.

A coronary precaution that must always be taught in the acute period is the importance of avoiding the Valsalva maneuver, defined as forced expiration against a closed glottis. This can be explained as "bearing down" when going to the bathroom or breath holding when repositioning in bed. The Valsalva maneuver has been associated with changes in blood pressure and heart rate because the increase in intrathoracic pressure decreases venous return to the right side of the heart.[40]

Patient education

The patient who comes into the emergency room within 6 hours of onset of chest pain immediately receives education about possible therapies to salvage the threatened myocardium, such as thrombolytic therapy or emergency percutaneous transluminal coronary angioplasty (PTCA). If the patient is admitted to the hospital beyond the window of time when the myocardium can be saved, he or she is admitted to the critical care unit and will have lost myocardial tissue. In the acute period the patient receives education about the reasons he or she is in the critical care unit and the importance of avoiding straining when coughing, moving, or using the commode or bathroom. Once the acute phase has passed, education for the patient and family is focused on risk factor reduction, manifestations of angina, when to call a physician or emergency services, medications, and resumption of physical and sexual activity.[41] If possible, a referral is made to a cardiac rehabilitation program so that this education can be reinforced outside the acute care hospital environment.[31]

HEART FAILURE

Description and Etiology

The National Heart, Lung, and Blood Institute estimates that more than 2 million Americans have heart failure (HF) and that about 400,000 new cases are diagnosed each year.[42] The heart failure rate is higher in men than in women for all age groups. The 5-year mortality rate in men is about 60%, whereas in women it is about 45%.[43] Heart failure is the most common cause of in-hospital mortality for patients with cardiac disease and is responsible for one third of the deaths of patients with an acute MI.

Heart failure is covered under DRG 127 (Heart Failure and Shock), with an anticipated length of stay of 5.8 days.[2]

Heart failure is a response to cardiac dysfunction, a condition in which the heart cannot pump blood at a volume required to meet the body's needs.[42] The cardiac dysfunction associated with heart failure is the result of conditions that cause abnormal cardiac muscle contraction or relaxation or both, an excessive pressure or volume load, and limit ventricular filling[43] (Box 10-10). For many years heart failure was known as congestive heart failure (CHF). However, because the patient in heart failure does not always have pulmonary congestion, the terms *acute heart failure* and *chronic heart failure* are increasingly being used.

BOX 10-10

PRECIPITATING CAUSES OF HEART FAILURE

ABNORMAL CARDIAC MUSCLE CONTRACTION AND RELAXATION OR BOTH

Myocardial infarction/ischemia
Dilated cardiomyopathy
Arrhythmias
Coronary artery disease
Myocarditis
Metabolic heart disease
Endocrine heart disease
Long-term alcohol consumption

EXCESSIVE PRESSURE OR VOLUME LOAD

Hypertension
Aortic stenosis
Mitral or tricuspid regurgitation
Intraventricular shunts (congenital heart disease)
High output states (thyrotoxicosis, anemia)

LIMITED VENTRICULAR FILLING

Mitral or tricuspid stenosis
Constrictive pericarditis
Restrictive cardiomyopathy
Hypertrophic obstructive cardiomyopathy

From Piano MR, Bondmass M, Schwertz DW: The molecular and cellular pathophysiology of heart failure, *Heart Lung* 27:3, 1998.

TABLE 10-2

NEW YORK HEART ASSOCIATION FUNCTIONAL CLASSIFICATION OF HEART FAILURE

CLASS	DEFINITION
I	Normal daily activity does not initiate symptoms
II	Normal daily activity initiates onset of symptoms, but symptoms subside with rest
III	Minimal activity initiates symptoms; patients are usually symptom free at rest
IV	Any type of activity initiates symptoms, and symptoms are present at rest

Pathophysiology

The function of the heart is to transfer blood coming into the ventricles from the venous system into the arterial system. Impaired cardiac function results in failure to empty the venous system and reduced delivery of blood to the pulmonary and arterial circulations—hence, heart failure. When the heart begins to fail and the cardiac output is no longer sufficient to meet the metabolic needs of the tissues, the body activates major compensatory mechanisms such as the sympathetic nervous system, the renin-angiotensin-aldosterone system, and the development of ventricular hypertrophy.

Sympathetic nervous system

This particular compensatory mechanism results in increased heart rate, contractility, and blood pressure. Although initially helpful, sinus tachycardia eventually becomes a negative factor because it increases myocardial oxygen demand while shortening the amount of time for coronary artery perfusion. This imbalance can lead to myocardial ischemia, which may decrease ventricular contraction, reduce ventricular filling, and necessitate a higher filling pressure. In addition, increased levels of circulating catecholamines cause a redistribution of regional blood flow, leading to shunting of blood from nonvital organs, such as the skin, to vital organs, such as the heart and brain.[43]

Renin-angiotensin-aldosterone system

Activation of the renin-angiotensin-aldosterone system promotes fluid retention in an attempt to maintain cardiac output. It causes constriction of the renal arterioles, decreased glomerular filtration, and increased reabsorption of sodium from the proximal and distal tubules. In addition, diminished hepatic metabolism of aldosterone increases the antidiuretic hormone (ADH) level and enhances water retention, which promotes the development of pulmonary and peripheral edema.[43]

Ventricular hypertrophy

Ventricular hypertrophy is the final compensatory mechanism. Initially, myocardial hypertrophy increases the force of contraction and helps the ventricle overcome an increase in afterload. Eventually, however, myocardial oxygen demand starts to exceed myocardial oxygen supply and subendocardial ischemia and myocardial necrosis occur.[43]

Assessment and Diagnosis

Heart failure is described in many ways, including (1) using the New York Heart Association (NYHA) classification (Table 10-2), (2) as primary ventricular involvement—right or left, (3) as progressing forward or backward, or (4) as primarily systolic or diastolic LV dysfunction. However heart failure is classified, it is important to remember that the ventricles do not function in isolation. They have a common septal wall and are encircled and bound together by continuous muscle fibers. Thus any interruption or damage to one chamber eventually affects all the chambers.

Right heart failure

Failure of the right side of the heart is defined as ineffective right ventricular contractile function. Pure failure of the right side of the heart may result from an acute condition such as a pulmonary embolus or a right ventricular infarction, but it is most commonly caused by failure of the left side of the heart or the backing up of blood behind the left ventricle. Its common manifestations are weakness, peripheral or sacral edema, jugular venous distention, hepatomegaly, jaundice, liver tenderness, and elevated central venous pressure (CVP). If peripheral perfusion is greatly compromised, cyanosis may be present. Gastrointestinal symptoms include anorexia, nausea, and a feeling of fullness (Table 10-3).

Left heart failure

Failure of the left side of the heart is defined as a disturbance of the contractile function of the left ventricle, resulting in pulmonary congestion and edema or decreased cardiac output, or both.[42] Most frequently it occurs in patients with left ventricular infarctions, hypertension, and aortic and/or mitral valve disease. Classic clinical manifestations include decreased peripheral perfusion, such as weak or diminished pulses; cool, pale extremities; and peripheral cyanosis (Table 10-3). Over time with progression of the disease state, the fluid accumulation behind the dysfunctional left ventricle produces dysfunction of the right ventricle, resulting in failure of the right side of the heart with its manifestations.

Forward heart failure

Forward heart failure is defined as inadequate delivery of blood into the arterial system. It occurs when systemic vascular resistance (afterload) is increased, producing decreased flow of blood out of the ventricles. This decrease results in a reduced cardiac output and hypoperfusion of vital organs. Forward failure often occurs with aortic stenosis or systemic hypertension.

Backward heart failure

Backward heart failure is defined as failure of the ventricle to empty. This is usually a result of left ventricular systolic dysfunction caused by myocardial infarction or cardiomyopathy. Backward heart failure results in a decreased systolic ejection fraction (EF), usually less than 30%, that causes an accumulation of fluid and elevation of pressure in all the chambers and in the venous system behind the ventricle. When the left ventricle pumps inef-

fectively, blood pools within the LV and left ventricular end-diastolic pressure (LVEDP) increases. As the mitral valve opens, the increased LVEDP results in increased atrial pressure, which is transmitted back into the pulmonary circuit, increasing pulmonary pressures.[42,44]

Acute versus chronic heart failure

Acute versus chronic heart failure refers to the rapidity with which the syndrome develops, the presence and activation of compensatory mechanisms, and the presence or absence of fluid accumulation in the interstitial space. Acute heart failure has a sudden onset, with no compensatory mechanisms. The patient may experience acute pulmonary edema, low cardiac output, or even cardiogenic shock. Patients with chronic heart failure are hypervolemic, have sodium and water retention, and have structural heart chamber changes such as dilation or hypertrophy. Chronic failure is ongoing, with symptoms that may be made tolerable by medication, diet, and a low activity level. A change to acute failure, however, can be precipitated by the onset of dysrhythmias, acute ischemia, sudden illness, or cessation of medications.

Clinical manifestations

The clinical manifestations of acute heart failure result from tissue hypoperfusion and organ congestion (Table 10-3). The severity of clinical manifestations progresses as heart failure worsens. Initially, manifestations appear only with exertion but eventually occur at rest.

Shortness of breath. The patient experiences the feeling of shortness of breath first with exertion, but as heart failure worsens, symptoms are present at rest. Breathlessness in heart failure is described by the following terms *dyspnea, orthopnea, paroxysmal nocturnal dyspnea,* and *cardiac asthma.* Dyspnea is the subjective sensation of shortness of breath. It results from pulmonary vascular congestion and decreased lung compliance. Orthopnea describes difficulty in breathing when lying flat because of an increase in venous return that occurs in the supine position. Paroxysmal nocturnal dyspnea is a severe form of orthopnea in which the patient awakens from sleep

---

TABLE 10-3

CLINICAL MANIFESTATIONS OF FAILURE OF RIGHT AND LEFT SIDES OF HEART

LEFT VENTRICULAR FAILURE		RIGHT VENTRICULAR FAILURE	
SIGNS	**SYMPTOMS**	**SIGNS**	**SYMPTOMS**
Tachypnea	Fatigue	Peripheral edema	Weakness
Tachycardia	Dyspnea	Hepatomegaly	Anorexia
Cough	Orthopnea	Splenomegaly	Indigestion
Bibasilar crackles	Paroxysmal nocturnal	Hepatojugular reflux	Weight gain
Gallop rhythms (S_3 and S_4)	dyspnea	Ascites	Mental changes
Increased pulmonary artery pressures	Nocturia	Jugular venous distention	
Hemoptysis		Increased central venous pressure	
Cyanosis		Pulmonary hypertension	
Pulmonary edema			

gasping for air. Cardiac asthma is dyspnea with wheezing, a nonproductive cough, and pulmonary crackles that progress to the gurgling sounds of pulmonary edema.

Pulmonary edema. Pulmonary edema, or fluid in the alveoli, inhibits gas exchange by impairing the diffusion pathway between the alveolus and the capillary. It is caused by increased left atrial and ventricular pressures and results in an excessive accumulation of serous or serosanguineous fluid in the interstitial spaces and alveoli of the lungs. This may be coughed up as a frothy, pink sputum. Two stages mark the formation of pulmonary edema. Stage I is characterized by interstitial edema, engorgement of the perivascular and peribronchial spaces, and increased lymphatic flow. Stage II is characterized by alveolar edema resulting from fluid moving into the alveoli from the interstitium. Eventually, blood plasma moves into the alveoli faster than the lymphatic system can clear it, interfering with diffusion of oxygen, depressing the arterial partial pressure of oxygen (PaO_2), and leading to tissue hypoxia (Fig. 10-9).

With acute onset, patients are extremely breathless and anxious with a sensation of suffocation. They expectorate pink, frothy liquid and feel as if they are drowning. They may sit bolt upright, gasp for breath, or thrash about. The respiratory rate is elevated, and accessory muscles of ventilation are used, with nasal flaring and bulging neck muscles. Respirations are characterized by loud inspiratory and expiratory gurgling sounds. Diaphoresis is profuse; and the skin is cold, ashen, and cyanotic, reflecting low cardiac output, increased sympathetic stimulation, peripheral vasoconstriction, and desaturation of arterial blood.

Arterial blood gases in pulmonary edema. Arterial blood gas (ABG) values are variable. In the early stage of pulmonary edema, respiratory alkalosis may be present because of hyperventilation, which eliminates CO_2. As the pulmonary edema progresses and as gas exchange becomes impaired, acidosis (pH less than 7.35) and hypoxemia ensue. A chest x-ray usually confirms an enlarged cardiac silhouette, pulmonary venous congestion, and interstitial edema.

Medical Management

The goals of medical management of heart failure are to relieve heart failure symptoms, enhance cardiac performance, and identify and correct the precipitating causes of acute heart failure.

Relieve symptoms and enhance cardiac performance

In the acute phase, the patient usually has a pulmonary artery catheter in place so that LV function can be followed closely. Control of symptoms involves management of fluid overload and improvement of cardiac output by decreasing systemic vascular resistance and increasing contractility. Diuretics are administered to decrease preload and to eliminate fluid from the body. If

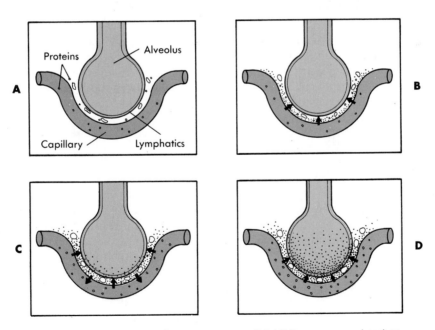

Fig. **10-9** As pulmonary edema progresses, it inhibits oxygen and carbon dioxide exchange at the alveolar capillary interface. **A,** Normal relationship. **B,** Increased pulmonary capillary hydrostatic pressure causes fluid to move from the vascular space into the pulmonary interstitial space. **C,** Lymphatic flow increases in an attempt to pull fluid back into the vascular or lymphatic space. **D,** Failure of lymphatic flow and worsening of left-sided heart failure results in further movement of fluid into the interstitial space and the alveoli.

pulmonary edema develops, additional diuretics are used. Morphine is given to facilitate peripheral dilatation and decrease anxiety. Afterload is decreased by vasodilators, such as sodium nitroprusside and nitroglycerin. Nitrates are used to decrease preload and vasodilate the coronary arteries if CAD is an underlying cause of the acute heart failure.[45] For some patients an intraaortic balloon pump (IABP) is also required. Contractility is increased by digitalis and positive inotropic agents, such as dopamine or dobutamine. Angiotensin-converting enzyme (ACE) inhibitors may alter chamber remodeling and slow the decline in contractility.[46]

Correct precipitating causes

Once symptoms of heart failure are controlled, diagnostic studies such as cardiac catheterization, echocardiogram, and thallium scan are undertaken to uncover the cause of the heart failure and tailor long-term management to treat the cause. Some structural problems such as valvular disease may require surgical correction.

Nursing Management

Nursing management of the patient with heart failure incorporates a variety of nursing diagnoses (Box 10-11). **Nursing priorities are directed toward optimizing cardiopulmonary function, providing rest periods, providing comfort and emotional support, and maintaining surveillance for complications.**

Optimizing cardiopulmonary function

The patient's ECG is evaluated for any dysrhythmias that may be present or that may develop as a result of drug toxicity or electrolyte imbalance. Patients experiencing heart failure are prone to digoxin toxicity secondary to decreased renal perfusion as well as to electrolyte imbalances. Breath sounds are auscultated frequently to determine adequacy of respiratory effort and to assess for onset or worsening of congestion. Oxygen through a nasal cannula is administered to relieve dyspnea. Diuretics or vasodilators are used to decrease excessive preload and afterload. If the patient is not hypotensive, morphine may be administered to decrease hyperventilation and anxiety. If the patient's ventilatory status worsens, the nurse must be prepared for endotracheal intubation and mechanical ventilation. Obtaining daily weights is important until the weight stabilizes at a "dry" weight. Generally, the daily weight is used in fluid management, and a weekly weight is used for tracking body weight (muscle, fat).

Promoting comfort and emotional support

During periods of breathlessness, activity must be restricted; bedrest usually is prescribed for the patient, who is positioned with the head of the bed elevated to allow for maximal lung expansion. The arms can be supported on pillows so that there is no undue stress placed on the shoulder muscles. The legs may be placed in a dependent position to encourage venous pooling,

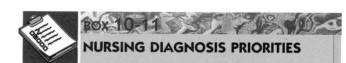

BOX 10-11

NURSING DIAGNOSIS PRIORITIES

Acute Heart Failure

- Impaired Gas Exchange related to ventilation/perfusion mismatching or intrapulmonary shunting, p. 476
- Decreased Cardiac Output related to alterations in preload, pp. 467-468
- Decreased Cardiac Output related to alterations in contractility, p. 469
- Activity Intolerance related to cardiopulmonary dysfunction, p. 465
- Ineffective Individual Coping related to situational crisis and personal vulnerability, pp. 453-455
- Knowledge Deficit: Medications related to lack of previous exposure to information, p. 433

thereby decreasing venous return. Rest periods must be carefully planned and adhered to, while independence within the patient's activity prescription is fostered.[47] Vital signs are recorded before an activity is begun and after it is completed. Signs of activity intolerance, such as dyspnea, fatigue, sustained increase in pulse, and onset of dysrhythmias, are documented and reported to the physician. Activity is gradually increased according to patient tolerance.

Patient education

The nurse assesses the patient's understanding of conservation of energy in planning activities and collaborates with the patient in organizing the day's schedule. Other topics to cover include the importance of a low-salt diet and the multiple medications used to control the symptoms of heart failure.

CARDIOMYOPATHY

Description and Etiology

Cardiomyopathy is a disease of the heart muscle. Cardiomyopathies are described as primary or secondary and further classified on the basis of associated structural abnormalities. These categories are hypertrophic, restrictive, and dilated cardiomyopathy (Fig. 10-10).

Cardiomyopathy falls under two different DRGs depending on whether the patient develops complications or comorbid conditions (CC). These are DRG 144 (Other Circulatory System Diagnoses with CC) and DRG 145 (Other Circulatory System Diagnoses without CC) with average lengths of stay of 5.4 days and 3.0 days, respectively.[2]

Primary cardiomyopathy

Primary, or idiopathic, cardiomyopathy is defined as a heart muscle disease of unknown cause, although both viral infections and autoimmune disorders have been implicated.

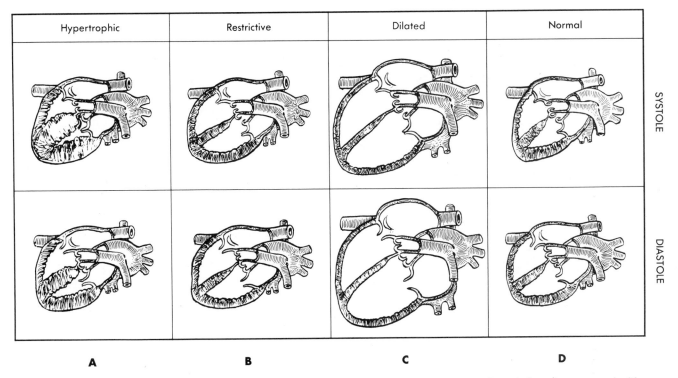

Fig. 10-10 Types of cardiomyopathies and the differences in ventricular diameter during systole and diastole compared with a normal heart. **A,** Hypertrophic. **B,** Restrictive. **C,** Dilated. **D,** Normal.

Secondary cardiomyopathy

Secondary cardiomyopathy is defined as heart muscle disease resulting from some other systemic disease, such as coronary artery disease, valvular heart disease, severe hypertension, alcohol abuse, or known autoimmune disease.

Pathophysiology and Medical Management

Hypertrophic cardiomyopathy

Hypertrophic cardiomyopathy (HCM) is characterized by stiff, noncompliant myocardial muscle with left ventricular hypertrophy and bizarre cellular hypertrophy of the upper ventricular septum. This septal hypertrophy results in obstruction of the aortic valve outflow tract (Fig. 10-10, *A*). It also pulls the papillary muscle out of alignment, causing mitral regurgitation. This disorder used to be known as idiopathic hypertrophic subaortic stenosis (IHSS); however, because IHSS described only 25% of affected patients, the more general term of HCM is now used.[48,49] Symptoms include exertional dyspnea, myocardial ischemia, supraventricular tachycardia (SVT), VT, syncope, and heart failure. Sudden cardiac death occurs in 2% to 3% of adults with HCM per year.[50] Medical management includes limitation of physical activity, beta-blockers, calcium channel blockers, antidysrhythmic therapy, treatment of heart failure, and for some patients an implantable cardioverter defibrillator (ICD), surgical myectomy, or mitral valve replacement.[48]

Restrictive cardiomyopathy

Restrictive cardiomyopathy (Fig. 10-10, *B*) is the least common form and is characterized by abnormal diastolic function. This cardiomyopathy results in ventricular wall rigidity as a consequence of myocardial fibrosis. The overall effect is the obstruction of ventricular filling. Restrictive cardiomyopathy may be misdiagnosed as constrictive pericarditis. Backward heart failure, low cardiac output, dyspnea, orthopnea, and liver engorgement are the most common clinical manifestations of restrictive cardiomyopathy. Medical management is directed toward the improvement of pump function, removal of excess fluid, and a low-sodium diet.

Dilated cardiomyopathy

Dilated cardiomyopathy is characterized by grossly dilated ventricles without muscle hypertrophy (Fig. 10-10, *C*). The muscle fibers contract poorly, resulting in global left ventricular dysfunction, low cardiac output, atrial and ventricular dysrhythmias, blood pooling that leads to ventricular clots and embolic episodes, and finally, refractory heart failure and premature death. The goals of medical management of dilated cardiomyopathy are improvement of pump function, removal of excess fluid, control of heart failure, and prevention of sudden cardiac death and other complications.[51]

Nursing Management

Nursing management of the patient with cardiomyopathy incorporates a variety of nursing diagnoses (Box

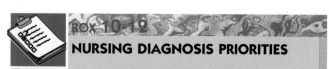

10-12). **Nursing priorities are individualized according to the type of cardiomyopathy and are directed toward maintaining fluid balance, monitoring pharmacologic therapy, providing comfort and emotional support, and maintaining surveillance for complications.**

Maintaining fluid balance

Patients are monitored for clinical manifestations of worsening heart failure, such as tissue edema, increased ventricular filling pressures, neck vein engorgement, pulmonary congestion, weight gain, increased fatigue, and onset of gallop rhythms. Daily weight and strict fluid restriction with accurate intake and output records are required.

Monitoring pharmacologic therapy

The patient with cardiomyopathy usually takes a wide range of medications that includes diuretics, calcium channel blockers, beta-blockers, vasodilators, anticoagulant or antiplatelet agents, and antidysrhythmics. Often the transition from IV to oral administration is supervised by the critical care nurse, and knowledge of appropriate and unwanted side effects is essential. For example, patients with cardiomyopathy are prone to digoxin toxicity related to decreased excretion of the drug secondary to a decreased glomerular filtration rate.

Patient education

Topics of education include all of those applicable to acute heart failure. Also, assessment of the patient's understanding of this illness, adaptive coping mechanisms, and support systems must be incorporated into the teaching plan. Patients and families need to know what support services are available. Most cardiomyopathies have only palliative treatments, and patients may need to be educated for several possible outcomes, including heart transplantation, cardiac disability, or sudden cardiac death.

ENDOCARDITIS

Description and Etiology

Infection by a microorganism of a platelet-fibrin vegetation on the endothelial surface of the heart results in infective endocarditis. Acute and subacute endocarditis is covered under DRG 126, with an anticipated length of stay of 13.1 days.[2]

Development of endocarditis depends on two factors: (1) a susceptible lesion in the vascular endothelium and (2) an organism to establish the infection.[52] The source of the organism may be unknown, or it may be traced to an invasive procedure, such as a biopsy, cannulation of the veins or arteries, urogenital procedures, dental work, or intravenous drug use.[53] Almost any bacterium or fungus can infect a susceptible site. In Western Europe and North America, streptococci and staphylococci account for 75% to 85% of all endocarditis cases. For this reason aggressive treatment of all streptococcal pharyngitis cases is encouraged.[54]

Pathophysiology

Endocarditis begins after the onset of bacteremia and the colonization of thrombotic vegetation. The bacteria is then encased in a platelet and fibrin shell, which protects it from destruction by phagocytic neutrophils, leading to a zone of localized agranulocytosis. It is because of this extensive protective mechanism, which restricts the body's normal response to infection, that antibiotic therapy must be so intensive and prolonged.

Assessment and Diagnosis

Endocarditis may be described as either acute or subacute. Acute infection develops on normal valves, progresses rapidly, causes severe destruction, and may be fatal if the patient is not treated. Subacute infection occurs on damaged heart valves and progresses much more slowly. The term *subacute bacterial endocarditis (SBE)* is not always accurate because, although most infections are bacterial, some are caused by yeast or fungus. It is much more useful to classify the disease according to the causative microorganism. Clinical manifestations of endocarditis are listed in Box 10-13.

Medical Management

Treatment requires prolonged parenteral therapy with adequate doses of bactericidal antibiotics. An increasing number of patients are being discharged home earlier than in the past and continue the parenteral therapy via a long-term venous access at home. In cases of prosthetic valve endocarditis, antibiotics are usually not a sufficient

CLINICAL MANIFESTATIONS OF ENDOCARDITIS

Fever
Splenomegaly
Hematuria
Petechiae
Cardiac murmurs
Easy fatigability
Osler's nodes (small, raised, tender areas most commonly found in pads of fingers and toes)
Splenic hemorrhages
Roth's spots (round or oval spots consisting of coagulated fibrin; seen in the retina and leading to hemorrhage)

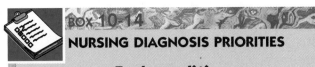

BOX 10-14

NURSING DIAGNOSIS PRIORITIES

Endocarditis

- Activity Intolerance related to cardiopulmonary dysfunction, p. 465
- Acute Pain related to transmission and perception of cutaneous, visceral, muscular, or ischemic impulses, pp. 461-464
- Risk for Infection, pp. 494-495
- Anxiety related to threat to biologic, psychologic, and/or social integrity, pp. 448-450
- Knowledge Deficit: Discharge Regimen related to lack of previous exposure to information, p. 443

BOX 10-15

ETIOLOGY OF VALVULAR HEART DISEASE

Rheumatic fever
Infective endocarditis
Inborn defects of connective tissue
Dysfunction or ruptures of the papillary muscles
Congenital malformations
Aging valve tissue

treatment, and surgical replacement of the valve is required.[55]

Nursing Management

Nursing management of the patient with endocarditis incorporates a variety of nursing diagnoses (Box 10-14). **Nursing priorities are directed toward monitoring for further infection, preventing the spread of infection, providing comfort and emotional support, and maintaining surveillance for complications.** In addition, the patient's response to the antibiotic therapy should be monitored for adverse effects.

Monitoring for further infection

Endocarditis requires a long course of intravenous antibiotics, usually 6 weeks. This is begun in the hospital and continued at home with an indwelling central catheter. Nursing assessment includes monitoring for signs of worsening infection, such as temperature elevation, malaise, weakness, easy fatigability, and night sweats.

Preventing the spread of infection

Prevention should be directed at eradicating pathogens from the environment and interrupting the spread of organisms from person to person. Possible sources include indwelling lines and the urinary drainage catheter. These invasive tools must be given proper aseptic care. Proper hand-washing technique is the single most important measure available to prevent the spread of bacteria from person to person.

Maintaining surveillance for complications

The patient with infective endocarditis is at risk for embolic events, either cerebral or pulmonary. Therefore level of consciousness, visual changes, and headache are assessed. As valvular dysfunction accelerates, acute heart failure develops. Cardiac assessment includes auscultation of heart sounds to detect the presence or change in a cardiac murmur. Shortness of breath or chest pain with hemoptysis must be reported. This could be caused either by worsening heart failure or by pulmonary emboli.

Patient education

The patient needs to know the manifestations of infection, how to take an oral temperature, activities that increase risk of a recurrence of the endocarditis, the necessity of providing other health care professionals such as the dentist or podiatrist with the endocarditis history, and information on how to obtain Medic Alert bracelets and cards if required.

VALVULAR HEART DISEASE

Description and Etiology

Valvular heart disease describes structural and/or functional abnormalities of single or multiple cardiac valves. The result is alteration in blood flow across the valve. Valvular diseases can be classified as either stenosis or regurgitation (insufficiency).

In the past in the United States, most valvular lesions were rheumatic in origin; that is, damage was a direct result of group A beta-hemolytic streptococcal pharyngitis. Today, with the aging population, degenerative valve changes are equally important (Box 10-15).

Pathophysiology and Assessment

Stenosis refers to a narrowing of the valve resulting in the need for a greater pressure to open the valve and main-

TABLE 10-4

VALVULAR DYSFUNCTION

	PATHOPHYSIOLOGY	CLINICAL MANIFESTATIONS	PHYSICAL SIGNS
A Mitral valve stenosis ⇣ indicates stenosis	**MITRAL VALVE STENOSIS** Left atrium must generate more pressure to propel blood beyond the lesion Rise in left atrial pressure and volume reflected retrograde into pulmonary vessels Right ventricular hypertrophy Right ventricular failure	Dyspnea on exertion Fatigue and weakness Pronounced respiratory symptoms—orthopnea, paroxysmal nocturnal dyspnea Mild hemoptysis with bronchial capillary rupture Susceptibility to pulmonary infections	Chest radiograph—pulmonary congestion, redistribution of blood flow to upper lobes ECG—atrial fibrillation and other atrial dysrhythmias Auscultation—diastolic murmur, accentuated S_1, opening snap Catheterization—elevated pressure gradient across valve; increased left atrial pressure, pulmonary artery wedge pressure, and pulmonary artery pressure; low cardiac output
B Mitral valve regurgitation ↑ indicates stenosis of the valve 🌿 indicates backward flow from a valve that is leaking or regurgitant	**MITRAL VALVE REGURGITATION** Left ventricular dilation and hypertrophy Left atrial dilation and hypertrophy	Weakness and fatigue Exertional dyspnea Palpitations Severe symptoms precipitated by left ventricular failure, with consequent low output and pulmonary congestion	Chest radiograph—left atrial and left ventricular enlargement, variable pulmonary congestion ECG—P-mitrale, left ventricular hypertrophy, atrial fibrillation Auscultation—murmur throughout systole Catheterization—opacification of left atrium during left ventricular injection, V waves, increased left atrial and left ventricular pressures Variable elevations of pulmonary pressures
C Aortic valve stenosis ↑ indicates stenosis	**AORTIC VALVE STENOSIS** Left ventricular hypertrophy Progressive failure of ventricular emptying Pulmonary congestion Failure of right side of heart, with systemic venous congestion	Exertional dyspnea Exercise intolerance Syncope Angina Heart failure (left ventricular failure)	Chest radiograph—poststenotic aortic dilation, calcification ECG—left ventricular hypertrophy Auscultation—systolic ejection murmur Catheterization—significant pressure gradient, increased left ventricular end-diastolic pressure
		Sudden cardiac death	

---

tain blood flow through the valve. Regurgitation refers to an incompetent valve resulting in bidirectional blood flow through the valve.

Mitral valve stenosis

Mitral stenosis describes a progressive narrowing of the mitral valve orifice from the normal size of 4 to 6 cm to less than 1.5 cm. This narrowing is usually caused by aging valve tissue or by acute rheumatic valvulitis (Table 10-4, *A*). Diffuse valve leaflet fibrosis and fusion of one or both commissures reduces leaflet mobility. Also the chordae tendineae may be thickened, shortened, and fused—further contributing to the stenotic mitral orifice. As a result, the mitral valve no longer can open and close passively in response to chamber pressure changes, and blood flow across the valve is impeded.[56,57]

TABLE 10-4

VALVULAR DYSFUNCTION—cont'd

	PATHOPHYSIOLOGY	CLINICAL MANIFESTATIONS	PHYSICAL SIGNS

AORTIC VALVE REGURGITATION

| | Increased volume load imposed on left ventricle
Left ventricular dilation and hypertrophy | Fatigue
Dyspnea on exertion
Palpitations | Chest radiograph—boot-shaped elongation of cardiac apex
ECG—left ventricular hypertrophy
Auscultation—diastolic murmur
Catheterization—opacification of left ventricle during aortic injection
Peripheral signs—hyperdynamic myocardial action and low peripheral resistance |

RA LA
RV LV
D

Aortic valve regurgitation

↑ **indicates stenosis of the valve**

indicates backward flow from a valve that is leaking or regurgitant

TRICUSPID VALVE STENOSIS

| | Right atrium must generate higher pressure to eject blood beyond the lesion
Right atrial dilation
Systemic venous engorgement
Increased venous pressures | Venous distention
Peripheral edema
Ascites
Hepatic engorgement
Anorexia | Chest radiograph—right atrial enlargement
ECG—right atrial enlargement (P-pulmonale)
Auscultation—diastolic murmur
Catheterization—elevated right atrial pressure with large a waves; pressure gradient across the tricuspid valve |

RA LA
RV LV
E

Tricuspid valve stenosis

↓ **indicates stenosis**

TRICUSPID VALVE REGURGITATION

| | Right ventricular hypertrophy and dilation | Decreased cardiac output
Neck vein distention
Hepatic engorgement
Ascites
Edema
Pleural effusions | Chest radiograph—right atrial and ventricular enlargement
ECG—right ventricular hypertrophy and right atrial enlargement, atrial fibrillation
Auscultation—murmur throughout systole
Catheterization—elevated right atrial pressure and V waves |

RA LA
RV LV
F

Tricuspid valve regurgitation

↑ **indicates stenosis of the valve**

indicates backward flow from a valve that is leaking or regurgitant

Mitral valve regurgitation

Mitral valve regurgitation may occur secondary to rheumatic disease or aging of the valve, or it can be caused by endocarditis, papillary muscle dysfunction, or a number of other events (Table 10-4, *B*). In mitral valve regurgitation the valve annulus, leaflets, commissures, chordae tendineae, and papillary muscles may all be dysfunctional or the dysfunction may be isolated to just one component of the valve. Mitral valve regurgitation results in retrograde flow of blood into the left atrium with each ventricular contraction. The left atrium dilates to accommodate this additional volume, whereas the left ventricle hypertrophies as it tries to maintain forward flow and an adequate stroke volume. Acute mitral valve regurgitation caused by papillary muscle rupture secondary to acute MI is a medical emergency. This condition is not tolerated without aggressive medical therapy to stabilize the patient's condition, which frequently includes the use of an intraaortic balloon pump. Once the patient's condition has been stabilized, surgical replacement of the incompetent valve is performed.[58]

Aortic valve stenosis

Aortic valve stenosis can result from aging, calcification of a congenital bicuspid valve, or rheumatic valvulitis (Table 10-4, *C*). Irrespective of its cause, the effect is the impedance of ejection of blood from the left ventricle into the aorta, resulting in increased left ventricular systolic pressure, left ventricular hypertrophy, and eventually, at end-stage disease, left ventricular dilation. In addition, when the increase in volume and pressure are communicated back to the atrial and pulmonary vasculature, the result is an increase in left atrial pressure and volume, elevated pulmonary venous pressure, and pulmonary congestion. The goal of medical and surgical management is to prevent left ventricular damage from occurring.[59]

Aortic valve regurgitation

Aortic valve regurgitation or insufficiency can occur as a result of rheumatic fever, systemic hypertension, Marfan's syndrome, syphilis, rheumatoid arthritis, aging valve tissue, or discrete subaortic stenosis (Table 10-4, *D*). Aortic valve incompetence results in reflux of blood back into the left ventricle during ventricular diastole. To accommodate this extra volume, the left ventricle initially dilates and then hypertrophies in an attempt to empty more completely and to meet the needs of the peripheral circulation. Recent research indicates that women, because of their smaller left ventricular size, may benefit from earlier aortic valve repair surgery than do men.[60]

Tricuspid valve stenosis

Tricuspid stenosis is rarely an isolated lesion; it frequently occurs in conjunction with mitral or aortic disease, or both. Its origin most often is rheumatic fever (Table 10-4, *E*). Tricuspid stenosis increases the pressure work of the usually low-pressure right atrium, resulting in right atrial hypertrophy. In addition, the right atrium dilates in an attempt to accommodate the residual right atrial volume and the incoming venous return. As a result, systemic venous congestion occurs—the consequences of which include jugular venous congestion, liver failure, hepatomegaly, ascites, and peripheral edema.[61,62]

Tricuspid valve regurgitation

Tricuspid valve regurgitation usually results from severe pulmonary hypertension or advanced failure of the left side of the heart, which eventually affects the right side of the heart (backward heart failure)[61,62] (Table 10-4, *F*).

Pulmonic valve disease

Pulmonic valve disease is not a common disorder in adults. It is most often related to congenital anomalies and produces failure of the right side of the heart.

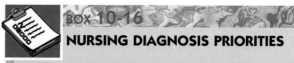

BOX 10-16

NURSING DIAGNOSIS PRIORITIES

Valvular Heart Disease

Decreased Cardiac Output related to alterations in preload, pp. 467-468
Decreased Cardiac Output related to alterations in afterload, pp. 468-469
Decreased Cardiac Output related to alterations in contractility, p. 469
Decreased Cardiac Output related to alterations in heart rate or rhythm, p. 470
Activity Intolerance related to cardiopulmonary dysfunction, p. 465
Ineffective Individual Coping related to situational crisis and personal vulnerability, pp. 453-455
Knowledge Deficit: Discharge Regimen related to lack of previous exposure to information, p. 443

Mixed valvular lesions

Many persons have mixed lesions (i.e., an element of both stenosis and regurgitation). Mixed lesions can accentuate the severity of a condition. For example, when combined, aortic stenosis and aortic regurgitation increase left ventricular volume and pressure and thereby multiply the degree of left ventricular work.

Medical Management

Management of valvular disorders includes pharmacologic therapy to control symptoms of heart failure, balloon dilatation, or cardiac surgical repair or replacement.

Nursing Management

Nursing management of the patient with valvular disease incorporates a variety of nursing diagnoses (Box 10-16). **Nursing priorities are directed toward optimizing cardiac output, maintaining fluid balance, providing comfort and emotional support, and maintaining surveillance for complications.**

Optimizing cardiac output

Low cardiac output is a common finding in patients with valvular heart disease. It can occur because of decreased forward flow through a stenotic valve or because of bidirectional flow across an incompetent valve. Vital signs and the effect of positive inotropic and afterload-reducing agents are assessed and documented. If the patient has hemodynamic catheters, cardiac output and hemodynamic parameters are measured and evaluated. Patient care activities are carefully planned to provide adequate rest periods to prevent fatigue.

Maintaining fluid balance

Fluid status is assessed by auscultating breath and heart sounds. The appearance of pulmonary crackles or an S_3 may indicate volume overload. The jugular vein may be assessed for signs of increased distention. Diuretics and vasodilators are administered, if required. The patient is weighed daily, and fluid intake and output is monitored and recorded.

Patient education

Patient education includes information related to diet and/or fluid restrictions, actions and side effects of heart failure medications, the need for prophylactic antibiotics before undergoing any invasive procedures such as dental work,[52] and when to call the health care provider to report a change in cardiac symptoms.

ATHEROSCLEROTIC DISEASES OF THE AORTA

Description and Etiology

Two atherosclerotic aortic conditions are described—aortic aneurysm and aortic dissection. An aortic aneurysm is a localized dilation of the arterial wall that results in an alteration in vessel shape and blood flow. Fig. 10-11 displays the four types of aneurysms. An aortic dissection occurs when a column of blood separates the vascular layers. This creates a false lumen, which communicates with the true lumen through a tear in the intima.[63]

The incidence of aortic aneurysm is higher in men than in women, and it is diagnosed most commonly after the fifth decade of life. Abdominal aortic aneurysm is four times more common than is thoracic aneurysm. Most patients with an aortic aneurysm (90%) have a history of systemic hypertension. Other causes of aortic aneurysm include (1) atherosclerotic changes in the thoracic and abdominal aorta, (2) blunt trauma, (3) Marfan's syndrome, (4) pregnancy, and (5) iatrogenic injury or dissection.[63]

Aortic aneurysm and aortic dissection fall under two different DRGs depending on whether the patient develops complications or comorbid conditions (CC). DRG 130 (Peripheral Vascular Disorders with CC) and DRG 131 (Peripheral Vascular Disorders without CC) have average lengths of stay of 6.3 days and 4.9 days, respectively.[2] If the patient has surgery, then two other DRGs are used, depending on the condition. These are DRG 110 (Major Cardiovascular Procedures with CC) and DRG 111 (Major Cardiovascular Procedures without CC) with average lengths of stay of 10.2 days and 6.2 days, respectively.[2]

Assessment and Diagnosis

An aortic aneurysm does not always have symptoms. It may be detected during routine abdominal examination as a palpable, pulsatile mass located in the umbilical region of the abdomen to the left of the midline. A thoracic aneurysm may be identified on a routine chest x-ray film. An aortic dissection is usually identified emergently by the onset of acute pain.

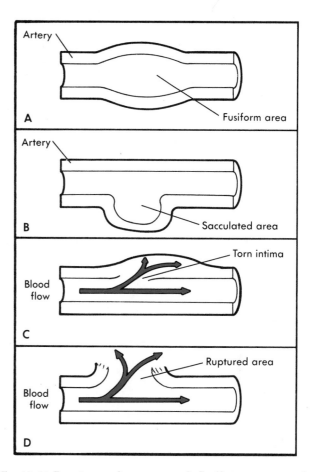

Fig. **10-11** Four types of aneurysms. **A,** Fusiform aneurysm, in which an entire segment of an artery is dilated, thus taking on a spindle or bulbous shape. Fusiform aneurysms occur most often in the abdominal aorta secondary to atherosclerosis. **B,** Sacculated aneurysm, which involves only one side of an artery and usually is located in the ascending aorta. **C,** Dissecting aneurysm, which occurs because of a tear in the intima, resulting in the shunting of blood between the intima and media of a vessel. **D,** Pseudoaneurysm, which results from a ruptured artery.

Aortic aneurysm

An aneurysm less than 4 cm in diameter can be managed on an outpatient basis with frequent blood pressure monitoring and ultrasound testing to document any changes in the aneurysm's size. The patient is encouraged to lose weight if obesity is a factor, and hypertension is treated to decrease hemodynamic stress on the site. An aneurysm greater than 5 cm usually requires surgical intervention (Box 10-17). After surgical repair, the patient generally is admitted to the critical care unit.

Aortic dissection

Aortic dissection is classified according to the site of the tear. There are two classification systems used in clinical practice. These use either the letters *A* and *B* or numerals *I, II,* or *III,* as shown in Fig. 10-12. The classic clinical manifestation of dissection is the sudden onset of intense, severe, tearing pain, which may be localized initially in the chest, abdomen, or back. As dissection ex-

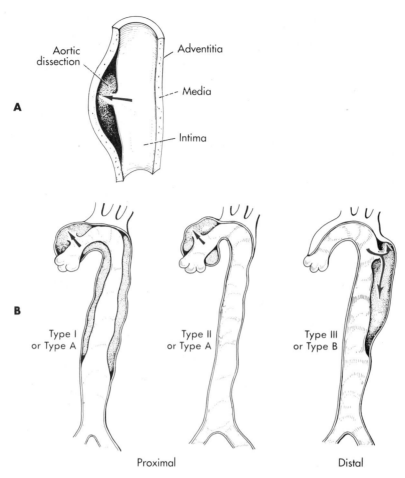

Fig. **10-12** Aortic dissection. **A,** Separation of vascular layers. **B,** Classification of aortic dissection. (Modified from Price SA, Wilson LM: *Pathophysiology: clinical concepts of disease processes,* ed 4, St Louis, 1992, Mosby.)

BOX 10-17

INDICATIONS FOR AORTIC ANEURYSM REPAIR

Aneurysm greater than 5 cm
Aneurysm progressively increasing in size
Impending rupture
Symptoms resulting from cerebral or coronary ischemia
Pericardial tamponade
Uncontrollable pain
Aortic insufficiency

---

tends, pain radiates to the back or distally toward the lower extremities. Cardiovascular signs may include severe hypertension, acute neurologic deficits, fleeting peripheral pulses, or a new murmur indicative of aortic regurgitation. The location of the dissection may be established by the site of the pain. A descending aortic dissection usually is accompanied by pain that radiates to the back, abdomen, or legs. An ascending aortic dissec-

tion produces central chest pain. Invasive diagnostic procedures that may be performed include an aortogram (aortic angiogram with radioopaque contrast), magnetic resonance imaging (MRI), and a computed tomographic (CT) scan using contrast.[64]

Medical Management

Medical management of an aortic aneurysm involves controlling hypertension and educating the patient about the need for corrective surgery if the aneurysm is more than 5 cm. Medical management of acute aortic dissection involves control of hypertension with intravenous agents and control of pain with narcotics such as morphine. Progression of the dissection is evaluated by the patient's report of worsening or new pain. Surgery to prevent death from cardiac tamponade is usually performed for dissections that involve the ascending aorta. This includes Type A, or Types I and II, dissections. The surgical procedure includes resection of the affected area, followed by graft placement and restoration of blood flow to major branches of the aorta. Replacement of the aortic valve may be performed if the dissection involves

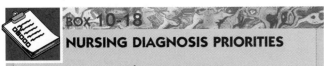

BOX 10-18

NURSING DIAGNOSIS PRIORITIES

Aortic Aneurysm and Aortic Dissection

- Decreased Cardiac Output related to alterations in preload, pp. 467-468
- Acute Pain related to transmission and perception of cutaneous, visceral, muscular, or ischemic impulses, pp. 461-464
- Altered Peripheral Tissue Perfusion related to decreased peripheral blood flow, p. 467
- Anxiety related to threat to biologic, psychologic, and/or social integrity, pp. 448-450
- Altered Renal Tissue Perfusion related to decreased renal blood flow, p. 485
- Knowledge Deficit: Discharge Regimen related to lack of previous exposure to information, p. 443

the valve.[64] Dissections that involve the descending aorta (Type B or Type III) do not always require surgery.

Nursing Management

Nursing management of the patient with aortic aneurysm or aortic dissection incorporates a variety of nursing diagnoses (Box 10-18). **Nursing priorities are directed toward controlling hypertension, facilitating pain management, providing comfort and emotional support, and maintaining surveillance for complications.**

Controlling hypertension

Cardiovascular status is assessed hourly, including monitoring blood pressure in both arms, checking peripheral pulses bilaterally, auscultating for an aortic murmur, and monitoring the ECG for ischemic changes or dysrhythmias. Patients usually require an arterial line and receive potent vasodilators such as labetalol or sodium nitroprusside.

Facilitating pain management

Acute pain is a classic sign of aortic dissection. Analgesics are given to control pain, decrease anxiety, and increase comfort. Because analgesics can mask the pain of further dissection, they are administered judiciously. The patient's neurovascular status is assessed hourly. Documentation includes the presence and distribution of pain, pallor, paresthesia, paralysis, and pulselessness.

HYPERTENSIVE CRISIS

Description and Etiology

Hypertensive crises are relatively uncommon, but when they do occur they are life threatening and demand early recognition and management to minimize morbidity and mortality. There are two types of hypertensive crises: (1) hypertensive emergencies, which develop rapidly over hours to days and place the patient at risk for end-organ damage; and (2) hypertensive urgencies, which develop over days to weeks and are characterized by a serious elevation in blood pressure but do not put the patient at risk for end-organ damage. Hypertensive crisis is characterized by a rise in diastolic blood pressure to greater than 120 to 130 mm Hg.[65]

Hypertensive crisis falls under DRG 134 (Hypertension) with an average length of stay of 3.6 days.[2]

Pathophysiology

Hypertensive crisis may occur in patients with no history of the condition or it can be precipitated by noncompliance with medical therapy or diet, or both, or by inadequate treatment. In patients with no known history of hypertension, common causes of crisis include (1) acute renal failure, (2) acute central nervous system (CNS) events, (3) drug-induced hypertension, (4) ingestion of tyramine-containing foods or beverages (beer or cheese) during treatment with a monoamine oxidase inhibitor (MAOI), and (5) pregnancy-induced eclampsia. The exact mechanism of hypertensive crisis is not known, but it is characterized by fibrinoid necrosis of the arterioles.

Assessment and Diagnosis

Hypertensive crisis is manifested by CNS compromise (headache, papilledema, coma), cardiovascular compromise (angina, myocardial infarction), acute renal failure, and a history consistent with catecholamine excess. Other symptoms include nausea and vomiting, confusion, lethargy, altered mental status, and blurring of vision. Worsening of such symptoms may indicate hypertensive encephalopathy. Table 10-5 lists symptoms and clinical findings associated with hypertensive emergencies.

Diagnostic studies include blood pressure measurement in both arms and placement of an intraarterial line for close monitoring of blood pressure. A 12-lead ECG is taken to evaluate for evidence of acute MI or left ventricular hypertrophy. Other pathologic diseases associated with acute hypertension include aortic dissection, stroke, acute heart failure, and acute renal failure.

Medical Management

Hypertensive emergencies necessitate admission of the patient to the critical care unit, where antihypertensive therapy can be administered parenterally and blood pressure monitored continuously by means of an arterial line. Several intravenous medications, in several different drug classes, are available for acute reduction of blood pressure. Medications include vasodilators such as sodium nitroprusside (SNP), nitroglycerin (NTG), hydralazine, and diazoxide. Short-acting effective beta-blockers are labetalol and esmolol. Beta-blockers are especially effective if aortic dissection is present. The intravenous

TABLE 10-5

HYPERTENSIVE EMERGENCIES

EMERGENCY	EXAMPLES OF CAUSES
CARDIOVASCULAR COMPROMISE	
Chest pain	Unstable angina, myocardial infarction, aortic dissection
Acute heart failure	Myocardial infarction, severe hypertension
Hypertension after vascular surgery	Aortic aneurysmectomy, carotid endarterectomy, coronary artery bypass grafting
CENTRAL NERVOUS SYSTEM (CNS) COMPROMISE	
Papilledema	Increased intracranial pressure—mass lesion Malignant hypertension—any cause
Headache, agitation, lethargy, confusion	Hypertensive encephalopathy—any cause, subarachnoid hemorrhage, cerebrovascular accident (CVA)
Coma	CVA, advanced hypertensive encephalopathy, trauma, tumor
Seizures	Advanced hypertensive encephalopathy, CNS tumor, eclampsia, CVA (less common)
Focal neurologic deficit	CVA, CNS tumor, hypertensive encephalopathy
ACUTE RENAL FAILURE	Malignant hypertension, vasculitis, scleroderma, glomerulonephritis
CATECHOLAMINE EXCESS	Pheochromocytomas, monoamine oxidase inhibitor (MAOI) in combination with certain drugs and foods, clonidine and guanabenz withdrawal

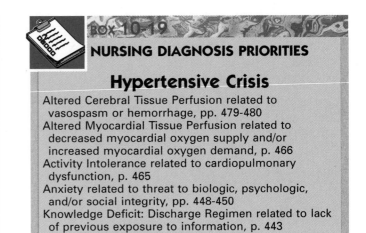

BOX 10-19

NURSING DIAGNOSIS PRIORITIES

Hypertensive Crisis

Altered Cerebral Tissue Perfusion related to vasospasm or hemorrhage, pp. 479-480
Altered Myocardial Tissue Perfusion related to decreased myocardial oxygen supply and/or increased myocardial oxygen demand, p. 466
Activity Intolerance related to cardiopulmonary dysfunction, p. 465
Anxiety related to threat to biologic, psychologic, and/or social integrity, pp. 448-450
Knowledge Deficit: Discharge Regimen related to lack of previous exposure to information, p. 443

Other oral drugs that may be used include clonidine, guanabenz, prazosin, and minoxidil. A loop diuretic (furosemide) is generally prescribed in addition to the antihypertensive agents.[65]

Hypertensive crisis with current therapy is associated with a 25% mortality 1 year after the event and 50% 5 years after the event. The most common causes of death are uremia, myocardial infarction, heart failure, and cerebrovascular accident.

Nursing Management

Nursing management of the patient with hypertensive crisis incorporates a variety of nursing diagnoses (Box 10-19). **Nursing priorities are directed toward normalizing blood pressure, providing comfort and emotional support, and maintaining surveillance for complications.**

Normalizing blood pressure

When short-acting intravenous antihypertensive agents are administered, blood pressure is closely monitored. If potent antihypertensive drugs such as sodium nitroprusside or labetalol are being used, an arterial line must be inserted and the drugs infused through an infusion pump.

Maintaining surveillance for complications

During the acute phase, the patient is closely observed for clinical manifestations in other organ systems, including the neurologic, cardiac, and renal systems. Neurologic compromise may be manifested by mental confusion, stupor, seizures, coma, or stroke. Cardiac compromise may be exhibited by aortic dissection, myocardial ischemia, or dysrhythmias. Acute renal failure may not be evident immediately, but urine output, blood urea nitrogen (BUN), and serum creatinine values are evaluated over several days to determine whether the kidneys were affected by the hypertensive episode.

ACE inhibitor enalapril will also lower blood pressure. Sometimes, combinations of the aforementioned agents are used to more effectively bring the hypertension under control.[65,66] An intravenous diuretic (furosemide) is used if fluid retention is present. It is important to be aware that cerebral hypoperfusion can occur if mean blood pressure is lowered too rapidly. During the first 24 hours of treatment, it is recommended that mean arterial pressure be decreased by no more than 20 to 30 mm Hg. Once the blood pressure is stabilized, oral antihypertensive therapy is initiated to achieve blood pressure values of less than 140/90 mm Hg.[7]

Hypertensive urgencies may not necessitate admission to a critical care unit because they can be treated with rapid-acting oral antihypertensive agents. The agent of choice is the calcium channel blocker nifedipine. A single 5 or 10 mg dose, when the capsule is bitten and then swallowed, will reduce blood pressure within 20 to 30 minutes. Captopril (25 mg), an ACE inhibitor, is also highly effective at lowering blood pressure. The beta-blocker labetalol can also be prescribed in oral doses.

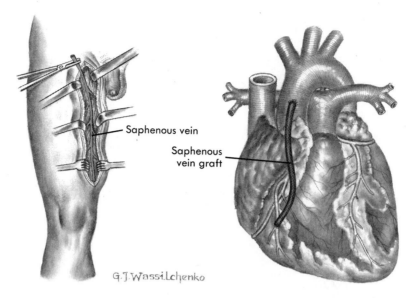

Saphenous vein

Saphenous vein graft

G.J.Wassilchenko

Fig. **10-13** Saphenous vein graft.

Patient education

Patient education during the acute phase is limited to an explanation of the need to control blood pressure and the purpose of the equipment used in the critical care unit. Once the hypertensive crisis is resolved, the focus of education is on life-style changes related to risk factor modification. Hypertension is emphasized as a risk factor for CAD, peripheral vascular disease, and cerebrovascular disease.

CARDIAC SURGERY

The following discussion introduces basic cardiac surgical techniques and the principles of cardiopulmonary bypass and highlights the key points about postoperative care of the adult patient who requires either valve replacement or coronary artery revascularization.

Coronary Artery Bypass Surgery

Since its introduction more than 2 decades ago, coronary artery bypass surgery has proved both safe and effective in relieving medically uncontrolled angina pectoris in most patients. With improved medical management of coronary artery disease (CAD), however, much debate has been generated regarding the efficacy of medical versus surgical therapy for CAD.

The combined results of three major randomized trials continue to support the view that coronary artery bypass grafting (CABG) affords dramatic symptomatic improvement and an improved quality of life.[67] CABG is more effective than medical therapy for improving survival in patients with left main–vessel or triple-vessel disease or with double-vessel disease involving the left anterior descending artery (LAD) as well as for relieving exercise-induced ischemia or chronic ischemia leading to left ventricular

(LV) dysfunction. Medical therapy is recommended when ischemia is prevented by antianginal drugs that are well-tolerated by the patient.[67]

Coronary artery bypass surgery falls under two different DRGs depending on whether the patient has a cardiac catheterization during the same hospital stay as the surgery. DRG 106 (Coronary Bypass with Cardiac Catheterization) and DRG 107 (Coronary Bypass without Cardiac Catheterization) have average lengths of the stay of 11.1 days and 8.3 days, respectively.[2]

Conduits

Myocardial revascularization involves the use of a conduit, or channel, designed to bypass an occluded coronary artery. Currently, the two most common conduits are the saphenous vein graft and the internal mammary artery (IMA). Saphenous vein graft (SVG) involves the anastomosis of an excised portion of the saphenous vein proximal to the aorta and distal to the coronary artery below the obstruction (Fig. 10-13). The IMA, which usually remains attached to its origin at the subclavian artery, is swung down and anastomosed distal to the coronary artery (Fig. 10-14). Both the right IMA (RIMA) and the left IMA (LIMA) may be used as conduits. Of note, urgent coronary artery bypass surgery may preclude the use of the IMA because of the extra time required to mobilize the artery, as well as the inability to effect cardioplegia through this conduit. The current trend, however, is to use arterial conduits such as the IMA when possible, because their long-term patency rates are superior to those of the SVG.[68] The right gastroepiploic artery (GEA) can also be used an alternate conduit for CABG. The GEA, which is a branch of the gastroduodenal artery, is pulled up to the pericardial cavity and anastomosed to a distal portion of the coronary artery. Although it is a little smaller in diameter than the IMA, studies indicate that patency rates

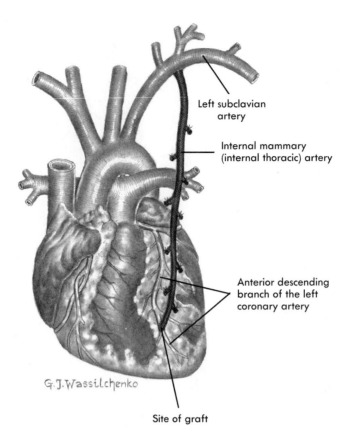

Left subclavian
artery

Internal mammary
(internal thoracic) artery

Anterior descending
branch of the left
coronary artery

G.J.Wassilchenko

Site of graft

Fig. **10-14** Internal mammary artery graft.

are excellent.[69,70] Because of its size and anatomic location, the GEA is well-suited for bypassing the right coronary artery and the posterior descending artery.[71] The technical aspects of obtaining this conduit, however, may limit its widespread use.

Valvular Surgery

Valvular disease results in various hemodynamic dysfunctions that usually can be managed medically as long as the patient remains symptom free. There is reluctance to intervene surgically early in the course of this disease because of the surgical risks and long-term complications associated with prosthetic valve replacement. These consequences, however, must be weighed against the possibility of irreversible deterioration in left ventricular function that may develop during the compensated asymptomatic phase.

Surgical therapy for aortic valve disease is limited at this time to aortic valve replacement (AVR). Three surgical procedures, however, are available to treat mitral valve disease: commissurotomy, valve repair, and valve replacement. Commissurotomy is performed for mitral stenosis and involves incising fused leaflets and debriding calcium deposits to increase valve mobility. In the setting of mitral regurgitation, valve repair may be at-

tempted, often with the use of a ring to reduce the size of the dilated mitral annulus, thus enhancing leaflet coaptation (annuloplasty). Both forms of valve reconstruction avoid the complications inherent with a prosthetic valve and may obviate the need for long-term anticoagulation.[72] If reconstruction of the mitral valve is not possible, it is replaced (mitral valve replacement [MVR]).

Valvular surgery falls under two different DRGs depending on whether the patient has a cardiac catheterization during the same hospital stay as the surgery. DRG 104 (Cardiac Valve Procedures with Cardiac Catheterization) and DRG 105 (Cardiac Valve Procedures without Cardiac Catheterization) have average lengths of the stay of 13.3 days and 10.2 days, respectively.[2]

Prosthetic valves

There are two categories of prosthetic valves: mechanical and biologic, or tissue, valves. Mechanical valves are made from combinations of metal alloys, pyrolite carbon, Dacron, and Teflon (Fig. 10-15). Their construction renders them highly durable, but all patients with mechanical valves require anticoagulation to reduce the incidence of thromboembolism. On the other hand, biologic, or tissue, valves, because of their low thrombogenicity, offer the patient freedom from therapeutic anticoagulation. Their durability, however, is limited by their

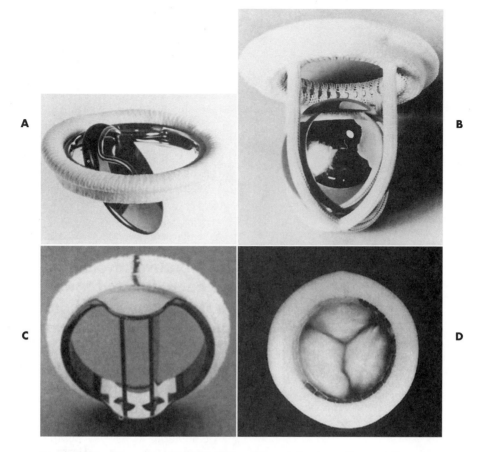

Fig. **10-15** Cardiac valves. **A,** Björk-Shiley tilting-disk valve with pyrolytic-carbon disk, Stellite cage, and Teflon cloth sewing ring, with valve that opens to 60 degrees. **B,** Starr-Edwards caged-ball valve model 6320 with completely cloth-covered Stellite cage and hollow Stellite ball, with specific gravity close to that of blood. **C,** St. Jude Medical mechanical heart valve, a mechanical central flow disk. **D,** Hancock II porcine aortic valve. The flexible Derlin stent and sewing ring are covered in Dacron cloth. (**A, B,** and **D** from Eagle K, et al: *The practice of cardiology,* ed 2, Boston, 1989, Little, Brown; **C** courtesy St. Jude Medical, Inc, Copyright 1993, St Paul, Minn.)

tendency toward early calcification. Box 10-20 gives a description of various valvular prostheses. Biologic valves are usually constructed from animal or human cardiac tissue.

The choice of a valvular prosthesis depends on many factors. Because mechanical valves are more durable, for example, they may be chosen over a tissue valve for a young person who is anticipated to have a relatively long life span ahead. Similarly, a bioprosthesis (tissue valve) may be chosen for an older patient (older than 65 years); even though the valve has a reduced longevity, the patient has a decreased life expectancy.[73] For patients with medical contraindications to anticoagulation or for patients whose past compliance with drug therapy has been questionable, a tissue valve is selected. Technical considerations, such as the size of the annulus (or anatomic ring in which the valve sits), can also influence the choice of valve (a bioprosthesis may be too big for a small aortic root).

Cardiopulmonary Bypass

Cardiopulmonary bypass (CPB) is a mechanical means of circulating and oxygenating a patient's blood while diverting most of the circulation from the heart and lungs during cardiac surgical procedures. The extracorporeal circuit consists of cannulas that drain off venous blood, an oxygenator that oxygenates the blood by one of several methods, and a pump head that pumps the arterialized blood back to the aorta through a single cannula. The patient is systemically heparinized before initiation of bypass to prevent clotting within the bypass circuit.

Hypothermia

Systemic hypothermia during bypass can reduce tissue oxygen requirements to 50% of normal, which affords the major organs additional protection from ischemic injury. Lowering the body temperature to about 28° C (82.4° F) is accomplished through a heat exchanger incorporated into

CLASSIFICATION OF PROSTHETIC CARDIAC VALVES

MECHANICAL VALVES

Tilting-disk: a free-floating, lens-shaped disk mounted on a circular sewing ring
   Björk-Shiley
   Omniscience (Lillehei-Kaster)
   Medtronic-Hall (Hall-Kaster)
Caged-ball: a ball moves freely within a three- or four-sided metallic cage mounted on a circular sewing ring
   Starr-Edwards
Bileaflet: two semicircular leaflets, mounted on a circular sewing ring, that open centrally
   St. Jude Medical

BIOLOGIC (TISSUE) VALVES (BIOPROSTHESES)

Porcine heterograft: a porcine aortic valve mounted on a semiflexible stent and preserved with glutaraldehyde
   Hancock
   Carpentier-Edwards
Bovine pericardial heterograft: bovine pericardium fashioned into three identical cusps that are then mounted on a cloth-covered frame
   Ionescu-Shiley
Homograft: a human heart valve (aortic or pulmonic) harvested from a donated heart and cryopreserved; may or may not be mounted on a support ring

---

TABLE **10-6**

PHYSIOLOGIC EFFECTS OF CARDIOPULMONARY BYPASS (CPB)

EFFECTS	CAUSES
Intravascular fluid deficit (hypotension)	Third spacing Postoperative diuresis Sudden vasodilation (drugs, rewarming)
Third spacing (weight gain, edema)	Decreased plasma protein concentration Increased capillary permeability
Myocardial depression (decreased cardiac output)	Hypothermia Increased systemic vascular resistance Prolonged CPB pump run Preexisting heart disease Inadequate myocardial protection
Coagulopathy (bleeding)	Systemic heparinization Mechanical trauma to platelets Depressed release of clotting factors from liver as a result of hypothermia
Pulmonary dysfunction (decreased lung mechanics and impaired gas exchange)	Decreased surfactant production Pulmonary microemboli Interstitial fluid accumulation in lungs
Hemolysis (hemoglobinuria)	Red blood cells damaged in pump circuit
Hyperglycemia (rise in serum glucose)	Decreased insulin release Stimulation of glycogenolysis
Hypokalemia (low serum potassium)	Intracellular shifts during bypass
Hypomagnesemia (low serum magnesium)	Postoperative diuresis secondary to hemodilution
Neurologic dysfunction (decreased level of consciousness, motor/sensory deficits)	Inadequate cerebral perfusion Microemboli to brain (air, plaque fragments, fat globules)
Hypertension (transient rise in blood pressure)	Catecholamine release and systemic hypothermia causing vasoconstriction

---

the pump. The blood is warmed back up to normal body temperature before the bypass is discontinued.

Hemodilution

The technique of hemodilution is also used to enhance tissue oxygenation by improving blood flow through the systemic and pulmonary microcirculation during bypass. Hemodilution refers to the dilution of autologous (patient's own) blood with the isotonic crystalloid solution used to prime the pump. Capillary perfusion is enhanced by hemodilution because the reduced viscosity (stickiness) of the blood decreases both resistance to flow through the capillaries and the possibility of microthrombi formation. At the completion of CPB, the large quantities of "pump blood" that remain in the bypass circuit can be collected and used for initial postoperative volume replacement.

In response to findings that the low cardiac output syndrome often seen postoperatively might be a result of intraoperative myocardial ischemia or necrosis, efforts have been directed toward providing additional protection to the myocardium during bypass. Rapidly stopping the heart in diastole by perfusing the coronary arteries with a cold potassium cardioplegic ("heart-paralyzing") agent has been the method of choice for intraoperative myocardial protection. Continued research in this area has resulted in the emergence of blood as a vehicle for the cardioplegic components to enhance the supply of oxygen

and nutrients to the arrested myocardial cells.[74] Warm (normothermic) cardioplegia is also being investigated and is believed by some to result in less ventricular dysfunction postoperatively.[75] Regardless of the type of cardioplegic solution used, it must be reinfused at regular intervals during bypass to keep the heart in an arrested state and to minimize myocardial oxygen requirements.

Numerous clinical sequelae can result from CPB (Table 10-6). Knowledge of these physiologic effects allows the nurse to anticipate problems and intervene effectively.

Postoperative Management

Nursing management of the patient undergoing cardiac surgery incorporates a variety of nursing diagnoses (Box

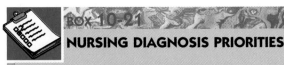

NURSING DIAGNOSIS PRIORITIES

Cardiac Surgery

Decreased Cardiac Output related to alterations in preload, pp. 467-468
Decreased Cardiac Output related to alterations in afterload, pp. 468-469
Decreased Cardiac Output related to alterations in contractility, p. 469
Decreased Cardiac Output related to alterations in heart rate, p. 470
Acute Pain related to transmission and perception of cutaneous, visceral, muscular, or ischemic impulses, pp. 461-464
Anxiety related to threat to biologic, psychologic, and/or social integrity, pp. 448-450
Knowledge Deficit: Discharge Regimen related to lack of previous exposure to information, p. 443

10-21). **Nursing priorities are directed toward optimizing cardiac output, correcting hypothermia, maintaining chest tube patency, facilitating early extubation, providing comfort and emotional support, and maintaining surveillance for complications.**

Optimizing cardiac output

Postoperative cardiovascular support often is indicated because of a low output state resulting from preexisting heart disease, a prolonged CPB pump run, and/or inadequate myocardial protection. Cardiac output can be maximized by adjustments in heart rate, preload, afterload, and contractility.

Heart rate. In the presence of low cardiac output, the heart rate can be appropriately regulated by means of temporary pacing or drug therapy. Temporary epicardial pacing usually is instituted when the heart rate of the adult patient who has had cardiac surgery drops to less than 80 beats per minute. In the case of tachycardia, intravenous beta-blockers (esmolol) or calcium channel blockers (diltiazem) may be used to slow supraventricular rhythms with a ventricular response that exceeds 110 beats per minute. Because ventricular ectopy can result from hypokalemia, serum potassium levels are maintained in the high-normal range (4.5 to 5.0 mEq/L) to provide some margin for error. Maintaining serum magnesium in a therapeutic range (2.0 mEq/L) has also been shown to reduce the incidence of dysrhythmias in the postoperative period.[76,77]

Preload. In most patients, reduced preload is the cause of low postoperative cardiac output. If a pulmonary artery catheter has been inserted during surgery, monitoring pulmonary artery wedge pressure (PAWP) can provide a more convenient and accurate guide to left ventricular preload than can monitoring central venous pressure (CVP) alone. To enhance preload, volume may be administered in the form of crystalloid, colloid, or packed red cells. It is not uncommon to achieve the greatest hemodynamic stability in cardiac surgery patients when filling pressures (pulmonary artery diastolic or PAWP) are in the range of 18 to 20 mm Hg (normally 5 to 12 mm Hg).

Afterload. Partly as a result of the peripheral vasoconstrictive effects of hypothermia, many patients who have had cardiac surgery demonstrate postoperative hypertension. Although it is transient, postoperative hypertension can precipitate or exacerbate bleeding from the mediastinal chest tubes. In addition, the high systemic vascular resistance (afterload) resulting from intense vasoconstriction can increase left ventricular workload. Therefore vasodilator therapy with intravenous sodium nitroprusside often is used to reduce afterload and thus control hypertension and improve cardiac output.

The use of warm cardioplegia may alter the traditional hemodynamic picture of postoperative cardiac surgery patients. These patients may have peripheral vasodilation, associated with hypotension and a low systemic vascular resistance. Therapy for these patients usually includes volume loading and vasopressors such as phenylephrine or dopamine to tighten the peripheral vasculature and maintain an adequate mean arterial pressure.[78]

Contractility. If these adjustments in heart rate, preload, and afterload fail to produce significant improvement in cardiac output, contractility can be enhanced with positive inotropic support or intraaortic balloon pumping (IABP), thus augmenting circulation.

Correcting hypothermia

Hypothermia can contribute to depressed myocardial contractility in the patient who has had cardiac surgery. To prevent subsequent excessive temperature elevations while hyperthermia blankets are used to warm the patient, care must be taken to remove the blankets promptly when the patient's temperature reaches 98.4° F (36.9° C).

Maintaining chest tube patency

Chest tube stripping to maintain patency of the tubes is controversial because of the high negative pressure generated by routine methods of stripping. It is believed to result in tissue damage that can actually contribute to bleeding. This risk, however, must be carefully weighed against the very real danger of cardiac tamponade if blood is not effectively drained from around the heart. Therefore chest tube stripping frequently is advocated in instances of excessive postoperative bleeding. The technique of "milking" the chest tubes, however, may be more advisable for routine postoperative care, because this technique generates less negative pressure and decreases the risk of bleeding.[79]

Facilitating early extubation

Until recently, overnight intubation to facilitate lung expansion and optimize gas exchange was common in patients who had had cardiac surgery. Newer protocols facilitating early extubation (within the first 4 to 8 hours) have now been implemented in many institutions.[80-81] Early extubation requires a multidisciplinary approach that incorporates anesthesiologists, surgeons, nurses, and respiratory therapists. Potential candidates must be identified preoperatively so that the anesthetic regimen can be modified to support early extubation. Generally, short-acting anesthetic agents such as propofol are used at the end of the surgery, and narcotics are minimized. Postoperatively, patients are evaluated for hemodynamic stability, adequate control of bleeding, and normothermia. Once these criteria are met, the patient is weaned off propofol and ventilator weaning can begin. If needed, narcotics are given in small increments to manage pain and anxiety. Patients who exhibit hemodynamic instability or intraoperative complications or who have underlying pulmonary disease related to long-term valvular dysfunction may require longer periods of mechanical ventilation. After extubation, supplemental oxygen is administered, and patients are medicated for incisional pain to facilitate adequate coughing and deep breathing.

Maintaining surveillance for complications

Complications of cardiac surgery include postoperative bleeding, postcardiotomy psychosis, infection, and acute tubular necrosis.

Postoperative bleeding. Postoperative bleeding from the mediastinal chest tubes can be caused by inadequate hemostasis, disruption of suture lines, or coagulopathy associated with CPB. Bleeding is more likely to occur with IMA grafts as a result of the extensive chest-wall dissection required to free the IMA. If bleeding in excess of 150 ml/hour occurs early in the postoperative period, clotting factors (fresh-frozen plasma and platelets) and additional protamine (used to reverse the effects of heparin) may be administered, along with prompt blood replacement.

The use of prophylactic positive end-expiratory pressure (PEEP) in conjunction with mechanical ventilation may be helpful in controlling bleeding in some cases by increasing intrathoracic pressure enough to effect tamponade of oozing mediastinal blood vessels. Rewarming the patient reverses the depressed manufacture and release of clotting factors that result from hypothermia. Persistent mediastinal bleeding, however—usually in excess of 500 ml in 1 hour or 400 ml/hour for 2 consecutive hours despite normalization of clotting studies—is an indication for reexploration of the surgical site.

Postcardiotomy psychosis. The transient neurologic dysfunction often seen in patients who have had cardiac surgery probably can be attributed to decreased cerebral perfusion and to cerebral microemboli, both related to the CPB pump run. Compounding these are environmental factors, such as sensory deprivation and sensory overload associated with being in a critical care unit. The term *postcardiotomy psychosis* has been used to describe this postoperative syndrome that initially may be seen as only a mild impairment of orientation but that may progress to agitation, hallucinations, and paranoid delusions.[82] Patients and family members need to be reassured that postcardiotomy psychosis is a temporary phenomenon that will resolve quickly. Meanwhile, every effort must be made to keep the patient informed of all that is going on in the surroundings so that unfamiliar sights, sounds, and smells are not overwhelming and confusing. Painful stimuli are kept to a minimum, and meaningful stimuli, such as touching, are encouraged. Nursing management is organized to maximize optimal sleep patterns whenever possible.

Infection. Postoperative fever is fairly common after CPB. However, persistent temperature elevation to more than 101° F (37.8° C) must be investigated. Sternal wound infections and infective endocarditis are the most devastating infectious complications, but leg wound infection, pneumonia, and urinary tract infection can also occur.[83]

Acute tubular necrosis. Hemolysis caused by trauma to the red blood cells in the extracorporeal circuit results in hemoglobinuria, which can damage renal tubules. Therefore small amounts of furosemide (Lasix) usually are given to promote urine flow if the urine output is low (less than 25 to 30 ml/hour) and "pink-tinged."

Patient education

Patient education includes information related to the surgical procedure as well as content related to risk factor management for the prevention of atherosclerosis. Patients who have undergone valve surgery may also require information regarding the need for antibiotic prophylaxis before invasive procedures as well as specifics pertaining to their anticoagulation regimen.

References

1. Kelly DT: Our future society: a global challenge, *Circulation* 95:2459, 1997.
2. *St. Anthony's DRG guidebook 1998,* Reston, Va, 1997, St. Anthony.
3. Teplitz L, Siwik DA: Cellular signals in atherosclerosis, *J Cardiovasc Nurs* 8(3):28, 1994.
4. Effat MA: Pathophysiology of ischemic heart disease: an overview, *AACN Clin Issues Crit Care Nurs* 6:369, 1995.
5. Hunink MG, et al: The recent decline in mortality from coronary heart disease, 1980-1990, *JAMA* 277:535, 1997.
6. Njølstad I, Arnesen E, Lund-Larsen PG: Smoking, serum lipids, blood pressure, and sex differences in myocardial infarction: a 12-year follow-up of the Finnmark study, *Circulation* 93:450, 1996.
7. Expert Panel on Detection, Evaluation, and Treatment of High Blood Cholesterol in Adults: Summary of the second report of the National Cholesterol Education Program (Adult Treatment Panel II), *JAMA* 269:3015, 1993.
8. Dietary Guidelines For Healthy American Adults: A statement for health professionals from the Nutrition Committee, American Heart Association, *Circulation* 94:1795, 1996.
9. Boushey CJ, et al: A quantitative assessment of plasma homocystine as a risk factor for vascular disease, *JAMA* 274:1049, 1995.
10. Nygård O, et al: Total plasma homocystine and cardiovascular risk profile: the Hordaland Homocystine Study, *JAMA* 274:1526, 1995.

11. Joint National Committee on Detection, Evaluation, and Treatment of High Blood Pressure: The fifth report of the Joint National Committee on Detection, Evaluation and Treatment of High Blood Pressure, *Arch Intern Med* 153:154, 1993.

12. Sytkowski PA, et al: Secular trends in long-term sustained hypertension, long-term treatment, and cardiovascular mortality: the Framingham Heart Study, 1950 to 1990, *Circulation* 93:697, 1996.

13. Stamler J, et al: MRFIT 12-year follow-up: diabetes and mortality, *Diabetes Care* 16:434, 1993.

14. Kawachi I, et al: Symptoms of anxiety and risk of coronary heart disease: the normative aging study, *Circulation* 90:2225, 1994.

15. Allison TG: Identification and treatment of psychosocial risk factors for coronary artery disease, *Mayo Clin Proc* 71:817, 1996.

16. Fuster V, et al: The pathogenesis of coronary artery disease and the acute coronary syndromes. II, *N Engl J Med* 326:310, 1992.

17. Fuster V, et al: The pathogenesis of coronary artery disease and the acute coronary syndromes. I, *N Engl J Med* 326:242, 1992.

18. Fuster V: Elucidation of the role of plaque instability and rupture in acute coronary events, *Am J Cardiol* 76:24C, 1995.

19. Fishbein MC, Siegel RJ: How big are coronary atherosclerotic plaques that rupture? *Circulation* 94:2662, 1996.

20. Waters D: Plaque stabilization: a mechanism for the beneficial effect of lipid-lowering therapies in angiography studies, *Prog Cardiovasc Dis* 27(3):107, 1994.

21. Superko HR, Krauss RM: Coronary artery disease regression: convincing evidence of the benefit of aggressive lipoprotein management, *Circulation* 90:1056, 1994.

22. Lamarche B, et al: Apolipoprotein A-I and B levels and risk of ischemic heart disease during a five-year follow-up of men in the Québec Cardiovascular Study, *Circulation* 94:273, 1996.

23. Braunwald E, et al: *Unstable angina: diagnosis and management, Clinical practice guideline No 10,* AHCPR Publ No 94-0602, Rockville, Md, 1994, Agency for Health Care Policy and Research and the National Heart, Lung, and Blood Institute, Public Health Service, US Department of Health and Human Services.

24. Catherwood E, O'Rourke DJ: Critical pathway management of unstable angina, *Prog Cardiovasc Dis* 27(3):121, 1994.

25. Bankwala Z, Swenson LJ: Unstable angina pectoris: what is the likelihood of further cardiac events? *Postgrad Med* 98(6):155, 1995.

26. Cohn P: Silent ischemia. In Fuster V, Ross R, Topol EJ, editors: *Atherosclerosis and coronary artery disease,* vol 2, New York, 1996, Lippincott-Raven.

27. Pepine CJ: Prognostic implications of silent myocardial ischemia, *N Engl J Med* 334:113, 1996.

28. Pilote L, et al: Regional variation across the United States in the management of acute myocardial infarction, *N Engl J Med* 333:565, 1995.

29. Ryan TJ, et al: ACC/AHA Guidelines for the Management of Patients with Acute Myocardial Infarction: a report of the American College of Cardiology/American Heart Association Task Force on Practice Guidelines (Committee on Management of Acute Myocardial Infarction), *J Am Coll Cardiol* 28:1328, 1996.

30. Hearns PA: Differentiating ischemia, injury, infarction: expanding the 12-lead electrocardiogram, *DCCN* 13:172, 1994.

31. Wang WWT: The educational needs of myocardial infarction patients, *Prog Cardiovasc Nurs* 9(4):28, 1994.

32. Antiplatelet Trialist's Collaboration: Collaborative overview of randomized trials of antiplatelet therapy: prevention of death, myocardial infarction, and stroke by prolonged antiplatelet therapy in various categories of patients, *Br Med J* 308:81, 1994.

33. Schühlen H, et al: Major benefit from antiplatelet therapy for patients at high risk for adverse cardiac events after coronary Palmaz-Schatz stent placement, *Circulation* 95:2015, 1996.

34. Azar AJ, et al: Optimal intensity of oral anticoagulant therapy after myocardial infarction, *J Am Coll Cardiol* 27:1349, 1996.

35. Cairns JA, et al: Antithrombotic agents in coronary artery disease, *Chest* 108(suppl 4):380S, 1995.

36. Kuhn FE, Gersh BJ: Mechanical complications of acute myocardial infarction. In Fuster V, Ross R, Topol EJ, editors: *Atherosclerosis and coronary artery disease,* vol 2, New York, 1996, Lippincott-Raven.

37. Van Dantzig JM, et al: Pathogenesis of mitral regurgitation in acute myocardial infarction: importance of changes in left ventricular shape and regional function, *Am Heart J* 131:865, 1996.

38. Becker RC, et al: A composite view of cardiac wall rupture in the United States National Registry of Myocardial Infarction, *J Am Coll Cardiol* 27:1321, 1996.

39. Pierce CD: Acute post-MI pericarditis, *J Cardiovasc Nurs* 6(4):46, 1992.

40. Riegel B, et al: Are nurses still practicing coronary precautions? A national survey of nursing care of myocardial infarction patients, *Am J Crit Care* 5(2):91, 1996.

41. Steinke EE, Patterson P: Sexual counselling of MI patients, *J Cardiovasc Nurs* 10(1):81, 1995.

42. Konstam M, et al: *Heart failure: evaluation and care of patients with left-ventricular systolic dysfunction,* Clinical practice guideline No 11, AHCPR Publ No 94-0612, Rockville, Md, 1994, Agency for Health Care Policy and Research and the National Heart, Lung, and Blood Institute, Public Health Service, US Department of Health and Human Services.

43. Piano MR, Bondmass M, Schwertz DW: The molecular and cellular pathophysiology of heart failure, *Heart Lung* 27:3, 1998.

44. Funk M: Epidemiology of heart failure, *Crit Care Nurs Clin North Am* 5:569, 1993.

45. Elkayam U: Nitrates in the treatment of congestive heart failure, *Am J Cardiol* 77:41C, 1996.

46. The SOLVD Investigators: Effect of enalapril on survival in patients with reduced left ventricular ejection fraction and congestive heart failure, *N Engl J Med* 325:293, 1991.

47. Schaefer KM, Polylycki MJS: Fatigue associated with congestive heart failure: use of Levine's Conservation Model, *J Adv Nurs* 18:260, 1993.

48. Louie EK, Edwards LC: Hypertrophic cardiomyopathy, *Prog Cardiovasc Dis* 36(4):275, 1994.

49. Uszenski HJ, et al: Hypertrophic cardiomyopathy: medical, surgical and nursing management, *J Cardiovasc Nurs* 7(2):13, 1993.

50. Chang AC, McAreavery D, Fananapazir L: Identification of patients with hypertrophic cardiomyopathy at high risk for sudden death, *Curr Opin Cardiol* 10(1):9, 1995.

51. Larsen L, Markham J, Haffajee CI: Sudden death in idiopathic dilated cardiomyopathy: role of ventricular arrhythmias. I, *Pacing Clin Electrophysiol* 16:1051, 1995.

52. Dajac AS, et al: Prevention of bacterial endocarditis: recommendations by the American Heart Association, *Circulation* 96:358, 1997.

53. Steckelberg JM, Wilson WR: Risk factors for infective endocarditis, *Infect Dis Clin North Am* 7:9, 1993.

54. Dajani A, et al: Treatment of acute streptococcal pharyngitis and prevention of rheumatic fever: a statement for health professionals, *Pediatrics* 96:758, 1995.

55. Wolff M, et al: Prosthetic valve endocarditis in the ICU, *Chest* 108:688, 1995.
56. Walter BF, Howard J, Fess S: Pathology of mitral valve stenosis and pure mitral regurgitation. I, *Clin Cardiol* 17:330, 1994.
57. Walter BF, Howard J, Fess S: Pathology of mitral valve stenosis and pure mitral regurgitation. II, *Clin Cardiol* 17:395, 1994.
58. Ling LH, et al: Clinical outcome of mitral regurgitation due to flail leaflet, *N Engl J Med* 335:1417, 1996.
59. Carabello BA: Indications for valve surgery in asymptomatic patients with aortic and mitral stenosis, *Chest* 108:1678, 1995.
60. Klodas E, et al: Surgery for aortic regurgitation in women: contrasting indications and outcomes compared with men, *Circulation* 94:2472, 1996.
61. Walter BF, Howard J, Fess S: Pathology of tricuspid valve stenosis and pure tricuspid regurgitation. I, *Clin Cardiol* 18:97, 1995.
62. Walter BF, Howard J, Fess S: Pathology of tricuspid valve stenosis and pure tricuspid regurgitation. II, *Clin Cardiol* 18:167, 1995.
63. House-Fancher MA: Aortic dissection: pathophysiology, diagnosis, and acute care management, *AACN Clin Issues Crit Care Nurs* 6:602, 1995.
64. Guilmet D, et al: Aortic dissection: anatomic types and surgical approaches, *J Cardiovasc Surg* 34(1):23, 1993.
65. Porsche R: Hypertension: diagnosis, acute anti-hypertensive therapy, and long-term management, *AACN Clin Issues Crit Care Nurs* 6:515, 1995.
66. Ram CV: Immediate management of severe hypertension, *Cardiol Clin* 13:579, 1995.
67. Kirklin JW, et al: ACC/AHA guidelines and indications for CABG surgery, *Circulation* 83:1125, 1991.
68. Alfieri O, Lorusso R: Developments in surgical techniques for coronary revascularization, *Curr Opin Cardiol* 10:556, 1995.
69. Jegaden O, et al: Technical aspects and late functional results of gastroepiploic bypass grafting (400 cases), *Eur J Cardiothorac Surg* 9:575, 1995.
70. Pym J, et al: Right gastroepiploic-to-coronary artery bypass: the first decade of use, *Circulation* 92(suppl 9):II45, 1995.
71. Dietl CA, et al: Which is the graft of choice for the right coronary and posterior descending arteries? Comparison of the right internal mammary artery and the right gastroepiploic artery, *Circulation* 92(suppl 9):II92, 1995.
72. Atunes MJ: Mitral valve repair in the 1990s, *Eur J Cardiothorac Surg* 6(suppl 1):S13, 1992.
73. Jamieson WR: Modern cardiac valve devices—bioprostheses and mechanical prostheses: state of the art, *J Card Surg* 8:89, 1993.
74. Brown KK: Surgical therapy of chronic heart failure and severe ventricular dysfunction, *Crit Care Nurs Q* 18:45, 1995.
75. Buckberg GD: Update on current techniques of myocardial protection, *Ann Thorac Surg* 60:805, 1995.
76. Colquhoun IW, et al: Arrhythmia prophylaxis after coronary artery surgery: a randomized controlled trial of intravenous magnesium chloride, *Eur J Cardiothorac Surg* 7:520, 1993.
77. Casthely PA, et al: Magnesium and arrhythmias after coronary artery bypass surgery, *J Cardiothorac Vasc Anesth* 8:188, 1994.
78. Barden C, Hansen M: Cold versus warm cardioplegia: recognizing hemodynamic variations, *DCCN* 14:114, 1995.
79. Gross SB: Current challenges, concepts, and controversies in chest tube management, *AACN Clin Issues Crit Care Nurs* 4:260, 1993.
80. Riddle MM, Dunstan JL, Castanis JL: A rapid recovery program for cardiac surgery patients, *Am J Crit Care* 5:152, 1996.
81. Maxam-Moore VA, Goedecke RS: The development of an early extubation algorithm for patients after cardiac surgery, *Heart Lung* 25:61, 1996.
82. Leahy NM: Neurologic complications after open heart surgery, *J Cardiovasc Nurs* 7(2):41, 1993.
83. Vaska PL: Sternal wound infections, *AACN Clin Issues Crit Care Nurs* 4:475, 1993.

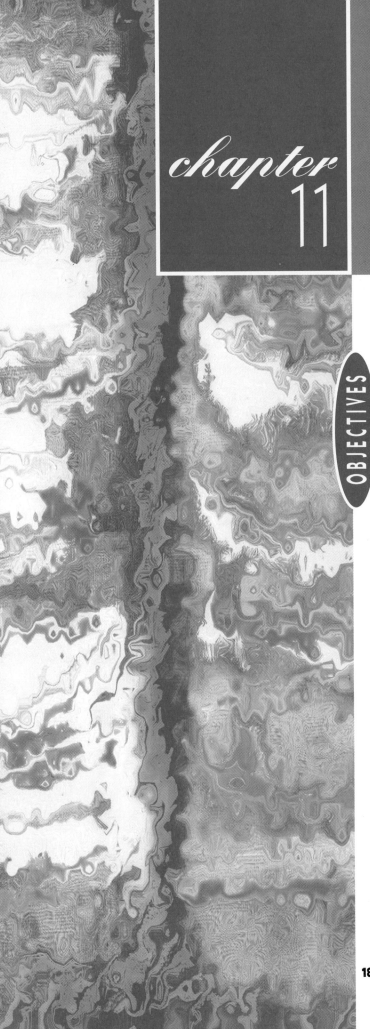

chapter 11

Cardiovascular Therapeutic Management

Joni Dirks

OBJECTIVES

● Describe the functions of a temporary pacemaker and an implantable cardioverter defibrillator.

● Outline the medical and nursing management of a patient undergoing cardiac surgery and cardiac interventional procedures.

● Identify the signs of reperfusion in a patient undergoing thrombolytic therapy.

A wide variety of therapeutic interventions are employed in the management of the patient with cardiovascular dysfunction. This chapter focuses on the priority interventions used to manage cardiovascular disorders in the critical care setting.

TEMPORARY PACEMAKERS

Pacemakers are electronic devices that can be used to initiate the heartbeat when the heart's intrinsic electrical system is unable to effectively generate a rate adequate to support cardiac output. Pacemakers can be used temporarily, either supportively or prophylactically, until the condition responsible for the rate or conduction disturbance resolves. Pacemakers also can be used on a permanent basis if the patient's condition persists despite adequate therapy.

Indications

The clinical indications for instituting temporary pacemaker therapy are outlined in Box 11-1. Dysrhythmias that are unresponsive to drug therapy and result in compromised hemodynamic status are a definite indication

INDICATIONS FOR TEMPORARY PACING

Bradydysrhythmias
   Sinus bradycardia and arrest
   Sick sinus syndrome
   Heart blocks
Tachydysrhythmias
   Supraventricular
   Ventricular
Permanent pacemaker failure
Support of cardiac output after cardiac surgery
Diagnostic studies
   Electrophysiology studies (EPS)
   Atrial electrograms (AEG)

for pacemaker therapy. The goal of therapy in the case of bradydysrhythmia is to increase the ventricular rate and thus enhance cardiac output. Alternately "overdrive" pacing can be used to decrease the rate of a rapid supraventricular or ventricular rhythm. This rapid pacing of the heart, or overdrive pacing, functions either to prevent the "breakthrough" ectopy that can result from a slow rate or to "capture" an ectopic focus and allow the natural pacemaker to regain control. Temporary pacing may be used in the treatment of symptomatic bradycardia or progressive heart block that occurs secondary to myocardial ischemia or drug toxicity. After cardiac surgery, temporary pacing can be used to improve a transiently depressed, rate-dependent cardiac output. In addition, conduction disturbances that can occur after valvular surgery can be managed effectively with temporary pacing.

Pacemaker System

A pacemaker system is a simple electrical circuit consisting of a pulse generator and a pacing lead (an insulated electrical wire) with either one or two electrodes.

Pulse generator

The pulse generator is designed to generate an electrical current that travels through the pacing lead and exits through an electrode (exposed portion of the wire) that is in direct contact with the heart. This electrical current initiates a myocardial depolarization. The current then seeks to return by one of several ways to the pulse generator to complete the circuit. The power source for a temporary external pulse generator is the standard 9-volt alkaline battery inserted into the generator.

Pacing lead

The pacing lead used for temporary pacing may be bipolar or unipolar. In a bipolar system, two electrodes (positive and negative) are located within the heart, whereas in a unipolar system only one electrode (negative) is in direct contact with the myocardium. In both unipolar and bipolar systems the current flows from the negative terminal of the pulse generator, down the pacing lead to the negative electrode, and into the heart. The current is then picked up by the positive electrode (ground) and flows back up the lead to the positive terminal of the pulse generator.

The bipolar lead used in transvenous pacing has two electrodes on one catheter (Fig. 11-1, *D*). The distal, or negative, electrode is at the tip of the pacing lead and is in direct contact with the heart, usually inside the right atrium or ventricle. Approximately 1 cm from the negative electrode is a positive electrode. The negative electrode is attached to the negative terminal, and the positive electrode is attached to the positive terminal of the pulse generator, either directly or via a bridging cable (see Fig. 11-1).

An epicardial lead system is frequently used for temporary pacing after cardiac surgery. The bipolar epicardial lead system has two separate insulated wires (one negative and one positive electrode) that are loosely secured with sutures to the cardiac chamber to be paced. Both leads are in contact with the myocardial tissue, so either wire may be used as the negative, or pacing, electrode. The remaining wire is then used as the positive, or ground, electrode.

A unipolar pacing system (epicardial or transvenous) has only one electrode (the negative electrode) making contact with the heart. In the case of a permanent pacemaker, the positive electrode can be created by the metallic casing of the subcutaneously implanted pulse generator. Or as is the case with a unipolar epicardial lead system, the positive electrode can be formed by a piece of surgical steel wire sewn into the subcutaneous tissue of the chest or the metal portion of a surface ECG electrode.

There are advantages and disadvantages to both systems. Because the unipolar pacing system has a wide sensing area as a result of the relatively large distance between the negative and positive electrodes, it has better sensing capabilities than does a bipolar system. This feature, however, makes the unipolar system more susceptible to sensing extraneous signals, such as the electrical artifact created by normal muscle movements (myopotentials) or external electromagnetic interference (EMI), that may result in inappropriate inhibition of the pacing stimulus.[1]

Pacing Routes

Several routes are available for temporary cardiac pacing. Transcutaneous cardiac pacing involves the use of two large skin electrodes, one placed anteriorly and the other posteriorly on the chest, connected to an external pulse generator. It is a rapid, noninvasive procedure that nurses can perform in the emergency setting and is recommended as a primary intervention in the Advanced Cardiac Life Support (ACLS) algorithm for the treatment of bradycardia.[2] Improved technology related to stimulus delivery and the development of large electrode pads

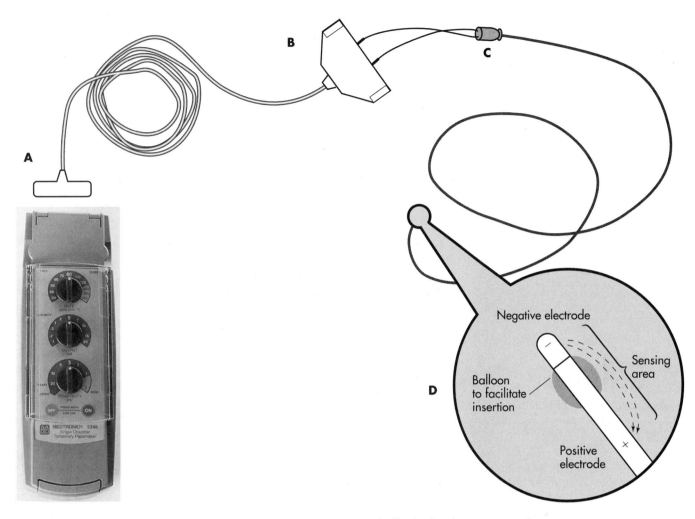

Fig. **11-1** The components of a temporary bipolar transvenous system. **A,** Single-chamber temporary (external) pulse generator. **B,** Bridging cable. **C,** Pacing lead. **D,** Enlarged view of the pacing lead tip.

that help disperse the energy have helped reduce the pain associated with cutaneous nerve and muscle stimulation.[1] Discomfort may still be an issue in some patients, particularly when higher energy levels are required to achieve capture. This route is generally used as a short-term therapy until the situation resolves or another route of pacing can be established (Appendix A.)

The insertion of temporary epicardial pacing wires has become a routine procedure during most cardiac surgical cases. Ventricular, and in many cases atrial, pacing wires are loosely sewn to the epicardium. The terminal pins of these wires are pulled through the skin before the chest is closed. If both chambers have pacing wires attached, the atrial wires exit subcostally to the right of the sternum and the ventricular wires exit in the same region but to the left of the sternum.[3] These wires can be removed several days after surgery by gentle traction at the skin surface with minimal risk of bleeding.

Temporary transvenous endocardial pacing is accomplished by advancing a pacing electrode wire through a vein, often the subclavian or internal jugular, and into the right atrium or right ventricle. Insertion can be facilitated either through direct visualization with fluoroscopy or by the use of the standard ECG. In some cases the pacing wire is inserted through a special pulmonary artery catheter via a port that exits in the right ventricle.

Five-Letter Pacemaker Codes

In 1974 the Inter-Society Commission for Heart Disease (ICHD) adopted a three-letter code for describing the various pacing modalities available. The code has since undergone several revisions, including the addition of two more letters representing programming characteristics and antitachycardia functions, to accommodate the development of newer devices that are rate-responsive or that combine pacing and cardioversion/defibrillation capabilities (Table 11-1 gives a description of the five-letter code).[4] The original three-letter code, however, remains adequate to describe temporary pacemaker function.

The original code is based on three categories, each represented by a letter. The first letter refers to the cardiac

---

TABLE 11-1

NASPE/BPEG GENERIC (NBG) CODE

POSITION	I	II	III	IV	V
	CHAMBER(S) PACED	**CHAMBER(S) SENSED**	**RESPONSE TO SENSING**	**PROGRAMMABILITY**	**ANTITACHYDYSRHYTHMIA FUNCTION(S)**
	0 = None A = Atrium	0 = None A = Atrium	0 = None T = Triggered	0 = None P = Simple programmability (rate, output, sensitivity)	0 = None P = Pacing (antitachy-dysrhythmia)
	V = Ventricle	V = Ventricle	I = Inhibited	M = Multiprogrammability	S = Shock
	D = Dual (A + V) S* = Single (A or V)	D = Dual (A + V) S = Single (A or V)	D = Dual (T + I)	C = Communicating R = Rate modulation (rate responsive)	D = Dual (P + S)

Modified from Bernstein AD, et al: The NASPE/BPEG generic pacemaker code for antibradycardia and adaptive rate pacing and antiachyarrhythmia devices, *PACE* 10:794, 1987.
*Used by manufacturer only.
NOTE: Positions I through III are used exclusively for antibradydysrhythmia function.
NASPE, North American Society of Pacing and Electrophysiology; *BPEG,* British Pacing and Electrophysiology Group; *NBG,* North American British Generic.

TABLE 11-2

EXAMPLES OF TEMPORARY PACING MODES

PACING MODE	DESCRIPTION
FIXED RATE	
AOO	Atrial pacing, no sensing
VOO	Ventricular pacing, no sensing
DOO	Atrial and ventricular pacing, no sensing
DEMAND	
AAI	Atrial pacing, atrial sensing, inhibited response to sensed P waves
VVI	Ventricular pacing, ventricular sensing, inhibited response to sensed QRS complexes
DVI	Atrial and ventricular pacing, ventricular sensing; both atrial and ventricular pacing are inhibited if a spontaneous ventricular depolarization is sensed
UNIVERSAL	
DDD	Both chambers are paced and sensed; inhibited response of the pacing stimuli to sensed events in their respective chamber; triggered response to sensed atrial activity to allow for rate-responsive ventricular pacing

---

chamber that is paced. The second letter designates which chamber is sensed, and the third letter indicates the pacemaker's response to the sensed event. These three letters are used to describe the mode of pacing. For example, a VVI pacemaker paces the ventricle when the pacemaker fails to sense an intrinsic ventricular depolarization. Sensing of a spontaneous ventricular depolarization, however, inhibits ventricular pacing. On the other hand, a VOO pacemaker paces the ventricle at a fixed rate and has no sensing capabilities. Table 11-2 gives a description of temporary pacing modes.

Physiologic pacing modes are those in which the normal physiologic, or sequential, relationship between atrial and ventricular stimulation and contraction is maintained. Atrioventricular (AV) synchrony increases the volume in the ventricle before contraction and thus helps to improve cardiac output. This may be achieved with atrial pacing in patients who have an intact conduction system, where each atrial pacing stimuli depolarizes the atria and is then conducted through to the ventricles. When atrial-to-ventricular conduction is impaired (i.e., during heart block), AV synchrony may be maintained via dual-chamber (i.e., both atrial and ventricular) pacing modes. The newest of these is the DDD mode, which is sometimes referred to as the "universal mode" because of its flexibility.[5] In DDD pacing, atrial and ventricular leads are used for both pacing and sensing. In response to sensed activity the pacemaker inhibits the pacing stimulus so that a sensed P wave in the atria will inhibit the atrial spike and a sensed R wave in the ventricle will inhibit the ventricular pacing spike. In addition, a sensed P wave may also be used to "trigger" a ventricular pacing stimulus when normal conduction through the AV node is impaired. Although the DDD mode is more complicated to program and interpret than earlier modes, it offers the most options for maintaining physiologic pacing.

Pacemaker Settings

The controls on all external temporary pulse generators are similar, and their function must be thoroughly understood so that pacing can be initiated quickly in an emergency situation, and troubleshooting can be facilitated should problems with the pacemaker arise.

The rate control (see Fig. 11-2) regulates the number of impulses that can be delivered to the heart per minute. The rate setting depends on the physiologic needs of the patient, but in general it is maintained between 60 and 80 beats per minute. Pacing rates for overdrive suppression of tachydysrhythmias may greatly exceed these values. Some generators have special controls for overdrive pacing that allow for rates of up to 800 stimuli per minute. If the pacemaker is operating in a dual-chamber mode, the ventricular rate control also regulates the atrial rate.

The output dial regulates the amount of electrical current (measured in milliamperes [mA]) that is delivered to the heart to initiate depolarization. The point at which depolarization occurs is termed the *pacing threshold* and is indicated by a myocardial response to the pacing stimulus (capture). Threshold can be determined by gradually decreasing the output setting until 1:1 capture is lost. The output, however, is set two to three times higher than the pacing threshold because thresholds tend to fluctuate over time. Separate output controls for both the atrium and the ventricle are used with a dual-chamber pulse generator.

The sensitivity control regulates the ability of the pacemaker to detect the heart's intrinsic electrical activity. Sensitivity is measured in millivolts (mV) and determines the size of the intracardiac signal that the generator will recognize. If the sensitivity is adjusted to its most sensitive setting—a setting of 1 mV—the pacemaker can respond even to low-amplitude electrical signals coming from the heart. This is referred to as *synchronous* or *demand pacing*. On the other hand, turning the sensitivity to its least sensitive setting (adjusting the dial to a setting of 20 mV or to the area labeled *async*) will result in the inability of the pacemaker to sense any intrinsic electrical activity and cause the pacemaker to function at a fixed rate. This is referred to as *asynchronous* or *fixed-rate pacing*. A sense indicator (often a light) on the pulse generator signals each time intrinsic cardiac electrical activity is sensed. A pulse generator may be designed to sense atrial or ventricular activity, or both. The sensitivity is set at half the value of the sensitivity threshold, to ensure that all appropriate intrinsic cardiac signals are sensed. The sensitivity threshold is the point at which the pacemaker is no longer able to sense the intrinsic activity of the heart. For example, if the measured sensitivity threshold is 3 mV, the generator is set at 1.5 mV. The pacemaker's sensing ability can be quickly evaluated by observing for a change in pacing rhythm in response to spontaneous depolarizations.

The AV interval control (available only on dual-chamber generators) regulates the time interval between the atrial and ventricular pacing stimuli. This interval is analogous to the PR interval that occurs in the intrinsic ECG. Proper adjustment of this interval to between 150 to 250 msec preserves AV synchrony and permits maximal ventricular stroke volume and enhanced cardiac output.

Temporary DDD pacemakers have several other digital controls that are unique to this newer type of temporary pulse generator (Fig. 11-2, *B*). The lower rate, or base rate, determines the rate at which the generator will pace when intrinsic activity falls below the set rate of the pacemaker. The upper rate determines the fastest ventricular rate the pacemaker will deliver in response to sensed atrial activity. This setting is needed to protect the patient's heart from being paced in response to rapid atrial dysrhythmias.[6] The pulse width, which can be adjusted from 0.05 to 2.0 msec, controls the length of time that the pacing stimulus is delivered to the heart. There also is an atrial refractory period, programmable from 150 to 500 msec, which regulates the length of time after either a sensed or paced ventricular event during which the pacemaker cannot respond to another atrial stimulus. An emergency button is also available on some models to allow for rapid initiation of asynchronous (DOO) pacing during an emergency.

Finally, on all temporary pacemakers, an on/off switch is provided with a safety feature that prevents the accidental termination of pacing.

Pacing Artifacts

All patients with temporary pacemakers require continuous ECG monitoring. The pacing artifact is the spike that is seen on the ECG tracing as the pacing stimulus is delivered to the heart. A P wave is visible after the pacing artifact if the atrium is being paced (Fig. 11-3, *A*). Similarly, a QRS complex follows a ventricular pacing artifact (Fig. 11-3, *B*). With dual-chamber pacing, a pacing artifact precedes both the P wave and the QRS complex (Fig. 11-3, *C*).

Not all paced beats look alike. For example, the artifact (spike) produced by a unipolar pacing electrode is larger than that produced by a bipolar lead (Fig. 11-4). Furthermore, the QRS complex of paced beats appears different, depending on the location of the pacing electrode. If the pacing electrode is positioned in the right ventricle, a left bundle branch block (LBBB) pattern is displayed on the ECG. On the other hand, a right bundle branch block (RBBB) pattern is visible if the pacing stimulus originates from the left ventricle.

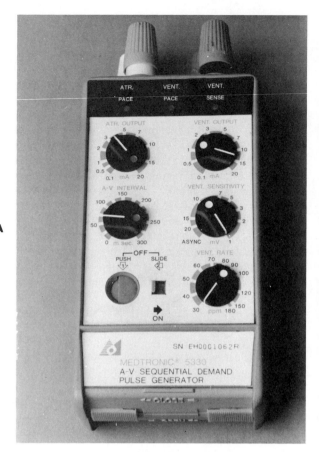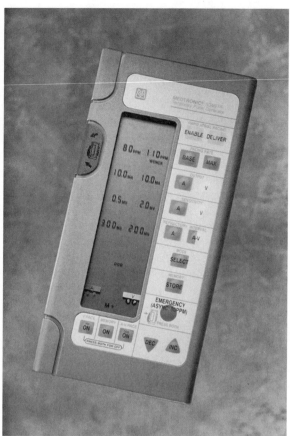

Fig. **11-2** Temporary dual-chamber pulse generators (external). (An example of a temporary single-chamber pulse generator is shown in Figure 11-1.) **A,** Older model AV sequential demand pulse generator. **B,** Newer model DDD pulse generator. (Courtesy Medtronic Inc., Minneapolis.)

Pacemaker Malfunctions

Most pacemaker malfunctions can be categorized as abnormalities of either pacing or sensing.

Pacing malfunctions

Problems with pacing can involve the failure of the pacemaker to deliver a pacing stimulus (failure to pace) or failure of a pacing stimulus to depolarize the heart (failure to capture). Another phenomenon, commonly referred to as *runaway pacemaker,* results in the firing of the pacemaker stimulus at rates greater than the set rate. This malfunction, which is caused by failure of the pulse generator's circuitry, necessitates replacement.

Failure to pace. Failure of the pacemaker to deliver the pacing stimulus results in the disappearance of the pacing artifact, even though the patient's intrinsic rate is less than the set rate on the pacer (Fig. 11-5). This can occur either intermittently or continuously and can be attributed to failure of the pulse generator or its battery, a loose connection between the various components of the pacemaker system, broken lead wires, or stimulus inhibition as a result of EMI. Tightening connections, replacing the batteries or the pulse generator itself, or removing the source of EMI may restore pacemaker function.[3]

Failure to capture. If the pacing stimulus fires but fails to initiate a myocardial depolarization, a pacing artifact will be present but will not be followed by the expected P wave or QRS complex, depending on the chamber being paced (Fig. 11-6). Failure to capture can most often be attributed to either displacement of the pacing electrode or to an increase in the pacing threshold as a result of drugs, metabolic disorders, electrolyte imbalances, or fibrosis or myocardial ischemia at the site of electrode placement. In many cases, increasing the output (mA) may elicit capture.[3] For transvenous leads, repositioning the patient to the left side may improve lead contact and restore capture.

Sensing malfunctions

Problems with sensing can involve the inability of the pacemaker to sense spontaneous myocardial depolarizations (undersensing) or the inappropriate sensing of extraneous electrical signals (oversensing).

Undersensing. Undersensing results in competition between paced complexes and the heart's intrinsic rhythm. This malfunction can be demonstrated on the ECG by pacing artifacts that occur after or unrelated to spontaneous complexes (Fig. 11-7). Undersensing can

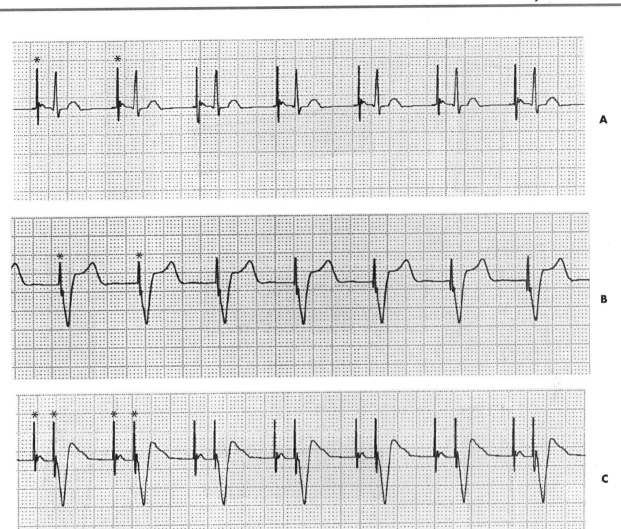

Fig. **11-3** Examples of paced rhythms. **A,** Atrial pacing. **B,** Ventricular pacing. **C,** Dual-chamber pacing. (The * represents a pacemaker impulse.)

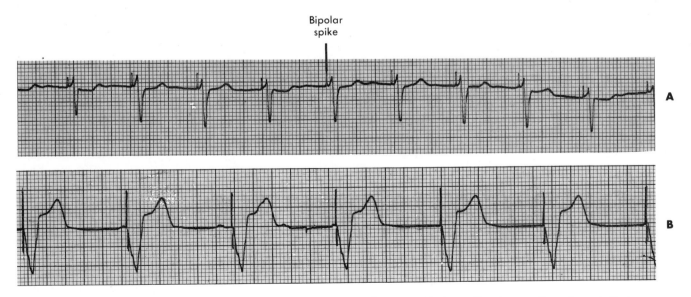

Fig. **11-4** Pacing artifact. **A,** Bipolar spikes. **B,** Unipolar spikes. (From Conover MB: *Understanding electrocardiography: arrhythmias and the 12-lead ECG,* ed 6, St Louis, 1992, Mosby.)

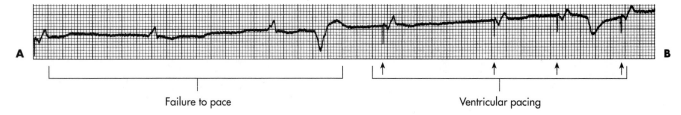

Failure to pace   Ventricular pacing

Fig. **11-5** Failure to pace. **A,** Patient with a transvenous pacemaker is turned onto the left side. Immediately there is a failure to pace (loss of pacer artifacts on ECG). The patient's heart rate is extremely low without pacemaker support. **B,** The nurse turns the patient onto the right side, the transvenous electrode floats into contact with the right ventricular wall, and pacing is resumed. (From Kesten KS, Norton CK: *Pacemakers: patient care, troubleshooting, rhythm analysis*, Baltimore, 1985, Resource Applications, Inc.)

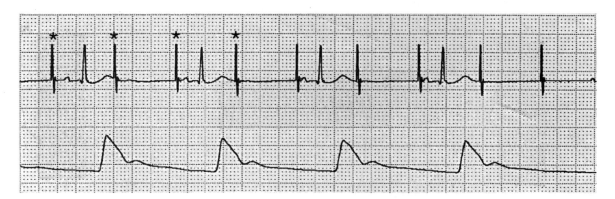

Fig. **11-6** Failure to capture. Atrial pacing and capture occur after pacer spikes(s) 1, 3, 5, and 7. The remaining pacer spikes fail to capture the tissue, resulting in loss of the P wave, no conduction to the ventricles, and no arterial waveform. (The * represents a pacemaker impulse.)

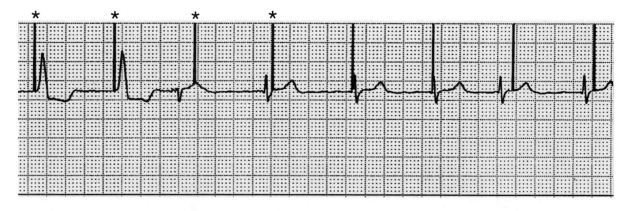

Fig. **11-7** Undersensing. Notice that after the first two paced beats there is a series of intrinsic beats. Failure of the pacemaker unit to sense these intrinsic QRS complexes leads to inappropriate pacemaker spikes(s), which fall on top of or after the intrinsic QRS complexes. These spikes do not capture the ventricle because they occur during the refractory period of the cardiac cycle. (The * represents a pacemaker impulse.)

result in the delivery of pacing stimuli into a relative refractory period of the cardiac depolarization cycle. Ventricular pacing stimuli delivered into the downslope of the T wave (R-on-T phenomenon) is a real danger with this type of pacer aberration because it may precipitate a lethal dysrhythmia. The nurse must act quickly to determine the cause and initiate appropriate interventions. Often the cause can be attributed to inadequate wave amplitude (or height of the P or R wave). If this is the case, the situation can be promptly remedied by increasing the sensitivity (moving the sensitivity dial toward its lowest setting). Other possible causes include inappropriate (i.e., asynchronous) mode selection, lead displacement or fracture, loose cable connections, and pulse generator failure.[3]

Oversensing. Oversensing can lead to unnecessary triggering or inhibiting of stimulus output, depending on the pacer mode. The source of these electrical signals can range from the presence of tall, peaked T waves to EMI in the critical care environment. Because most temporary pulse generators are programmed in demand modes, oversensing results in unexplained pauses in the ECG tracing as the extraneous signals are sensed and inhibit pacing. Often, simply moving the sensitivity dial toward 20 mV stops the pauses.[3]

Medical Management

The physician determines the pacing route, based on the patient's clinical situation. Generally transcutaneous pacing is used in emergent situations, until a transvenous lead can be secured. If the patient is undergoing heart surgery, epicardial leads may be electively placed at the end of the operation. The physician places the transvenous or epicardial pacing lead(s), repositioning as needed to obtain adequate pacing and sensing thresholds. Decisions regarding lead placement may later limit the pacing modes available to the clinician. For example, to perform dual-chamber pacing, both atrial and ventricular leads must be placed. In emergent situations, however, interventions are focused on establishing ventricular pacing, and atrial lead placement may not be feasible. After lead placement, the initial settings for output and sensitivity are determined, the pacing rate and mode are selected, and the patient's response to pacing is evaluated.

Nursing Management

Nursing priorities for managing the patient with a temporary pacemaker include preventing pacemaker malfunction, protecting the patient against microshock, and maintaining surveillance for complications.

Preventing pacemaker malfunction

Continuous ECG monitoring is essential to facilitate prompt recognition of and appropriate intervention for pacemaker malfunction. In addition, proper care of the pacing system can do a great deal to prevent pacing abnormalities.

The temporary pacing lead and bridging cable must be properly secured to the body with tape to prevent the accidental displacement of the electrode, which can result in failure to pace or sense. The external pulse generator can be secured to the patient's waist with a strap or placed in a telemetry bag for the mobile patient. For the patient on a regimen of bedrest, the pulse generator can be suspended with twill tape from an intravenous (IV) pole mounted overhead on the ceiling, which not only will prevent tension on the lead while the patient is moved (given adequate length of bridging cable) but also will alleviate the possibility of accidental dropping of the pulse generator. The nurse inspects for loose connections between the lead(s) and pulse generator on a regular basis. In addition, replacement batteries and pulse generators must always be available on the unit. Although the

battery has an anticipated life span of 1 month, it probably is sound practice to change the battery if the pacemaker has been operating continually for several days. Newer generators provide a low battery signal 24 hours before complete loss of battery function to prevent inadvertent interruptions in pacing. The pulse generator must always be labeled with the date that the battery was replaced.

Protecting the patient against microshock

It is important to be aware of all sources of electromagnetic interference (EMI), which, within the critical care environment, could interfere with the pacemaker's function. Sources of EMI in the clinical area include electrocautery, defibrillation current, radiation therapy, magnetic resonance imaging devices, and transcutaneous electrical nerve stimulation (TENS) units. In most cases, if EMI is suspected of precipitating pacemaker malfunction, converting to the asynchronous mode (fixed rate) will maintain pacing until the cause of the EMI is removed. Because the pacing electrode provides a direct, low-resistance path to the heart, the nurse takes special care while handling the external components of the pacing system to avoid conducting stray electrical current from other equipment. Even a small amount of stray current transmitted via the pacing lead could precipitate a lethal dysrhythmia. The possibility of "microshock" can be minimized by the wearing of rubber gloves when handling the pacing wires and by proper insulation of terminal pins of pacing wires when they are not in use. The latter can be accomplished either by using caps provided by the manufacturer or by improvising with a needle cover or section of disposable rubber glove. The wires are to be taped securely to the patient's chest to prevent accidental electrode displacement. Additional safety measures include using a nonelectric or a properly grounded electric bed, keeping all electrical equipment away from the bed, and permitting the use of only rechargeable electric razors.

Maintaining surveillance for complications

Complications of temporary pacing include infection and myocardial perforation. The site(s) is carefully inspected for purulent drainage, erythema, and edema, and the patient is observed for signs of systemic infection. Site care is performed according to the institution's policy and procedure. Although most infections remain localized, endocarditis can occur in patients with endocardial pacing leads. A less common complication associated with transvenous pacing is myocardial perforation, which can result in rhythmic hiccoughs or cardiac tamponade.

IMPLANTABLE CARDIOVERTER DEFIBRILLATOR

If a ventricular tachydysrhythmia is not amenable to surgical or radiofrequency ablation or to antidysrhythmic drugs, an implantable cardioverter defibrillator (ICD) may be inserted. The ICD is capable of identifying and terminating life-threatening ventricular dysrhythmias. A recent clinical trial suggests that ICD therapy may be the preferred treatment for patients at increased risk for sudden cardiac death. Researchers found that patients who received an ICD had a decreased mortality when compared with those who received antidysrhythmic therapy with amiodarone.[7]

ICD System

The ICD system contains sensing electrodes to recognize the dysrhythmia and defibrillation electrodes or patches that are in contact with the heart and can deliver a "shock." These electrodes are connected to a generator that is surgically placed in the subcutaneous tissue in the upper left abdominal quadrant (Fig. 11-8). The early model generators could defibrillate or cardiovert only lethal dysrhythmias. Recent improvements in ICD treatment include the use of "tiered" therapy generators that incorporate antitachycardia pacing, bradycardia back-up pacing, low-energy cardioversion, and high-energy defibrillation options. With tiered therapy, antitachycardia pacing is used as the first line of treatment in some cases of ventricular tachycardia (VT). If the VT can be pace-terminated successfully, the patient will not receive a "shock" from the generator and may not even realize that the ICD terminated the dysrhythmia. If programmed bursts of pacing do not terminate the VT, the ICD will "cardiovert" the rhythm. If the dysrhythmia deteriorates into ventricular fibrillation (VF), the ICD is programmed to defibrillate at a higher energy. If the dysrhythmia terminates spontaneously, the device will not discharge (see Figure 11-8). Occasionally, the electrical rhythm may deteriorate to asystole or a slow idioventricular rhythm. In such cases the bradycardia back-up pacing function is activated.

ICD Insertion

Initially, all ICDs were implanted surgically either during open heart surgery, with electrode patches sewn directly onto the epicardium, or by means of a thoracotomy incision, with the electrode patches attached to the outside of the pericardium. Recently, several new devices have become available that obviate the need for a thoracic surgical intervention. Transvenous electrode leads are inserted into the subclavian vein and advanced into the right side of the heart where contact with the endocardium is achieved. To improve defibrillation efficacy, an additional subcutaneous patch may be placed with some models. The endocardial leads are used for sensing, pacing, and cardioversion/defibrillation. They are connected to the generator by tunneling through the subcutaneous tissue; thus thoracotomy is avoided. The endocardial lead system offers several advantages: it is less invasive, requires shorter hospitalization, and is associated with significantly lower implantation mortality.[8] Technical advances

and the development of smaller ICDs have made it feasible to implant these devices in the pectoral position, similar to that used for permanent pacemakers.[9]

Medical Management

Medical management of the ICD patient begins before implantation, with a thorough evaluation of the patient's dysrhythmia and underlying cardiac function. A number of noninvasive studies are available to help identify patients at risk for sudden cardiac death (SCD). These include signal averaged electrocardiography, echocardiography, baroreceptor sensitivity testing, and heart rate variability studies. Generally, patients identified at risk for SCD undergo an electrophysiology study to identify the origin of the dysrhythmia and to determine the effect of antidysrhythmic agents in suppressing or altering the rate of the dysrhythmia. Further assessment of cardiac status is made to determine whether additional interventions (cardiac surgery, angioplasty) are indicated to improve cardiac function. This part of the work-up may include cardiac catheterization, stress testing, and echocardiography. Based on the aforementioned evaluation, decisions are made regarding the implantation approach (i.e., thoracotomy at the time of surgery or nonthoracotomy) as well as the type of therapy required (antitachypacing, cardioversion, defibrillation).

ICD programming

Initial programming of the device is generally performed by an electrophysiologist at the time of implantation. During implantation, defibrillation threshold measurements are obtained. This involves inducing the dysrhythmia and then evaluating the device's ability to terminate the dysrhythmia. Once it is determined that the ICD functions adequately, further follow-up is conducted on an outpatient basis to monitor the number of discharges and the battery life of the device.

Nursing Management

Nursing priorities for managing the patient with an ICD include monitoring for dysrhythmias and maintaining surveillance for complications. If the ICD system was implanted during open heart surgery, the nursing management is similar to that for any patient undergoing cardiac surgery. If an endocardial lead system is implanted, the nursing management is less intense and the hospital stay is shorter.[10]

Monitoring for dysrhythmias

In the case of a ventricular dysrhythmia, it is important to know the type of ICD implanted, how the device functions, and whether it is activated. Most patients will continue to take some antidysrhythmic medications to decrease the frequency of VT or VF and thus decrease the number of "shocks" required and prolong the battery life of the device.[8] Patients with new ICDs have continuous

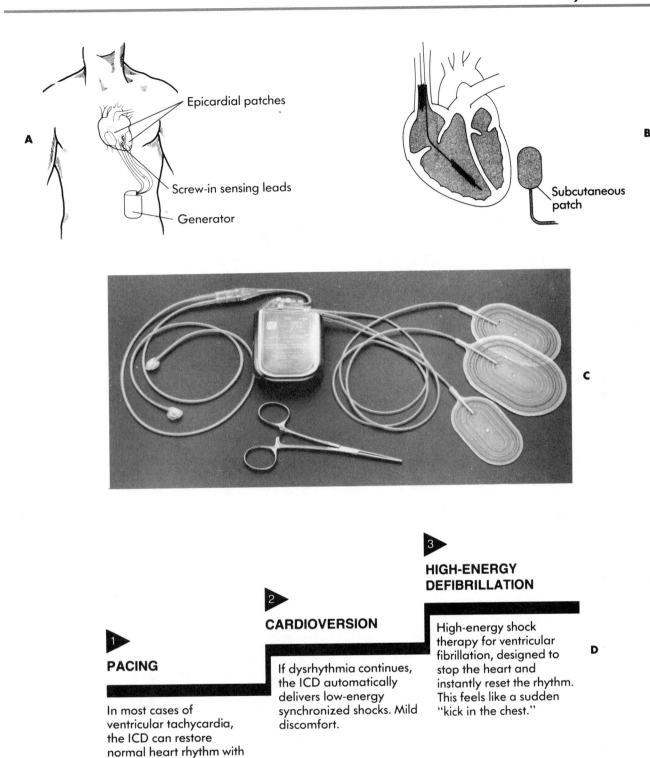

Fig. **11-8** Implantable cardioverter defibrillator (ICD). **A,** Placement of an ICD and epicardial lead system. The generator is placed in a subcutaneous "pocket" in the left upper abdominal quadrant. The epicardial screw-in sensing leads monitor the heart rhythm and connect to the generator. If a life-threatening dysrhythmia is sensed, the generator can pace-terminate the dysrhythmia or deliver electrical cardioversion or defibrillation through the epicardial patches. With this system, the leads/patches must be placed during open-chest (sternal or thoracotomy) surgery. **B,** In the transvenous lead system, open-chest surgery is not required. The pacing/cardioversion/defibrillation functions are all contained in a lead (or leads) inserted into the right atrium and ventricle. A subcutaneous patch may be placed under the skin. **C,** An example of an ICD tiered therapy generator (Medtronic PCD) with epicardial screw-in sensing leads and patches. **D,** Tiered therapy is designed to use increasing levels of intensity to terminate ventricular dysrhythmias. (Courtesy Medtronic Inc., Minneapolis.)

ECG monitoring to detect correct ICD function in the event of a dysrhythmia. During an episode of VT or VF, the patient is monitored to ensure that the device terminates the dysrhythmia successfully.

Maintaining surveillance for complications

Complications associated with the ICD include infection from the implanted system, broken leads, and the sensing of supraventricular tachydysrhythmias resulting in unneeded discharges.[11]

Patient education

To facilitate a positive psychologic adjustment to the ICD, education of the patient and family about the device is vital. Preoperative teaching for the ICD patient includes information about how the device works and what to expect during the implantation procedure. After implantation, education is focused on aspects of living with an ICD. Patients need information pertaining to scheduled device follow-up and instructions about what to do if they experience a "shock." Many institutions also have successfully used family support groups for this patient population.

CARDIAC INTERVENTIONAL PROCEDURES

Percutaneous Transluminal Coronary Angioplasty

Percutaneous transluminal coronary angioplasty (PTCA) involves the use of a balloon-tipped catheter that, when advanced through an atherosclerotic lesion (atheroma), can be inflated intermittently for the purpose of dilating the stenotic area and improving blood flow through

it (Fig. 11-9). The high balloon-inflation pressure stretches the vessel wall, fractures the plaque, and enlarges the vessel lumen. A successful angioplasty procedure is one in which the stenosis is reduced to less than 50% of the vessel lumen diameter, although most clinicians aim for less than 30% final diameter stenosis.[12] Procedural success is influenced by patient variables such as age, cardiac function, and co-morbidities such as diabetes as well as by characteristics of the lesion itself. Lesions that are discrete (less than 1 cm in length), concentric, easily accessible, and have little or no calcification are most likely to be treated successfully with PTCA.[12] PTCA is also a valuable adjunct to thrombolytic therapy in terms of reducing a severe stenosis that persists after thrombolysis.[13] The advantages of PTCA included avoiding the risks involved with cardiac surgery (general anesthesia, thoracotomy, extracorporeal circulation, and mechanical ventilation) and significantly decreasing convalescence time. Disadvantages included acute complications related to the procedure itself, late restenosis, and difficulty in accessing certain lesions.

Procedure

PTCA is performed in the cardiac catheterization laboratory under fluoroscopy. Introducer catheters or "sheaths" are inserted percutaneously into the femoral artery and vein. The venous sheath can be used to perform a right heart catheterization with a pulmonary artery (PA) catheter or to insert a pacing catheter, or both. A catheter with pacing capabilities may be indicated if dilation of the right coronary artery or circumflex artery is anticipated because the blood supply to the conduction system of the heart may be interrupted, requiring emergency pacing. The pacing catheter also serves as an anatomic landmark for locating the lesions to be dilated. The

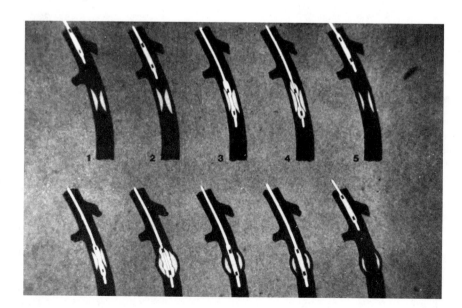

Fig. **11-9** Balloon compression of an atherosclerotic lesion. (From Kinney M, et al: *Comprehensive cardiac care*, ed 8, St Louis, 1996, Mosby.)

patient is systemically heparinized to prevent clots from forming on or in any of the catheters. A special guiding catheter designed to engage the coronary ostia is inserted through the arterial sheath and advanced in a retrograde manner through the aorta. Nitroglycerin or calcium channel blockers may be given at this time to prevent coronary artery spasm and to maximize coronary vasodilation during the procedure. A guidewire is then advanced down the coronary artery and negotiated across the occluding atheroma. The balloon catheter is advanced over this guidewire and positioned across the lesion. The balloon is inflated and deflated repetitively (each inflation not to exceed 90 seconds) until evidence of dilation is demonstrated on an angiogram. In cases that require prolonged balloon inflations, however, an autoperfusion angioplasty catheter is available with side holes that allow passive blood flow through the central lumen to the distal coronary artery if adequate systemic blood pressure is present.

Medical management

The patient is transferred to the coronary care or angioplasty unit for overnight care and observation. The introducer sheaths are left in place for several reasons. First, the intravenous infusion of heparin is continued for 6 to 24 hours after PTCA to prevent clot formation on the roughened endothelium at the site of dilation.[14] Therefore removal of the sheaths during this time causes a predisposition to bleeding. Second, it allows for rapid vascular access should redilation become necessary. The arterial sheath must be attached to a continuous heparinized saline flush, however, and intravenous fluids must be infused through the venous sheath to maintain luminal patency. If the patient's postangioplasty course is uneventful, the heparin infusion is discontinued and the sheaths are removed within 24 hours of the procedure. After sheath removal, the patient may be discharged home 6 to 12 hours later.

Complications. Serious complications can result from angioplasty that necessitate emergency CABG surgery. These complications include persistent coronary artery spasm, myocardial infarction, and acute coronary occlusion. Abciximab (Reopro) has recently been approved by the Food and Drug Administration (FDA) as an adjunct to PTCA for the prevention of abrupt closure of arteries in high-risk patients. When administered as a bolus and followed with a continuous infusion for 12 hours after angioplasty, Reopro was found to decrease the risk of reocclusion. The major complication of Reopro is bleeding.[15] Other complications that can occur in the period immediately after angioplasty include bleeding and hematoma formation at the site of vascular cannulation, compromised blood flow to the involved extremity, allergic reaction to radioopaque contrast dye, dysrhythmias, and vasovagal response (hypotension, bradycardia, and diaphoresis) during manipulation or removal of introducer sheaths. Restenosis can occur up to 6 months after angioplasty; however, this late complication typically is amenable to repeat angioplasty. The mechanism involved in restenosis remains unclear, but it is thought to be related to intimal hyperplasia, as well as to platelet deposition and thrombus formation. For this reason, patients are started on a regimen of antiplatelet drugs (e.g., a combination of aspirin and dipyridamole or ticlopidine).

Although PTCA has relatively high success rates in initially opening occluded vessels, this technique has major limitations, including a high frequency of restenosis and abrupt vessel closure. The fact that angioplasty does not remove the occlusive material but rather compresses it to widen the vessel lumen is thought to contribute to the rate of restenosis. Coronary atherectomy, laser angioplasty, and placement of endovascular prostheses (stents) are interventional technologies developed to address the problems of acute closure and restenosis associated with PTCA.[12]

Atherectomy

Atherectomy is the excision and removal of the atherosclerotic plaque by cutting, shaving, or grinding; specialized coronary catheters are used to achieve a more controlled mechanism of injury, with the hope of fewer complications.[16] Three atherectomy devices are described in Table 11-3.[17] All three devices are FDA-approved for use in coronary as well as peripheral arteries. Because these devices use different mechanisms, they may offer special advantages for different types of lesions.

Laser Angioplasty

Laser is an acronym for "light amplification by stimulated emission of radiation." Laser plaque ablation in coronary arteries, using the excimer laser, is currently being studied in clinical trials. The excimer laser is a contact cutter, meaning that it only ablates tissue that it touches. The catheter is advanced by a guidewire system similar to that used in angioplasty. The excimer laser, which uses high-energy pulsed ultraviolet light—so-called cold laser—to vaporize plaque, is particularly suited for distal disease and occluded saphenous vein grafts.[18]

Coronary Stents

Another major coronary technology is the coronary stent prosthesis. This is a self-expanding or balloon-expandable stent that is introduced into the coronary artery over a guidewire in a region that has been previously dilated with PTCA to prevent acute closure and restenosis as well as to obtain a larger vascular lumen diameter.[18,19] The procedure for stent placement is similar to that used in other catheter interventions. Access to the coronary arteries is obtained via a femoral sheath, which allows for placement of a catheter over a guidewire. A stent is positioned at the target side, is expanded, and the catheter is removed, leaving the stent in place. At present, approved indications for stents include threatened or

TABLE 11-3

ATHERECTOMY DEVICES

DEVICE	DESIGN	USES
Directional atherectomy (Simpson Atherocath)	Rotating cup-shaped cutter within a windowed cylindric housing; plaque that protrudes into window is shaved off and collected within nose cone of cutter housing	Ostial lesions SVG Eccentric lesions in large vessels Proximal, discrete lesions
Rotational ablation (Rotablator)	Rotating diamond-studded burr; "sanding effect"; generates microparticles that pass distally into microcirculation	Distal lesions Long, diffuse lesions Tortuous vessels Calcified lesions Eccentric lesions Ostial lesions Small vessels
Transluminal extraction catheter (TEC)	Motorized cutting head with triangular blades; excised plaque removed by suction	Diffuse disease SVG

SVG, Saphenous venous graft.

abrupt vessel closure ("failed" angioplasty or atherectomy) and primary stenting as an alternative to angioplasty or bypass surgery.[20]

Because the stent is a foreign object (generally made of stainless steel) in the bloodstream, the stent's presence in the coronary artery activates the coagulation cascade. To prevent acute thrombosis of the stent, intense anticoagulation and antiplatelet therapy was initially used during and after stent placement. This consisted of preprocedure aspirin and dypyridamole and the administration of IV heparin both during and after the procedure to prevent acute thrombosis of the stent. Consequently, bleeding was a major complication of stent placement. Recent studies have indicated that reduced anticoagulation may be sufficient to maintain stent patency. Many physicians now use heparin only during the procedure and remove access sheaths as soon as the activated clotting time (ACT) returns to normal.[20] Aspirin is continued indefinitely, and ticlopidine and/or low molecular weight heparin are commonly prescribed after stent placement.

Balloon Valvuloplasty

After the development of percutaneous balloon angioplasty for coronary artery disease, it became reasonable to consider adaptation of this technique as a nonsurgical intervention for stenotic cardiac valves. Although long-term results are not promising at this point, especially for aortic valvuloplasty, balloon valvuloplasty can provide palliation and short-term symptomatic relief in selected patient populations.[21] Balloon valvuloplasty is performed in the cardiac catheterization laboratory. The procedure is similar to a routine cardiac catheterization, including cannulation of the femoral artery and vein with percutaneous introducer sheaths. The balloon dilation catheter is then threaded over a guidewire across the stenotic valvular orifice. The valves may be approached either retrograde via the aorta or antegrade across the interatrial septum. In the

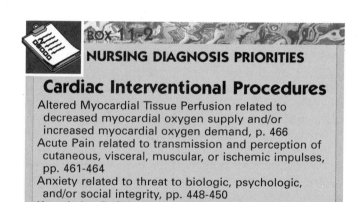

BOX 11-2

NURSING DIAGNOSIS PRIORITIES

Cardiac Interventional Procedures

Altered Myocardial Tissue Perfusion related to decreased myocardial oxygen supply and/or increased myocardial oxygen demand, p. 466
Acute Pain related to transmission and perception of cutaneous, visceral, muscular, or ischemic impulses, pp. 461-464
Anxiety related to threat to biologic, psychologic, and/or social integrity, pp. 448-450
Knowledge Deficit: Discharge Regimen related to lack of previous exposure to information, p. 443

antegrade transseptal approach, the balloon catheter is passed across the interatrial septum, which results in the creation of a small atrial septal defect.[22] Subsequent inflations of the balloon increase the valve opening by separating fused commissures, cracking calcified leaflets, and stretching valve structures. Inflations are continued until the balloon "waist" disappears which indicates full inflation.[23] Regurgitant flow can result, particularly after mitral valvuloplasty. The risks of balloon valvuloplasty, which are similar to those inherent in most catheterization procedures, include damage to the valve, cardiac perforation, thromboembolic events, dysrhythmias, hypotension, and bleeding.[22,23]

Nursing Management

Nursing management of the patient undergoing a cardiac interventional procedure incorporates a variety of nursing diagnoses (Box 11-2). **Nursing priorities are directed toward monitoring for recurrent chest pain, managing the introducer sheaths, providing comfort** and emotional support, and maintaining surveillance for complications.

Monitoring for recurrent chest pain

It is essential that the patient is observed for recurrent angina, a clinical indication of myocardial ischemia. Angina may be accompanied by elevated ST segments on the bedside monitor or the 12-lead ECG. Angina during interventional cardiology procedures is an expected occurrence at the time of balloon inflation or manipulation within the coronary artery. Intraprocedure angina is caused by the temporary interruption of blood flow through the involved artery, which should subside with deflation or removal of the balloon or nitroglycerin administration, or both. Angina after a coronary interventional procedure may be a result of transient coronary vasospasm, or it may signal the more serious complication of acute thrombosis. Initial treatment usually consists of the administration of intravenous nitroglycerin. Continued angina despite maximal vasodilator therapy generally rules out transient coronary vasospasm as the source of ischemic pain, and redilation or emergency coronary artery bypass surgery must be considered.

Managing the introducer sheaths

The introducer sheaths are left in place for 6 to 24 hours after the procedure. During that time the patient is instructed to keep the involved leg straight and not to elevate the head of the bed any more than 30 degrees (to prevent dislodgment) and for several hours after its removal (to prevent bleeding). The arterial sheath should be treated as an arterial line and the venous sheath as a central line. Use of an eggcrate mattress may help alleviate the lower back pain many patients experience while immobile after an interventional procedure. After sheath removal, direct pressure is applied to the puncture site for 15 to 30 minutes; a sandbag may be ordered if direct pressure is inadequate for hemostasis. For stents or atherectomy, which require a larger sheath size, a femoral artery compression device may be used to apply continued pressure for 1 to 2 hours to ensure adequate hemostasis. The patient usually is allowed to resume ambulation 6 to 8 hours later, depending on institutional protocol. Excessive bleeding or hematoma formation can become a serious problem because it may result in hypotension or compromised blood flow to the involved extremity. For this reason, pulses are usually monitored every 15 minutes for the first couple of hours immediately after the procedure, and then every 1 to 2 hours until the sheaths are removed. After sheath removal, pulses are again monitored at 15-minute intervals for a brief period.

Maintaining surveillance for complications

While the sheath is in place or after its removal, bleeding or hematoma at the sheath insertion site may occur as a result of the effects of heparin. The patient is observed for bleeding or swelling at the puncture site and for adequacy of circulation to the involved extremity. The patient is also assessed for back pain, which can indicate retroperitoneal bleeding from the internal arterial puncture site.

Patient education

All patients require education about their medication regimen and about risk-factor modification. Because of the abbreviated hospital stay, the nurse often has insufficient time to do more than identify the offending risk factors and initiate basic instruction. Patients are referred to local cardiac rehabilitation centers for more extensive teaching and follow-up to facilitate understanding and compliance with risk factor modification. Another point of instruction that must be addressed is the patient's knowledge deficit related to discharge medications. Patients frequently are sent home on a regimen of antiplatelet drugs as well as a nitrate such as isosorbide to promote vasodilation. In addition, if the patient has demonstrated evidence of a vasospastic component to the disease, calcium channel blockers are prescribed. It is essential that the patient clearly understand the rationale for therapy as well as potential side effects of each drug. It is important that patients be provided with written information as well as a number to call if problems occur.[24]

THROMBOLYTIC THERAPY

Thrombolytic therapy is an important clinical intervention for the patient experiencing acute myocardial infarction (AMI). Before the introduction of thrombolytic agents, the management of AMI was focused on decreasing myocardial oxygen demands to minimize myocardial necrosis. Today efforts to limit the size of infarction are directed toward the timely reperfusion of the jeopardized myocardium. The use of thrombolytic therapy to accomplish this objective is predicated on the prevailing theory that the significant event in most transmural infarctions is the rupture of an atherosclerotic plaque with thrombus formation. The administration of a thrombolytic agent results in the lysis of the acute thrombus, thus opening the obstructed coronary artery and restoring blood flow to the affected tissue. However, residual coronary stenosis resulting from the atherosclerotic process remains even after successful thrombolysis. This residual coronary stenosis can cause rethrombosis. Therefore thrombolytic therapy is recognized as an emergency procedure to restore patency until more definitive therapy can be initiated to effectively reduce the degree of stenosis (interventional catheter procedure) or to bypass the offending occlusion (coronary artery bypass surgery). The optimal timing of these interventions is yet to be determined.

Eligibility Criteria

Certain criteria have been developed to determine the patient population that would most likely benefit from the administration of thrombolytic therapy. In general, patients with recent onset of chest pain (less than 6 hours'

BOX 11-3

THROMBOLYTIC THERAPY SELECTION CRITERIA

No more than 6 hours from onset of chest pain and less if possible
ST-segment elevation on ECG
Ischemic chest pain of 30 minutes' duration
Chest pain unresponsive to sublingual nitroglycerin or nifedipine
No conditions that might cause a predisposition to hemorrhage

BOX 11-4

NONINVASIVE EVIDENCE OF REPERFUSION

Cessation of chest pain
Reperfusion dysrhythmias, primarily ventricular
Return of elevated ST segments to baseline
Early and marked peaking of creatine kinase (CK)

duration) are candidates. Research suggests that the earlier the treatment is instituted, the higher the likelihood of successful reperfusion. Patients with persistent ST-segment elevation despite sublingual nitroglycerin or nifedipine, a sign of impending transmural infarction, are considered candidates for therapy. Patients with abnormal Q waves are not excluded from therapy because this finding is not necessarily evidence of a completed infarction. Exclusion criteria is usually based on the increased risk of bleeding incurred by the use of thrombolytics. Patients who have stable clots that might be disrupted by thrombolytic therapy (secondary to recent surgery or a recent cerebrovascular accident) are generally not considered candidates for thrombolytic therapy. Other common criteria for the use of thrombolytic therapy are included in Box 11-3.

Thrombolytic Agents

Five thrombolytic agents are currently available for either intracoronary or intravenous treatment of acute myocardial infarction. Although these agents differ in their mechanism of clot lysis, all have been found effective in lysing clots and restoring perfusion. A comparison of these agents is provided in Table 11-4.[25,26] Because patients with an area of plaque disruption are still at risk for clot formation and reocclusion, intravenous heparin and oral aspirin are prescribed either during or immediately after thrombolytic therapy. The timing of these interventions may vary, based on the specific thrombolytic agent used and institutional protocols. Heparin therapy is usually continued for 24 to 72 hours, whereas daily aspirin is continued indefinitely.

Nursing Management

Nursing management of the patient undergoing thrombolytic therapy begins with identifying potential candidates. In many institutions, checklists are used to facilitate rapid identification of patients who are candidates for thrombolytics. The nurse prepares the patient for thrombolytic therapy by starting intravenous lines and obtaining base-

line laboratory values and vital signs. **Nursing priorities for managing the patient receiving thrombolytic therapy include monitoring for signs of reperfusion and maintaining surveillance for complications.**

Monitoring for signs of reperfusion

Several phenomena may be observed after the reperfusion of an artery that has been completely occluded by a thrombus (Box 11-4).

Cessation of chest pain and reperfusion dysrhythmias. Initially, when there is reperfusion there is an abrupt cessation of ischemic chest pain as blood flow is restored. Another reliable indicator of reperfusion is the appearance of various "reperfusion" dysrhythmias. Premature ventricular contractions, bradycardias, heart block, ventricular tachycardia, and, rarely, ventricular fibrillation may occur. The reason for the occurrence of these dysrhythmias remains unclear, but they are thought to be the result of restored flow to ischemic tissue. Generally, reperfusion dysrhythmias are self-limiting or nonsustained, and aggressive antidysrhythmic therapy is not required. Vigilant monitoring of the patient's ECG is essential, however, because a stable condition may deteriorate rapidly, and the dysrhythmias may require emergency treatment.

Normalization of the ST segment. Another noninvasive marker of reperfusion is the rapid resolution of the previously elevated ST segments, which indicates restoration of blood flow to previously ischemic myocardial tissue. For this reason a monitoring lead should be chosen that clearly demonstrates ST elevation before initiation of therapy.[27]

Creatine kinase washout. The serum concentration of creatine kinase (CK) rises rapidly and markedly after reperfusion of the ischemic myocardium. This phenomenon is termed *washout*, because it is thought to result from the rapid readmission of creatine kinase—an enzyme released by damaged myocardial cells—into the circulation after restoration of blood flow to previously unperfused areas of the heart.

Maintaining surveillance for complications

The most common complication related to thrombolysis is bleeding, not only as a result of the thrombolytic therapy itself but also because patients routinely receive anticoagulation therapy for several days to minimize the possibility of rethrombosis. Therefore the nurse must

TABLE 11-4

THROMBOLYTIC AGENTS APPROVED BY THE FDA FOR USE IN ACUTE MYOCARDIAL INFARCTION

DRUG	DOSAGE	ACTIONS	SPECIAL CONSIDERATIONS
Anistreplase (APSAC)	30 mg via slow IV bolus over 2-5 min	A molecular combination of streptokinase and plasminogen with actions similar to streptokinase Has systemic lytic effects	May cause allergic reactions and hypotension Long half-life, so heparin is usually started 4-6 hr after APSAC Aspirin begun with treatment and continued q day
rPA (reptelase)	IV: 10 million U given as a bolus, repeated in 30 min	Binds to fibrin at the clot and promotes activation of plasminogen to plasmin	Heparin started with administration of the drug and continued for 24 hr Aspirin begun with treatment and continued q day
Streptokinase	IV: 1.5 million U given over 60 min	Catalyzes the conversion of plasminogen to plasmin, which causes lysis of fibrin Has systemic lytic effects	May cause allergic reactions and hypotension Heparin may be administered IV or SQ Aspirin begun with treatment and continued q day May be administered intracoronary
t-PA (alteplase)	Conventional IV: 100 mg over 3 hr, with the first 10 mg given as a bolus, followed by 40 mg the first hour and 20 mg/hr for the second and third hr Front-loaded IV: 100 mg over 1.5 hr, with the first 15 mg given as a bolus Accelerated-dose IV: 100 mg over 90 min with the first 15 mg given as a bolus	Binds to fibrin at the clot (clot-specific) and promotes activation of plasminogen to plasmin	Short half-life, so heparin is usually started with the t-PA as a bolus and then followed with an infusion Aspirin begun with treatment and continued q day
Urokinase	IV: 2 million U over 1 hr IC: 4000-6000 U/min, average dose 500,000 U	Non-selective thrombolysis when given IV	No allergic side effects (nonantigenic) May be administered intracoronary Aspirin begun with treatment and continued q day

continually monitor for clinical manifestations of bleeding. Mild gingival bleeding and oozing around venipuncture sites are common and not a cause for concern. Should serious bleeding occur, such as intracranial or internal bleeding, all fibrinolytic and heparin therapies are discontinued, and volume expanders or coagulation factors, or both, are administered. In addition to accurate assessment of the patient for evidence of bleeding, nursing management includes preventative measures to minimize the potential for bleeding. For example, patient handling is limited, injections are avoided if at all possible, and additional pressure is provided to ensure hemostasis at venipuncture and arterial puncture sites. Intravenous lines are placed before administering lytic therapy, and a heparin lock may be used for obtaining laboratory specimens during treatment. Antacids can be given prophy-

lactically, especially if the patient complains of gastric discomfort.

INTRAAORTIC BALLOON PUMP

The intraaortic balloon pump (IABP) currently is the most widely used temporary mechanical circulatory assist device to support failing circulation (Box 11-5). Its therapeutic effects are based on the hemodynamic principles of diastolic augmentation and afterload reduction. The most commonly used intraaortic balloon consists of a single sausage-shaped polyurethane balloon that is wrapped around the distal end of a vascular catheter and positioned in the descending thoracic aorta just distal to the takeoff of the left subclavian artery. The second generation of intraaortic balloon catheters is more flexible and can be wrapped to a smaller diameter than their predecessors and therefore can be inserted into the femoral artery percutaneously rather than surgically. Contraindications to balloon pumping include aortic aneurysm, aortic valve insufficiency, and severe peripheral vascular disease.

BOX **11-5**

INDICATIONS FOR THE USE OF INTRAAORTIC BALLOON PUMP

Left ventricular failure after cardiac surgery
Unstable angina refractory to medications
Recurrent angina after AMI
Complications of AMI
   Cardiogenic shock
   Papillary muscle dysfunction/rupture with mitral regurgitation
   Ventricular septal defect
   Refractory ventricular dysrhythmias

Physiologic Effects

When attached to a bedside pumping console and properly synchronized to the patient's cardiac cycle, the intraaortic balloon inflates during diastole and deflates just before systole. Initially, as the balloon is inflated in diastole concurrent with aortic valve closure, the blood in the aortic arch above the level of the balloon is displaced retrograde (backward) toward the aortic root, augmenting diastolic coronary arterial blood flow and increasing myocardial oxygen supply (Fig. 11-10, *A*). The blood volume in the aorta below the level of the balloon is propelled forward toward the peripheral vascular system, which may enhance renal perfusion. Subsequently, the deflation of the balloon just before the opening of the aortic valve creates a potential space or vacuum in the aorta, toward which blood flows unimpeded during ventricular ejection (Fig. 11-10, *B*). This decreased resistance to left ventricular ejection, or decreased afterload, facilitates ventricular emptying and reduces myocardial oxygen demands. The overall physiologic effect of IABP therapy is

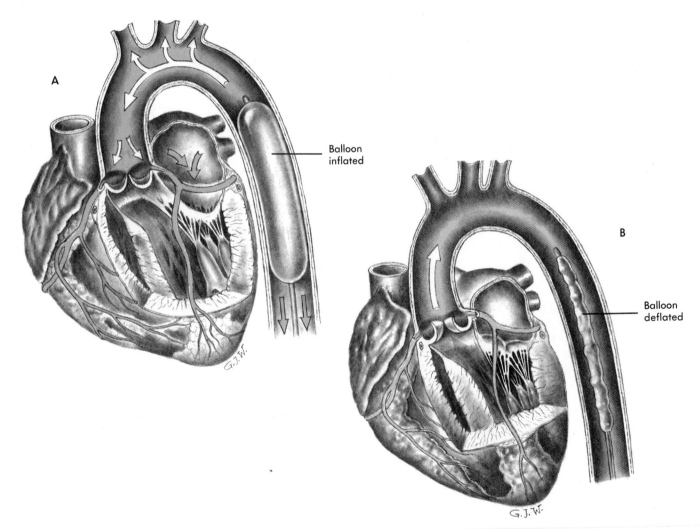

Fig. **11-10** Mechanisms of action of intraaortic balloon pump. **A,** Diastolic balloon inflation augments coronary blood flow. **B,** Systolic balloon deflation decreases afterload.

an improvement in the balance between myocardial oxygen supply and demand.[28]

Insertion

The intraaortic balloon may be inserted in the operating room, the cardiac catheterization laboratory, or the critical care unit. The IAB is usually inserted percutaneously through the femoral artery and advanced to the correct position in the descending thoracic aorta. The physician may insert the balloon through an introducer sheath, or perform a sheathless insertion to minimize the degree of vessel occlusion created by the catheter. If percutaneous catheter placement is not feasible, the catheter may be placed via surgical cutdown or a direct thoracic approach. After insertion, the balloon is attached to the console and filled with the prescribed volume of helium, and pumping is initiated. If the balloon fails to unwrap completely during filling, the physician may rapidly inflate and deflate the balloon manually, using a syringe.

Nursing Management

Nursing priorities for managing the patient requiring an intraaortic balloon pump include assessing balloon timing, ensuring proper balloon placement, weaning from IABP support, and maintaining surveillance for complications.

Assessing balloon timing

The ECG and arterial pressure tracing are constantly monitored to verify the timing and effect of balloon counterpulsations (Fig. 11-11). For counterpulsation to occur, the pump must receive a trigger signal to identify the beginning of a new cardiac cycle. The trigger can be the R wave of the ECG, the upstroke of the arterial pressure waveform, or a pacemaker spike.[29] Dysrhythmias can adversely affect the timing of balloon inflation and deflation; thus rhythm disturbances must be detected and treated promptly. Mean arterial pressure is ideally maintained at about 80 mm Hg with adequate pumping.

Ensuring proper balloon placement

The balloon catheter must be maintained in proper position to optimize its effectiveness and minimize complications. The balloon may migrate proximally and occlude the left subclavian artery, or it may move distally, compromising renal circulation. Therefore careful assessment of the left radial pulse and urinary output is essential. Measures to prevent accidental displacement of the balloon catheter include ensuring that the patient observes complete bedrest, with the head of the bed elevated no

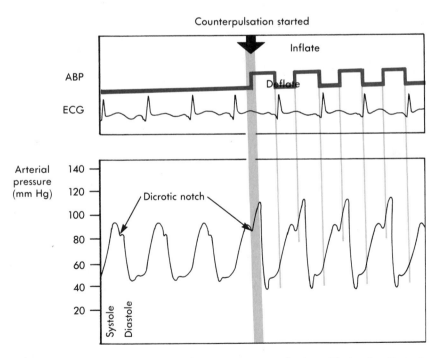

Fig. **11-11** The timing and effect of balloon counterpulsations. Timing is adjusted by synchronizing balloon inflation with the dicrotic notch on the arterial waveform, resulting in an elevated diastolic pressure. Inflation is maintained throughout diastole, to augment coronary perfusion. Deflation occurs just before the next systole, resulting in a reduced systolic pressure and decreased afterload. (From Guzzetta CE, Dossey BM: *Cardiovascular nursing: holistic practice*, St Louis, 1992, Mosby.)

more than 30 degrees, and avoiding any flexion of the involved hip.

Maintaining surveillance for complications

Complications of IABP therapy include peripheral ischemia, balloon perforation, bleeding and infection.

Peripheral ischemia. The most common complication of IABP is lower extremity ischemia secondary to occlusion of the femoral artery, either by the catheter itself or by emboli from thrombus formation on the balloon.[30] Consequently, the presence and quality of peripheral pulses distal to the catheter insertion site are assessed frequently, along with color, temperature, and capillary refill of the involved extremity. Doppler localization of peripheral pulses may be required if pulses are difficult to palpate on the cannulated extremity. Signs of diminished perfusion must be reported immediately. Anticoagulation, such as a heparin infusion, may be prescribed to decrease the incidence of thrombosis. Other vascular complications of IABP include acute aortic dissection and the development of pseudoaneurysms at the catheter insertion site.

Balloon perforation. Another potential complication of IAB therapy is balloon perforation. Perforation occurs secondary to repeated contact of the balloon membrane with calcified plaque in the aorta as the balloon inflates and deflates. The patient is monitored for evidence of a balloon leak, such as a gas leak alarm from the pump console and the presence of blood in the IAB tubing. If a balloon leak is detected, pumping is stopped, and the physician is immediately notified so that the balloon can be removed. If the balloon isn't promptly removed or pumping is attempted after the perforation, the IAB may become entrapped as the blood hardens within the catheter, creating a mass. If this occurs, the balloon must be surgically removed.

Bleeding and infection. Log rolling, in which the patient is moved from side to side every 2 hours, is used to maintain skin integrity and to prevent pulmonary atelectasis. Some institutional protocols call for implementation of continuous lateral rotation therapy to help facilitate pulmonary toilet in the IAB patient. Since thrombocytopenia may occur as a result of mechanical destruction of the platelets by the pumping action of the balloon, platelet counts are closely monitored and the patient is observed for evidence of bleeding. Because infection of the insertion site is a potential complication, the IAB dressing is changed in accordance with the hospital policy for other invasive lines.

Weaning from IABP support

Weaning from the balloon pump is considered when hemodynamic stability has been achieved with no, or only minimal, pharmacologic support. One weaning procedure consists of slowly decreasing the pumping frequency from every beat to every eighth beat, as tolerated. Decreasing balloon volume is another method of weaning.[30] To prevent thrombus formation on the balloon surface, the IABP must remain at a minimal pumping ratio

(or volume) until its removal. Dependence on the balloon for more than 48 hours, indicative of severe cardiac dysfunction, usually is associated with a poor prognosis.

VENTRICULAR ASSIST DEVICES

The ventricular assist device (VAD) is designed to support a failing natural heart with flow assistance. Diversion of varying amounts of systemic blood flow around a failing ventricle by means of an extracorporeal pump reduces cardiac workload while maintaining the circulation. VADs also can maintain adequate perfusion during periods of cardiac arrest.[31] Device selection is based on individual VAD capabilities and institutional preference (Table 11-5).

The VAD currently is indicated for two types of clinical applications. The first category of patients includes those who, despite aggressive medical therapy, continue to demonstrate persistent cardiac failure but who have the potential for regaining normal heart function if the heart is given time to rest. This category, termed *pending recovery,* consists of patients who either cannot be weaned from cardiopulmonary bypass or are in refractory cardiogenic shock after AMI. The second category, termed *bridge to transplant,* includes those patients who need circulatory support until heart transplantation can be performed.[32]

The left ventricular assist device (LVAD) is used most commonly because left ventricular (LV) failure occurs more often than does right ventricular (RV) failure. Use of biventricular support (bi-VAD) is becoming more common because RV failure often follows LV failure.[33] Outflow cannulas that divert blood from the heart to the LVAD for LV support are surgically placed in either the left atrium or LV apex depending on the indication for the device. For example, if the patient is "pending recovery" of the natural heart, preservation of LV function mandates left atrial cannulation. The right atrium is cannulated for outflow for right ventricular support. Inflow back to the heart from the pump is accomplished by cannulation of the aorta or femoral artery for the LVAD and pulmonary artery for the right ventricular assist device (RVAD). Flow rates between 1 and 6 L/minute are used to maintain adequate cardiac output while decreasing ventricular workload.

Nursing Management

Nursing priorities for managing the patient requiring a ventricular assist device include optimizing cardiac output, weaning from VAD support, and maintaining surveillance for complications.

Optimizing cardiac output

The same interventions to optimize cardiac output by manipulation of heart rate, preload, afterload, and contractility that are used with cardiac surgery patients apply to patients with a VAD. Adequate filling volumes are required to maintain pump flow. Afterload reduction

TABLE 11-5

VENTRICULAR ASSIST DEVICES

TYPE	EXAMPLE	USE	DESCRIPTION	INSERTION
Centrifugal	Biomedicus	Univentricular or biventricular support	Blood is diverted to a cone-shaped pump head where blades rotate and propel blood back through return cannula via continuous (non-pulsatile) flow	Cannulate LA or femoral artery to aorta for LVAD Cannulate RA and PA for RVAD
Rotary	Hemopump	LV support	A propeller housed in the LV cannula draws blood from the LV and propels it into the aorta	Via femoral artery, across aortic valve, and into LV
Pneumatic	Thoratec	Univentricular or biventricular support	External pulsatile pump that uses a pressurized air sac to eject blood through outflow cannula	Cannulate LA and aorta for LVAD Cannulate RA and PA for RVAD Inflow through ventricular apex when cardiotomy is expected
	Abiomed BVS 5000	Univentricular or biventricular support	A two-chamber external pump with bladders that fill by gravity; blood pumps are positioned at a level relative to the patient	Cannulate LA and aorta for LVAD Cannulate RA and PA for RVAD
	TCI Heartmate	LVAD	A pneumatically driven, totally implantable pump with external drive console	Inflow from LV apex with outflow to aorta via graft
Electric	Novacor	LVAD	An electrically driven pulsatile pump that is implanted in an upper abdominal quadrant	Via LV apex and ascending aorta
	TCI Heartmate Vented Electric	LVAD	Totally implantable pump, powered by two 12-volt batteries or a direct power source	LV to aorta
Cardiopulmonary support	Bard CPS	Emergency resuscitation (e.g., supported angioplasty)	Femoral-femoral bypass; venous blood delivered to centrifugal pump that passes through normothermic heat exchanger to membrane oxygenator and back to patient	Percutaneous or cutdown insertion of catheters into femoral vein and femoral artery

may be needed to improve output from the unassisted ventricle when univentricular support is used.

Weaning from VAD support

Weaning is accomplished by gradually decreasing flow rates to allow the patient's ventricle to contribute more to total blood flow. Controversy exists with regard to anticoagulation; however, during weaning of VAD flow rates to less than 2 L/minute, ACTs are maintained between 160 and 480 seconds with heparin, depending on institutional protocols. This minimizes the potential for thrombus formation in the extracorporeal circuit during weaning but also increases the risk of bleeding and therefore necessitates close monitoring.

Maintaining surveillance for complications

Complications of a VAD include device failure, bleeding, emboli, and infection.

Device failure. Because of the life-saving nature of this therapy, device failure is a life-threatening event. Since VAD designs vary considerably, troubleshooting methods for device failure are unique to each device.

Bleeding and emboli. The requirement for anticoagulation varies with the type of VAD, the flow rate, and institutional protocol. If patients are anticoagulated with heparin, nurses are responsible for maintaining the activated clotting time (ACT) within a therapeutic range and monitoring for complications of bleeding. If bleeding occurs, additional coagulation studies, such as partial thromboplastin time (PTT), prothrombin time (PT), and fibrinogen and platelet counts, may be performed. Continued bleeding may necessitate holding the heparin infusion and administering fresh frozen plasma and platelets. If patients are not anticoagulated, the risk of thrombi obstructing a VAD cannula increases, as does the risk of an embolic event.

Infection. Patients with a VAD are at considerable risk for infection. The most common infection is pneumonia secondary to immobility and the need for ventilatory support. Other infectious risks are posed by the presence of invasive catheters and the surgically implanted VAD. Infection is prevented by using strict aseptic technique with all invasive tubing and dressing changes. Site care varies, depending on institutional protocols and the type of ventricular assist device that is used. Nurses monitor patients for infection by obtaining temperatures, inspecting insertion sites and incisions, and following daily leukocyte counts. If an infection is suspected, pan-cultures (blood, urine, and sputum) are taken to guide appropriate antibiotic therapy.

CARDIOVASCULAR DRUGS

Multiple medications are used in the treatment of critically ill cardiovascular patients. **Nursing priorities are directed toward ensuring the medications are administered safely and properly, monitoring the patient's response to the medications and maintaining surveillance for adverse drug reactions.** The critical care nurse is responsible for preparation and administration of these drugs and often is required to titrate the dose on the basis of the patient's hemodynamic response. An understanding of the effects of the medications on the patient's heart rate and rhythm, vital signs, and hemodynamic pressures is critical. The following discussion provides an overview of the intravenous medications commonly administered to support cardiovascular function in the critical care setting.

Antidysrhythmic Drugs

Antidysrhythmic drugs comprise a diverse category of pharmacologic agents used to terminate or prevent an array of abnormal cardiac rhythms. These drugs commonly are classified according to their primary effect on the action potential of cardiac cells. The classification scheme shown in Table 11-6 is the most commonly used system. Classification of newer agents becomes more difficult because some of these agents have characteristics of more than one class and others have no characteristics of the current system.

Antidysrhythmic drugs carry the risk of serious side effects, some of which may be life threatening. The most severe complication is the potential for a "prodysrhythmic" effect. This may result in a worsening of the underlying dysrhythmia, the occurrence of a new dysrhythmia, or the development of a bradydysrhythmia. Torsades de pointes is a prodysrhythmia caused by Class IA agents.

Class I drugs

Class I agents are sodium channel blockers that decrease the influx of sodium ions through "fast" channels during phase 0 depolarization. This prolongs the absolute (effective) refractory period, thus decreasing the risk of premature impulses from ectopic foci. In addition, these drugs depress automaticity by slowing the rate of spontaneous depolarizations of pacemaker cells during the resting phase.

Class I drugs can be further subdivided into three groups, according to their potency as sodium channel inhibitors and their effect on phase 3 repolarization.[34] Class IA agents (e.g., quinidine, procainamide, and disopyramide) block not only the fast sodium channels but also

---

TABLE 11-6

CLASSIFICATION OF ANTIDYSRHYTHMIC AGENTS

CLASS	ACTION	DRUGS
I	Blocks sodium channels ("stabilizes" cell membrane)	—
IA	Blocks sodium channels and delays repolarization, thus lengthening the duration of the action potential	Quinidine Procainamide Disopyramide
IB	Blocks sodium channels and accelerates repolarization, thus shortening the duration of the action potential	Lidocaine Mexiletine Tocainide
IC	Blocks sodium channels and slows conduction through the His-Purkinje system, thus prolonging the QRS duration	Flecainide Encainide Propafenone
II	Blocks beta receptors	Esmolol Metoprolol Propranolol
III	Slows repolarization and prolongs the duration of the action potential	Amiodarone Ibutilide Sotalol
IV	Blocks calcium channels	Diltiazem Verapamil

phase 3 repolarization and thereby prolong the action potential duration. Clinically, this may result in measurable increases in the QRS duration and the QT interval. All class IA agents may depress myocardial contractility, with disopyramide having the most potent negative inotropic effect.[35] Class IB agents (e.g., lidocaine, mexiletine, and tocainide) have only a moderate effect on sodium channels and actually accelerate phase 3 repolarization to shorten the action potential duration. Class IC agents (e.g., encainide, flecainide, and propafenone) are the most potent sodium channel blockers, with little effect on repolarization. These agents increase both the PR and the QRS intervals. The results of the Cardiac Arrhythmia Suppression Trial (CAST) indicated that treatment with encainide and flecainide may be associated with increased mortality and the results have thus decreased the use of these agents in clinical practice.[36]

Class II drugs

Class II drugs are beta-adrenergic blockers (betablockers). These agents inhibit dysrhythmias mediated by the sympathetic nervous system by competing with endogenous catecholamines for available receptor sites. As a result, spontaneous depolarization during the resting phase is depressed and atrioventricular conduction is slowed.

Drugs in this class can be further subdivided into cardioselective (those that block only beta$_1$ receptors) and noncardioselective (those that block both beta$_1$ and beta$_2$ receptors). Knowledge of the effects of adrenergic-receptor stimulation allows for anticipation not only of the therapeutic responses brought about by beta-blockade but also the potential adverse effects of these agents (see Table 11-7). Beta-blockers also are negative inotropes and must be used cautiously in patients with left ventricular dysfunction. Although numerous beta-blockers are available, only esmolol, metoprolol, and propranolol are available as intravenous agents for the treatment of acute dysrhythmias. Of these, esmolol offers significant advantages in the critically ill patient because of its short half-life (approximately 9 minutes). It is used in the treatment of supraventricular tachycardias, such as atrial fibrillation and atrial flutter.

Class III drugs

Class III agents (e.g., amiodarone, bretylium, ibutilide, and sotalol) markedly slow the rate of phase 3 repolarization, increasing the effective refractory period and the action potential duration. Although their effect on the action potential is similar, these drugs differ greatly in their mechanism of action and their side effects. Bretylium is used in the treatment of life-threatening ventricular dysrhythmias that are refractory to other antidysrhythmic agents, such as lidocaine and procainamide.[2] Amiodarone is considered a second-line therapy for serious ventricular dysrhythmias that are refractory to other medications.[37] Ibutilide is a short-term antidysrhythmic agent

used for the rapid conversion of acute atrial fibrillation or atrial flutter to sinus rhythm. The drug is administered as a 10-minute infusion in a carefully monitored clinical setting. The most serious side effect of ibutilide is its potential for inducing life-threatening dysrhythmias, especially torsades de pointes.[38]

Class IV drugs

Class IV agents (e.g., verapamil and diltiazem) are calcium channel blockers that inhibit the influx of calcium through slow calcium channels during the plateau phase. This effect occurs primarily in tissue in which slow calcium channels predominate, primarily in the sinus and atrioventricular (AV) nodes and the atrial tissue. Verapamil depresses sinus and AV node conduction and is effective in terminating supraventricular tachycardias caused by AV nodal reentry. Studies suggest that diltiazem may be as effective as verapamil in treating supraventricular dysrhythmias, with fewer hypotensive side effects.[39]

Unclassified antidysrhythmics

Adenosine is a newer antidysrhythmic agent that remains unclassified under the current system. Adenosine occurs endogenously in the body as a building block of adenosine triphosphate (ATP). Given in intravenous boluses, adenosine slows conduction through the AV node, causing transient AV block. It is used clinically to convert supraventricular tachycardias and to facilitate differential diagnosis of rapid dysrhythmias. Because of its short half-life, the drug is administered intravenously as a rapid bolus, followed by a saline flush. The bolus is delivered as centrally as possible, so that the drug reaches the heart before it is metabolized.[40] Side effects are transient because the drug is rapidly taken up by the cells and is cleared from the body within 10 seconds.

Magnesium is also unclassified under the present system. Although its action as an antidysrhythmic agent is not entirely understood, clinical studies suggest that it may reduce the incidence of both ventricular and supraventricular dysrhythmias in selected patient populations. It is considered the treatment of choice in patients with torsades de pointes. For acute treatment, 1 to 2 g of magnesium is administered over 1 to 2 minutes. In patients with confirmed hypomagnesemia, this bolus may be followed with a 24-hour infusion.[41]

Vasoactive Drugs

Inotropic agents

Critically ill patients with compromised cardiac function frequently require the use of medications to enhance myocardial contractility (positive inotropes). Clinically available inotropes include cardiac glycosides, sympathomimetics, and phosphodiesterase inhibitors. These agents increase myocardial contractility, resulting in improved cardiac output, more complete emptying of the ventricles, and decreased filling pressures.

Cardiac glycosides. Cardiac glycosides include digitalis and its derivatives. Although these drugs have been used for centuries, their slow onset of action and risk of toxicity make them more appropriate for the management of chronic heart failure. Because digoxin also causes slowing of the sinus rate and a decrease in AV conduction, it may be administered intravenously in the acute care setting to control supraventricular dysrhythmias.

Sympathomimetics. Sympathomimetic agents stimulate adrenergic receptors, thereby simulating the effects of sympathetic nerve stimulation. Included in this category are naturally occurring catecholamines (epinephrine, dopamine, and norepinephrine), as well as synthetic catecholamines (dobutamine and isoproterenol). The cardiovascular effects of these drugs, which vary according to their selectivity for specific receptor sites (Table 11-7), are often dose-dependent as well.[42] Table 11-8 describes the cardiovascular effects of sympathomimetic drugs at various dosages.

Dopamine. Dopamine is one of the most widely used drugs in the critical care setting. It is a chemical precursor of norepinephrine, which, in addition to both alpha- and beta-receptor stimulation, can activate dopaminergic receptors in the renal and mesenteric blood vessels. The actions of this drug are entirely dose-related.[2] At low dosages of 1 to 2 μg/kg/min, dopamine stimulates dopaminergic receptors, causing renal and mesenteric vasodilation. The resultant increase in renal perfusion increases urinary output. Moderate dosages result in stimulation of beta$_1$ receptors to increase myocardial contractility and improve cardiac output. At dosages greater than 10 μg/kg/min, dopamine predominantly stimulates alpha receptors, resulting in vasoconstriction that often negates both the beta-adrenergic and dopaminergic effects.

Dobutamine. Dobutamine is a synthetic catecholamine with predominantly beta$_1$ effects. It also produces some beta$_2$ stimulation, resulting in a mild vasodilation. Dobutamine is as effective as dopamine in increasing myocardial contractility, but it lacks the dopaminergic effects of that drug. Dobutamine is useful in the treatment of heart failure, especially in hypotensive patients who cannot tolerate vasodilator therapy. The usual dosage range is 2.5 to 20 μg/kg/min, titrated on the basis of hemodynamic parameters.

TABLE 11-7

EFFECTS OF ADRENERGIC RECEPTORS

RECEPTOR	LOCATION	RESPONSE TO STIMULATION
Alpha	Vessels of skin, muscles, kidneys, and intestines	Vasoconstriction of peripheral arterioles
Beta$_1$	Cardiac tissue	Increased heart rate Increased conduction Increased contractility
Beta$_2$	Vascular and bronchial smooth muscle	Vasodilation of peripheral arterioles Bronchodilation

TABLE 11-8

PHYSIOLOGIC EFFECTS OF SYMPATHOMIMETIC AGENTS

DRUG	DOSAGE	RECEPTOR ACTIVATED				CARDIOVASCULAR EFFECTS		
		ALPHA	BETA$_1$	BETA$_2$	DOPA	CO	HR	SVR
Dobutamine	<5 μg/kg/min	0	↑↑↑	↑	0	↑↑	↑	0/↓
	5-20 μg/kg/min	0	↑↑↑	↑↑	0	↑↑↑	↑↑	↓
	>20 μg/kg/min	0	↑↑↑	↑↑	0	↑↑↑	↑↑↑	↓↓
Dopamine	<3 μg/kg/min	0	↑	↑	↑↑↑	0/↑	0/↑	0
	3-10 μg/kg/min	↑	↑↑↑	↑	↑↑↑	↑↑↑	↑	↑
	11-20 μg/kg/min	↑↑↑	↑↑↑	↑	↑↑	↑↑	↑↑	↑↑↑
	>20 μg/kg/min	↑↑↑↑	↑↑	↑	↑	↑	↑	↑↑↑↑
Epinephrine	<2 μg/min	0	↑	↑↑	0	0/↑	0/↑	↓
	2-8 μg/min	↑↑	↑↑↑	↑↑	0	↑↑↑	↑	↑
	9-20 μg/min	↑↑↑	↑↑	↑↑	0	↑↑	↑↑	↑↑
Isoproterenol	1-7 μg/min	0	↑↑↑	↑↑↑	0	↑↑↑	↑↑↑	↓↓↓
Norepinephrine	<2 μg/min	↑↑↑	↑↑	0	0	↑	0/↓	↑↑↑
	2-16 μg/min	↑↑↑↑	↑↑	0	0	↓	↓	↑↑↑↑
Phenylephrine	10-100 μg/min	↑↑↑↑	0	0	0	0/↓	↓	↑↑↑

NOTE: Refer to Table 11-7 for actions of receptors.
CO, Cardiac output; *HR,* heart rate; *SVR,* systemic vascular resistance; *0,* no effect; ↑, increased; ↓, decreased (the number of arrows indicates the degree of effect [e.g., ↑ = mild and ↑↑↑↑ = strong effect]).

Epinephrine. Epinephrine is produced by the adrenal gland as part of the body's response to stress. This agent has the ability to stimulate both alpha and beta receptors, depending on the dose administered. At doses of 1 to 2 μg/min, epinephrine binds with beta receptors to increase heart rate, cardiac conduction, contractility, and vasodilation, thereby increasing cardiac output. As the dosage is increased, alpha receptors are stimulated, resulting in increased vascular resistance and blood pressure. At these doses, epinephrine's impact on cardiac output depends on the heart's ability to pump against the increased afterload. Epinephrine accelerates the sinus rate and may precipitate ventricular dysrhythmias in the ischemic heart. Other side effects include restlessness, angina, and headache.

Norepinephrine. Norepinephrine is similar to epinephrine in its ability to stimulate $beta_1$ and alpha receptors, but it lacks the $beta_2$ effects. At low infusion rates, $beta_1$ receptors are activated to produce increased contractility and thus augment cardiac output. At higher doses the inotropic effects are limited by marked vasoconstriction mediated by alpha receptors. Clinically, norepinephrine is used most often as a vasopressor to elevate blood pressure in shock states.

Isoproterenol. Isoproterenol is a pure beta-receptor stimulant with no alpha effects. It produces dramatic increases in heart rate, conduction, and contractility via $beta_1$ stimulation and vasodilation via $beta_2$ stimulation. Isoproterenol also produces vasodilation of the pulmonary arteries and bronchodilation. It greatly increases the automaticity of cardiac cells and frequently precipitates dysrhythmias, such as premature ventricular contractions and even ventricular tachycardia. These effects limit its usefulness in the compromised heart. Its most common use is as a temporary treatment for symptomatic bradycardia until a pacemaker is available.

Phosphodiesterase inhibitors. Phosphodiesterase inhibitors are a new group of inotropic agents that also are potent vasodilators. Drugs in this classification inhibit the enzyme phosphodiesterase, resulting in increased levels of cyclic adenosine monophosphate (AMP) and intracellular calcium. Amrinone and milrinone were the first of these agents approved for use in the United States. Increases in cardiac output occur as a result of increased contractility (inotropic effects) and decreased afterload (vasodilative effects). Filling pressures tend to decrease, whereas the heart rate and blood pressure remain fairly constant. Amrinone may cause thrombocytopenia, so platelet counts are monitored and patients are observed for hemorrhagic complications.[42] Milrinone is associated with a lower rate of thrombocytopenia but can induce ventricular dysrhythmias (premature ventricular complexes, ventricular tachycardia) in a significant number of patients.

Vasodilator agents

Vasodilators are pharmacologic agents that improve cardiac performance by various degrees of arterial or venous dilation or both. The goal of vasodilator therapy may be a reduction of preload or afterload or both. Afterload reduction is accomplished by vasodilation of arterial vessels. This results in decreased resistance to left ventricular ejection and may improve cardiac output without increasing myocardial oxygen demands. Reduction of preload is accomplished by dilating venous vessels to increase capacitance. This results in decreased filling pressures for a failing heart. These drugs may be classified into direct smooth muscle relaxants, calcium channel blockers, angiotensin-converting enzyme (ACE) inhibitors, and alpha-adrenergic blockers.

Direct smooth muscle relaxants. Direct-acting vasodilators include sodium nitroprusside, nitroglycerin, and hydralazine. These drugs produce relaxation of vascular smooth muscle, resulting in decreased peripheral vascular resistance. Hypotension may occur as a result of peripheral vasodilation, and headaches may be caused by cerebral vasodilation. Compensatory mechanisms can occur in response to the drop in blood pressure. These include baroreceptor activation that causes reflex tachycardia and activation of the renin-angiotensin-aldosterone system, with resultant sodium and water retention.[43]

Nitroprusside. Nitroprusside is a potent, rapidly acting venous and arterial vasodilator, particularly suitable for rapid reduction of blood pressure in hypertensive emergencies and perioperatively. It also is effective for afterload reduction in the setting of severe heart failure. The drug is administered by continuous intravenous infusion, with the dosage titrated to maintain the desired blood pressure and systemic vascular resistance (SVR). Prolonged administration can result in thiocyanate toxicity, manifested by nausea, confusion, and tinnitus.[42]

Nitroglycerin. Intravenous nitroglycerin causes both arterial and venous vasodilation, but its venous effect is more pronounced. It is used in the critical care setting for the treatment of acute heart failure (HF) because it reduces cardiac filling pressures, relieves pulmonary congestion, and decreases cardiac workload and oxygen consumption. In addition, nitroglycerin dilates the coronary arteries and is a useful adjunct in the treatment of unstable angina and acute myocardial infarction. Nitroglycerin also is administered prophylactically to prevent coronary vasospasm after coronary angioplasty, atherectomy, stent insertion, or thrombolytic therapy. The most common side effects of this drug include hypotension, flushing, and headache.[44]

Hydralazine. Hydralazine is a potent arterial vasodilator. It seldom is given as a continuous infusion but rather in intravenously administered dosages of 5 to 10 mg every 4 to 8 hours. Occasionally, hydralazine is given as an intermediate drug in the transition between the weaning of a continuous infusion and the initiation of oral antihypertensive medications. The major side effect is reflex tachycardia mediated by the sympathetic nervous system. This may be diminished by the concomitant administration of beta-blockers.

Calcium channel blockers. Calcium channel blockers include nifedipine, nicardipine, verapamil, and diltiazem. These are a chemically diverse group of drugs with differing pharmacologic effects.

Nifedipine and nicardipine. Nifedipine and nicardipine act as arterial vasodilators. These drugs reduce the influx of calcium in the arterial resistance vessels. Both coronary and peripheral arteries are affected. They are used in the critical care setting to treat hypertension. Nifedipine is available only in an oral form but often is prescribed sublingually. Although controversy exists over the absorption of sublingual nifedipine, studies indicate that if the drug is bitten before swallowing, the drug is absorbed more quickly.[45] Nicardipine is available in an intravenous form, and as such it offers more accurate titration for effective control of hypertension.[46] Side effects of nifedipine and nicardipine are related to vasodilation and include hypotension, reflex tachycardia, flushing, headache, and ankle edema.

Verapamil and diltiazem. Verapamil and diltiazem are part of another group of calcium channel blockers with differing functions. These drugs dilate coronary arteries but have little effect on the peripheral vasculature. They are used in the treatment of angina, especially that which has a vasospastic component, and as antidysrhythmics in the treatment of supraventricular tachycardias.

ACE inhibitors. Angiotensin-converting enzyme (ACE) inhibitors produce vasodilation by blocking the conversion of angiotensin I to angiotensin II. Because angiotensin is a potent vasoconstrictor, limiting its production decreases peripheral vascular resistance. In contrast to the direct vasodilators and nifedipine, ACE inhibitors do not cause reflex tachycardia nor induce sodium and water retention. However, these drugs may cause a profound fall in blood pressure, especially in patients who are volume-depleted. Blood pressure must be monitored carefully, especially during initiation of therapy.[47] The only ACE inhibitor currently available in intravenous form is enalapril.

Alpha-adrenergic blockers. Peripheral adrenergic blockers block alpha receptors in the arteries and veins, resulting in vasodilation. Orthostatic hypotension is a common side effect and may result in syncope. Long-term therapy also may be complicated by fluid and water retention.[43]

Labetalol. Labetalol, a combined alpha- and beta-blocker, is used in the treatment of hypertensive emergencies. Because the blockade of beta$_1$ receptors permits the decrease of blood pressure without the risk of reflexive tachycardia and increased cardiac output, this drug also is useful in the treatment of acute aortic dissection.

Phentolamine. Phentolamine is a peripheral alpha-blocker that causes decreased afterload via arterial vasodilation. It is given as a continuous infusion at a rate of 1 to 2 mg/minute and is titrated to achieve the required reduction in blood pressure and SVR.[42] This drug also is used to treat the extravasation of dopamine. If this occurs, 5 to 10 mg is diluted in 10 ml normal saline and administered intradermally into the infiltrated area.

Vasoconstrictor agents

Vasoconstrictors are sympathomimetic agents that mediate peripheral vasoconstriction through stimulation of alpha-receptors (see Table 11-8). This results in increased systemic vascular resistance and thus elevates blood pressure. Some of these drugs (epinephrine and norepinephrine) also have the ability to stimulate beta receptors. Vasoconstrictors are not widely used in the treatment of critically ill cardiac patients because the dramatic increase in afterload is taxing to a damaged heart, although they are often used to maintain organ perfusion in shock states.

References

1. Moses HW, et al: *A practical guide to cardiac pacing*, ed 4, Boston, 1995, Little, Brown.
2. American Heart Association: *Textbook of advanced cardiac life support*, Dallas, 1997, The Association.
3. Stausmire JM: *Temporary epicardial pacing: a practical guide for nurses*, Aliso Viejo, CA, 1998, American Association of Critical Care Nurses.
4. Bernstein AD, et al: The NASPE/BPEG generic pacemaker code for antibradycardia and adaptive rate pacing and antitachyarrhythmia devices, *Pacing Clin Electrophysiol* 10:794, 1987.
5. Vlay SC: *A practical approach to cardiac arrhythmias*, ed 4, Boston, 1995, Little, Brown.
6. Witherell CL: Cardiac rhythm control devices, *Crit Care Nurs Clin North Am* 6:85, 1994.
7. Moss AJ, et al: Improved survival with an implanted defibrillator in patients with coronary disease at high risk for ventricular arrhythmia, *N Engl J Med* 335:1933, 1996.
8. Jordaens L, et al: A new transvenous internal cardioverter defibrillator: implantation technique, complications, and short-term follow-up, *Am Heart J* 129:251, 1995.
9. Akhtar M, et al: Role of implantable cardioverter defibrillator therapy in the management of high-risk patients, *Circulation* 85(suppl 1):I131, 1992.
10. Knight I, et al: Caring for patients with third generation implantable cardioverter defibrillators: from decision to implant to patient's return home, *Crit Care Nurs* 17(5):46, 1997.
11. Burke LR, Rodgers BL, Jenkins LS: Living with recurrent ventricular dysrhythmias, *Focus Crit Care* 19(1):60, 1992.
12. Ryan TJ, et al: Guidelines for percutaneous transluminal coronary angioplasty, *J Am Coll Cardiol* 22:2033, 1993.
13. Holmes DR, et al: Emergency "rescue" percutaneous transluminal coronary angioplasty after failed thrombolysis with streptokinase: early and late results, *Circulation* 81(suppl 3):51, 1990.
14. Murphy MC, et al: Differences in symptoms during post-PTCA versus rotational ablation, *Prog Cardiovasc Nurs* 9(2):4, 1994.
15. EPIC Investigators: Use of monoclonal antibody directed against platelet glycoprotein IIb/IIIa receptor in high risk coronary angioplasty, *N Engl J Med* 330:956, 1994.
16. Perra BM: Managing coronary atherectomy patients in a special procedure unit, *Crit Care Nurs* 15(3):57, 1995.
17. Fogarty, et al: Atherectomy: a review of current devices and methods. In Kerstein MD, White JV, editors: *Alternatives to open vascular surgery*, Philadelphia, 1995, Lippincott.
18. Albert NM: Laser angioplasty and intracoronary stents: going beyond the balloon, *AACN Clin Issues Crit Care Nurs* 5:15, 1994.
19. Bevans M, McLimore E: Intracoronary stents: a new approach to coronary artery dilation, *J Cardiovasc Nurs* 7:34, 1992.

20. Pepine CJ, et al: Coronary artery stents (ACC Expert Concensus Document), *J Am Coll Cardiol* 28:782, 1996.
21. Oakley CM: Management of valvular stenosis, *Curr Opin Cardiol* 10:117, 1995.
22. Kawaniski DT, Rahimtoola SH: Catheter balloon commissurotomy for mitral stenosis: complications and results, *J Am Coll Cardiol* 19:192, 1992.
23. Holloway S, Feldman T: An alternative to valvular surgery in the treatment of mitral stenosis: balloon mitral valvotomy, *Crit Care Nurs* 17(3):27, 1997.
24. Gardner E, et al: Intracoronary stent update: focus on patient education, *Crit Care Nurs* 16(2):65, 1995.
25. Majoros KA: Comparisons and controversies in clot buster drugs, *Crit Care Nurs Q* 16:46, 1993.
26. Habib GB: Current status of thrombolysis in acute myocardial infarction. I. Optimal drug selection and delivery of a thrombolytic drug, *Chest* 107:225, 1995.
27. Drew BJ, Tisdale LA: ST segment monitoring for coronary artery reocclusion following thrombolytic therapy and coronary angioplasty: identification of optimal bedside monitoring leads, *Am J Crit Care* 2:280, 1993.
28. Wojner AJ: Assessing the five points of intra-aortic balloon pump waveform, *Crit Care Nurs* 14(3):48, 1994.
29. Cadwell CA, Quaal SJ: Intra-aortic balloon counterpulsation timing, *Am J Crit Care* 5:254, 1996.
30. Shinn AE, Joseph D: Concepts on intraaortic balloon pulsation, *J Cardiovasc Nurs* 8(2):45, 1994.
31. Moroney DA, Reedy JE: Understanding ventricular assist devices: a self-study guide, *J Cardiovasc Nurs* 8(2):1, 1994.
32. Vaca KJ, Lohmann DP, Moroney DA: Current status and future trends of mechanical circulatory support, *Crit Care Nurs Clin North Am* 7:249, 1995.
33. Emery RW, Joyce LD: Directions in cardiac assistance, *J Cardiac Surg* 6:400, 1991.
34. Stier F: Antidysrhythmic agents, *AACN Clin Issues Crit Care Nurs* 3:483, 1992.
35. Weiner B: Hemodynamic effects of antidysrhythmic drugs, *J Cardiovasc Nurs* 5(4):39, 1991.
36. Bennett B, Singh S: Management of ventricular arrhythmias: then and now, *Am J Crit Care* 1(3):107, 1992.
37. Levine JH, et al: Intravenous amiodarone for recurrent sustained hypotensive ventricular tachyarrhythmias, *J Am Coll Cardiol* 27:67, 1996.
38. Ellenbogen KA, et al: Efficacy of intravenous ibutilide for rapid termination of atrial fibrillation and flutter: a dose response study, *J Am Coll Cardiol* 28:130, 1996.
39. Peitz TJ: Intravenous diltiazem hydrochloride rather than verapamil for resistant paroxysmal supraventricular tachycardia, *West J Med* 19:598, 1993.
40. Morton PG: Update on new antiarrhythmic drugs, *Crit Care Nurs Clin North Am* 6:69, 1994.
41. Lefor N, Cardello FP, Felicetta JV: Recognizing and treating torsades de pointes, *Crit Care Nurs* 12(6):23, 1992.
42. Clements JV: Sympathomimetics, inotropics, and vasodilators, *AACN Clin Issues Crit Care Nurs* 3:395, 1992.
43. Deglin JH, Deglin S: Hypertension: current trends and choices in pharmacotherapeutics, *AACN Clin Issues Crit Care Nurs* 3:507, 1992.
44. Kuhn M: Nitrates, *AACN Clin Issues Crit Care Nurs* 3:409, 1992.
45. Schumann D: Sublingual nifedipine controversy in drug delivery, *DCCN* 10:314, 1991.
46. Halpern NA, et al: Postoperative hypertension: a multicenter, prospective, randomized comparison between intravenous nicardipine and sodium nitroprusside, *Crit Care Med* 20:1637, 1992.
47. Kuhn M: Angiotensin-converting enzyme inhibitors, *AACN Clin Issues Crit Care Nurs* 3:461, 1992.

UNIT FOUR

PULMONARY ALTERATIONS

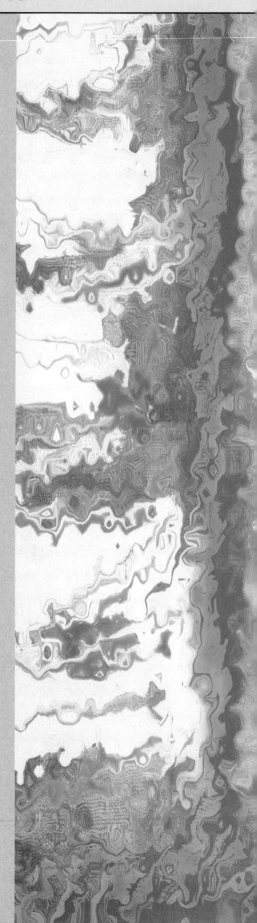

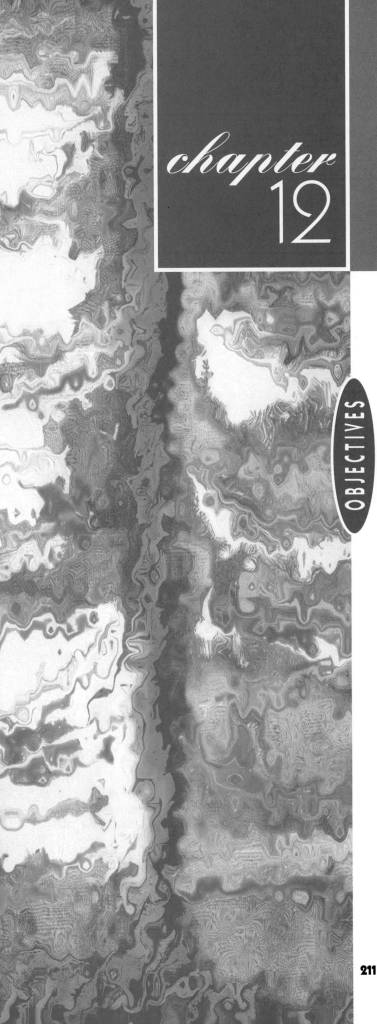

chapter 12

Pulmonary Assessment and Diagnostic Procedures

Kathleen M. Stacy
and Jeanne M. Maiden

OBJECTIVES

- **Identify the components of a pulmonary history.**

- **Describe inspection, palpation, percussion, and auscultation of the patient with pulmonary dysfunction.**

- **Outline the steps in analyzing an arterial blood gas.**

- **Identify key diagnostic procedures used in assessment of the patient with pulmonary dysfunction.**

- **Discuss the nursing management of a patient undergoing a pulmonary diagnostic procedure.**

- **Delineate the use of pulse oximetry for bedside monitoring.**

Assessment of the patient with pulmonary dysfunction is a systematic process that incorporates both a history and a physical examination. The purpose of the assessment is twofold: (1) to recognize changes in the patient's pulmonary status that would necessitate nursing or medical intervention and (2) to determine the ways in which the patient's pulmonary dysfunction is interfering with self-care activities.[1] To complete the assessment, the patient's laboratory studies and diagnostic tests must be reviewed. This chapter focuses on priority clinical assessments, laboratory studies, and diagnostic tests for the critically ill patient with pulmonary dysfunction.

HISTORY

The initial presentation of the patient determines the rapidity and direction of the interview. For a patient in acute distress, the history is curtailed to just a few questions about the patient's chief complaint and precipitating events. For a patient in no obvious distress, the history focuses on four different areas: (1) review of the patient's present illness, (2) overview of the patient's general respiratory status, (3) examination of the patient's general health status, and (4) survey of the patient's lifestyle.[2,3] Questions to be included in the interview are outlined in Box 12-1.

A description of the patient's current symptoms is also obtained. Symptoms that are common in the pulmonary patient include dyspnea, cough, wheezing, edema, palpitations, fatigue, chest pain,[4] hemoptysis, and sputum.[5] Information is elicited regarding the location, onset and duration, characteristics, setting, aggravating and alleviating factors, associated symptoms,[4] and efforts to treat the symptoms.[6] If the cough is productive, the patient is asked questions about the color, amount, odor, and consistency of the sputum.[7]

CLINICAL ASSESSMENT

Inspection

Inspection of the patient focuses on three priorities: (1) observation of the tongue and sublingual area, (2) assessment of chest-wall configuration, and (3) evaluation of respiratory effort. If possible, the patient is positioned upright, with the arms resting at the sides.[3]

Observation of the tongue and sublingual area

The patient's tongue and sublingual area are observed for a blue, gray, or dark purple tint or discoloration, indicating the presence of central cyanosis. Central cyanosis is a sign of hypoxemia, or inadequate oxygenation of the blood, and is considered to be life threatening. The fingers and toes may also appear discolored, an indication of the presence of peripheral cyanosis.[8]

Assessment of chest-wall configuration

The size and shape of the patient's chest wall are assessed for an increase in the anteroposterior (AP) diameter and for structural deviations. Normally the ratio of AP diameter to lateral diameter ranges from 1:2 to 5:7.[1,9,10] An increase in the AP diameter is suggestive of chronic obstructive pulmonary disease (COPD).[1] The shape of the chest is inspected for any structural deviations. Some of the more commonly seen abnormalities are pectus excavatum, pectus carinatum, barrel chest, and spinal deformities. In pectus excavatum (funnel chest), the sternum and lower ribs are displaced posteriorly, creating a funnel or pit-shaped depression in the chest. This causes a decrease in the AP diameter of the chest and may interfere with respiratory function. In pectus carinatum (pigeon breast), the sternum projects forward, causing an increase in the AP diameter of the chest. A barrel chest also results in an increase in AP diameter of the chest and is characterized by displacement of the sternum forward and the ribs outward. Spinal deformities such as kyphosis, lordosis, and scoliosis may also be present and can interfere with respiratory function.[9-11]

Evaluation of respiratory effort

The patient's respiratory effort is evaluated for rate, rhythm, symmetry, and quality of ventilatory movements.[1] Normal breathing at rest is effortless and regular and occurs at a rate of 12 to 20 breaths per minute.[3] Some of the more commonly seen patterns in patients with pulmonary dysfunction are tachypnea, hyperventilation, and air trapping. Tachypnea is manifested by an increase in the rate and decrease in the depth of ventilation. Hyperventilation is manifested by an increase in both the rate and depth of ventilation. Patients with COPD often experience obstructive breathing, or air trapping. As the patient breathes, air becomes trapped in the lungs and ventilations become progressively shallower until the patient actively and forcefully exhales.[12]

Additional assessment areas

Other areas assessed are patient position, use of accessory muscles, presence of intercostal retractions, unequal movement of the chest wall, flaring of nares, and pausing midsentence to take a breath.[1,10] The presence of other iatrogenic features, such as chest tubes, central venous

---

BOX 12-1

PULMONARY HISTORY QUESTIONS

PRESENT ILLNESS

What brought you to the hospital?
What were the precipitating events?
When did the problem start?

RESPIRATORY STATUS

Do you currently have a chronic lung disease, such as asthma, bronchitis, and emphysema?
Do you have a history of any lung disease, such as chronic respiratory infections and tuberculosis?
Have you had any chest surgery?

GENERAL HEALTH STATUS

Do you have any other chronic disease or illness?
Do you have a history of any other disease, illness, or surgery?
Are you currently taking any medications, prescription or nonprescription?

LIFESTYLE

Do you smoke or have you smoked in the past?
Have you been exposed to secondhand smoke?
Have you ever been exposed to lung irritants or cancer-causing agents, such as asbestos, chemicals, fumes, beryllium, coal or stone quarry dust, or Agent Orange?

lines, artificial airways, and nasogastric tubes, should be noted as they may affect assessment findings.

Palpation

Palpation of the patient focuses on three priorities: (1) confirmation of tracheal position, (2) assessment of respiratory excursion, and (3) evaluation of fremitus. In addition, the thorax is assessed for any areas of tenderness, lumps, or bony deformities. The anterior, posterior, and lateral areas of the chest are evaluated in a systematic fashion.[9,11]

Confirmation of tracheal position

The patient's tracheal position is confirmed at midline. It is assessed by placing the fingers in the suprasternal notch and moving upward.[12] Deviation of the trachea to either side can indicate pneumothorax, unilateral pneumonia, diffuse pulmonary fibrosis, a large pleural effusion, or severe atelectasis. With atelectasis, the trachea shifts to the same side as the problem, and with pneumothorax the trachea shifts to the opposite side of the problem.[11]

Assessment of respiratory excursion

The patient's respiratory excursion is assessed for the degree and symmetry of movement. It is evaluated by placing the hands on the anterolateral chest with the thumbs extended along the costal margin, pointing to the xiphoid process, or by placing the hands on the posterolateral chest with the thumbs on either side of the spine at the level of the tenth rib. The patient is instructed to take a few normal breaths, then a few deep breaths. Chest movement is assessed for equality, which signifies symmetry of thoracic expansion.[3,10,11] Asymmetry is an abnormal finding that can occur with pneumothorax, pneumonia, or other disorders that interfere with lung inflation. The degree of chest movement is felt to ascertain the extent of lung expansion. The thumbs should separate 3 to 5 cm during deep inspiration.[11] Lung expansion of a hyperinflated chest is less than that of a normal one.[4,9]

Evaluation of tactile fremitus

Assessment of tactile fremitus is performed to identify, describe, and localize any areas of increased or decreased fremitus. Fremitus refers to the palpable vibrations felt through the chest wall when the patient speaks. It is assessed by placing the palmar surface of the hands against opposite sides of the chest wall and having the patient repeat the word "ninety-nine." The hands are moved systematically around the thorax until the anterior, posterior, and both lateral areas have been assessed.[10,11] Fremitus varies from patient to patient and depends on the pitch and intensity of the voice. Fremitus is described as normal, decreased, or increased. With normal fremitus, vibrations can be felt over the trachea but are barely palpable over the periphery. With decreased fremitus, there is interference with the transmission of vibrations. Ex-

amples of disorders that decrease fremitus include pleural effusion, pneumothorax, bronchial obstruction, pleural thickening, and emphysema. With increased fremitus, there is an increase in the transmission of vibrations. Examples of disorders that increase fremitus include pneumonia, lung cancer, and pulmonary fibrosis.[3]

Percussion

Percussion of the patient focuses on two priorities: (1) evaluation of the underlying lung structure and (2) assessment of diaphragmatic excursion. Although not an often used technique, percussion is useful for confirming suspected abnormalities.

Evaluation of underlying lung structure

The patient's underlying lung structure is evaluated to estimate the amounts of air, liquid, or solid material present. It is performed by placing the middle finger of the nondominant hand on the chest wall. The distal portion, between the last joint and the nailbed, is then struck with the middle finger of the dominant hand. The hands are moved side-to-side, systematically around the thorax, to compare similar areas, until the anterior, posterior, and both lateral areas have been assessed. Five different tones can be elicited: resonance, hyperresonance, tympany, dullness, and flatness. These tones are distinguished by differences in intensity, pitch, duration, and quality. Table 12-1 describes the different percussion tones and their associated conditions.[1,9,12]

TABLE 12-1

PERCUSSION TONES AND THEIR ASSOCIATED CONDITIONS

TONE	DESCRIPTION	CONDITION
Resonance	Intensity—loud Pitch—low Duration—long Quality—hollow	Normal lung Bronchitis
Hyperresonance	Intensity—very loud Pitch—very low Duration—long Quality—booming	Asthma Emphysema Pneumothorax
Tympany	Intensity—loud Pitch—musical Duration—medium Quality—drumlike	Large pneumothorax Emphysematous blebs
Dullness	Intensity—medium Pitch—medium-high Duration—medium Quality—thudlike	Atelectasis Pleural effusion Pulmonary edema Pneumonia Lung mass
Flatness	Intensity—soft Pitch—high Duration—short Quality—extremely dull	Massive atelectasis Pneumonectomy

Assessment of diaphragmatic excursion

Diaphragmatic excursion is assessed by measuring the difference in the level of the diaphragm on inspiration and expiration. It is performed by instructing the patient to inhale and hold the breath. The posterior chest is percussed downward, over the intercostal spaces, until the dull sound produced by the diaphragm is heard. The spot is marked. The patient is then instructed to take a few breaths in and out, exhale completely, and then hold his or her breath. The posterior chest is percussed again, and the new area of dullness over the diaphragm is then located and marked. The difference between the two spots is noted and measured. Normal diaphragmatic excursion is 3 to 5 cm.[9,11] It is decreased in disorders or conditions such as ascites, pregnancy, hepatomegaly, and emphysema. It is increased in pleural effusion or disorders that elevate the diaphragm, such as atelectasis or paralysis.[4]

Auscultation

Auscultation of the patient focuses on three priorities: (1) evaluation of normal breath sounds, (2) identification of abnormal breath sounds, and (3) assessment of voice sounds. Auscultation requires a quiet environment, proper positioning of the patient, and a bare chest.[13] Breath sounds are best heard with the patient in the upright position.[5]

Evaluation of normal breath sounds

The patient's breath sounds are auscultated to evaluate the quality of air movement through the pulmonary system and to identify the presence of abnormal sounds. It is performed by placing the diaphragm of the stethoscope against the chest wall and instructing the patient to breathe in and out slowly with his or her mouth open. Both the inspiratory and expiratory phases are assessed. Auscultation is done in a systematic sequence—side to side, top to bottom, posteriorly, laterally, and anteriorly[5,9,11] (Fig. 12-1).

Normal breath sounds are different, depending on their location. They are classified into three categories: bronchial, bronchovesicular, and vesicular. Table 12-2 describes the characteristics of normal breath sounds.[3,9,12,13]

Identification of abnormal breath sounds

Abnormal breath sounds are identified once the normal breath sounds have been clearly delineated. There are three categories of abnormal breath sounds: absent or diminished breath sounds, displaced bronchial breath sounds, and adventitious breath sounds. Table 12-3 describes the various abnormal breath sounds and their associated conditions.[3,7,13]

An absent or diminished breath sound indicates that there is little or no airflow to a particular portion of the lung (either a small segment or an entire lung).[13] Displaced bronchial breath sounds are normal bronchial sounds heard in the peripheral lung fields instead of over the trachea. This condition is usually indicative of fluid or exudate present in the alveoli.[13]

Adventitious breath sounds are extra or added sounds heard in addition to the other sounds already discussed. They are classified as crackles, rhonchi, wheezes, and

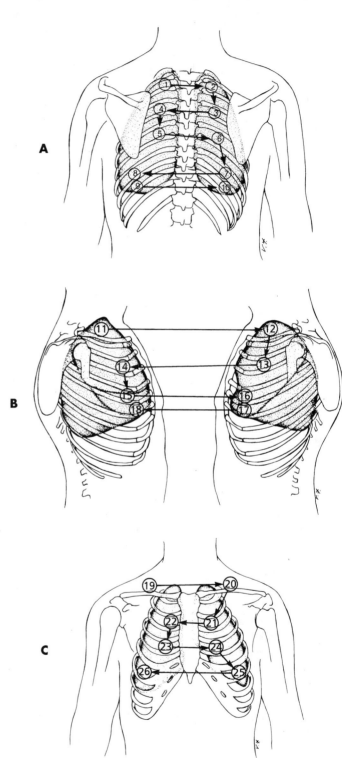

Fig. **12-1** Auscultation sequence. **A,** Posterior. **B,** Lateral. **C,** Anterior. (From Perry AG, Potter PA: *Clinical nursing skills and techniques,* ed 3, St Louis, 1994, Mosby.)

friction rubs. Crackles (also called rales) are short, discrete, popping or crackling sounds produced by fluid in the small airways or alveoli or by the snapping open of collapsed airways during inspiration. They are mainly heard on inspiration and are usually unchanged with coughing.[11] Crackles can be further classified as fine, medium, or coarse, depending on pitch.[13] Rhonchi are coarse, rumbling, low-pitched sounds produced by airflow over secretions in the larger airways or by narrowing of the large airways. They are mainly heard on expiration and are usually changed with coughing.[11] Rhonchi can further be classified as bubbling, gurgling, or sonorous, depending on the characteristics of the sound.[13] Wheezes are high-pitched, squeaking, whistling sounds produced by airflow through narrowed small airways. They are mainly heard on expiration but may be heard throughout the ventilatory cycle.[11] Depending on their severity, wheezes can be further classified as mild, moderate, or severe.[13] Pleural friction rubs are creaking, leathery, loud, dry, coarse sounds produced by irritated pleural surfaces rubbing together. They are usually heard best in the lower anterolateral chest area during the latter portion of inspiration and the beginning of expiration. Pleural friction rubs are caused by inflammation of the pleura.[3,7,10,11]

Assessment of voice sounds

Assessment of the patient's voice sounds is particularly useful in detecting lung consolidation or lung compression. Three abnormal types of voice sounds are bronchophony, whispering pectoriloquy, and egophony.

TABLE 12-2

CHARACTERISTICS OF NORMAL BREATH SOUNDS

SOUND	CHARACTERISTICS
Vesicular	Heard over most of lung field; low pitch; soft and short exhalation and long inhalation
Bronchovesicular	Heard over main bronchus area and over upper right posterior lung field; medium pitch; exhalation equals inhalation
Bronchial	Heard only over trachea; high pitch; loud and long exhalation

Modified from Thompson JM, et al: *Mosby's clinical nursing,* ed 3, St Louis, 1993, Mosby.

TABLE 12-3

ABNORMAL BREATH SOUNDS AND THEIR ASSOCIATED CONDITIONS

ABNORMAL SOUND	DESCRIPTION	CONDITION
Absent breath sounds	No airflow to particular portion of lung	Pneumothorax Pneumonectomy Emphysematous blebs Pleural effusion Lung mass Massive atelectasis Complete airway obstruction
Diminished breath sounds	Little airflow to particular portion of lung	Emphysema Pleural effusion Pleurisy Atelectasis Pulmonary fibrosis
Displaced bronchial sounds	Bronchial sounds heard in peripheral lung fields	Atelectasis with secretions Lung mass with exudate Pneumonia Pleural effusion Pulmonary edema
Crackles (rales)	Short, discrete, popping or crackling sounds	Pulmonary edema Pneumonia Pulmonary fibrosis Atelectasis Bronchiectasis
Rhonchi	Coarse, rumbling, low-pitched sounds	Pneumonia Asthma Bronchitis Bronchospasm
Wheezes	High-pitched, squeaking, whistling sounds	Asthma Bronchospasm
Pleural friction rub	Creaking, leathery, loud, dry, coarse sounds	Pleural effusion Pleurisy

Bronchophony describes a condition in which the spoken voice is heard on auscultation with higher intensity and clarity than usual. Normally the spoken word is muffled when heard through the stethoscope. It is assessed by placing the diaphragm of the stethoscope against the posterior side of the patient's chest and instructing the patient to say "ninety-nine." Bronchophony is present when the sound heard is clear, distinct, and loud. Whispering pectoriloquy describes a condition of unusually clear transmission of the whispered voice on auscultation. Normally the whispered word is unintelligible when heard through the stethoscope. It is assessed by placing the stethoscope against the posterior side of the patient's chest and instructing the patient to whisper "one, two, three." Whispering pectoriloquy is present when the sound heard is clear and distinct. Egophony describes a condition in which the voice sounds increase in intensity and develop a nasal bleating quality on auscultation. It is assessed by placing the stethoscope against the posterior side of the patient's chest and instructing the patient to say "e-e-e." Egophony is present when the "e" sound changes to an "a" sound.[11,13]

LABORATORY STUDIES

Arterial Blood Gases

Interpretation of arterial blood gas (ABG) levels can be difficult, especially if one is under pressure to do it quickly and accurately. One method that can help ensure accuracy when analyzing arterial blood gas levels is to follow the same steps of interpretation each time. A specific method to be used each time that blood gas values must be interpreted is presented in brief in Box 12-2.

Step 1: Look at the PaO_2 level and answer the question, "Does the PaO_2 level show hypoxemia?" The PaO_2 is a measure of the partial pressure of oxygen dissolved in arterial blood plasma, with *P* standing for *partial pressure* and *a* standing for *arterial*. It is reported in millimeters of mercury (mm Hg). PaO_2 reflects 3% of total oxygen in the blood.[14]

The normal range in PaO_2 for persons breathing room air at sea level is 80 to 100 mm Hg. However, the normal range is age-dependent in two groups: infants and persons 60 years and older. The normal level for infants breathing room air is 40 to 70 mm Hg.[15] The normal level for persons 60 years and older decreases with age as changes occur in the ventilation/perfusion (V/Q) matching in the aging lung.[14] The correct PaO_2 for older persons can be ascertained as follows: 80 mm Hg (the lowest normal value) minus 1 mm Hg for every year that a person is over the age of 60. Using this formula, a 65-year-old individual can have a PaO_2 as low as 75 mm Hg and still be within the normal range (formula for 5 years over 60 years of age: 80 mm Hg − 5 mm Hg = 75 mm Hg). An acceptable range for an 80-year-old person is 60 mm Hg (formula for 20 years over the age of 60: 80 mm Hg − 20 mm Hg = 60 mm Hg). At any age, a PaO_2 lower than 40

mm Hg represents a life-threatening situation that requires immediate action.[14] In addition, a PaO_2 less than the predicted lowest value indicates hypoxemia, which means that a lower-than-normal amount of oxygen is dissolved in plasma.

Step 2: Look at the pH level and answer the question, "Is the pH on the acid or alkaline side of 7.40?" The pH is the hydrogen ion (H^+) concentration of plasma. Calculation of pH is accomplished by using the partial pressure of carbon dioxide ($PaCO_2$) and the plasma bicarbonate level (HCO_3^-).[16]

The normal pH of arterial blood is 7.35 to 7.45, with the mean being 7.40. If the pH level is less than 7.40, it is on the acid side of the mean. A pH level less than 7.35 is known as *acidemia,* and the overall condition is called *acidosis.* If the pH level is greater than 7.40, it is on the alkaline side of the mean. A pH level greater than 7.45 is known as *alkalemia,* and the overall condition is called *alkalosis.*[14]

Step 3: Look at the $PaCO_2$ level and answer the question, "Does the $PaCO_2$ show respiratory acidosis, alkalosis, or normalcy?" The $PaCO_2$ is a measure of the partial pressure of carbon dioxide dissolved in arterial blood plasma and is reported in mm Hg. It is the acid-base component that reflects the effectiveness of ventilation in relation to the metabolic rate.[14] In other words, the $PaCO_2$ value indicates whether the patient can ventilate well enough to rid the body of the carbon dioxide produced as a consequence of metabolism.

The normal range for $PaCO_2$ is 35 to 45 mm Hg. This range does not change as a person ages. A $PaCO_2$ value of

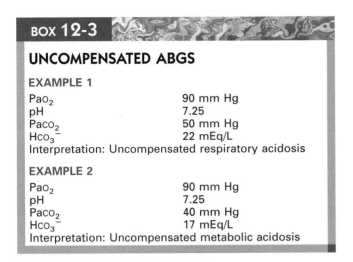

BOX 12-3

UNCOMPENSATED ABGS

EXAMPLE 1

PaO_2	90 mm Hg
pH	7.25
$PaCO_2$	50 mm Hg
HCO_3^-	22 mEq/L

Interpretation: Uncompensated respiratory acidosis

EXAMPLE 2

PaO_2	90 mm Hg
pH	7.25
$PaCO_2$	40 mm Hg
HCO_3^-	17 mEq/L

Interpretation: Uncompensated metabolic acidosis

BOX 12-4

COMPENSATED ABGS

EXAMPLE 1

PaO_2	90 mm Hg
pH	7.37
$PaCO_2$	60 mm Hg
HCO_3^-	38 mEq/L

Interpretation: Compensated respiratory acidosis with metabolic alkalosis. (The acidosis is considered the main disorder and the alkalosis the compensatory response because the pH is on the acid side of 7.40.)

EXAMPLE 2

PaO_2	90 mm Hg
pH	7.42
$PaCO_2$	48 mm Hg
HCO_3^-	35 mEq/L

Interpretation: Compensated metabolic alkalosis with respiratory acidosis. (The alkalosis is considered the main disorder and the acidosis the compensatory response because the pH is on the alkaline side of 7.40.)

greater than 45 mm Hg defines respiratory acidosis, which is caused by alveolar hypoventilation. Hypoventilation can result from COPD, oversedation, head trauma, anesthesia, drug overdose, neuromuscular disease, or hypoventilation with mechanical ventilation.[17] A $PaCO_2$ value that is less than 35 mm Hg defines respiratory alkalosis, which is caused by alveolar hyperventilation. Hyperventilation can result from hypoxia, anxiety, pulmonary embolism, pregnancy, and hyperventilation with mechanical ventilation or as a compensatory mechanism to metabolic acidosis.[17]

Step 4: Look at the HCO_3^- level and answer the question, "Does the HCO_3^- show metabolic acidosis, alkalosis, or normalcy?" The bicarbonate (HCO_3^-) is the acid-base component that reflects kidney function. The bicarbonate is reduced or increased in the plasma by renal mechanisms. The normal range is 22 to 26 mEq/L.[18] A bicarbonate level of less than 22 mEq/L defines metabolic acidosis, which can result from ketoacidosis, lactic acidosis, renal failure, or diarrhea. The cumulative effect is a gain of acids or a loss of base. A bicarbonate level that is greater than 26 mEq/L defines metabolic alkalosis, which can result from fluid loss from the upper gastrointestinal tract (vomiting or nasogastric suction), diuretic therapy, severe hypokalemia, alkali administration, or steroid therapy.[16,17]

Step 5: Look back at the pH level and answer the question, "Does the pH show a compensated or an uncompensated condition?" If the pH level is abnormal (less than 7.35 or greater than 7.45), the $PaCO_2$ value or the HCO_3^- level, or both, will also be abnormal. This is an uncompensated condition because there has not been enough time for the body to return the pH to its normal range (Box 12-3).[14,16] If the pH level is within normal limits and both the $PaCO_2$ value and the HCO_3^- level are abnormal, the condition is compensated because there has been enough time for the body to restore the pH to within its normal range.[16] Differentiating the primary disorder

from the compensatory response can be difficult. The primary disorder is the abnormality that caused the pH level to shift initially; thus, on whichever side of 7.40 the pH level occurs is considered the primary disorder (Box 12-4).[14] Partial compensation may also be present and is evidenced by abnormal pH, $PaCO_2$, and HCO_3^- levels, indications that the body is attempting to return the pH to its normal range.[17]

Table 12-4 summarizes the changes in the acid-base components that accompany various acid-base disorders.[14,17] In addition to the parameters previously discussed, other factors must be considered when reviewing a patient's ABGs, including oxygen saturation, oxygen content, expected PaO_2, and base excess and deficit.

Oxygen saturation

Oxygen saturation is a measure of the amount of oxygen bound to hemoglobin, compared with hemoglobin's maximal capability for binding oxygen. It can be assessed as a component of the ABG (SaO_2) or can be measured noninvasively using a pulse oximeter (SpO_2).[19] Oxygen saturation is reported as a percentage or as a decimal, with normal being greater than 95% on room air. Normally, the saturation level cannot reach 100% (on room air) because of the physiologic shunting.[14] However, when supplemental oxygen is administered, oxygen saturation may approach 100% so closely that it is reported as 100%.

Proper evaluation of the oxygen saturation level is vital. For example, an SaO_2 of 97% means that 97% of the available hemoglobin is bound with oxygen. The word *available* is essential to evaluating the SaO_2 level because

TABLE 12-4

SUMMARY OF ARTERIAL BLOOD GAS ASSESSMENT

DISORDER	pH	Paco$_2$	Hco$_3^-$
Respiratory acidosis			
Uncompensated	<7.35	>45 mm Hg	22-26 mEq/L
Partially compensated	<7.35	>45 mm Hg	26 mEq/L
Compensated	7.35-7.39	>45 mm Hg	26 mEq/L
Respiratory alkalosis			
Uncompensated	>7.45	<35 mm Hg	22-26 mEq/L
Partially compensated	>7.45	<35 mm Hg	22 mEq/L
Compensated	7.41-7.45	<35 mm Hg	22 mEq/L
Metabolic acidosis			
Uncompensated	<7.35	35-45 mm Hg	22 mEq/L
Partially compensated	<7.35	<35 mm Hg	22 mEq/L
Compensated	7.35-7.39	35 mm Hg	22 mEq/L
Metabolic alkalosis			
Uncompensated	>7.45	35-45 mm Hg	26 mEq/L
Partially compensated	>7.45	45 mm Hg	26 mEq/L
Compensated	7.41-7.45	45 mm Hg	26 mEq/L
Combined respiratory and metabolic acidosis	<7.35	45 mm Hg	22 mEq/L
Combined respiratory and metabolic alkalosis	>7.45	35 mm Hg	26 mEq/L

the hemoglobin level is not always within normal limits and oxygen can bind only with what is available. A 97% saturation level associated with 10 g of hemoglobin does not deliver as much oxygen to the tissues as does a 97% saturation associated with 15 g of hemoglobin. Thus assessing only the SaO$_2$ level and finding it within normal limits must not lead one to believe that the patient's oxygenation status is normal. The hemoglobin level must also be evaluated before a decision on oxygenation status can be made.[18]

Oxygen content

Oxygen content (CaO$_2$) is a measure of the total amount of oxygen carried in the blood, including the amount dissolved in plasma (measured by the PaO$_2$) and the amount bound to the hemoglobin molecule (measured by the SaO$_2$). CaO$_2$ is reported in milliliters (ml) of oxygen carried per 100 ml of blood. The normal value is 20 ml of oxygen per 100 ml of blood. To calculate the oxygen content, the PaO$_2$, the SaO$_2$, and the hemoglobin level are used (Appendix B). A change in any one of these parameters will affect the CaO$_2$.[1,8]

Expected PaO$_2$

When a patient receives supplemental oxygen, the PaO$_2$ level is expected to rise. Knowing the level to which the PaO$_2$ should rise in normal subjects on a given FIO$_2$ and comparing that with the level to which the PaO$_2$ actually does rise in patients with pulmonary disease has value because it illustrates how well the lung is functioning. Calculating the expected PaO$_2$ is accomplished by multiplying the FIO$_2$ value by 5.[14] Thus the expected PaO$_2$ on an FIO$_2$ of 30% is at least 150 mm Hg (30 × 5), whereas the expected PaO$_2$ on an FIO$_2$ of 50% is 250 mm Hg (50 × 5). These expected PaO$_2$ values represent the oxygen level

TABLE 12-5

GUIDELINES FOR ESTIMATING FIo$_2$ WITH LOW-FLOW OXYGEN DEVICES

100% O$_2$ FLOW RATE (L)	FIo$_2$ (%)
NASAL CANNULA OR CATHETER	
1	24
2	28
3	32
4	36
5	40
6	44
OXYGEN MASK	
5-6	40
6-7	50
7-8	60
MASK WITH RESERVOIR BAG	
6	60
7	70
8	80
9	90
10	99+

From Shapiro BA, Peruzzi WT, Kozelowski-Templin R: *Clinical application of blood gases*, ed 5, St Louis, 1994, Mosby.
NOTE: Normal ventilatory pattern assumed.

achievable with healthy lungs. Pulmonary disease can radically decrease the expected PaO$_2$ level. It is impossible to apply the "FIO$_2$ value × 5" rule to achieve the expected PaO$_2$ value when the patient is on a system that delivers oxygen by liters per minute. For these situations, Table 12-5 shows the FIO$_2$ levels that correspond to various oxygen delivery systems.

Classic Shunt Equation and Oxygen Tension Indices

The efficiency of oxygenation can be assessed by measuring the degree of intrapulmonary shunting that occurs in a patient at any one time, using the classic shunt equation and oxygen tension indices. *Intrapulmonary shunting* (QS/QT [the portion of cardiac output not exchanging with alveolar blood divided by the total cardiac output]) refers to venous blood that flows to the lungs without being oxygenated because of nonfunctioning alveoli.[14,19] Other names for this condition include *shunt effect, low V/Q, wasted blood flow,* and *venous admixture*.[15] Direct determination of intrapulmonary shunting requires the use of the classic shunt equation (Appendix B), which is both invasive and cumbersome. A shunt greater than 10% is considered abnormal and indicative of a shunt-producing disorder.[14]

Often times, intrapulmonary shunting is estimated by using the oxygen tension indices. One advantage to these methods is the ease of performance, though they have been found to be unreliable in critically ill patients.[14] An estimate of intrapulmonary shunting can be determined by computing the difference between the alveolar and arterial oxygen concentrations. Normally, alveolar and arterial P_{O_2} values are approximately equal.[19] When they are not, it indicates that venous blood is passing malfunctioning alveoli and returning unoxygenated to the left side of the heart.[20] The most common oxygen tension indices used to estimate intrapulmonary shunting are the Pa_{O_2}/FI_{O_2} ratio, the Pa_{O_2}/PA_{O_2} ratio, and the A-a gradient (see Appendix B for formulas).

Pa_{O_2}/FI_{O_2} ratio

The Pa_{O_2}/FI_{O_2} ratio is clinically the easiest formula to calculate because it does not call for the computation of the alveolar P_{O_2}. Normally, the Pa_{O_2}/FI_{O_2} ratio is greater than 286, with the lower the value the worse the lung function.[19]

Pa_{O_2}/PA_{O_2} ratio

The Pa_{O_2}/PA_{O_2} ratio (arterial/alveolar O_2 ratio) is normally greater than 60%. The disadvantage to using this formula is that it calls for the computation of the alveolar P_{O_2}, but the advantage is that it is unaffected by changes in the FI_{O_2} as long as the underlying lung condition is stable.[14]

Alveolar-arterial gradient

The A-a gradient ($P[A-a]_{O_2}$) is normally less than 20 mm Hg on room air for patients younger than 61 years old. This estimate of intrapulmonary shunting is the least reliable clinically but is frequently used in clinical decision-making. One of the major disadvantages to using this formula is that it is greatly influenced by the amount of oxygen the patient is receiving.[14,19]

Dead Space Equation

The efficiency of ventilation can be measured using the clinical dead space (V_D/V_T) equation (Appendix B). The formula measures the fraction of tidal volume not participating in gas exchange. Dead space greater than 0.6 indicates a dead space–producing disorder and is considered abnormal. The major limitations to using this formula are that it requires the measurement of exhaled carbon dioxide to complete and that the work of breathing by patients must remain stable during the collection.[14]

Sputum Studies

Careful analysis of sputum specimens is crucial for the rapid identification and treatment of pulmonary infections. The most difficult aspect of sputum examination is proper collection of the specimen. In general, collection of a good sputum sample requires a conscious, cooperative, sufficiently hydrated patient. When the patient has difficulty producing sputum, heated, nebulized saline may help to loosen secretions for expectoration.[21] Chest physiotherapy combined with nebulization can improve the success rate. Collection of a sputum specimen is best done in the morning because there is a greater volume of secretions as a result of nighttime pooling.[22]

Many critically ill patients cannot cough effectively, and thus sputum collection by other means is required. These methods include tracheobronchial aspiration, transtracheal aspiration, and the use of a fiberoptic bronchoscopy with a protected brush catheter. Because each method has its own benefits and risks, the patient's clinical condition determines the appropriate technique.[23]

Many critically ill patients have endotracheal or tracheostomy tubes already in place. Collecting sputum specimens from these patients requires special attention to technique (Box 12-5). Deep specimens are obtained to avoid collecting specimens that contain resident upper airway flora that may have migrated down the tube. Colonization of the lower airways with upper airway flora can occur within 48 hours of intubation.[24]

Once a sputum specimen is obtained, it is examined for volume, physical properties, mucopurulence, and color. Next, a microscopic examination is done to identify the source of the specimen. If a bacterial infection is suspected, a Gram stain followed by a culture and sensitivity (C&S) is performed.[24]

DIAGNOSTIC PROCEDURES

Table 12-6 presents an overview of the various diagnostic procedures used to evaluate the patient with pulmonary dysfunction.

Nursing Management

The nursing management of a patient undergoing a diagnostic procedure involves a variety of interventions. **Priorities are directed toward preparing the patient psy-**

BOX 12-5

PROCEDURE FOR COLLECTION OF TRACHEAL OR ENDOTRACHEAL SPECIMEN

- Clear the endotracheal or tracheostomy tube of all local secretions, avoiding deep airway penetration.
- Attach a sputum trap to a sterile suction catheter and advance the catheter into the trachea while trying to avoid contact with the endotracheal tube or tracheostomy tube.
- After the catheter is fully advanced, apply suction until secretions return to the sputum trap. When enough secretions are collected, discontinue suctioning and remove the catheter.
- Do not apply suction while the catheter is being withdrawn because this can contaminate the sample with sputum from the upper airway. Do not flush the catheter with sterile water because this dilutes the sample.
- If the catheter becomes plugged with secretions, place it in a sterile container and send it to the laboratory. The specimen must be transported immediately or refrigerated if a delay is necessary.

BOX 12-6

MANIFESTATIONS OF RESPIRATORY DECOMPENSATION

INADEQUATE AIRWAY

Stridor
Noisy respirations
Supraclavicular and intercostal retractions
Flaring of nares
Labored breathing with use of accessory muscles

INADEQUATE VENTILATION

Absence of air exchange at nose and mouth (breathlessness)
Minimal/absent chest-wall motion
Manifestations of obstructed airway
Central cyanosis
Decreased or absent breath sounds (bilateral, unilateral)
Restlessness, anxiety, confusion
Paradoxical motion involving significant portion of chest wall
Decreased PaO_2, increased $PaCO_2$, decreased pH

INADEQUATE GAS EXCHANGE

Tachypnea
Decreased PaO_2
Increased dead space
Central cyanosis
Chest infiltrates on x-ray evaluation

---

chologically and physically for the procedure, **monitoring the patient's responses to the procedure, and assessing the patient after the procedure.** Preparing the patient includes teaching the patient about the procedure, answering any questions, and transporting and/or positioning the patient for the procedure. Monitoring the patient's responses to the procedure includes observing the patient for signs of pain, anxiety, or respiratory decompensation (Box 12-6) and monitoring vital signs. Assessing the patient after the procedure includes observing for complications of the procedure and medicating the patient for any postprocedure discomfort. **Any evidence of respiratory distress should be immediately reported to the physician and emergency measures to maintain breathing must be initiated.**

BEDSIDE MONITORING

Bedside Pulmonary Function Tests

Pulmonary function tests (PFTs) are designed to quantify respiratory function and are an essential component of a thorough pulmonary evaluation. PFTs are used for a variety of purposes, including preoperative assessment, evaluating lung mechanics, diagnosing and tracking pulmonary diseases, and monitoring therapy. Results are individualized according to age, gender, and body size.[25] In the critically ill patient measurements of pulmonary function are usually limited to those areas that give the practitioner information about the patient's need for or ability to wean from mechanical ventilation. This section covers the areas most frequently tested at the bedside of critically ill individuals (Table 12-7).

Lung compliance should be measured on all patients on ventilators. Compliance is a measure of the distensibility of the lungs (how easily they are inflated) and an indicator of the improvement or worsening of the patient's lung disease. Dynamic compliance is measured during the breathing cycle. A value of 35 to 50 ml/cm H_2O is normal (Appendix B). It should be noted that measurement of dynamic compliance does not separate lung compliance and airway resistance forces; therefore, conditions that increase resistance of either force will alter the dynamic compliance value. Dynamic compliance decreases with any decrease in lung compliance or increase in airway resistance, such as occurs with bronchospasm and retained secretions. Static compliance is measured under no-flow conditions so that resistance forces are removed. Static compliance decreases with any decrease in lung compliance, such as occurs with pneumothorax, atelectasis, pneumonia, pulmonary edema, and chest-wall restrictions. A normal value is 60 to 100 ml/cm of H_2O[25] (Appendix B).

Assessment of inspiratory muscle strength can be evaluated through the measurement of *maximal inspiratory pressure (MIP)* and *negative inspiratory pressure (NIP)*. Both should be more negative than -20 to -25 cm H_2O. Other names for these same tests are *negative inspiratory effort (NIE)*, *peak inspiratory pressure (PIP)*, and *peak inspiratory force (PIF)*. Both the MIP and NIP require a coopera-

TABLE 12-6

PULMONARY DIAGNOSTIC PROCEDURES

PROCEDURES	EVALUATES	COMMENTS
Chest x-ray	• Detects lung pathology (e.g., pneumonia, pulmonary edema, atelectasis, tuberculosis) • Determines size and location of lung lesions and tumors • Verifies placement of endotracheal tube, central venous catheters, chest tubes	• Necessary to inquire about possibility of pregnancy • Noninvasive test with minimal radiation exposure • Posteroanterior (PA) and lateral films most common, but in critical care areas anteroposterior (AP) portable films frequently necessary because patient cannot be transported • Lateral decubitus films for identification of pleural effusion
Tomography	• Defines lesions, masses, cavities, or shadows seen on a normal chest x-ray • Evaluates tracheal or bronchial narrowing	• X-rays taken at different angles
Bronchography	• Detects obstruction or malformation of the tracheobronchial tree	• Inspiration of radioopaque substance before x-ray examination • Necessary to inquire about possibility of pregnancy
Laryngoscopy or bronchoscopy	• Obtains cytology specimen or biopsy • Identifies tumors • Evaluates lung changes • Is used therapeutically to remove secretions, foreign bodies, other contaminants	• Patient sedated before the procedure, usually with a benzodiazepine (e.g., diazepam, midazolam) • Patient monitored for subcutaneous emphysema after study; indicates tracheal or bronchial tear • Patient monitored for hemoptysis: some blood in sputum normal after biopsy, but frank hemoptysis requires immediate attention
Lung scan or ventilation-perfusion (V/Q) scan	• Diagnoses ventilation and perfusion abnormalities, including emphysema, pulmonary emboli	• Invasive test: radioisotope inspired and injected intravascularly • Necessary to inquire about possibility of pregnancy • Nuclear scan study: patient is assured that amount of radioactive material is minimal
Magnetic resonance imaging (MRI)	• Distinguishes tumors from other structures (e.g., tumor, pleural thickening, fibrosis)	• Noninvasive test • Contraindicated for patients with pacemakers or implanted metallic devices
Ultrasonography	• Evaluates pleural disease • Visualizes diaphragm and detects disease around diaphragm (e.g., subphrenic hematoma, abscess)	• Noninvasive test
Pulmonary angiography	• Detects changes in lung tissue (e.g., masses) • Diagnoses abnormalities in pulmonary vasculature, including thrombi and emboli • Identifies congenital abnormalities of the circulation	• Invasive test • Necessary to inquire about possibility of pregnancy • Contrast media injected into pulmonary artery: ensure adequate hydration after study • Necessary to monitor arterial puncture point for hematoma or hemorrhage
Thoracentesis	• Obtains pleural fluid specimen • Is used therapeutically to remove pleural fluid	• Necessary to monitor patient for indications of pneumothorax • Necessary to monitor for leakage from puncture point
Transthoracic needle lung biopsy	• Obtains specimen for cytology evaluation	• Necessary to perform under fluoroscopy; inquire about possibility of pregnancy

Modified from Dennison RD: *Pass CCRN!* St Louis, 1996, Mosby.

TABLE 12-7

BEDSIDE PULMONARY FUNCTION TESTS

TEST	DESCRIPTION
Respiratory rate (f)	Number of breaths per minute
Tidal volume (V_T)	Volume of air exhaled after a normal resting inhalation
Minute ventilation (V_E)	Volume of air expired per minute (tidal volume respiratory rate = minute ventilation)
Maximal voluntary ventilation (MVV)	Maximal amount of air that can be moved into and out of the lungs in 1 minute
Forced vital capacity (FVC)	Maximal amount of air that can be forcefully exhaled from the lungs after maximal inhalation
Maximal inspiratory pressure (MIP)	Maximal negative pressure generated on inhalation
Maximal expiratory pressure (MEP)	Maximal positive pressure generated on exhalation
Peak expiratory flow rate (PEFR)	Maximal flow rate achieved during forced exhalation
Forced expiratory flow at midpoint of vital capacity ($FEF_{25\%-75\%}$)	Measure of the average flow rate during the middle 50% of exhalation
Forced expiratory flow at 1 second (FEV_1)	Volume of air exhaled in first second of forced exhalation

tive patient and can provide useful information about spontaneous breathing ability.[25] Maximal expiratory pressure (MEP) can be measured to test the ability to cough in neuromuscular patient populations. Other common methods used to assess respiratory muscle strength are maximum voluntary ventilation (MVV), minute ventilation (V_E), and breathing pattern.

Dynamic pulmonary function tests are designed to evaluate the function of the respiratory muscles, thorax, and lungs. These tests are timed breathing studies that evaluate the degree of respiratory impairment and include forced vital capacity (FVC), peak expiratory flow rate (PEFR), forced expiratory volume in 1 second (FEV_1), and forced expiratory volume divided by the forced vital capacity (FEV_1/FVC). Forced expiratory flow ($FEF_{25\%-75\%}$) is the mean rate of air flow over the middle half of the FVC and is a good index of airway resistance. When these studies are performed at the bedside they require the use of spirometry for volume measurement. The tests can be performed with intubated or nonintubated patients. In the intubated patient, the spirometer is attached to the end of the endotracheal tube. In the nonintubated patient, a nose clip is placed on the patient and the patient is instructed to breathe through a spirometer tube. The patient is seated on the side of the bed if possible.[25]

Pulse Oximetry

Pulse oximetry is a noninvasive method for monitoring oxygen saturation (SpO_2). It is indicated in any situation in which the patient's oxygenation status requires continuous observation. It consists of a microprocessor and a probe that attaches to the patient (finger, ear, toe, or nose). The probe consists of two light-emitting diodes and a photodetector. The diodes transmit red and infrared light wavelengths through the pulsating vascular bed to the photodetector on the other side. The photodetector converts the light signals into an electric signal, which is then sent to the microprocessor, which converts it to a digital reading. The pulse oximeter is considered very accurate, within $\pm2\%$ at a saturation greater than 70%.[26]

Nursing priorities are directed toward minimizing the physiologic and technical factors that can limit the monitoring system.

Physiologic limitations

Physiologic limitations include elevated levels of abnormal hemoglobins, presence of vascular dyes, and poor tissue perfusion. The pulse oximeter cannot differentiate between normal and abnormal hemoglobin. Elevated levels of abnormal hemoglobin falsely elevate the SpO_2. Vascular dyes, such as methylene blue, indigo carmine, indocyanine green, and fluorescein, also interfere with pulse oximetry and can lead to falsely low readings. Poor tissue perfusion to the area with the probe leads to loss of pulsatile flow and signal failure.[26]

Technical limitations

Technical limitations include bright lights, excessive motion, and incorrect placement of the probe. Bright lights may interfere with the photodetector and cause inaccurate results. The probe must be covered to limit optical interference. Excessive motion can mimic arterial pulsations and can lead to false readings. Incorrect placement of the probe can lead to inaccurate results because part of the light can reach the photodetector without having passed through blood (optical shunting). Interventions to limit these problems include using the proper probe in the appropriate spot (e.g., not using a finger probe on the ear), applying the probe according to the directions, and ensuring that the area being monitored has adequate perfusion.[26]

References

1. Rokosky JS: Assessment of the individual with altered respiratory function, *Nurs Clin North Am* 16:195, 1981.
2. Gehring PE: Physical assessment begins with a history, *RN* 54(11):26, 1991.
3. Brenner M, Welliver J: Pulmonary and acid-base assessment, *Nurs Clin North Am* 25:761, 1990.
4. Dettenmeier PA: *Pulmonary nursing care*, St Louis, 1992, Mosby.
5. Wilkins RL: Bedside assessment of the patient. In Scanlan CL, Spearman CB, Sheldon RL, editors: *Egan's fundamentals of respiratory care*, ed 6, St Louis, 1995, Mosby.
6. Wilson SF, Thompson JM: *Respiratory disorders*, St Louis, 1990, Mosby.

7. Stiesmeyer JK: A four-step approach to pulmonary assessment, *Am J Nurs* 93(8):22, 1993.

8. Carpenter KD: A comprehensive review of cyanosis, *Crit Care Nurs* 13(4):66, 1993.

9. King C: Examining the thorax and respiratory system, *RN* 45(8):55, 1982.

10. Kuhn KW, McGovern M: Respiratory assessment of the elderly, *J Gerontol Nurs* 18(5):40, 1992.

11. Barkauskas V, et al: *Health and physical assessment*, ed 2, St Louis, 1998, Mosby.

12. Seidel HM, et al: *Mosby's guide to physical examination*, ed 3, St Louis, 1995, Mosby.

13. Boyda EK, et al: *Pulmonary auscultation*, St Paul, 1987, 3M Health Care Group.

14. Shapiro BA, Peruzzi WT, Kozelowski-Templin R: *Clinical application of blood gases*, ed 5, St Louis, 1994, Mosby

15. Hazinski MF: *Nursing care of the critically ill child*, ed 2, St Louis, 1992, Mosby.

16. McCance KL, Huether SE: *Pathophysiology: the biologic basis for disease in adults and children*, ed 3, St Louis, 1998, Mosby.

17. Haber RJ: A practical approach to acid-base disorders, *West J Med* 155:146, 1991.

18. Ahern J: A guide to blood gases, *Nurs Stand* 9:50, 1995.

19. Ahrens T: Respiratory monitoring in critical care, *AACN Clin Issues Crit Care Nurs* 4:56, 1993.

20. Pier AF: Using mixed venous oxygen saturation to trend overall oxygenation in cardiothoracic surgical patients, *Crit Care Nurs Q* 16:72, 1993.

21. Fink J: Humidity and aerosol therapy. In Scanlan CL, Spearman CB, Sheldon RL, editors: *Egan's fundamentals of respiratory care*, ed 6, St Louis, 1995, Mosby.

22. Lewis SM, Collier IC, Heitkemper MM: *Medical-surgical nursing*, ed 4, St Louis, 1996, Mosby.

23. MacLeod JA: Collecting specimens for laboratory analysis, *Nurs Stand* 5:36, 1992.

24. Midha NK, Stratton CW: Laboratory tests in critical care, *Crit Care Clin* 1:15, 1998.

25. Douce FH: Basic pulmonary function measurements. In Scanlan CL, Spearman CB, Sheldon RL, editors: *Egan's fundamentals of respiratory care*, ed 6, St Louis, 1995, Mosby.

26. Grap, MJ: *Pulse oximetry*, Aliso Viejo, CA, 1996, American Association of Critical Care Nurses.

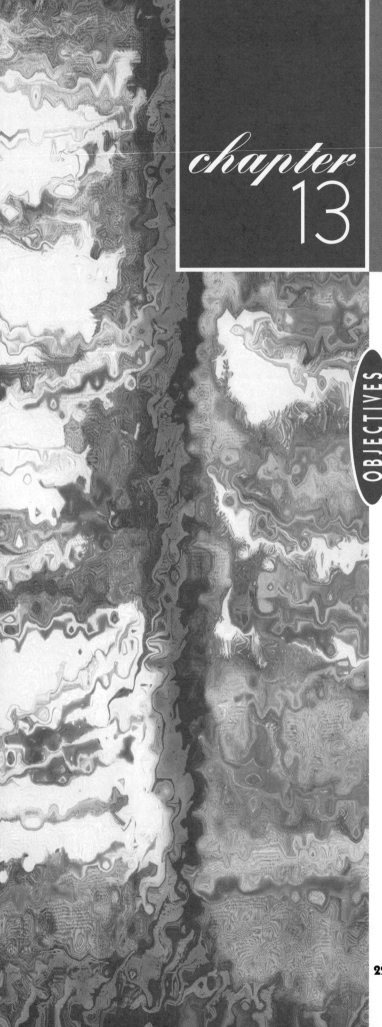

chapter 13

Pulmonary Disorders

Kathleen M. Stacy

- Describe the etiology and pathophysiology of selected pulmonary disorders.
- Identify the clinical manifestations of selected pulmonary disorders.
- Explain the treatment of selected pulmonary disorders.
- Discuss the nursing priorities for managing the patient with selected pulmonary disorders.

Understanding the pathology of the a disease, the areas of assessment on which to focus, and the usual medical management allows the critical care nurse to more accurately anticipate and plan nursing interventions. This chapter focuses on pulmonary disorders commonly seen in the critical care environment.

ACUTE RESPIRATORY FAILURE

Description and Etiology

Acute respiratory failure (ARF) is a clinical condition in which the pulmonary system fails to maintain adequate gas exchange.[1] It is probably the most prevalent problem seen in critical care today.[2] ARF can be classified as hypoxemic normocapnic respiratory failure (Type I) or hypoxemic hypercapnic respiratory failure (Type II), depending on the patient's arterial blood gases (ABGs). In Type I respiratory failure the patient presents with a low PaO_2 and a normal $PaCO_2$, whereas in Type II respiratory failure PaO_2 is low and $PaCO_2$ is high.[3]

Although any number of Diagnosis Related Groups (DRGs) may apply to the patient with ARF, depending on the underlying cause and subsequent treatment, usually DRG 475 (Respiratory System Diagnosis with Ventilator

Support) is used with an anticipated length of stay of 11.6 days.[4]

ARF results from a deficiency in the performance of the pulmonary system.[1-3] It usually occurs secondary to another disorder that has altered the normal function of the pulmonary system in such a way as to decrease the ventilatory drive, decrease muscle strength, decrease chest wall elasticity, decrease the lung's capacity for gas exchange, increase airway resistance, or increase metabolic oxygen requirements.[5]

The etiologies of ARF may be classified as extrapulmonary or intrapulmonary, depending on the component of the respiratory system that is affected. Extrapulmonary causes include disorders that affect the brain, spinal cord, neuromuscular system, thorax, pleura, and upper airways. Intrapulmonary causes include disorders that affect the lower airways and alveoli, pulmonary circulation, and alveolar-capillary membrane.[6] Table 13-1 lists the different etiologies of ARF and their associated disorders.

Pathophysiology

Hypoxemia is the result of impaired gas exchange and is the hallmark of acute respiratory failure. Hypercapnia may be present, depending on the underlying cause of the problem. The main causes of hypoxemia are alveolar hypoventilation, ventilation/perfusion (V/Q) mismatching, and intrapulmonary shunting.[7] Type I respiratory failure usually results from V/Q mismatching and intrapulmonary shunting while Type II respiratory failure usually results from alveolar hypoventilation, which may or may not be accompanied by V/Q mismatching and intrapulmonary shunting.[1]

Alveolar hypoventilation

Alveolar hypoventilation occurs when the amount of oxygen being brought into the alveoli is insufficient to meet the metabolic needs of the body.[6] This can be the result of increasing metabolic oxygen needs or decreasing ventilations.[5] Hypoxemia caused by alveolar hypoventilation is often associated with hypercapnia and commonly results from extrapulmonary disorders.[1,7]

Ventilation/perfusion (V/Q) mismatching

V/Q mismatching occurs when ventilation and blood flow are mismatched in various regions of the lung in excess of what is normal. Blood passes through alveoli that are underventilated for the given amount of perfusion, leaving these areas with a lower-than-normal amount of oxygen. V/Q mismatching is the most common cause of hypoxemia and is usually the result of alveoli that are partially collapsed or partially filled with fluid.[7,8]

Intrapulmonary shunting

The extreme form of V/Q mismatching, intrapulmonary shunting, occurs when blood reaches the arterial system without participating in gas exchange. The mixing of unoxygenated (shunted) blood and oxygenated

TABLE **13-1**	
ETIOLOGIES OF ACUTE RESPIRATORY FAILURE	
AFFECTED AREA	**DISORDERS***
EXTRAPULMONARY	
Brain	Drug overdose
	Central alveolar hypoventilation syndrome
	Brain trauma or lesion
	Postoperative anesthesia depression
Spinal cord	Guillain-Barré syndrome
	Poliomyelitis
	Amyotrophic lateral sclerosis
	Spinal cord trauma or lesion
Neuromuscular system	Myasthenia gravis
	Multiple sclerosis
	Neuromuscular-blocking antibiotics
	Organophosphate poisoning
	Muscular dystrophy
Thorax	Massive obesity
	Chest trauma
Pleura	Pleural effusion
	Pneumothorax
Upper airways	Sleep apnea
	Tracheal obstruction
	Epiglottitis
INTRAPULMONARY	
Lower airways and alveoli	Chronic obstructive pulmonary disease (COPD)
	Asthma
	Bronchiolitis
	Cystic fibrosis
	Pneumonia
Pulmonary circulation	Pulmonary emboli
Alveolar-capillary membrane	Pulmonary edema
	Acute respiratory distress syndrome (ARDS)
	Inhalation of toxic gases
	Near-drowning

*Not an inclusive list.

blood lowers the average level of oxygen present in the blood. Intrapulmonary shunting occurs when blood passes through a portion of a lung that is not ventilated. This may be the result of alveolar collapse (e.g., atelectasis), alveolar consolidation (e.g., pneumonia), or excessive mucus accumulation (e.g., chronic bronchitis).[7,8]

Complications

If allowed to progress, hypoxemia can result in a deficit of oxygen at the cellular level. As the tissue demands for oxygen continue and the supply diminishes, an oxygen supply/demand imbalance occurs and tissue hypoxia develops. Decreased oxygen to the cells contributes to impaired tissue perfusion and the development of lactic acidosis and multiple organ dysfunction syndrome.[8]

Assessment and Diagnosis

The patient with ARF may experience a variety of clinical manifestations, depending on the underlying cause and the extent of tissue hypoxia. The clinical manifestations commonly seen in the patient with ARF are usually related to the development of hypoxemia, hypercapnia, and acidosis. Because the clinical symptoms are so varied, they are not considered reliable in predicting the degree of hypoxemia or hypercapnia.[8-10]

Diagnosing and following the course of respiratory failure is best accomplished by arterial blood gas (ABG) analysis. ABG analysis confirms the level of $PaCO_2$, PaO_2, and blood pH. ARF is generally accepted as being present when the PaO_2 is less than 50 mm Hg and/or the $PaCO_2$ is greater than 50 mm Hg.[2,3] In patients with chronically elevated $PACO_2$ levels, these criteria must be broadened to include a pH less than 7.35.[5]

Medical Management

Medical management of the patient with ARF is aimed at treating the underlying cause, promoting adequate gas exchange, correcting acidosis, and preventing complications.[5] Medical interventions to promote gas exchange are aimed at improving oxygenation and ventilation.

Oxygenation

Actions to improve oxygenation include supplemental oxygen administration and the use of positive airway pressure. The purpose of oxygen therapy is to correct hypoxemia and although the absolute level of hypoxemia varies in each patient, most treatment approaches aim to keep the oxygen saturation at 90% or above. The goal is to keep the tissues' needs satisfied but not produce hypercapnia or oxygen toxicity.[5] Supplemental oxygen administration is effective in treating hypoxemia related to alveolar hypoventilation and V/Q mismatching. When intrapulmonary shunting exists, supplemental oxygen alone is ineffective.[11] In this situation, positive pressure—in the form of constant positive airway pressure (CPAP) or positive end-expiratory pressure (PEEP)—is necessary to open collapsed alveoli and facilitate their participation in gas exchange. Positive pressure may be delivered noninvasively via a mask[12] or invasively via an endotracheal tube.[13]

Ventilation

Interventions to improve ventilation include intubation and mechanical ventilation. Intubation can be accomplished either orally or nasally. If prolonged intubation is required, a tracheostomy should be considered. Once intubated, the patient is placed on a positive-pressure ventilator. The selection of mode and settings depends on the patient's underlying condition, severity of respiratory failure, and body size. In the patient with chronic hypercapnia, the settings should be adjusted to maintain a normal pH level as opposed to $PaCO_2$ level.[14]

Pharmacology

Medications to facilitate removal of secretions and dilate airways may also be of benefit in the treatment of the patient with ARF. Mucolytics are administered to help liquefy secretions, which facilitates their removal. Bronchodilators, such as xanthines (e.g., theophylline and aminophylline), beta$_2$ agonists (e.g., albuterol, bitolterol, isoetharine, metaproterenol, terbutaline), and anticholinergic agents (e.g., ipratropium), aid in smooth muscle relaxation and are of particular benefit to patients with airflow limitations. Steroids are also often administered to decrease airway inflammation and enhance the effects of the beta$_2$ agonists.[5,14]

Sedation is necessary in many patients to assist with maintaining adequate ventilation. It can be used to comfort the patient and decrease the work of breathing, particularly if the patient is fighting the ventilator. Analgesics should be administered for pain control.[14] In some patients, sedation does not decrease spontaneous respiratory efforts enough to allow adequate ventilation. Neuromuscular paralysis may be necessary to facilitate optimal ventilation. Paralysis also may be necessary to decrease oxygen consumption in the severely compromised patient. Three neuromuscular blocking agents commonly used are pancuronium (Pavulon), vecuronium (Norcuron), and atracurium (Tracrium).[15]

Acidosis

Acidosis may occur in the patient for a number of reasons. Hypoxemia causes impaired tissue perfusion, which leads to the production of lactic acid and the development of metabolic acidosis. Impaired ventilation leads to the accumulation of carbon dioxide and the development of respiratory acidosis. Once the patient is adequately oxygenated and ventilated, the acidosis should correct itself. Bicarbonate administration may be necessary if the acidosis persists or is severe (pH <7.2).[5]

Complications

The patient with acute respiratory failure may experience a number of complications including cardiac dysrhythmias, pulmonary embolism, gastrointestinal bleeding, and problems associated with mechanical ventilation. Dysrhythmias can be precipitated by hypoxemia, acidosis, electrolyte imbalances, and the administration of beta$_2$ agonists and xanthines. Maintaining oxygenation, normalizing electrolytes, and monitoring drug levels should assist in the prevention of dysrhythmias. Symptomatic dysrhythmias should be treated in the conventional manner. Pulmonary embolism can be prevented through the use of deep vein thrombosis prophylaxis with heparin. In addition, the patient should be placed on stress ulcer prophylaxis, with a histamine blocker or sucralfate, to prevent gastrointestinal bleeding.[5]

Nursing Management

Nursing management of the patient with acute respiratory failure incorporates a variety of nursing diagnoses

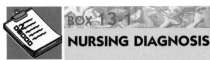

NURSING DIAGNOSIS PRIORITIES

Acute Respiratory Failure

- Impaired Gas Exchange related to alveolar hypoventilation, pp. 476-477
- Impaired Gas Exchange related to ventilation/perfusion mismatching or intrapulmonary shunting, p. 476
- Altered Nutrition: Less than Body Requirements related to lack of exogenous nutrients or increased metabolic demand, p. 460
- Acute Confusion related to sensory overload, sensory deprivation, and sleep pattern disturbance, pp. 444-448
- Knowledge Deficit: Discharge Regimen related to lack of previous exposure to information, p. 443

(Box 13-1). **Nursing priorities are directed toward optimizing oxygenation and ventilation, facilitating nutritional support, providing comfort and emotional support, and maintaining surveillance for complications.**

Optimizing oxygenation

Nursing interventions to optimize oxygenation and ventilation include positioning, preventing desaturation, and promoting secretion clearance.

Positioning. Positioning of the patient with ARF depends on the type of lung injury. The goal of positioning is to facilitate or optimize V/Q matching and thus help to alleviate hypoxemia. Patients with unilateral lung disease should be positioned with the good lung down.[16-18] Patients with diffuse lung disease should be positioned prone with the right lung down and/or should be continuously turned. Some patients benefit from nonrecumbent positions, such as sitting or a semierect position.[18] Although not often used, the prone position has also been shown to increase oxygenation in patients with severe respiratory failure.[16,17]

Preventing desaturation. A number of activities can prevent desaturation from occurring. These include performing procedures only as needed, hyperoxygenating the patient before suctioning, providing adequate rest and recovery time between various procedures,[18,19] and minimizing oxygen consumption.[20] Interventions to minimize oxygen consumption include limiting the patient's physical activity, administering sedation to control anxiety, and providing measures to control fever.[20] The patient should be continuously monitored with a pulse oximeter to warn of signs of desaturation.[19]

Promoting secretion clearance. Interventions to promote secretion clearance include those that prevent secretion retention and those that facilitate secretion removal. Actions to prevent secretion retention include providing adequate systemic hydration, humidifying supplemental oxygen, and preventing hypoventilation. Activities to facilitate secretion removal include suctioning (endotracheal or nasotracheal) and chest physical therapy (percussion, vibration, postural drainage, and coughing).[19]

Preventing hypoventilation. To facilitate deep breathing, the patient's thorax should be maintained in alignment and the head of the bed elevated at least 30 degrees. This position best accommodates diaphragmatic descent and intercostal muscle action. Frequent repositioning (at least every 2 hours) or lateral rotation therapy is essential because it results in a change in ventilatory pattern and V/Q matching.[19]

Once the patient is extubated, deep breathing and incentive spirometry should be started as soon as possible. Deep breathing involves having the patient take a deep breath and hold it for approximately 3 seconds or longer. Incentive spirometry involves having the patient take at least 10 deep, effective breaths per hour using an incentive spirometer. These actions help prevent atelectasis and reexpand any collapsed lung tissue. The chest should be auscultated during inflation to ensure that all dependent parts of the lung are well ventilated and to help the patient understand the depth of breath necessary for optimal effect. Coughing should be avoided unless secretions are present because it promotes collapse of the smaller airways.[19]

Facilitating nutritional support

The initiation of nutritional support is of utmost importance in the management of the patient with ARF. The goals of nutritional support are to improve the patient's overall nutritional status, enhance the immune system, and promote respiratory muscle function. Because of the severity of the patient's illness, initially the patient may be started on total parenteral nutrition (TPN) with the goal to change to enteral feedings as soon as the patient is able to tolerate them.[7,10]

Patient education

Early in the patient's hospital stay, the patient and family should be taught about acute respiratory failure, its etiologies and its treatment. As the patient moves toward discharge, teaching should focus on the interventions necessary for preventing the reoccurrence of the precipitating disorder. If the patient smokes, he or she should be encouraged to stop smoking and should be referred to a smoking cessation program. In addition, the importance of participating in a pulmonary rehabilitation program should be stressed.

ACUTE RESPIRATORY DISTRESS SYNDROME

Description and Etiology

Acute (formerly called "adult") respiratory distress syndrome (ARDS)[20] is an inflammatory syndrome marked by disruption of the alveolar-capillary membrane.[21] A number of theories postulate that ARDS is part of the multisystem response to injury. Instead of multiple organ dysfunction syndrome (MODS) being the consequence of

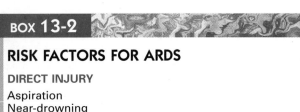

RISK FACTORS FOR ARDS

DIRECT INJURY

Aspiration
Near-drowning
Toxic inhalation
Pulmonary contusion
Pneumonia
Oxygen toxicity
Transthoracic radiation

INDIRECT INJURY

Sepsis
Nonthoracic trauma
Hypertransfusion
Cardiopulmonary bypass
Severe pancreatitis
Embolism—air, fat, amniotic fluid
Disseminated intravascular coagulation (DIC)
Shock states

ARDS, newer theories indicate that ARDS starts from the same inflammatory–immune-mediated response and is part of MODS. ARDS appears to occur first because of the immediate nature of impaired gas exchange.[22] The mortality rate from ARDS has been declining over the last several years, but it still ranges from 23% to 57%, depending on the initiating event.[23]

Although any number of DRGs may apply to the patient with ARDS, depending on the underlying cause and subsequent treatment, usually DRG 475 (Respiratory System Diagnosis with Ventilator Support) is used with an anticipated length of stay of 11.6 days.[4]

A wide variety of clinical conditions are associated with the development of ARDS[20,24,25] (Box 13-2). They can be divided into direct and indirect injuries, depending on the primary event or site of injury. Sepsis, aspiration of gastric contents, pulmonary contusion, pneumonia and near drowning have been found to be major risk factors.[24]

Pathophysiology

Although the exact cause of ARDS is unclear, it is generally believed that stimulation of the inflammatory-immune system initiates a systemic response that includes the sequestering of neutrophils in the lungs, activation of alveolar macrophages, and the release of endotoxin (Fig. 13-1). Once stimulated, these cellular systems release a variety of mediators that result in increased capillary membrane permeability, changes in the diameter of the small airways, pulmonary vasoconstriction, injury to the pulmonary vasculature, and microemboli formation in the lungs. Several of the mediators implicated in this response are oxygen-free radicals, tumor necrosis factor, interleukin 1, proteases, platelet-activating factor, and eicosanoids.[24,26]

Permeability defect

Increased capillary membrane permeability results in a permeability defect, which allows leakage of fluid and protein in the pulmonary interstitium. As the fluid and protein accumulate in the interstitium, normal local controlling factors (e.g., oncotic pressure, capillary hydrostatic pressure, lymphatic drainage) are overwhelmed and damage to the type I alveolar epithelial cells occurs. Eventually, fluid and protein enter the alveoli and damage the type II alveolar epithelial cells, resulting in impaired surfactant production. Injury to the cells and the loss of surfactant leads to alveoli collapse, resulting in intrapulmonary shunting, V/Q mismatching, decreased functional residual capacity (FRC), and decreased lung compliance.[22,24,26]

Bronchoconstriction

Changes in the diameter of the small airways leads to bronchoconstriction, which results in increased airway resistance, decreased lung compliance, and increased V/Q mismatching. Hypoxemia and the work of breathing increases, leading to fatigue and hypoventilation, which further heightens hypoxemia.[24,26]

Pulmonary hypertension

Injury to the pulmonary vasculature leads to structural abnormalities and vascular remodeling, resulting in pulmonary hypertension. The formation of microemboli in the lungs and pulmonary artery vasoconstriction also contribute to the development of elevated pulmonary pressures. In addition, damage to the pulmonary circuit can lead to impairment of the compensatory response of hypoxic vasoconstriction. The end result is increased alveolar dead space, V/Q mismatching, and intrapulmonary shunting that further increase hypoxemia and the work of breathing. Pulmonary hypertension also increases right ventricular afterload and can lead to right ventricular dysfunction and decreased cardiac output.[26]

Assessment and Diagnosis

The patient with ARDS may present with a variety of clinical manifestations, depending on the precipitating event. Initially, the patient presents with tachypnea, restlessness, apprehension, and moderate accessory muscle use progressing to agitation, dyspnea, fatigue, excessive accessory muscle use and fine crackles as respiratory failure occurs.[24,26]

Arterial blood gas analysis reveals a low PaO_2, despite increases in supplemental oxygen administration (refractory hypoxemia).[25,26] Initially the $PaCO_2$ is low, as a result of hyperventilation, but eventually the $PaCO_2$ increases as the patient fatigues. The pH is high initially but decreases as respiratory acidosis develops.[21,25]

Initially the chest x-ray may be normal because changes in the lungs do not become evident for up to 24 hours. As the pulmonary edema becomes apparent, diffuse patchy interstitial and alveolar infiltrates appear.

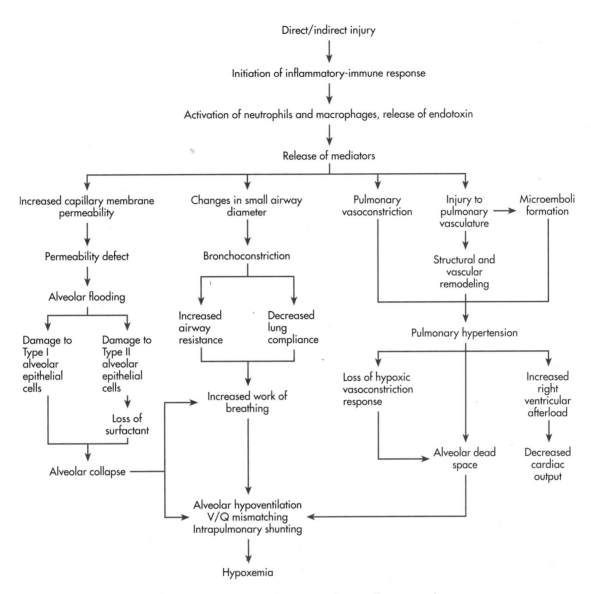

Fig. **13-1** Pathophysiology of acute respiratory distress syndrome.

This progresses to multifocal consolidation of the lungs, which appears as a "white out" on the chest x-ray.[24,27]

Many different criteria have been used to diagnose ARDS, which has led to confusion. In 1992, the American-European Consensus Committee on ARDS recommended defining ARDS as acute in onset, PaO_2/FIO_2 less than or equal to 200 mm Hg (regardless of PEEP level), bilateral infiltrates on chest radiography, and a pulmonary artery wedge pressure less than or equal to 18 mm Hg or no clinical evidence of left atrial hypertension.[20]

Medical Management

Medical management of the patient with ARDS involves a multifaceted approach. This strategy includes treating the underlying cause, promoting gas exchange, supporting tissue oxygenation, and monitoring for complications.[22,25] Medical interventions to promote gas exchange include supplemental oxygen administration, PEEP, intubation, and mechanical ventilation.[22,20]

Oxygenation

Oxygen should be administered at the lowest level possible to support tissue oxygenation. Continued exposure to high levels of oxygen can lead to oxygen toxicity, which further perpetuates the entire process. The goal of oxygen therapy is to maintain a SaO_2 of 90 mm Hg or greater using the lowest FIO_2. Because the hypoxemia that develops with ARDS is often refractory to oxygen therapy, it is usually necessary to facilitate oxygenation with PEEP.[22,25,27]

Ventilation

Intubation and mechanical ventilation are usually required to facilitate ventilation, particularly as fatigue develops and ventilatory failure occurs. During the acute phase of ARDS, the patient should receive complete ventilatory support. This allows the ventilator to do the majority of the work of breathing and the patient to rest. Usually the assist/control (also known as continuous mandatory ventilation) mode and the synchronized intermittent mandatory ventilation (SIMV) mode are used. The assist/control mode allows the patient to rest completely, thus decreasing the work of breathing. The SIMV mode allows the patient to be ventilated with lower mean airway pressures, thus reducing the incident of hemodynamic compromise and barotrauma.[27]

An alternative ventilatory modality that is also used in managing the patient with ARDS is inverse ratio ventilation (IRV), either pressure-controlled or volume-controlled. IRV prolongs the inspiratory (I) time and shortens the expiratory (E) time, thus reversing the normal I:E ratio. The effect is intentional air trapping, which increases functional residual capacity (FRC) and alveolar recruitment while maintaining lower airway pressures. Disadvantages to IRV include the development of auto-PEEP, which can cause hemodynamic compromise and worsening gas exchange. In addition, patients on IRV usually require neuromuscular blockade and sedation to prevent them from fighting the ventilator.[24,25,27]

Tissue perfusion

Interventions to support tissue perfusion include cautious fluid management and maintenance of CO. Newer approaches to fluid management include maintaining a very low intravascular volume (pulmonary artery wedge pressure of 5 to 8 mm Hg) with fluid restriction and diuretics while supporting the CO with vasoactive and inotropic medications. The goal is to decrease the amount of fluid leakage into the lungs.[22,25,27]

Nursing Management

Nursing management of the patient with ARDS incorporates a variety of nursing diagnoses (Box 13-3). **Nursing priorities are directed toward optimizing oxygenation and ventilation, maximizing tissue perfusion, facilitating nutritional support, providing comfort and emotional support, and maintaining surveillance for complications.**

Optimizing oxygenation and ventilation

Nursing interventions to optimize oxygenation and ventilation include positioning, preventing desaturation, and promoting secretion clearance. For further discussion on these interventions see section, Acute Respiratory Failure, Nursing Management.

Maximizing tissue perfusion

Adequate tissue perfusion depends on an adequate supply of oxygen being transported to the tissues. An adequate CO and hemoglobin level are critical to oxygen transport. CO depends on heart rate, preload, afterload,

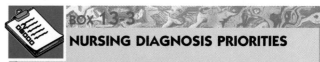

BOX 13-3

NURSING DIAGNOSIS PRIORITIES

Acute Respiratory Distress Syndrome

- Impaired Gas Exchange related to ventilation/perfusion mismatching or intrapulmonary shunting, p. 476
- Decreased Cardiac Output related to alterations in preload, pp. 467-468
- Altered Nutrition: Less than Body Requirements related to lack of exogenous nutrients or increased metabolic demand, p. 460
- Anxiety related to threat to biologic, psychologic, or social integrity, pp. 448-450
- Ineffective Family Coping: Compromised related to critically ill family member, pp. 452-453

and contractility. A variety of fluids and medications are used to manipulate this parameter. The types of fluids include both crystalloids and colloids. The types of medications include vasoconstrictors, vasodilators, positive inotropes, antidysrhythmics, and diuretics.[24,26]

Facilitating nutritional support

The initiation of nutritional support is of utmost importance in the management of the patient with ARDS. The goals of nutritional support are to improve the patient's overall nutritional status, enhance the immune system, and prevent the development of multiple organ dysfunction syndrome. Because of the severity of the patient's illness, initially the patient may be started on total parenteral nutrition (TPN) with the goal to change to enteral feedings as soon as the patient is able to tolerate them.[24,21]

PNEUMONIA

Description and Etiology

Pneumonia is an acute inflammation of the lung parenchyma caused by an infectious agent that can lead to alveolar consolidation. Pneumonia can be classified as community-acquired (CAP) or hospital-acquired (HAP) (nosocomial). Community-acquired is pneumonia acquired outside of the hospital and is usually less virulent than hospital-acquired pneumonia. CAP can be further classified as typical or atypical pneumonia. Typical pneumonia is an infection produced by bacterial organisms that normally inhabit the nasopharyngeal airway. Atypical pneumonia is an infection acquired from inhalation of organisms from the environment. Hospital-acquired (HAP) is pneumonia that is acquired inside the hospital and is usually much more serious than CAP as many of the causative agents are resistant to conventional antibiotic therapy.[28] Ventilator-associated pneumonia (VAP) is a subgroup of HAP that refers to an infection developed during mechanical ventilation more than 48 hours after intubation.[29]

Pneumonia falls under two different DRGs, depending on whether the patient develops complications or co-morbid conditions (CC). DRG 79 (Respiratory Infections and Inflammation, Age >17 Years with CC) and DRG 80 (Respiratory Infections and Inflammation, Age >17 Years Without CC) have average lengths of the stay of 8.7 days and 6.1 days respectively.[4] If the patient requires intubation, DRG 475 (Respiratory System Diagnosis with Ventilator Support) is then used with an expected length of stay of 11.6 days.[4]

The etiologies of pneumonia vary greatly with the type. Causes of typical CAP include *Streptococcus pneumoniae, Haemophilus influenzae,* and *Moraxella catarrhalis.*[30] Causes of atypical CAP include *Mycoplasma pneumoniae, Chlamydia pneumoniae,* and *Legionella pneumophila.*[30] *Pneumocystis carinii* is the predominate cause of pulmonary infection in patients with AIDS.[31] Nosocomial pneumonia is usually caused by *Pseudomonas aeruginosa, Haemophilus influenzae, Staphylococcus aureus, Klebsiella pneumoniae, Enterobacter* species, and *Escherichia coli.*[32] Often, institutions have their own resident flora that predominate in nosocomial infection. Usually the pathogens are the aerobic gram-negative bacilli[27] from the aquatic environment of the hospital.[30]

There are a number of conditions that predispose a patient to developing pneumonia, including depressed gag and cough reflexes, decreased ciliary activity, increased secretions, decreased lymphatic flow, atelectasis, fluid in the alveoli, immunologic defect, and impaired alveolar macrophages.[33] Table 13-2 lists the precipitating conditions and their causes.

Risk factors for these conditions are host-related, device-related, and personnel/procedure-related. Host-related factors include age greater than 65 years, underlying illness (e.g., COPD, immunosuppression, diabetes), alcoholism, smoking, depressed consciousness and malnutrition, and thoracic or abdominal surgery. Device-related factors include endotracheal intubation, mechanical ventilation, and gastric intubation with enteral feedings. Personnel/procedure-related factors include cross-contamination by hands, infected personnel, antibiotic therapy, and histamine blockers and antacid therapy.[32,34] Histamine blockers, antacid therapy, and enteral feedings elevate the pH of the stomach and promote bacterial overgrowth. The nasogastric tube acts as a wick, facilitating the movement of bacteria to the oropharynx where it can be aspirated.[28]

Pathophysiology

Development of acute pneumonia implies a defect in host defenses, a particularly virulent organism, or an overwhelming inoculation event. Bacterial invasion of the lower respiratory tract can occur by inhalation, aspiration, migration from adjacent sites or colonization, direct inoculation, exogenous penetration from an infected site, or hematogenous seeding from another site. The most common method appears to be microaspiration of bacteria colonized in the upper airway[35] (Figure 13-2).

The oropharynx has a stable population of resident flora that may be anaerobic or aerobic. When stress occurs, such as with illness, surgery, or a viral infection, pathogenic organisms replace normal resident flora. Previous antibiotic therapy affects the resident flora population, making replacement by pathologic organisms more likely. The pathogens are then able to invade the sterile lower respiratory tract. Critically ill patients usually have gram-negative bacteria present in the oropharynx. Disruption of the gag and cough reflexes, altered consciousness, abnormal swallowing, and artificial airways all predispose the patient to aspiration and colonization of the lungs and subsequent infection. Histamine blockers, antacids, and enteral feedings also contribute to this problem as they raise the pH of the stomach and promote bacterial overgrowth. The nasogastric tube then acts as a wick facilitating the movement of bacteria from the stomach to the pharynx where it can be aspirated.[32,36]

Infection results in pulmonary inflammation with or without significant exudates. Increased capillary permeability occurs with increased interstitial and alveolar

TABLE **13-2**	
PRECIPITATING CONDITIONS OF PNEUMONIA	
CONDITION	**ETIOLOGIES**
Depressed epiglottal and cough reflexes	Unconsciousness, neurologic disease, endotracheal or tracheal tubes, anesthesia, aging
Decreased cilia activity	Smoke inhalation, smoking history, oxygen toxicity, hypoventilation, intubation, viral infections, aging, COPD
Increased secretion	COPD, viral infections, bronchiectasis, general anesthesia, endotracheal intubation, smoking
Atelectasis	Trauma, foreign body obstruction, tumor, splinting, shallow ventilations, general anesthesia
Decreased lymphatic flow	CHF, tumor
Fluid in alveoli	CHF, aspiration, trauma
Abnormal phagocytosis and humoral activity	Neutropenia, immunocompetent disorders, patients receiving chemotherapy
Impaired alveolar macrophages	Hypoxemia, metabolic acidosis, cigarette smoking history, hypoxia, alcohol use, viral infections, aging

COPD, Chronic obstructive pulmonary disease; *CHF,* congestive heart failure.

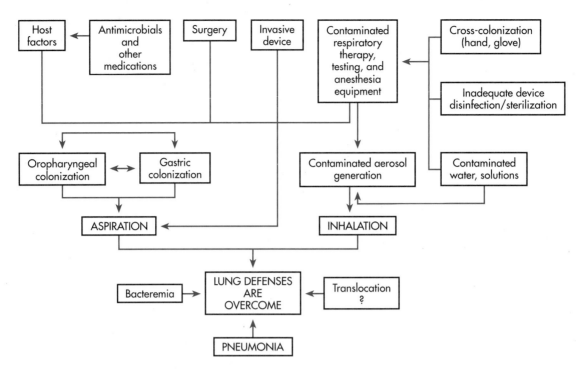

Fig. **13-2** Pathophysiology of pneumonia. (From Tablan OC, et al: Guideline for prevention of nosocomial pneumonia. Part 1. Issues on prevention of nosocomial pneumonia—1994, *Am J Infect Contr* 22:247, 1994.)

fluid. V/Q mismatching and intrapulmonary shunting occur, resulting in hypoxemia as lung consolidation progresses.

Untreated pneumonia can result in ARF and initiation of the inflammatory-immune response. In addition, the patient may develop a pleural effusion. This is the result of the vascular response to inflammation, whereby capillary permeability is increased and fluid from the pulmonary capillaries diffuses into the pleural space.[33]

Assessment and Diagnosis

The clinical manifestations of pneumonia will vary with the type of pneumonia. Typical pneumonia usually presents with fever and chills, productive cough, purulent sputum, crackles on auscultation, localized alveolar infiltrates on chest-ray, and leukocytosis. The diagnosis is usually made based on positive gram-stain and confirmed with positive cultures.[28]

Atypical pneumonia usually presents with flu-like symptoms, nonproductive cough, little sputum, crackles and rhonchi on auscultation, diffuse alveolar infiltrates on chest x-ray, and normal or slightly elevated WBC count. Sputum cultures usually fail to identify the offending organism, thus the diagnosis is usually made with a positive serology, although the test may take weeks to be diagnostic. Sputum gram-stains are usually negative also, although a variety of other staining techniques (e.g., direct fluorescent antibody, acid-fast stain, potassium hydroxide preparation) may be more helpful.[28]

The clinical manifestations of HAP are similar to those of CAP but will depend on the patient's underlying condition. Nosocomial pneumonia has an onset greater than 72 hours after hospitalization. Physical examination shows rales or dullness to percussion or an infiltrate on the chest x-ray and at least one of the following findings; purulent sputum, isolation of a pathogen from blood, transtracheal aspirate, biopsy specimen, or a bronchial brush specimen, isolation of a virus in respiratory secretions, diagnostic antibody titers, or histopathologic evidence of pneumonia.[36]

Medical Management

Medical management of the patient with pneumonia should include antibiotic therapy, oxygen therapy for hypoxemia, mechanical ventilation if acute respiratory failure develops, fluid management for hydration, nutritional support, and treatment of associated medical problems and complications. For patients having difficulty mobilizing secretions, mucolytics and therapeutic bronchoscopy may be necessary.

Antibiotic therapy

Although bacteria-specific antibiotic therapy is the goal, this may not always be possible because of difficulties in identifying the organism and the seriousness of the patient's condition. The time involved obtaining cultures should be balanced against the need to begin some treatment based on patient condition. Empirical therapy has

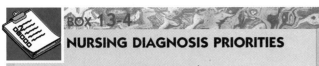

BOX 13-5

RISK FACTORS FOR ASPIRATION

Altered level of consciousness
Depressed gag, cough, or swallowing reflexes
Presence of feeding tubes (all types)
Presence of artificial airways
Ileus or gastric distention
History of gastrointestinal disorders
    Dysphagia
    Achalasia
    Gastroesophageal reflux disease
    Esophageal strictures

become a generally acceptable approach. In this approach, choice of antibiotic treatment is based on the most likely etiologic organism while avoiding toxicity, superinfection, and unnecessary cost. If available, gram stain results should be used to guide choices of antibiotics. Antibiotics should be chosen that offer broad coverage of the usual pathogens in the hospital or community. Failure to respond to such therapy may indicate that the chosen antibiotic regimen does not appropriately cover all of the etiologic pathogens or that a new source of infection has developed.[30]

Nursing Management

Nursing management of the patient with pneumonia incorporates a variety of nursing diagnoses (Box 13-4). **Nursing priorities are directed toward optimizing oxygenation and ventilation, preventing the spread of infection, providing comfort and emotional support, and maintaining surveillance for complications.** In addition, the patient's response to the antibiotic therapy should be monitored for adverse effects.

Optimizing oxygenation and ventilation

Nursing interventions to optimize oxygenation and ventilation include positioning, preventing desaturation, and promoting secretion clearance. For further discussion on these interventions, see the section Acute Respiratory Failure, Nursing Management.

Preventing the spread of infection

Prevention should be directed at eradicating pathogens from the hospital environment and interrupting the spread of organisms from person to person. Significant progress has been made in removing contaminants from the patient environment through proper disinfection of respiratory equipment and increased use of disposable supplies. Other possible environmental sources of pathogens include suctioning equipment and indwelling lines. These invasive tools must be given proper aseptic care. Proper hand-washing technique is the single most impor-

tant measure available to prevent the spread of bacteria from person to person.[35] In addition, meticulous oral care is critical in decreasing the bacterial colonization of the oropharynx.

ASPIRATION LUNG DISORDER

Description and Etiology

The presence of abnormal substances in the airways and alveoli as a result of aspiration is misleadingly called *aspiration pneumonia.* This term is misleading because the aspiration of toxic substances into the lung may or may not involve an infection. Aspiration lung disorder is a more accurate title because injury to the lung can result from the chemical, mechanical, and/or bacterial characteristics of the aspirate.

Aspiration lung disorder falls under two different DRGs, depending on whether the patient develops complications or comorbid conditions (CC). DRG 101 (Other Respiratory System Diagnoses With CC) and DRG 102 (Other Respiratory System Diagnoses Without CC) have average lengths of the stay of 4.7 days and 2.9 days, respectively.[4] If the patient requires intubation, DRG 475 (Respiratory System Diagnosis with Ventilator Support) is then used with an expected length of stay of 11.6 days.[4]

Etiology

A number of factors have been identified that place the patient at risk for aspiration (Box 13-5). Gastric contents and oropharyngeal bacteria are the most common things aspirated by the critically ill patient.[37] The effects of gastric contents on the lungs will vary based on the pH of the liquid. If the pH is less than 2.5, then the patient will develop a severe chemical pneumonitis resulting in hypoxemia.[38,39] If the pH is greater than 2.5, the immediate damage to the lungs will be lessened[38] but the elevated pH may indicate bacterial overgrowth of the stomach.[39] Once the gastric contents are aspirated into the lungs, overwhelming bacterial pneumonia can develop.[35,39]

Pathophysiology

The type of lung injury that develops after aspiration is determined by a number of factors, including the quality and volume of the aspirate and the status of the patient's respiratory defense mechanisms.

Nonacid liquid contents

The aspiration of nonacid (pH >2.5) liquid gastric contents is similar to acid liquid aspiration initially but with minimal structural damage occurring. Intrapulmonary shunting and V/Q mismatching usually start to reverse within 4 hours and hypoxemia clears within 24 hours.[38]

Nonacid food particles

The aspiration of nonacid (pH >2.5) nonobstructing food particles is similar to acid aspiration initially, with significant edema and hemorrhage occurring within 6 hours. After the initial reaction, the response changes to a foreign body-type reaction with granuloma formation occurring around the food particles within 1 to 5 days. In addition to hypoxemia, hypercapnia and acidosis occur as a result of hypoventilation.[38]

Acid liquid contents

The aspiration of acid (pH <2.5) liquid gastric contents results in the development of bronchospasm and atelectasis almost immediately. Over the next 4 hours, tracheal damage, bronchitis, bronchiolitis, alveolar-capillary breakdown, interstitial edema, and alveolar congestion and hemorrhage occurs. Severe hypoxemia develops as a result of intrapulmonary shunting and V/Q mismatching. The clinical course will follow one of three patterns: (1) rapid improvement in 1 week, (2) initial improvement followed by deterioration and development of ARDS or pneumonia, (3) rapid death from progressive ARF.[37-39]

Acid food particles

The aspiration of acid (pH <2.5) nonobstructing food particles can produce the most severe pulmonary reaction because of extensive pulmonary damage. Severe hypoxemia, hypercapnia, and acidosis occur.[38,39]

Assessment and Diagnosis

Clinically, the patient presents with signs of acute respiratory distress[37] and gastric contents may be present in the oropharynx.[38] The patient will have shortness of breath, coughing, wheezing, cyanosis, and signs of hypoxemia.[38] Tachypnea, tachycardia, hypotension, fever, and crackles also are present. Copious amounts of sputum are produced as alveolar edema develops.[37]

ABGs reflect severe hypoxemia. Chest x-ray changes appear 12 to 24 hours after the initial aspiration with no one pattern being diagnostic of the event. Infiltrates will appear in a variety of distribution patterns, depending on the position of the patient during aspiration and the volume of the aspiration. If bacterial infection becomes established, leukocytosis and positive sputum cultures occur.[37,39]

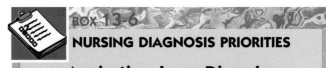

NURSING DIAGNOSIS PRIORITIES

Aspiration Lung Disorder

- Impaired Gas Exchange related to ventilation/perfusion mismatching or intrapulmonary shunting, p. 476
- Ineffective Airway Clearance related to excessive secretions or abnormal viscosity of mucus, pp. 472-473
- Risk for Aspiration, pp. 477-478
- Risk for Infection, pp. 494-495
- Ineffective Individual Coping related to situational crisis and personal vulnerability, pp. 453-455

Medical Management

Management of the patient with aspiration lung disorder includes both emergency and follow-up treatment. When aspiration is witnessed, emergency treatment should be instituted to secure the airway and minimize pulmonary damage. The patient should be placed in a slight (6 to 8 inches head-down) Trendelenburg position and turned to the right lateral decubitus position to aid drainage and avoid involvement of other lung areas. Oropharyngeal suctioning should immediately follow.[38] Direct visualization by bronchoscopy is indicated to remove large particulate aspirate or to confirm an unwitnessed aspiration event. Bronchoalveolar lavage is not recommended because this practice disseminates the aspirate in lungs and increases damage. Prophylactic antibiotics are not recommended either.[38]

After airway clearance, attention should be given to supporting oxygenation and hemodynamics. Hypoxemia should be corrected with supplemental oxygen or mechanical ventilation with PEEP, if necessary. Hemodynamic changes result from fluid shifts that can occur after massive aspirations, causing noncardiogenic pulmonary edema. Monitoring intravascular volume is essential, and judicious amounts of replacement fluids should be instituted to maintain adequate urinary output and vital signs.[37,38]

Nursing Management

Nursing management of the patient with aspiration lung disorder incorporates a variety of nursing diagnoses (Box 13-6). **Nursing priorities are directed toward optimizing oxygenation and ventilation, preventing further aspiration events, providing comfort and emotional support, and maintaining surveillance for complications.**

Optimizing oxygenation and ventilation

Nursing interventions to optimize oxygenation and ventilation include positioning, preventing desaturation, and promoting secretion clearance. For further discussion on these interventions, see section, Acute Respiratory Failure, Nursing Management.

Preventing aspiration

One of the most important interventions to prevent aspiration is identifying the patient at risk for aspiration. Actions to prevent aspiration include confirming feeding tube placement, checking for signs and symptoms of feeding intolerance and aspiration of gastric contents into lungs, elevating the head of the bed at least 30 degrees or turning patients on the right side if they must remain flat, ensuring proper inflation of artificial airway cuffs, and frequent suctioning of the oropharynx of intubated patients to prevent secretions from pooling above the cuff of the tube.[40]

PULMONARY EMBOLUS

Description and Etiology

A pulmonary embolus (PE) occurs when a clot (thrombotic emboli) or other matter (nonthrombotic emboli) lodges in the pulmonary arterial system, disrupting the blood flow to a region of the lungs. The majority of thrombotic emboli arise from the deep leg veins, particularly the iliac, femoral, and popliteal veins.[41] Other sources include the right ventricle, the upper extremities, and the pelvic veins. Nonthrombotic emboli arise from fat, tumors, amniotic fluid, air, and foreign bodies.[42] This section will focus on thrombotic emboli.

Pulmonary embolus falls under DRG 78 (Pulmonary Embolism) with an average length of the stay of 7.7 days.[4] If the patient requires intubation, DRG 475 (Respiratory System Diagnosis with Ventilator Support) is then used with an expected length of stay of 11.6 days.[4]

A number of predisposing factors and precipitating conditions put a patient at risk for developing a PE (Box 13-7). Of the three predisposing factors (e.g., hypercoagulability, injury to vascular endothelium, and venous stasis [Virchow's triad]), venous stasis appears to be the most significant.[43]

Pathophysiology

A massive PE occurs with the blockage of a lobar or larger artery, resulting in occlusion of more than 40% of the pulmonary vascular bed. Blockage of the pulmonary arterial system has both pulmonary and hemodynamic consequences. The effects on the pulmonary system are increased alveolar dead space, bronchoconstriction, and compensatory shunting. The hemodynamic effects include an increase in pulmonary vascular resistance and right ventricular workload.[44]

Increased dead space

An increase in alveolar dead space occurs because an area of the lung is receiving ventilation without being perfused. The ventilation to this area is known as wasted ventilation because it does not participate in gas exchange. This effect leads to alveolar dead-space ventilation and an increase in the work of breathing. To limit the amount of dead-space ventilation, localized bronchoconstriction occurs.[44]

BOX 13-7

RISK FACTORS FOR PULMONARY THROMBOEMBOLISM

PREDISPOSING FACTORS

Venous stasis
    Atrial fibrillation
    Decreased cardiac output (CO)
    Immobility
Injury to vascular endothelium
    Local vessel injury
    Infection
    Incision
    Atherosclerosis
Hypercoagulability
    Polycythemia

PRECIPITATING CONDITIONS

Previous pulmonary embolus
Cardiovascular disease
    Congestive heart failure
    Right ventricular infarction
    Cardiomyopathy
    Cor pulmonale
Surgery
    Orthopedic
    Vascular
    Abdominal
Cancer
    Ovarian
    Pancreatic
    Stomach
    Extrahepatic bile duct system
Trauma (injury or burns)
    Lower extremities
    Pelvis
    Hips
Gynecologic status
    Pregnancy
Postpartum period
Birth control pills
Estrogen replacement therapy

Bronchoconstriction

Bronchoconstriction develops as a result of alveolar hypocarbia, hypoxia, and the release of mediators. Alveolar hypocarbia occurs as a consequence of decreased carbon dioxide in the affected area and leads to constriction of the local airways, increased airway resistance, and redistribution of ventilation to perfused areas of the lungs. A variety of mediators are released from the site of the injury, either from the clot or the surrounding lung tissue, which further causes constriction of the airways.[44] Bronchoconstriction promotes the development of atelectasis.[43]

Compensatory shunting

Compensatory shunting occurs as a result of the unaffected areas of the lungs having to accommodate the entire cardiac output. This creates a situation where perfusion exceeds ventilation and blood is returned to the left side of the heart without participating in gas exchange. This leads to the development of hypoxemia.[44]

Hemodynamic consequences

The major hemodynamic consequence of a PE is the development of pulmonary hypertension, which is part of the effect of a mechanical obstruction when more than 50% of the vascular bed is occluded. In addition, the mediators released at the injury site and the development of hypoxia cause pulmonary vasoconstriction, which further exacerbates pulmonary hypertension. As the pulmonary vascular resistance increases, so does the workload of the right ventricle as reflected by a rise in PA pressures. Consequently, right ventricular failure occurs, which can lead to a decrease in left ventricular preload, decrease in cardiac output (CO), decrease in blood pressure, and shock.[44]

Assessment and Diagnosis

The patient with a PE may have any number of presenting clinical manifestations. Common symptoms include dyspnea, chest pain, cough, palpitations, apprehension, and diaphoresis. The chest pain is pleuritic in nature, with an abrupt onset, and is aggravated by deep breathing.[45,46] Syncope may be present if right ventricular failure occurs.[43]

Common signs include an increase in tachypnea, tachycardia, crackles, decreased breath sounds over the affected side, and low-grade fever.[45] If right ventricular failure occurs, distended neck veins and an S_3 on auscultation may be present. Additional signs that indicate right ventricular decompensation are fixed splitting of the second heart sound (P_2), resulting from delayed closure of the pulmonic valve, and a diastolic murmur, caused by pulmonic insufficiency.[46]

Initial laboratory studies that may be done are an ABG analysis, electrocardiogram (ECG), and chest radiography. ABGs may show a low PaO_2, indicating hypoxemia; a low $PaCO_2$, indicating hypocarbia; and a high pH, indicating a respiratory alkalosis. The hypocarbia with resulting respiratory alkalosis is caused by tachypnea.[45] Common ECG findings are transient ST segment depression and sinus tachycardia. The classic findings of P-pulmonale, S wave in lead I, and Q wave with inverted T wave in lead III are seen in less than 15% of the patients.[45] Chest x-ray findings vary from normal to abnormal with enlargement of the descending pulmonary artery, elevation of the diaphragm, and the presence of pleural effusion as the most common signs.[45]

Differentiating a PE from other illnesses can be difficult because many of its clinical manifestations are found in a variety of other disorders.[45] Thus a variety of other tests may be necessary, including a V/Q scan, pulmonary angiogram, and deep vein thrombosis (DVT) studies. A definitive diagnosis of a PE requires confirmation by a high probability V/Q scan, positive pulmonary angiogram, or strong clinical suspicion coupled with abnormal findings on lower extremity DVT studies.[44]

Medical Management

Prevention of PE is the first line of treatment for the disorder. Patients at risk for a thromboembolism should be placed on prophylactic anticoagulation with adjusted-dose heparin, low molecular weight heparin, or oral anticoagulants. High-risk patients should be anticoagulated to maintain the activated partial thromboplastin time (aPTT) in the high-normal range or an international normalization ratio (INR) of 2.0 to 2.5.[47]

Medical management for the patient with a PE includes both prophylactic and definitive measures and the correction of the hypoxemia.

Prophylactic measures

Prophylactic interventions are focused on preventing the recurrence of a PE and include the administration of heparin and warfarin (Coumadin) and interruption of the inferior vena cava.

Heparin is administered to prevent further clots from forming and has no effect on the existing clot. Heparin may be administered by continuous drip, intermittent intravenous injection, or subcutaneous injection. The heparin should be adjusted to maintain the aPTT at 1.5 to 2 times the control. Warfarin should be started at the same time, and, when the INR reaches 2.0 to 3.0, the heparin should be discontinued. The patient should remain on warfarin for at least 3 months.[47]

Interruption of the inferior vena cava is reserved for patients in whom anticoagulation is contraindicated. The procedure involves placement of a percutaneous venous filter into the vena cava usually below the renal arteries. The filter prevents further thrombotic emboli from migrating into the lungs.[44]

Definitive measures

Definitive actions are directed at treating the current PE and include the administration of thrombolytic agents and surgery to remove the clot. Measures to correct the hypoxemia include supplemental oxygen administration and intubation and mechanical ventilation.

The administration of thrombolytic agents in the treatment of PE has had limited success. Usually thrombolytic therapy is reserved for the patient with an acute massive PE and concomitant hemodynamic instability.[43] Either recombinant tissue-type plasminogen activator (rt-PA), streptokinase, or urokinase may be used. The therapeutic window for using thrombolytic therapy is 14 days.[48]

Surgical embolectomy is considered a last resort measure that involves the extraction of the embolus from the pulmonary arterial system. It is reserved for the patient with a massive PE refractory to all other measures. It is an extremely risky surgery with a high operative mortality.[44]

To reverse the hemodynamic effects of pulmonary hypertension, additional measures may be taken. These include the administration of inotropic agents and fluid. Fluids should be administered to increase right ven-

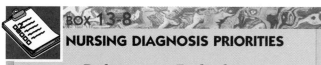

tricular preload, which will stretch the right ventricle and increase contractility, thus overcoming the elevated pulmonary arterial pressures. Inotropic agents also can be used to increase contractility to facilitate an increase in CO.[44]

Nursing Management

Prevention of PE should be a major nursing focus because the majority of critically ill patients are at risk for this disorder. **Nursing priorities are directed toward preventing the development of DVT, which is a major complication of immobility and a leading cause of PE.** These measures include the use of antiembolic stockings and/or pneumatic compression stockings, elevation of the legs, active/passive range of motion, adequate hydration, and progressive ambulation. Patients at risk should be routinely assessed for signs of a DVT, specifically, deep calf pain (Homan's sign), calf tenderness, or redness.[46]

Nursing management of the patient with a PE incorporates a variety of nursing diagnoses (Box 13-8). **Nursing priorities are directed toward optimizing oxygenation and ventilation, monitoring for bleeding, providing comfort and emotional support, and maintaining surveillance for complications.**

Optimizing oxygenation and ventilation

Nursing interventions to optimize oxygenation and ventilation include positioning, preventing desaturation, and promoting secretion clearance. For further discussion on these interventions, see section, Acute Respiratory Failure, Nursing Management.

Monitoring for bleeding

The patient receiving anticoagulant or thrombolytic therapy should be observed for signs of bleeding. The patient's gums, skin, urine, stool, and emesis should be screened for signs of overt or covert bleeding. In addition, following the patient's INR or aPTT is critical to managing the anticoagulation therapy.[46]

Patient education

Early in the patient's hospital stay, the patient and family should be taught about pulmonary embolus, its etiologies and its treatment. As the patient moves toward discharge, teaching should focus on the interventions necessary for preventing the reoccurrence of deep vein thrombosis and subsequent emboli, recognizing the signs and symptoms of deep vein thrombosis and anticoagulant complications, and adopting measures to prevent bleeding. If the patient smokes, he or she should be encouraged to stop smoking and referred to a smoking cessation program.

STATUS ASTHMATICUS

Description and Etiology

Acute asthma is a chronic obstructive pulmonary disease that is characterized by severe airflow obstruction as a result of bronchospasm, mucosal edema, and increased mucus production.[49] Status asthmaticus is a severe asthma attack that fails to respond to conventional therapy with bronchodilators and may result in acute respiratory failure.[50] The precipitating cause of the attack is usually an upper respiratory infection, allergen exposure, or a decrease in antiinflammatory medications.[50] Other factors that have been implicated include over-reliance on bronchodilators, environmental pollutants, lack of access to health care, failure to identify worsening airflow obstruction, and noncompliance with the health care regimen.[51]

Status asthmaticus falls under DRG 88 (Chronic Obstructive Pulmonary Disease) with an average length of the stay of 5.7 days, if the patient does not require intubation. If the patient does require intubation, DRG 475 (Respiratory System Diagnosis with Ventilator Support) is then used with an expected length of stay of 11.6 days.[4]

Pathophysiology

An asthma attack is initiated when exposure to a irritant or trigger occurs, resulting in the initiation of the inflammatory-immune response in the airways. Bronchospasm occurs along with increased vascular permeability and increased mucus production. Mucosal edema and thick tenacious mucus further increase airway responsiveness. The combination of bronchospasm, airway inflammation, and hyperresponsiveness results in narrowing of the airways and airflow obstruction.[49] These changes have significant effects on the pulmonary and cardiovascular system.

Pulmonary effects

As the diameter of the airway decreases, airway resistance increases, resulting in increased residual volume, hyperinflation of the lungs, increased work of breathing, and abnormal distribution of ventilation. V/Q mismatching occurs and results in hypoxemia. Alveolar dead space also increases as hypoxic vasoconstriction occurs and results in hypercapnia.[50]

Cardiovascular effects

Inspiratory muscle force also increases in an attempt to ventilate the hyperinflated lungs. This results in a significant increase in negative intrapleural pressure, leading to an increase in venous return and pooling of blood in the right ventricle. The stretched right ventricle causes the intraventricular septum to shift impinging on the left ventricle. In addition, the left ventricle has to work harder to pump blood from the markedly negative pressure in the thorax to elevated pressure in the systemic circulation. This leads to a decrease in cardiac output and a fall in systolic blood pressure on inspiration (pulsus paradoxus).[50]

Assessment and Diagnosis

Initially the patient may present with a cough, wheezing, and dyspnea. As the attack continues, the patient develops tachypnea, tachycardia, diaphoresis, increased accessory muscle use, and pulsus paradoxus greater than or equal to 25 mm Hg.[50] Decreased level of consciousness, inability to speak, significantly diminished or absent breath sounds, central cyanosis,[51] and inability to lie supine[52] herald the onset of acute respiratory failure.

Initial ABGs indicate hypocapnia and respiratory alkalosis caused by hyperventilation. As the attack continues and the patient starts to fatigue, hypoxemia and hypercapnia develop. Lactic acidosis may also occur from lactate overproduction of the respiratory muscles. The end result is the development of respiratory and metabolic acidosis.[50,51]

Deterioration of pulmonary function tests despite aggressive bronchodilator therapy is diagnostic of status asthmaticus and indicates a potential need for intubation. FEV_1 (maximum volume of gas that the patient can exhale in 1 second) and/or PEFR (maximum flow rate that the patient can generate) less than 30% to 50% of predicted or patient's personal best indicates severe airflow obstruction and the imminent need for intubation with mechanical ventilation.[52]

Medical Management

Medical management of the patient with status asthmaticus is directed toward supporting oxygenation and ventilation. Bronchodilators, corticosteroids, oxygen therapy, intubation, and mechanical ventilation are the mainstays of therapy.

Bronchodilators

Inhaled beta$_2$ agonists and anticholinergics are the bronchodilators of choice for status asthmaticus. Beta$_2$ agonists promote bronchodilation and can be administered by nebulizer or metered-dose inhaler (MDI).[49-52] Usually larger and more frequent doses are given,[52] and the drug is titrated to the patient's response.[50] Anticholinergics that inhibit bronchoconstriction are not very effective by themselves, but, in conjunction with beta$_2$ agonists, they have a synergistic effect and produce a greater improvement in airflow.[49-51] The routine use of xanthines is not recommended in the treatment of status asthmaticus because they have been shown to have no therapeutic benefit.[50,51]

Corticosteroids

Systemic corticosteroids are also used in the treatment of status asthmaticus. Their antiinflammatory effects limit mucosal edema, decrease mucus production, and potentiate beta$_2$ agonists. Inhaled corticosteroids should also be continued or started if the patient was not on them before the attack.[49,52] It usually takes 6 to 12 hours for the effects of the corticosteroids to become evident.[49-51]

Oxygen therapy

Initial treatment of hypoxemia is usually with supplemental oxygen. Low-flow oxygen therapy should be administered to keep the patient's SaO_2 greater than 92%.[50,52]

Intubation and mechanical ventilation

Indications for mechanical ventilation include cardiac or respiratory arrest,[51] disorientation,[52] failure to respond to bronchodilator therapy, and exhaustion.[50] A large endotracheal tube (≥ 8 mm) should be used to decrease airway resistance and to facilitate suctioning of secretions.[51,52] Ventilating the patient with status asthmaticus can be very difficult. High inflation pressures should be avoided as they can result in barotrauma. PEEP should also not be used as the patient is prone to developing air trapping. Patient-ventilator asynchrony can also be a major problem. Sedation and neuromuscular paralysis may be necessary to allow for adequate ventilation of the patient.[50-52]

Nursing Management

Nursing management of the patient with status asthmaticus incorporates a variety of nursing diagnoses (Box 13-9). **Nursing priorities are directed toward optimizing oxygenation and ventilation, providing comfort and emotional support, and maintaining surveillance for complications.**

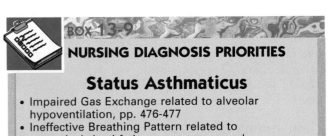

BOX 13-9

NURSING DIAGNOSIS PRIORITIES

Status Asthmaticus

- Impaired Gas Exchange related to alveolar hypoventilation, pp. 476-477
- Ineffective Breathing Pattern related to musculoskeletal fatigue or neuromuscular impairment, p. 474
- Ineffective Airway Clearance related to excessive secretions or abnormal viscosity of mucus, pp. 472-473
- Anxiety related to threat to biologic, psychologic, or social integrity, pp. 448-450
- Knowledge Deficit: Discharge Regimen related to lack of previous exposure to information, p. 443

Optimizing oxygenation and ventilation

Nursing interventions to optimize oxygenation and ventilation include positioning, preventing desaturation, and promoting secretion clearance. For further discussion on these interventions, see section Acute Respiratory Failure, Nursing Management.

Patient education

Early in the patient's hospital stay, the patient and family should be taught about asthma, its triggers and its treatment. As the patient moves toward discharge, teaching should focus on the interventions necessary to prevent the reoccurrence of status asthmaticus, early warning signs of worsening airflow obstruction, correct use of an inhaler and a peak flow meter, measures to prevent pulmonary infections, and signs and symptoms of a pulmonary infection. If the patient smokes, he or she should be encouraged to stop smoking and referred to a smoking cessation program. In addition, the importance of participating in a pulmonary rehabilitation program should be stressed.

THORACIC SURGERY

Types of Surgery

Thoracic surgery refers to a number of surgical procedures that involve opening the thoracic cavity (thoracotomy) and/or the organs of respiration. Indications for thoracic surgery range from tumors and abscesses to repair of the esophagus and thoracic vessels.[53] Table 13-3 describes a variety of thoracic surgical procedures and their indications.[54,55] This discussion focuses only on the surgical procedures that involve the removal of lung tissue.

Thoracic surgery falls under three different DRGs, depending on the type of surgery and whether the patient develops complications or comorbid conditions (CC). DRG 75 (Major Chest Procedures), DRG 76 (Other Respiratory System OR Procedures With CC), and DRG 77 (Other Respiratory System OR Procedures Without CC) have average lengths of the stay of 10.6 days, 11.7 days, and 5.1 days, respectively.[4]

Surgical Considerations

The type and location of surgery will dictate the type of surgical approach used. The most common approach is the posterolateral thoracotomy, which allows for exposure of both the lung and mediastinum. Other approaches that are used include anterolateral thoracotomy, axillary incision, and median sternotomy.[54]

Special care is taken to avoid drainage of blood or secretions into the unaffected lung during surgery because such an occurrence could cause hypoxemia and cardiac dysfunction. A double-lumen endotracheal tube is used during surgery to protect the unaffected lung from secretions and necrotic tumor fragments. In addition, the deflated lung is suctioned and ventilated every 20 to 30 minutes during the procedure.[55]

After a pneumonectomy, the mediastinal position requires evaluation. This is done on closure of the operative site and involves manometric measurement and a chest x-ray examination. With the patient lying in the supine position, pressure in the empty chest cavity should be -4 to -6 cm of H_2O pressure. When the pressure is abnormal, air or fluid can be added or withdrawn. If the abnormality is not corrected, a mediastinal shift can occur, resulting in hemodynamic compromise and cardiac dysfunction. A chest x-ray examination will show the location of the mediastinum.[54]

Complications and Medical Management

A number of complications are associated with a lung resection. These include acute respiratory failure, bronchopleural fistula, hemorrhage, cardiovascular disturbances, and mediastinal shift.

Bronchopleural fistula

Development of a postoperative bronchopleural fistula a major cause of mortality after a lung resection. A bronchopleural fistula develops when the suture line fails to secure occlusion of the bronchial stump and an opening develops. This can result from an imperfect stump closure, perforation of the stump (e.g., with a suction catheter), high pressure within the airways (e.g., caused by mechanical ventilation)[56] or infection.[57] During surgery, careful attention is given to isolating and closing the bronchus in an attempt to secure a lasting seal with subsequent stump healing.[54] In addition, early extubation is encouraged to eliminate the possibility of perforation of the stump and high airway pressures.[56] Clinical manifestations of a bronchopleural fistula include shortness of breath and coughing up serosanguineous sputum. Immediate surgery is usually necessary to close the stump to prevent flooding of the remaining lung with fluid from the residual space producing aspiration.[57] If this occurs, the patient should be placed with the operative side down (remaining lung up) and a chest tube should be inserted to drain the residual space.

Hemorrhage

Hemorrhage is an early, life-threatening complication that can occur after a lung resection. It can result from bronchial or intercostal artery bleeding or disruption of a suture or clip around a pulmonary vessel.[56] Excessive chest tube drainage can signal excessive bleeding. During the immediate postoperative period, chest tube drainage should be measured every 15 minutes, and this frequency decreased as the patient stabilizes. If chest tube loss is greater than 100 ml/hour, fresh blood is noted, or a sudden increase in drainage occurs, hemorrhage should be suspected.

Cardiovascular disturbances

Cardiovascular complications after thoracic surgery include dysrhythmias and pulmonary edema. Resections of a large lung area or a pneumonectomy may be

TABLE **13-3**

THORACIC SURGERIES

PROCEDURE	DEFINITION	INDICATIONS
Segmental resection (also called segmentectomy)	Resection of bronchovascular segment of lung lobe	Small peripheral lesions Patients with borderline lung function who would not tolerate a more extensive procedure
Wedge resection	Removal of small section of lung tissue	Small peripheral lesions (without lymph node involvement) Peripheral granulomas Pulmonary blebs
Lobectomy	Resection of one or more lobes of lung	Lesions confined to a single lobe Pulmonary tuberculosis Bronchiectasis Lung abscesses or cysts Trauma
Pneumonectomy	Removal of entire lung with or without resection of the mediastinal lymph nodes	Malignant lesions Unilateral tuberculosis Extensive unilateral bronchiectasis Multiple lung abscesses Massive hemoptysis Bronchopleural fistula
Bronchoplastic reconstruction (also called sleeve resection)	Resection of lung tissue and bronchus with end-to-end reanastomosis of bronchus	Small lesions involving the carina or major bronchus without evidence of metastasis May be combined with lobectomy
Decortication	Removal of fibrous membrane from pleural surface of lung	Fibrothorax resulting from hemothorax or empyema
Bullectomy	Resection of large bullae	Severe emphysema with large bullae compressing surrounding tissue
Lung reduction volume surgery (also called reduction pneumoplasty or pneumectomy)	Resection of the most damaged portions of lung tissue, allowing more normal chest-wall configuration	Emphysema
Tracheal resection	Resection of portion of trachea with end-to-end reanastomosis of trachea	Tracheal stenosis Tumors Trauma
Thoracoscopy	Endoscopic procedure performed through small incisions in the chest	Evaluation of pulmonary, pleural, mediastinal, or pericardial conditions Biopsy of lung, pleural, or mediastinal lesions Recurrent spontaneous pneumothorax Evacuation of emphysema, hemothorax, pleural effusion, or pericardial effusion Thymectomy Blebectomy/bullectomy Pleurodesis Sympathectomy Closure of bronchopleural fistula Lysis of adhesions

followed by a rise in central venous pressure. With the loss of one lung, the right ventricle must empty its stroke volume into a vascular bed that has been reduced by 50%. This means a higher pressure system is created, which increases right-ventricular workload, precipitating right ventricular failure. Depending on previous heart function, acute decompensation of both ventricles can result. Measures are aimed at supporting cardiac function and avoiding intravascular volume excess. These mea-

sures include optimizing preload, afterload, and contractility with vasoactive agents.[55,56]

Mediastinal shift

The pneumonectomy patient should be also monitored for a shift in the mediastinum. The mediastinal position can be determined by palpating for tracheal deviation, palpating and auscultating the position of the apex of the heart, and performing a chest x-ray examination. If

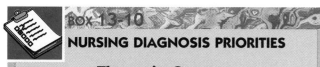

NURSING DIAGNOSIS PRIORITIES

Thoracic Surgery

- Ineffective Breathing Pattern related to decreased lung expansion, pp. 473-474
- Impaired Gas Exchange related to alveolar hypoventilation, pp. 476-477
- Acute Pain related to transmission and perception of cutaneous, visceral, muscular, or ischemic impulses, pp. 461-464
- Body Image Disturbance related to actual change in body structure, function, or appearance, p. 451
- Ineffective Family Coping: Compromised related to critically ill family member, pp. 452-453

BOX 13-10

a mediastinal shift occurs, it should be corrected by injecting or withdrawing air or fluid.[57]

Postoperative Nursing Management

Nursing care of the patient with thoracic surgery incorporates a number of nursing diagnoses (Box 13-10). **Nursing priorities are directed toward optimizing oxygenation and ventilation, preventing atelectasis, monitoring chest tubes, assisting the patient to return to an adequate activity level, and maintaining surveillance for complications.**

Optimizing oxygenation and ventilation

Nursing interventions to optimize oxygenation and ventilation include positioning, preventing desaturation during procedures, and promoting secretion clearance.

Preventing atelectasis

Nursing interventions to prevent atelectasis include proper patient positioning and early ambulation, deep breathing exercises, incentive spirometry (IS), and pain management. The goal is to promote maximal lung ventilation and prevent hypoventilation.

Patient positioning and early ambulation. The nurse should consider the surgical incision site and the type of surgery when positioning the patient. After a lobectomy, the patient should be turned onto the nonoperative side to promote V/Q matching. When the good lung is dependent, blood flow is greater to the area with better ventilation and V/Q matching is better. V/Q mismatching results when the affected lung is positioned down because of the increase in blood flow to an area with less ventilation. The patient should be turned frequently to promote secretion removal but should have the affected lung dependent as little as possible.[56] The patient who has had a pneumonectomy should be positioned supine or on the operative side during the initial period. Turning onto the operative side can result in disruption of the suture line and shifting of the mediasti-

num, which may compress the unaffected lung. In addition, this position promotes splinting of the incision and facilitates deep breathing exercises. Tilting the patient slightly toward the unaffected side is possible, but the surgeon should indicate when free side-to-side positioning is safe.[57]

When sitting at the bedside or ambulating, patients must be encouraged to keep the thorax in straight alignment while they breathe deeply. This position best accommodates diaphragmatic descent and intercostal muscle action. The sitting or standing position provides enhanced ventilation to areas of the lung that are dependent in the supine position, thus accommodating maximal inflation and promoting gas exchange. Ambulation is essential in restoring lung function and should be initiated as soon as possible.[58]

Deep breathing and incentive spirometry. Deep breathing and incentive spirometry should be performed regularly by patients who have undergone a thoracotomy. Deep breathing involves having the patient take a deep breath and hold it for approximately 3 seconds or longer. Incentive spirometry involves having the patient take at least 10 deep, effective breaths per hour using an incentive spirometer. These activities help reexpand collapsed lung tissue, thus promoting early resolution of the pneumothorax in patients with partial lung resections. The chest should be auscultated during inflation to ensure that all dependent parts of the lung are well ventilated and to help the patient understand the depth of breath necessary for optimal effect. Coughing, which should be encouraged only when secretions are present, assists in mobilizing secretions for removal.[58]

Pain management. Pain can be a major problem after thoracic surgery. Pain can increase the workload of the heart, precipitate hypoventilation, and inhibit mobilization of secretions. Clinical manifestations of pain include tachypnea, tachycardia, elevated blood pressure, facial grimacing, splinting of the incision, hypoventilation, moaning, and restlessness. There are several alternatives for pain management after thoracic surgery. The two most common methods are systemic narcotic administration or epidural narcotic administration. Systemic narcotics can be administered intravenously, intramuscularly, or via patient-controlled analgesia (PCA) method. In addition, the patient should be assisted with splinting the incision with a pillow or blanket when deep breathing and coughing. Splinting stabilizes the area and reduces pain when moving, deep breathing, or coughing.[56,57,59]

Maintaining the chest tube system

Chest tubes are placed after all thoracic surgical procedures (except a pneumonectomy) to remove air and fluid. The drainage will initially appear bloody, becoming serosanguinous and then serous over the first 2 to 3 days postoperatively. There will be approximately 100 to 300 ml of drainage during the first 2 hours postoperatively, which will decrease to less than 50 ml/hour over the next several hours. Routine milking or stripping of chest tubes is not recommended because excessive negative pressure can be generated in the chest. If blood clots are present in the drainage tubing or an obstruction is present, the chest tubes may be carefully milked.[59]

During auscultation of the lungs, air leaks should be evaluated. In the early phase, an air leak is commonly heard over the affected area because the pleura has not yet tightly sealed. As healing occurs, this leak should disappear. An increase in an air leak or appearance of a new air leak should prompt investigation of the chest drainage system to discover whether air is leaking into the system from outside or whether the leak is originating from the patient's incision. Increased air leaks not related to the thoracic drainage system may indicate disruption of sutures.[59]

Assisting the patient to return to adequate activity level

Within a few days after surgery, range of motion to the shoulder on the operative side should be performed. The patient frequently splints the operative side and avoids shoulder movement because of pain. If immobility is allowed, stiffening of the shoulder joint can result. This is referred to as frozen shoulder and may require physical therapy and rehabilitation to regain satisfactory range of motion of the shoulder joint.[54,57]

Usually on the day after surgery, the patient is able to sit in a chair. Activity should be systematically increased, with attention to the patient's activity tolerance. With adequate pulmonary function before surgery and a surgical approach designed to preserve respiratory function, full return to previous activity levels is possible. This may take as long as 6 months to 1 year, depending on the tissue resected and the patient's general condition.[57]

LONG-TERM MECHANICAL VENTILATION DEPENDENCE

Description

Long-term mechanical ventilation (LTMV) dependence is a secondary disorder that occurs when a patient requires assisted ventilation for more than 3 days. It is the result of complex medical problems, which do not allow the normal weaning process to take place in a timely manner and results in ventilator dependence. Ventilator dependence can be described as a state in which the patient is mechanically ventilated longer than expected given the patient's underlying condition[60] and in which the patient has failed at least one weaning attempt.[61]

Long-term mechanical ventilation comes under DRG 475 (Respiratory System Diagnosis With Ventilator Support) if the patient does not have a tracheostomy, and DRG 483 (Tracheostomy Except for Face, Mouth, and Neck Diagnoses) if the patient does have a tracheostomy, with anticipated lengths of the stay of 12.3 and 46.4 days, respectively.[4]

BOX 13-11

PHYSIOLOGIC FACTORS CONTRIBUTING TO THE DEVELOPMENT OF LTMV

Decreased gas exchange
  Ventilation/perfusion mismatching
  Intrapulmonary shunting
  Alveolar hypoventilation
  Anemia
  Acute heart failure
Increased ventilatory workload
  Decreased lung compliance
  Increased airway resistance
  Small endotracheal tube
  Decreased ventilator sensitivity
  Improper positioning
  Abdominal distension
  Dyspnea
Increased ventilatory demand
  Increased pulmonary dead space
  Increased metabolic demands
  Improper ventilator mode/settings
  Metabolic acidosis
  Overfeeding
Decreased ventilatory drive
  Respiratory alkalosis
  Metabolic alkalosis
  Hypothyroidism
  Sedatives
  Malnutrition
Increased respiratory muscle fatigue
  Increased ventilatory workload
  Increased ventilatory demand
  Malnutrition
  Hypokalemia
  Hypomagnesemia
  Hypophosphatemia
  Hypothyroidism
  Critical illness polyneuropathy
  Inadequate muscle rest

Etiology and Pathophysiology

There are a wide variety of physiologic and psychologic factors that contribute to the development of LTMV. Physiologic factors include those conditions that result in decreased gas exchange, increased ventilatory workload, increased ventilatory demand, decreased ventilatory drive, and increased respiratory muscle fatigue[60-65] (Box 13-11). Psychologic factors include those conditions that result in loss of breathing pattern control, lack of motivation and confidence, and delirium (Box 13-12).[62,66] The development of LTMV is also effected by the severity and duration of the patient's current illness and any underlying chronic health problems.[66]

Medical and Nursing Management

The goal of medical and nursing management of the patient requiring LTMV is successful weaning. The Third National Study Group on Weaning from Mechanical Ventilation, sponsored by the American Association of Criti-

BOX 13-12

PSYCHOLOGIC FACTORS CONTRIBUTING TO THE DEVELOPMENT OF LTMV

Loss of breathing pattern control
    Anxiety
    Fear
    Dyspnea
    Pain
    Ventilator asynchrony
    Lack of confidence in ability to breathe
Lack of motivation and confidence
    Inadequate trust in staff
    Depersonalization
    Hopelessness
    Powerlessness
    Depression
    Inadequate communication
Delirium
    Sensory overload
    Sensory deprivation
    Sleep deprivation
    Pain
    Medications

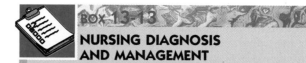

BOX 13-13

NURSING DIAGNOSIS AND MANAGEMENT

Long-Term Mechanical Ventilation

- Inability to Sustain Spontaneous Ventilation related to respiratory muscle fatigue or neuromuscular impairment, p. 475
- Dysfunctional Ventilatory Weaning Response related to physical, psychosocial, or situational factors, pp. 471-472
- Altered Nutrition: Less than Body Requirements related to lack of exogenous nutrients and increased metabolic demand, p. 460
- Risk for Infection, pp. 494-495
- Acute Confusion related to sensory overload, sensory deprivation, and sleep pattern disturbance, pp. 444-448
- Powerlessness related to lack of control over current situation or disease progression, pp. 455-456

---

cal Care Nurses, proposed a conceptual model (Weaning Continuum Model) that divides weaning into three stages; preweaning, weaning process, and weaning outcome.[67] It is within this framework that the management of the long-term ventilator-dependent patient is described. In addition, common nursing diagnoses for this patient population are listed in Box 13-13.

Preweaning stage

For the long-term ventilator patient, the preweaning stage consists of resolving the precipitating event that necessitated ventilatory assistance and preventing the physiologic and psychologic factors that can interfere with weaning. Before any attempts at weaning, the patient should be assessed for weaning readiness, an approach should be determined, and a method selected.[60]

Weaning preparedness. The patient should be physiologically and psychologically prepared to initiate the weaning process by addressing those factors that can interfere with weaning. Aggressive medical management to prevent and treat ventilation/perfusion mismatching, intrapulmonary shunting, anemia, cardiac failure, decreased lung compliance, increased airway resistance, acid-base disturbances, hypothyroidism, abdominal distension, and electrolyte imbalances should be initiated. In addition, interventions to decrease the work of breathing should be implemented, such as replacing a small endotracheal tube with a larger tube or a tracheostomy, suctioning airway secretions, administering bronchodilators, optimizing the ventilator settings and trigger sensitivity, and positioning the patient in straight alignment with the head of the bed elevated at least 30 degrees. Enteral or parenteral nutrition should be started, and the patient's

nutritional state optimized. Physical therapy should be initiated for the patient with critical illness polyneuropathy as increased mobility facilitates weaning. A means of communication should be established with the patient. Sedatives can be administered to provide anxiety control but the avoidance of respiratory depression is critical.[68,69]

Weaning readiness. Although a variety of different methods for assessing weaning readiness have been developed, none of them have proven to be very accurate in predicting weaning success in the patient requiring LTMV.[69] One study did indicate that the presence of left ventricular dysfunction, fluid imbalance, and nutritional deficiency did increase the duration of mechanical ventilation.[70] Another study suggested that the upward trending of the albumin level may be predictive of weaning success.[71] As so many variables can effect the patient's ability to wean, any assessment of weaning readiness should incorporate these variables.[72] Cardiac function, gas exchange, pulmonary mechanics, nutritional status, electrolyte and fluid balance, and motivation should all be considered when making the decision to wean. This assessment should be ongoing so as to reflect the dynamic nature of the process.

Weaning approach. Although weaning the patient requiring short-term mechanical ventilation is a relatively simple process that can usually be accomplished with a nurse and respiratory therapist, weaning the patient requiring LTMV is much more complex process that usually requires a multidisciplinary team approach.[60,69] Multidisciplinary weaning teams that use a coordinated and collaborative approach to weaning have demonstrated improved patient outcomes and decreased weaning times.[69] The team should consist of a physician, nurse, respiratory therapist, dietitian, physical therapist, and also a case manager, clinical outcomes manager, or a clinical nurse specialist. Additional members, if possible, should include an occupational therapist, speech therapist, discharge planner, and a social worker. Working together, the team members should develop for the patient a comprehensive plan of care that is efficient, consistent, progressive, and cost-effective.[69]

Weaning method. There are a variety of weaning methods available but no one method has consistently proven to be superior to the others.[69] The methods include T-tube (T-piece), constant positive airway pressure (CPAP), pressure support ventilation (PSV), and synchronized intermittent mandatory ventilation (SIMV).[60] One recent multicenter study provides evidence supporting the use of PSV for weaning over T-tube or SIMV weaning.[73] Often these weaning methods are used in combination with each other, such as SIMV with PSV, CPAP with PSV, or SIMV with CPAP.[60]

Weaning process stage

For the long-term ventilator patient, the weaning process stage consists of initiating the weaning method selected and minimizing the physiologic and psychologic factors that can interfere with weaning.[60] It is imperative that the patient not become exhausted during this stage because this can result in a setback in the weaning process.[74] During this stage, the patient is assessed for weaning progress and signs of weaning intolerance.[60]

Weaning initiation. Weaning should be initiated in the morning while the patient is rested. Before starting the weaning process, patients are provided with an explanation of how the process works, a description of the sensations that should be expected, and reassurance that they will be closely monitored and returned to the original ventilator mode and settings if they are having difficulty.[62] This information should be reinforced during each weaning attempt.

T-tube and CPAP weaning are accomplished by removing patients from the ventilator and placing them on a T-tube or by placing patients on CPAP mode for a specified duration of time, known as a weaning trial, for a specified number of times per day. When the weaning trial is over, the patient is placed on the assist-control mode (continuous mandatory ventilation mode on the Puritan-Bennett 7200 ventilator) and allowed to rest to prevent respiratory muscle fatigue. Gradually the duration of time spent weaning is increased as is the frequency until the patient is able to breath spontaneously for 24 hours. If PSV is used in conjunction with CPAP, the PSV is initially set to provide the patient with an assisted tidal volume of 10 to 12 ml/kg, and this is gradually weaned until a level of 6 to 8 cm H_2O of pressure support is achieved. SIMV and PSV weaning are accomplished by gradually decreasing the number of breaths or the amount of pressure support the patient receives by a specified amount until the patient is able to breath spontaneously for 24 hours.[74]

Weaning progress. Weaning progress can be evaluated using various methods. Evaluation of weaning progress when using a weaning method that gradually withdraws ventilatory support, such as SIMV or PSV, can be accomplished by measuring the percentage of minute ventilation requirement that is provided by the ventilator. If the percentage steadily decreases, weaning is progressing. Evaluation of weaning progress when using a weaning method that removes ventilatory support, such as T-tube or CPAP, can be accomplished by measuring the amount of time the patient remains free from support. If the time steadily increases, weaning is progressing.[60]

Weaning intolerance. Once the weaning process has begun, the patient should be continuously assessed for signs of intolerance. When present, these signs indicate the patient should be placed back on the ventilator or should be returned to previous ventilator settings. Commonly used indicators include dyspnea, accessory muscle use, restlessness, anxiety, change in facial expression, changes in heart rate and blood pressure, rapid, shallow breathing, and discomfort.[60,62,69]

Facilitative therapies

Additional therapies may be needed to facilitate weaning in the patient who is having difficulty making weaning progress. These therapies include ventilatory muscle training and biofeedback.[60,62,69] Inspiratory muscle training is used to enhance the strength and endurance of the respiratory muscles.[69,74] Biofeedback can be used to promote relaxation and assist in the management of dyspnea and anxiety.[68,69]

Weaning outcome stage

There are three possible outcomes for a patient requiring LTMV: weaning completed, incomplete weaning/partial support, incomplete weaning/full support.[67]

Weaning completed. Weaning is considered completed when a patient is able to breathe spontaneously for 24 hours without ventilatory support. Once this occurs, the patient may be extubated or decannulated at anytime, although this is not necessary for weaning to be considered completed.[60]

Incomplete weaning. Weaning is deemed incomplete when a patient has reached a plateau (5 days at the same ventilatory support without any changes) in the weaning process despite managing the physiologic and psychologic factors that impede weaning. Thus the patient is unable to breathe spontaneously for 24 hours without full or partial ventilatory support. Once this occurs, the patient should be placed in a subacute ventilator facility or discharged home on a ventilator with home care nursing follow-up.[60]

References

1. Op't Holt TB, Scanlan CL: Respiratory failure and the need for ventilatory support. In Scanlan CL, Spearman CB, Sheldon RL, editors: *Egan's fundamentals of respiratory care*, ed 6, St Louis, 1995, Mosby.
2. Bone RC: Acute respiratory failure. In Burton GG, Hodgkin JE, Ward JJ, editors: *Respiratory care: a guide to clinical practice*, ed 3, Philadelphia, 1991, JB Lippincott.

3. Balk R, Bone RC: Classification of acute respiratory failure, *Med Clin North Am* 67:551, 1983.

4. *St Anthony's DRG guidebook 1998*, Reston, VA, 1997, St Anthony Publishing, Inc.

5. Curtis JR, Hudson LD: Emergent assessment and management of acute respiratory failure in COPD, *Clin Chest Med* 15:481, 1994.

6. Pratter MR, Irwin RS: Extrapulmonary causes of respiratory failure, *J Intens Care Med* 1:197, 1986.

7. Green KE, Peters JI: Pathophysiology of acute respiratory failure, *Clin Chest Med* 15:1, 1994.

8. Misasi RS, Keyes JL: The pathophysiology of hypoxia, *Crit Care Nurs* 14(4):55, 1994.

9. Higgins TL, Yared JP: Clinical effects of hypoxemia and tissue hypoxia, *Respir Care* 38:603, 1993.

10. Vaughan P: Acute respiratory failure in the patient with chronic obstructive lung disease, *Crit Care Nurs* 1(6):46, 1981.

11. Misasi RS, Keyes JL: Matching and mismatching ventilation and perfusion in the lung, *Crit Care Nurs* 16(3):23, 1996.

12. Meduri GU, et al: Noninvasive positive pressure ventilation via face mask, *Chest* 109:179, 1996.

13. Slutsky AS, et al: American College of Chest Physicians' Consensus Conference: mechanical ventilation, *Chest* 104:1833, 1993.

14. American Thoracic Society: Standards for the diagnosis and care of patients with chronic obstructive pulmonary disease, *Am J Respir Crit Care Med* 152:S77, 1995.

15. Sapirstein A, Hurford WE: Neuromuscular blocking agents in the management of respiratory failure: indications and treatment guidelines, *Crit Care Clin* 10:831, 1994.

16. Doering LV: The effect of positioning on hemodynamics and gas exchange in the critically ill: a review, *Am J Crit Care* 2:208, 1993.

17. Lasater-Erhand M: The effect of patient position on arterial saturation, *Crit Care Nurs* 15(5):31, 1995.

18. Norton LC, Conforti C: The effect of body position on oxygenation, *Heart Lung* 14(1):45, 1985.

19. Cosenza JJ, Norton LC: Secretion clearance: state-of-the-art from a nursing perspective, *Crit Care Nurs* 6(4):23, 1986.

20. Bernard GR, et al: The American-European Consensus Conference on ARDS: definitions, mechanisms, relevant outcomes, and clinical trial coordination, *Am J Respir Crit Care Med* 149:818, 1994.

21. Hammer J: Challenging diagnosis: adult respiratory distress syndrome, *Crit Care Nurs* 15(5):46, 1995.

22. Luce JM: Acute lung injury and the acute respiratory distress syndrome, *Crit Care Med* 26:369, 1998.

23. Milberg JA, Davis DR, Steinberg KP, Hudson LD: Improved survival of patients with acute respiratory distress syndrome (ARDS): 1983-1993, *J Am Med Assoc* 273:306, 1995.

24. Brandstetter RD, et al: Adult respiratory distress syndrome: a disorder in need of improved outcome, *Heart Lung* 26:3, 1997.

25. Marinelli WA, Ingbar DH: Diagnosis and management of acute lung injury, *Clin Chest Med* 15:517, 1994.

26. Vollman KM: Adult respiratory distress syndrome, *Crit Care Nurs Clin North Am* 6:341, 1994.

27. Kollef MH, Schuster DP: The acute respiratory distress syndrome, *New Engl J Med* 332:27, 1995.

28. Gleeson K, Reynolds HY: Life-threatening pneumonia, *Clin Chest Med* 3:581, 1994.

29. Kollef MH, Silver P: Ventilator-associated pneumonia, *Respir Care* 40:1130, 1995.

30. Cunha B: Severe community-acquired pneumonia, *Crit Care Clin* 14:105, 1998.

31. Huang L, Stansell JD: AIDS and the lung, *Med Clin North Am* 80:775, 1996.

32. Lode HM, et al: Nosocomial pneumonia in the critical care unit, *Crit Care Clin* 14:119, 1998.

33. Nelson S, Mason CM, Kolls J, Summer WR: Pathophysiology of pneumonia, *Clin Chest Med* 16:1, 1995.

34. Tablan OC, et al: Guideline for prevention of nosocomial pneumonia. Part 1. Issues on prevention of nosocomial pneumonia—1994, *Am J Infect Control* 22:247, 1994.

35. American Thoracic Society: Hospital-acquired pneumonia in adults: diagnosis, assessment of severity, initial antimicrobial therapy, and preventable strategies—a consensus statement, *Am J Respir Crit Care Med* 153:1711, 1995.

36. Dal Nogare AR: Nosocomial pneumonia in the medical surgical patient, *Med Clin North Am* 78:1081, 1994.

37. DePaso WJ: Aspiration pneumonia, *Clin Chest Med* 12:269, 1991.

38. Tietjen PA, Kaner RJ, Quinn CE: Aspiration emergencies, *Clin Chest Med* 15:117, 1994.

39. Shifrin RY, Choplin RH: Aspiration in patient in critical care units, *Radiol Clin North Am* 34:83, 1996.

40. Goodwin RS: Prevention of aspiration pneumonia: a research-based protocol, *Dimen Crit Care Nurs* 15(2):58, 1996.

41. Wagenvoort CA: Pathology of pulmonary thromboembolism, *Chest* 107:11S, 1995.

42. King MB, Harmon KR: Unusual forms of pulmonary embolism, *Clin Chest Med* 15:561, 1994.

43. Cowen JC, Kelley MA: An organized approach to detecting pulmonary embolism in the critically ill, *J Crit Ill* 9:551, 1994.

44. Kelley MA, Abbuhl S: Massive pulmonary embolism, *Clin Chest Med* 15:547, 1994.

45. Manganelli D, Palla A, Donnamaria V, Guintini C: Clinical features of pulmonary embolism: doubts and certainties, *Chest* 107:25S, 1995.

46. Davis LA, O'Rouke NC: Pulmonary embolism: early recognition and management in the postanesthesia care unit, *J Post Anesth Nurs* 8:338, 1993.

47. Agnelli G: Anticoagulation in the prevention and treatment of pulmonary embolism, *Chest* 107:39S, 1995.

48. Daniels LB, et al: Relation of duration of symptoms with response to thrombolytic therapy in pulmonary embolism, *Am J Cardiol* 80:184, 1997.

49. Cohen NH, Eigen H, Shaughnessy TE: Status asthmaticus, *Crit Care Clin* 13:459, 1997.

50. Abou-Shala N, MacIntyre N: Emergency management of acute asthma, *Med Clin North Am* 80:677, 1996.

51. Leatherman J: Life-threatening asthma, *Clin Chest Med* 15:453, 1994.

52. Corbridge TC, Hall JB: The assessment and management of adults with status asthmaticus, *Am J Respir Crit Care Med* 151:1296, 1995.

53. Litwack K: Practical points in the care of the thoracic surgery patient, *Post Anesth Nurs* 5:276, 1990.

54. Langston W: Surgical resection of lung cancer, *Nurs Clin North Am* 27:665, 1992.

55. Boysen PG: Perioperative management of the thoracotomy patient, *Clin Chest Med* 14:321, 1993.

56. Daitch JS: Post-anesthesia care after thoracic surgery. In Frost EAM, editor: *Post-anesthesia care unit: current practices*, ed 2, St Louis, 1990, Mosby.

57. Brenner Z, Addona C: Caring for the pneumonectomy patient: challenges and changes, *Crit Care Nurs* 15(5):65, 1995.

58. Brooks-Braun, JA: Postoperative atelectasis and pneumonia, *Heart Lung* 24:94, 1995.

59. Whitman GR, Weber MM: Postoperative care after thoracic surgery, *Curr Rev PACU* 14:137, 1992.

60. Knebel AR, et al: Weaning from mechanical ventilation: concept development, *Am J Crit Care Nurs* 3:416, 1994.

61. Pierson DJ: Long-term mechanical ventilation and weaning, *Respir Care* 40:289, 1995.

62. Knebel AR: When weaning from mechanical ventilation fails, *Am J Crit Care* 1(3):19, 1992.

63. MacIntyre NR: Respiratory factors in weaning from mechanical ventilatory support, *Respir Care* 40:244, 1995.

64. Pierson DJ: Nonrespiratory aspects of weaning from mechanical ventilation, *Respir Care* 40:263, 1995.

65. Hund EF, et al: Critical illness polyneuropathy: clinical findings and outcomes of a frequent cause of neuromuscular weaning failure, *Crit Care Med* 24:1328, 1996.

66. MacIntyre NR: Psychological factors in weaning from mechanical ventilatory support, *Respir Care* 40:277, 1995.

67. Knebel A, et al: Weaning from mechanical ventilatory support: refinement of a model, *Am J Crit Care* 7:149, 1998.

68. Criner GJ, Tzouanakis A, Kreimer DT: Overview of improving tolerance of long-term mechanical ventilation, *Crit Care Clin* 10:845, 1994.

69. Burns SM, et al: Weaning from long-term mechanical ventilation, *Am J Crit Care* 4:4, 1995.

70. Clochesy JM: Weaning chronically critically ill adults from mechanical ventilatory support: a descriptive study, *Am J Crit Care* 4:93, 1995.

71. Sapijaszko MJA, et al: Nonrespiratory predictor of mechanical ventilation dependency in intensive care unit patients, *Crit Care Med* 24:601, 1996.

72. Ingersoll GL, et al: Measurement issues in mechanical ventilation weaning research, *Online J Knowledge Synthesis Nurs* 2:(12):24, 1995.

73. Brochard L, et al: Comparison of three methods of gradual withdrawal from ventilatory support during weaning from mechanical ventilation, *Am J Respir Crit Care Med* 150:898, 1994.

74. Brochard LJ, Lessard MR: Weaning form ventilatory support, *Clin Chest Med* 17:475, 1996.

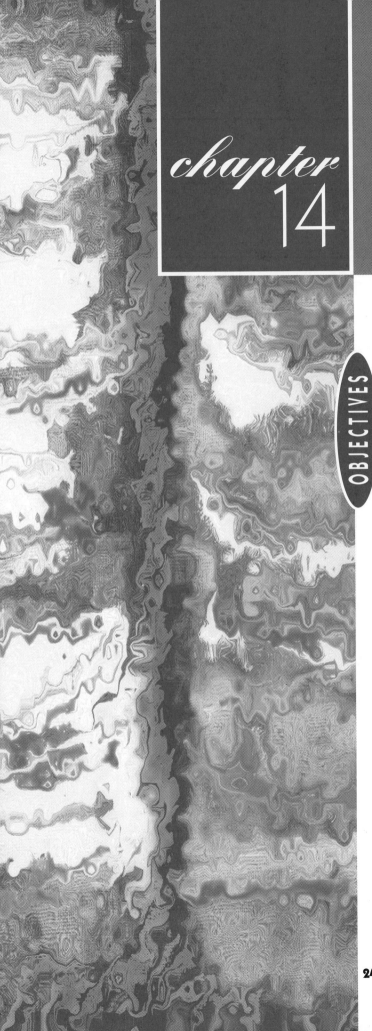

chapter 14

Pulmonary Therapeutic Management

Kathleen M. Stacy

OBJECTIVES

- Describe nursing management of a patient receiving oxygen therapy.
- List the indications and complications of the different artificial airways.
- Outline the principles of airway management.
- Discuss the various modes of invasive and noninvasive mechanical ventilation.
- Describe the management of a patient on mechanical ventilation.

A wide variety of therapeutic interventions are employed in the management of the patient with pulmonary dysfunction. This chapter focuses on the priority interventions used to manage pulmonary disorders in the critical care setting.

OXYGEN THERAPY

Normal cellular function depends on an adequate supply of oxygen to meet metabolic needs. The primary indications for oxygen administration are hypoxemia and tissue hypoxia. The goal of oxygen administration is to provide a sufficient concentration of inspired oxygen to permit full use of the oxygen-carrying capacity of the arterial blood, thus ensuring adequate tissue oxygenation if the cardiac output (CO) is adequate and if the hemoglobin (Hgb) concentration and structure are normal.[1,2]

Oxygen is an atmospheric gas that must also be considered a drug, because—like most other drugs—oxygen has both detrimental and beneficial effects. Oxygen is one of the most commonly used and misused drugs. As a drug, it must be administered for good reason and in a

TABLE 14-1

OXYGEN ADMINISTRATION DEVICES

EQUIPMENT	OBJECTIVE	L/MIN	FIo$_2$ (%)	ADVANTAGES/DISADVANTAGES
LOW FLOW-SYSTEMS				
Nasal cannula	Provides oxygen through a low-flow oxygen delivery system	1 2 3 4 5 6	24 28 32 36 40 44	Can be used with mouth breathers Convenient Comfortable Good low flow Allows for talking and eating FIo$_2$ not really accurate because it depends on patient's respiratory pattern May cause sinus pain >2 L/min requires added humidity Easily displaced Nasal passages must be patent
Simple face mask*	Provides oxygen through a mask and low-flow oxygen delivery system	5 6 8	40 50 60	Simple set-up; good for emergency situations Can get uncomfortable Poor patient tolerance FIo$_2$ not really accurate because it depends on patient's respiratory pattern Cannot provide enough humidity for prolonged use Must be removed at meals Tight fitting mask can cause pressure sores Aspiration of vomitus is a potential problem
Partial re-breathing mask	Provides a high oxygen concentration through a low-flow delivery system	6 8 10-15	35 45-50 In excess of 60, depending on patient's ventilatory pattern	Simple set-up; good in emergency situations Can be uncomfortable Does not provide adequate humidity for long-term use
Nonrebreathing mask	Provides high oxygen concentration	6 8 10-15	55-60 60-80 80-90	Delivers the highest possible oxygen concentration (55%-90%) possible with a low-flow system Good for short-term therapy and transport Has three one-way valves Requires a tight seal May irritate skin

From Flynn JBM, Bruce NP: *Introduction to critical care nursing skills,* St Louis, 1993, Mosby.
*A minimum flow rate of 5 L/min to flush expired carbon dioxide from the mask is needed.

proper, safe manner. Oxygen is generally ordered in liters per minute (L/min), as a concentration of oxygen expressed as a percent such as 40%, or as a fraction of inspired oxygen (FIo$_2$), such as 0.4.[3]

The amount of oxygen administered depends on the pathophysiologic mechanisms affecting the patient's oxygenation status. In most cases the amount required should provide an arterial partial pressure of oxygen (Pao$_2$) of 60 to 90 mm Hg, so that a Hgb saturation (Sao$_2$) of greater than 90% is achieved.[3] The concentration of oxygen given to an individual patient is a clinical judgment based on many factors that influence oxygen transport, such as Hgb concentration, CO, and the arterial oxygen tension.[1,2]

Once oxygen therapy has begun, the patient should continuously be assessed for level of oxygenation and the factors affecting it. The patient's oxygenation status should be evaluated several times daily until the desired oxygen level is reached and has stabilized. If the desired

response to the amount of oxygen delivered is not achieved, the oxygen supplementation should be adjusted and the patient's condition reevaluated. It is important to use this dose-response method, so that the lowest possible level of oxygen is administered that will still achieve a satisfactory Pao$_2$ or Sao$_2$.[3]

Methods of Delivery

Oxygen therapy can be delivered by many different devices (Table 14-1). These devices are classified as either low-flow or high-flow delivery systems. A low-flow system supplies an amount of oxygen that is insufficient to meet all inspiratory volume requirements and depends on the existence of a reservoir of oxygen, dilution with room air, and the patient's ventilatory pattern. The anatomic reservoir in this case is composed of the nasopharynx and the oropharynx. As the patient's ventilatory pattern changes, the inspired oxygen concentra-

TABLE 14-1

OXYGEN ADMINISTRATION DEVICES—cont'd

EQUIPMENT	OBJECTIVE	L/MIN	FIo$_2$ (%)	ADVANTAGES/DISADVANTAGES
HUMIDIFYING SYSTEMS				
Aerosol mask (high humidity face mask)	Delivers a specific FIo$_2$ through an aerosol device		28-100 (variable)	High humidity Accurate FIo$_2$ Does not dry mucous membranes Can be uncomfortable May need extra equipment for higher FIo$_2$ Moisture build-up in tube
Face tent	Delivers high humidity		21-55	Used for patients with facial trauma Does not dry mucous membranes Can function as high-flow system when attached to Venturi system Interferes with eating and talking Impractical for long-term use Possible to rebreathe CO_2
Trach mask T-tube	Delivers a specific FIo$_2$ through an aerosol system		28-100 (variable)	High humidity Accurate FIo$_2$ Can control oxygen Does not need vent May need extra equipment for higher FIo$_2$
HIGH-FLOW SYSTEMS				
Air-entrainment (Venturi) mask†	Provides high-flow oxygen with a precise FIo$_2$ in a selected range	Blue-4 Yellow-4 White-6 Green-8 Pink-8	24 28 31 35 40	Can provide humidity Accurate oxygen levels Simple set-up; good for emergency situations Well-tolerated Can only have FIo$_2$ in selected range Hot and confining Must fit snugly
CONSTANT POSITIVE AIRWAY PRESSURE (CPAP)				
CPAP mask	Provides continual positive airway pressure through a mask without the use of a ventilator		30-100	Do not need ventilator Do not need to be intubated Can get gastric distention Mask is uncomfortable Not useful if patient becomes apneic

†Jet adapters on Venturi masks are color coded.

tion varies because of differing amounts of air mixing with the reservoir gas and the constant flow of oxygen. With a high-flow system, the oxygen flows out of the device into the patient's airway in amounts sufficient to meet all inspiratory volume requirements. This type of system is not affected by the patient's ventilatory pattern. Examples of low-flow systems are nasal cannulas, simple oxygen masks, partial rebreathing masks, and nonrebreathing masks. An air-entrainment (Venturi) mask is an example of a high-flow oxygen delivery system.[1,3,4]

Complications of Oxygen Therapy

Oxygen, like most drugs, has adverse effects and complications associated with its use. The old adage "if a little is good, a lot is better" does not apply to oxygen. The lung is designed to handle a concentration of 21% oxygen, with some adaptability to higher concentrations, but ad-verse effects and oxygen toxicity can result if a high concentration is administered for too long.[2]

Oxygen toxicity

The most detrimental effect of breathing a high concentration of oxygen is the development of oxygen toxicity. It can occur in any patient breathing oxygen concentrations of greater than 50% for more than 24 hours. Patients most likely to develop oxygen toxicity are those who require intubation, mechanical ventilation, and high oxygen concentrations for extended periods.[1,3,5]

Hyperoxia, or the administration of higher-than-normal oxygen concentrations, produces an overabundance of oxygen-free radicals. These radicals are responsible for the initial damage to the alveolar-capillary membrane. Oxygen-free radicals are toxic metabolites of oxygen metabolism. Normally, enzymes neutralize the radicals, which prevents any damage from occurring. During the administration of high levels of oxygen, the large number of oxygen-free radicals produced exhausts the supply of neutralizing enzymes. Thus damage to the lung parenchyma and vasculature occurs.[1,5]

The pathologic features of oxygen toxicity can be divided into an early exudative stage and a late proliferative stage. Within 24 to 48 hours of oxygen exposure, exudative changes appear. Initially, the capillary endothelial cells become damaged, and they leak serum protein and fluid into the interstitial space of the alveolar wall. This fluid is collected by the lymphatic system, which empties it into the general circulation. As the capillary damage progresses, the flow of fluid out of the capillaries increases and exceeds the lymphatic system's ability to drain it. With continued exposure to hyperoxia, the type I alveolar cells become damaged, allowing the escaped alveolar-capillary fluid to pass directly into the alveolar spaces and causing "flooding" of the alveoli and severe gas exchange impairment.[5]

The lung will respond with cellular proliferation if it survives the aforementioned process and the disease process originally responsible for the hypoxemia. Cellular proliferation occurs in an attempt to repair the alveolar damage, and the alveolar walls become filled with fibroblasts. Alveolar type II cells, which are relatively tolerant to hyperoxia, replicate and reestablish the damaged alveolar wall. Endothelial cell repair and replacement occurs, and the pulmonary edema is reabsorbed. The final result is irregular scarring that can lead to pulmonary fibrosis.[5]

A number of clinical manifestations are associated with oxygen toxicity. The first symptom is substernal chest pain that is exacerbated by deep breathing. A dry cough and tracheal irritation follow. Eventually, definite pleuritic pain occurs on inhalation, followed by dyspnea. Upper airway changes may include a sensation of nasal stuffiness, sore throat, and eye and ear discomfort. Chest radiographs and pulmonary function tests show no abnormalities until symptoms are severe. Complete, rapid reversal of these symptoms occurs as soon as normal oxygen concentrations return.[5]

As oxygen toxicity progresses, objective pulmonary damage becomes evident. A chest radiograph reveals atelectatic streaks and patches of bronchopneumonia, and bronchoscopy reveals tracheobronchitis but no infection. As atelectasis develops, there is evidence of decreased vital capacity, decreased compliance, reduced functional residual capacity, and increased intrapulmonary shunting. These abnormalities are reversible several days after normal oxygen concentrations return. If high oxygen concentrations are still needed, permanent damage may occur.[5]

Carbon dioxide retention

In patients with severe chronic obstructive pulmonary disease (COPD), carbon dioxide (CO_2) retention may occur as a result of administering oxygen in higher concentrations. There are a number of possible theories for this phenomena. One theory states that in patients with COPD the normal stimulus to breathe (increasing CO_2 levels) is muted and decreasing oxygen levels become the stimulus to breathe. When oxygen is administered and hypoxemia corrected, the stimulus to breathe is abolished and hypoventilation develops, resulting in a further increase in the arterial partial pressure of carbon dioxide ($PaCO_2$).[2,3] Another theory is that the administration of oxygen abolishes the compensatory response of hypoxic pulmonary vasoconstriction. This results in an increase in perfusion of underventilated alveoli and the development of dead space, producing ventilation/perfusion mismatching. As alveolar dead space increases so does the retention of CO_2.[3,6] A third theory states the rise in CO_2 is related to the proportion of deoxygenated hemoglobin to oxygenated hemoglobin (Haldane effect). As deoxygenated hemoglobin carries more CO_2 than oxygenated hemoglobin, when oxygen is administered it increases the amount of oxygenated hemoglobin, resulting in an increase in the release of CO_2 at the lung level.[6] Because of the risk of CO_2 accumulation, all chronically hypercapnic patients require careful low-flow oxygen administration.[2]

Absorption atelectasis

Another adverse effect of high concentrations of oxygen is absorption atelectasis. Breathing high concentrations of oxygen washes out the nitrogen that normally fills the alveoli and helps hold them open (residual volume). As oxygen replaces the nitrogen in the alveoli, the alveoli start to shrink and collapse because oxygen is absorbed into the bloodstream faster than it can be replaced in the alveoli, particularly in areas of the lungs that are minimally ventilated.[1]

Nursing Management

Nursing priorities for the patient receiving oxygen include ensuring the oxygen is being administered as ordered and observing for complications of the therapy. Confirming that the oxygen therapy device is properly positioned and replacing it after removal is important. During meals an oxygen mask should be changed to a nasal cannula if the patient can tolerate one. The patient on oxygen therapy should also be transported with the oxygen. In addition, the oxygen saturation should be periodically monitored using a pulse oximeter.

ARTIFICIAL AIRWAYS

Oropharyngeal and Nasopharyngeal Airways

Pharyngeal airways are made of rubber or plastic and are used to maintain airway patency by keeping the tongue from obstructing the upper airway. An oral airway is placed by inserting it upside down and rotating it 180 degrees as it is passed into the mouth. It should be used only in an unconscious patient who has an absent or diminished gag reflex. A nasal airway is placed by lubricating the tube and inserting it midline along the floor of the nares into the posterior pharynx. Respirations should be assessed after placement of either airway to ensure proper position. Complications of these airways include trauma to the oral or nasal cavity, obstruction of the airway, laryngospasm, and gagging and vomiting.[7-9]

Endotracheal Tubes

An endotracheal tube (ETT) is the most commonly used artificial airway for providing short-term airway management. Indications for endotracheal intubation include airway maintenance and protection, secretion control, oxygenation, and ventilation.[10] An endotracheal tube may be placed through the orotracheal or nasotracheal route. In most situations involving emergency placement, the orotracheal route is used because the approach is simpler and affords use of a larger diameter endotracheal tube. A larger diameter tube facilitates secretion removal, decreases the work of breathing, and allows for fiberoptic bronchoscopy, if necessary. The orotracheal route also avoids nasal and sinus complications. Nasotracheal intubation provides greater patient comfort over time and is preferred in situations in which the patient has a jaw fracture.[9-11]

ETTs are available in a variety of sizes, according to the inner diameter of the tube, and have a radioopaque marker that runs the length of the tube. On one end of the tube is a cuff that is inflated using the pilot balloon. Because of the high incidence of the cuff-related problems, low-pressure, high-volume cuffs are preferred. On the other end of the tube is a 15-mm adaptor that facilitates the connection of the tube to a manual resuscitation bag (MRB), T-tube, or ventilator[12] (Fig. 14-1).

Intubation

Before intubation, equipment should be organized to facilitate the procedure. Equipment that should be readily available includes a suction system with catheters and tonsil suction, an MRB with a mask connected to 100% oxygen, a laryngoscope handle with assorted blades, a variety of sizes of ETTs, and a stylet. Before the procedure is initiated, all equipment should be inspected to ensure it is in working order. The patient should be prepared for the procedure if possible with an intravenous catheter in place and be monitored with a pulse oximeter. The patient should be sedated before the procedure and a topical anesthetic applied to facilitate placement of the tube. In some cases a paralytic agent may be necessary if the patient is extremely agitated.[7-9]

The procedure is initiated by positioning the patient with the neck flexed and head slightly extended in the "sniff" position. The oral cavity and pharynx should be suctioned and any dental devices removed. The patient should be preoxygenated and ventilated using the MRB and mask with 100% oxygen. Each intubation attempt should be limited to 30 seconds. Once the ETT is inserted, the patient should be assessed for bilateral breath sounds and chest movement. A disposable end-tidal CO_2 detector can be used to initially verify correct airway placement.[10] after which the cuff of the tube should then be inflated, the tube secured, and a chest radiograph obtained to confirm placement.[7,9,10] The tip of the endotracheal tube should be approximately 5 to 7 cm above the carina when the patient's head is in the neutral position.[13] Once final adjustment of the position is complete, the level of insertion (marked in centimeters on side of tube) should be noted.[10]

Complications. There are a number of complications with intubation. These include gastric intubation; right mainstem bronchus intubation; vomiting with aspiration; trauma to the mouth, nose, pharynx, trachea, esophagus, eyes, or facial tissue; laryngospasm; hypoxemia; and hypercapnia. Hypoxemia and hypercapnia can cause bradycardia, tachycardia, dysrhythmias, hypertension, and hypotension.[7,10,14]

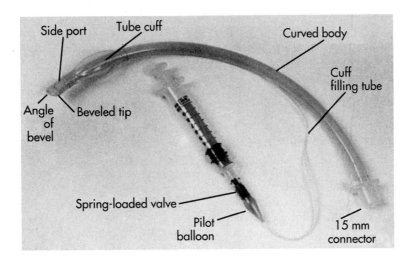

Fig. **14-1** Endotracheal tube. (From Simmons K: Airway care. In Scanlan CL, Spearman CB, Sheldon RL, editors: *Egan's fundamentals of respiratory care,* ed 6, St Louis, 1995, Mosby.)

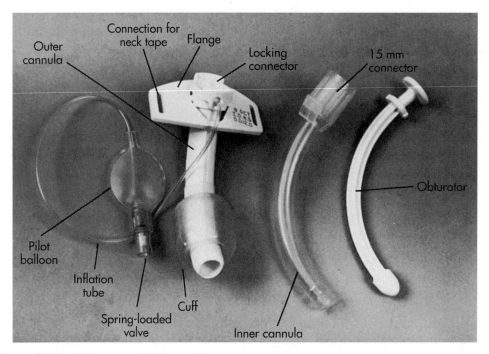

Fig. **14-2** Tracheostomy tube. (From Simmons K: Airway care. In Scanlan CL, Spearman CB, Sheldon RL, editors: *Egan's fundamentals of respiratory care,* ed 6, St Louis, 1995, Mosby.)

Complications

A number of factors predispose a patient to the development of complications while he or she is intubated, particularly with prolonged intubation. Complications that can occur include tube obstruction and displacement, sinusitis, nasal injury, and tracheoesophageal fistulas (Table 14-2). A number of complications can occur days to weeks after the ETT is removed. These include mucosal lesions, laryngeal and/or tracheal stenosis, and cricoid abscess. Delayed complications usually require some form of surgical intervention to correct.[14]

Tracheostomy Tubes

A tracheostomy tube is the preferred method of airway maintenance in the patient requiring intubation for more than 21 days. It is also indicated in several other situations. These include upper airway obstruction or malformation, failed intubation, repeated intubations, presence of complications of endotracheal intubation, glottic incompetence, sleep apnea, and chronic inability to clear secretions.[9,11,15]

A tracheostomy tube provides the best route for long-term airway maintenance and avoids the oral, nasal, pharyngeal, and laryngeal complications of endotracheal intubation. The tube is shorter, of wider diameter, and less curved than is the endotracheal tube; thus the resistance to air flow is less, and breathing is easier. Tracheostomy has other advantages over endotracheal intubation, including easier secretion removal, increased patient acceptance and comfort, the possibility of the patient's eating and talking, and the facilitation of ventilator weaning be-

cause a tracheostomy tube is easier to breathe through when the patient is off the ventilator.[9,15]

Tracheostomy tubes are made of plastic or metal and may be single-lumen or double-lumen tubes. Single-lumen tubes consist of the tube and a built-in cuff, which is connected to a pilot balloon for inflation purposes and an obturator, which is used during tube insertion. The double-lumen tubes consist of the tube with the attached cuff, the obturator, and an inner cannula that can be removed for cleaning and reinserted or, if disposable, replaced by a new sterile inner cannula. The inner cannula can quickly be removed if it becomes obstructed, making the system safer for patients with significant secretion problems. Single-lumen tubes provide a larger inside diameter for air flow than do double-lumen tubes, thus reducing air-flow resistance and allowing the patient to ventilate through the tube with greater ease. Plastic tracheostomy tubes also have a 15-mm adaptor on the end[16] (Fig. 14-2).

Complications

Tracheostomy tubes are inserted either surgically or percutaneously. Placement complications include hemorrhage, pneumothorax, pneumomediastinum, tracheoesophageal fistula, laryngeal nerve injury, and cardiopulmonary arrest. Immediate postprocedural complications include hemorrhage, wound infection, subcutaneous emphysema, tube obstruction, and displacement of the tube[10,17] (Table 14-3). Later complications of a tracheotomy include tracheal stenosis, tracheoesophageal fistula, tracheoinnominate artery fistula, and tracheocutaneous fistula[10,18] (see Table 14-3).

TABLE **14-2**

ENDOTRACHEAL TUBES: COMPLICATIONS, CAUSES, AND TREATMENT

COMPLICATIONS	CAUSES	PREVENTION/TREATMENT

Tube obstruction	Patient biting tube
	Tube kinking during repositioning
	Cuff herniation
	Dried secretions, blood, or lubricant
	Tissue from tumor
	Trauma
	Foreign body
		Prevention:
		  Place bite block
		  Sedate patient PRN
		  Suction PRN
		  Humidify inspired gases
		Treatment:
		  Replace tube

Tube displacement	Movement of patient's head
	Movement of tube by patient's tongue
	Traction on tube from ventilator tubing
	Self-extubation
		Prevention:
		  Secure tube to upper lip
		  Restrain patient's hands
		  Sedate patient PRN
		  Ensure that only 2 inches of tube extend beyond lip
		  Support ventilator tubing
		Treatment:
		  Replace tube

Sinusitis and nasal injury	Obstruction of the paranasal sinus drainage
	Pressure necrosis of nares
		Prevention:
		  Avoid nasal intubations
		  Cushion nares from tube and tape/ties
		Treatment:
		  Remove all tubes from nasal passages
		  Administer antibiotics

Tracheoesophageal fistula	Pressure necrosis of posterior tracheal wall, resulting from overinflated cuff and rigid nasogastric tube	*Prevention:*
		  Inflate cuff with minimal amount of air necessary
		  Monitor cuff pressures every 8 hours
		Treatment:
		  Position cuff of tube distal to fistula
		  Place gastrostomy tube for enteral feedings
		  Place esophageal tube for secretion clearance proximal to fistula

Mucosal lesions	Pressure at tube and mucosal interface	*Prevention:*
		  Inflate cuff with minimal amount of air necessary
		  Monitor cuff pressures every 8 hours
		  Use appropriate size tube
		Treatment:
		  May resolve spontaneously
		  Perform surgical intervention

Laryngeal or tracheal stenosis	Injury to area from end of tube or cuff, resulting in scar tissue formation and narrowing of airway	*Prevention:*
		  Inflate cuff with minimal amount of air necessary
		  Monitor cuff pressures every 8 hours
		  Suction area above cuff frequently
		Treatment:
		  Perform tracheostomy
		  Place laryngeal stent
		  Perform surgical repair

Cricoid abscess	Mucosal injury with bacterial invasion	*Prevention:*
		  Inflate cuff with minimal amount of air necessary
		  Monitor cuff pressures every 8 hours
		  Suction area above cuff frequently
		Treatment:
		  Perform incision and drainage of area
		  Administer antibiotics

TABLE 14-3

TRACHEOSTOMY TUBES: COMPLICATIONS, CAUSES, AND TREATMENT

COMPLICATION	CAUSES	PREVENTION/TREATMENT

Hemorrhage	Vessels' opening after surgery
	Vessel erosion caused by tube
		Prevention:
		  Use appropriate size tube
		  Treat local infection
		  Suction gently
		  Humidify inspired gases
		  Position tracheal window not lower than third tracheal ring
		Treatment:
		  Pack lightly
		  Perform surgical intervention

Wound infection	Colonization of stoma with hospital flora	*Prevention:*
		  Perform routine stoma care
		Treatment:
		  Remove tube, if necessary
		  Perform aggressive wound care and debridement
		  Administer antibiotics

Subcutaneous emphysema	Positive pressure ventilation
	Coughing against a tight, occlusive dressing or sutured or packed wound
		Prevention:
		  Avoid suturing or packing wound closed around tube
		Treatment:
		  Remove any sutures or packing if present

Tube obstruction	Dried blood or secretions
	False passage into soft tissues
	Opening of cannula positioned against tracheal wall
	Foreign body
	Tissue from tumor
		Prevention:
		  Suction PRN
		  Humidify inspired gases
		  Use double-lumen tube
		  Position tube so that opening does not press against tracheal wall
		Treatment:
		  Remove/replace inner cannula
		  Replace tube

Tube displacement	Patient movement
	Coughing
	Traction on ventilatory tubing
		Prevention:
		  Tie tapes to allow only one finger width between the tape and neck
		  Suture tube in place
		  Use tubes with adjustable neck plates for patients with short necks
		  Support ventilator tubing
		  Sedate patient PRN
		  Restrain patient PRN
		Treatment:
		  Cover stoma and manually ventilate patient via mouth
		  Replace tube

Tracheal stenosis	Injury to area from end of tube or cuff, resulting in scar tissue formation and narrowing of airway	*Prevention:*
		  Inflate cuff with minimal amount of air necessary
		  Monitor cuff pressures every 8 hours
		Treatment:
		  Perform surgical repair

Tracheoesophageal fistula	Pressure necrosis of posterior tracheal wall, resulting from overinflated cuff and rigid nasogastric tube	*Prevention:*
		  Inflate cuff with minimal amount of air necessary
		  Monitor cuff pressures every 8 hours
		Treatment:
		  Perform surgical repair

Tracheoinnominate artery fistula	Direct pressure from the elbow of the cannula against the innominate artery
	Placement of tracheal stoma below fourth tracheal ring
	Downward migration of the tracheal stoma, resulting from traction on tube
	High-lying innominate artery
		Prevention:
		  Position tracheal window not lower than third tracheal ring
		Treatment:
		  Hyperinflate cuff to control bleeding
		  Remove tube and replace with endotracheal tube and apply digital pressure through stoma against the sternum
		  Perform surgical repair

Tracheocutaneous fistula	Failure of stoma to close after removal of tube	*Treatment:* Perform surgical repair

Nursing Management

The patient with an endotracheal or tracheostomy tube requires some additional measures to address the effects associated with tube placement on the respiratory and other body systems.

Nursing priorities in the management of the patient with an artificial airway include humidification, cuff management, suctioning, and communication. Because the tube bypasses the upper airway system, warming and humidifying of air must be performed by external means. Because the cuff of the tube can cause damage to the walls of the trachea, proper cuff inflation and management is imperative. In addition, the normal defense mechanisms are impaired and secretions may accumulate; thus suctioning may be needed to promote secretion clearance. Because the tube does not allow air flow over the vocal cords, developing a method of communication is also very important. Lastly, observing the patient to ensure proper placement of the tube and patency of the airway is essential. **In the event of unintentional extubation or decannulation, the patient's airway should be opened with the head-tilt/chin lift maneuver and maintained with an oropharyngeal or nasopharyngeal airway. If the patient is not breathing, he or she should be manually ventilated with an MRB and face mask with 100% oxygen. In the case of a tracheostomy, the stoma should be covered to prevent air from escaping through it.**

Humidification

Humidification of air normally is performed by the mucosal layer of the upper respiratory tract. When this area is bypassed, such as occurs in endotracheal intubation and tracheostomy or when supplemental oxygen is used, humidification by external means is necessary. Various humidification devices add water to inhaled gas to prevent drying and irritation of the respiratory tract, to prevent undue loss of body water, and to facilitate secretion removal.[19]

Bubble humidifiers commonly are used to provide moisture to inhaled gas. They may be warm or cold humidifiers. With a cold humidifier, the gas diffuses out of a stem submerged in water, breaks into small bubbles, and vaporizes. At room temperature, the gas provides only approximately 50% of the humidification needed by the body. Therefore this method of humidification can lead to drying and irritation of mucous membranes when used for a significant time. Bubble humidifiers cannot humidify gas adequately at higher rates of flow, making them more suitable for low-flow oxygen delivery over short time spans. Cold humidifiers are relatively simple and reliable devices and are available as disposable units, thus decreasing maintenance time and eliminating the potential for infection associated with reusable equipment. Warm humidifiers provide better humidification than do cold humidifiers because warm humidification supplies both heat and moisture and breaks gas into smaller particles at higher flow rates. Heated cascade humidifiers are pre-ferred for use with intubated patients, because 100% humidification of inhaled gas can be ensured.[19]

Cuff management

Because the cuff of the endotracheal or tracheostomy tube is a major source of the complications associated with artificial airways, proper cuff management is essential. To prevent the complications associated with cuff design, only low-pressure, high-volume cuffed tubes should be used in clinical practice.[9,20] Even with these tubes, cuff pressures can be generated that are high enough to lead to tracheal ischemia and injury. Both cuff-inflation techniques and cuff-pressure monitoring are critical components to the care of the patient with an artificial airway.[20]

Cuff-inflation techniques. Two different cuff-inflation techniques are currently being used: the minimal leak (ML) technique and the minimal occlusion volume (MOV) technique. The ML technique consists of injecting air into the cuff until no leak is heard and then withdrawing the air until a small leak is heard on inspiration.[21] Problems with this technique include difficulty maintaining positive end-expiratory pressure (PEEP),[9] aspiration around the cuff,[9,21] and increased movement of the tube in the trachea.[21] The MOV technique consists of injecting air into the cuff until no leak is heard, then withdrawing the air until a small leak is heard on inspiration, and then adding more air until no leak is heard on inspiration.[21] The problem with this technique is that it generates higher cuff pressures than does the ML technique.[22] The selection of one technique over the other should be determined for the individual patient. If the patient needs a seal to provide adequate ventilation and/or is at high risk for aspiration, the MOV technique should be used. If these are not concerns, the ML technique should be used.[22]

Cuff pressure monitoring. Cuff pressures should be monitored at least every 8 hours with a mercury or aneroid manometer.[9,21,22] Cuff pressures should be maintained at 18 to 22 mm Hg (25 to 30 cm H_2O) because greater pressures decrease blood flow to the capillaries in the tracheal wall and lesser pressures increase the risk of aspiration. Pressures in excess of 22 mm Hg (30 cm H_2O) should be reported to the physician. In addition, cuffs should not be routinely deflated because this increases the risk of aspiration.[22]

Foam cuff tracheostomy tubes. One tracheostomy tube on the market has a cuff made of foam that is self-inflating. It is deflated during insertion after which the pilot port is opened to atmospheric pressure (room air) and the cuff self-inflates. Once inflated the foam cuff conforms to the size and shape of the patient's trachea, thereby reducing the pressure against the tracheal wall. The pilot port is either left open to atmospheric pressure or attached to the mechanical ventilator tubing, thus allowing the cuff to inflate and deflate with the cycling of the ventilator. Routine maintenance of a foam cuff tracheostomy tube includes aspirating the pilot port every 8 hours to measure cuff volume, removing any condensation from the cuff area, and assessing the integrity of the cuff. Removal of the tube is accomplished by deflating the cuff and can be complicated if the plastic sheath covering the foam is perforated. When perforation occurs, the foam may not be deflatable because the air cannot be totally aspirated.[23]

Suctioning

Suctioning is often required to maintain a patent airway in a patient with an endotracheal or tracheostomy tube. Suctioning is a sterile procedure that should be performed only when the patient needs it and not on a routine schedule. Indications for suctioning include coughing, respiratory distress, presence of rhonchi on auscultation, increased peak airway pressures on the ventilator, and decreasing SaO_2 or PaO_2.[24] A number of complications are associated with suctioning, including hypoxemia, atelectasis, bronchospasm, cardiac dysrhythmias, hemodynamic alteration, increased intracranial pressure,[25] and airway trauma.[9]

Complications. Hypoxemia can result from disconnecting the oxygen source from the patient and/or removing oxygen from the patient's airways when suction is applied.[25] Atelectasis is thought to occur when the suction catheter is larger than one half of the diameter of the ETT. Excessive negative pressure occurs when suction is applied, promoting collapse of the distal airway.[25] Bronchospasm is the result of the stimulation of the airway with the suction catheter.[25] Cardiac dysrhythmias, particularly bradycardias, are attributed to vagal stimulation.[26]

Some hemodynamic alterations—such as increases in mean arterial pressure, cardiac output, and pulmonary artery pressure—can result from lung hyperinflation during the procedure.[27] Airway trauma occurs with impaction of the catheter in the airway and excessive negative pressure applied to the catheter.[25]

Suctioning protocol. A number of protocols regarding suctioning have been developed. Several different practices have been found helpful in limiting the complications of suctioning. Hypoxemia can be minimized by giving the patient three hyperoxygenation breaths (breaths at 100% FIO_2) with the ventilator before the procedure and after each pass of the suction catheter.[28] If the patient exhibits signs of desaturation, hyperinflation (breaths at 150% tidal volume) should be added to the procedure.[29] Atelectasis can be avoided by using a suction catheter with an external diameter less than one half of the internal diameter of the ETT.[24,25] Using 100 mm Hg of suction or a flow rate of 15 to 20 L/min will decrease the chances of hypoxemia and airway trauma.[18] Limiting the duration of each suction pass to 10 seconds and the number of passes to three or less will also help minimize hypoxemia, airway trauma, cardiac dysrhythmias, and hemodynamic alterations.[25,30] The process of applying intermittent, instead of continuous, suction has been shown to be of no benefit.[31] In addition, the instillation of normal saline to help remove secretions has not proven to

be of any benefit[32] and may actually contribute to lower airway colonization and development of nosocomial pneumonia.[33]

Closed tracheal suction system. One of the newer devices to facilitate suctioning a patient on a ventilator is the closed tracheal suction system (CTSS). This device consists of a suction catheter in a plastic sleeve that attaches directly to the ventilator tubing. It allows the patient to be suctioned while remaining on the ventilator. Advantages of CTSS include the maintenance of oxygenation and positive end-expiratory pressure (PEEP) during suctioning, the reduction of hypoxemia-related complications, and the protection of staff members from the patient's secretions. CTSS is convenient to use, requiring only one person to perform the procedure. Concerns related to CTSS include autocontamination, inadequate removal of secretions, and increased risk of unintentional extubation, resulting from the extra weight of the system on the ventilator tubing. Autocontamination has been shown not to be an issue if the catheter is cleaned properly after every use and is changed every 24 hours. Inadequate removal of secretions may or may not be a problem, and further investigation is required to settle this issue.[34]

Communication

One of the major stressors for the patient with an artificial airway is impaired communication. This is related to the inability to speak, insufficient explanations from staff members, inadequate understanding, fear of being unable to communicate, and difficulty with communication methods.[35] A number of interventions can facilitate communication in the patient with an endotracheal or tracheostomy tube. These include performing a complete assessment of the patient's ability to communicate, teaching the patient how to communicate, using a variety of methods to communicate, and facilitating the patient's ability to communicate by providing the patient with his or her eyeglasses or hearing aid.[36]

A number of methods are available to facilitate communication in this patient population. These include the use of verbal and nonverbal language and a variety of devices to assist the short-term and long-term ventilator-assisted patient. Nonverbal communication may include the use of sign language, gestures, lip reading, pointing, facial expressions, or eye blinking. Simple devices available include pencil and paper; magic slates; magnetic boards with plastic letters; picture, alphabet, or symbol boards; and flash cards. More sophisticated devices include typewriters, computers, talking tracheostomy and endotracheal tubes, and external handheld vibrators. Regardless of the method selected, the patient must be taught how to use the device.[36] Patients with ETTs should be encouraged to communicate in writing because attempts at speech cause tube movement and increase tracheal injury.[9]

Passy-Muir valve. One of the newer devices to assist the mechanically ventilated patient with a tracheostomy to speak is the Passy-Muir valve. This one-way valve opens on inhalation, allowing air to enter the lungs through the tracheostomy tube, and closes on exhalation, forcing air over the vocal cords and out the mouth, thus permitting the patient to speak. Before placing the valve on a tracheostomy tube, the cuff must be deflated to allow air to pass around the tube while the tidal volume of the ventilator has to be increased to compensate for the air leak. In addition to assisting the patient to communicate, the Passy-Muir valve can assist the ventilator-dependent patient with relearning normal breathing patterns. The valve is contraindicated in patients with laryngeal and pharyngeal dysfunction, excessive secretions, and/or poor lung compliance.[37]

Extubation

Once the airway is no longer needed, it is removed. Extubation is the process of removing an endotracheal tube. It is a simple procedure that can be accomplished at the bedside.[9] Complications of extubation include glottic edema, laryngeal dysfunction, sore throat and hoarseness, and vocal cord paralysis. Decannulation is the process of removing a tracheostomy tube. It is also a simple process that can be performed at the bedside. After the removal of a tracheostomy tube, the stoma is usually covered with a dry dressing with the expectation that it should close within several days.[38]

INVASIVE MECHANICAL VENTILATION

Indications

Mechanical ventilation is indicated for a variety of physiologic and clinical reasons. Physiologic objectives include supporting cardiopulmonary gas exchange (alveolar ventilation and arterial oxygenation), increasing lung volume (end-expiratory lung inflation and functional residual capacity), and reducing the work of breathing. Clinical objectives include reversing hypoxemia and acute respiratory acidosis, relieving respiratory distress, preventing or reversing atelectasis, reversing ventilatory muscle fatigue, permitting sedation and/or neuromuscular blockade, decreasing systemic or myocardial oxygen consumption, reducing intracranial pressure, and stabilizing the chest wall.[39]

Types of Ventilators

The two main types of ventilators currently available are positive-pressure ventilators and negative-pressure ventilators. Negative-pressure ventilators are applied externally to the patient and decrease the atmospheric pressure surrounding the thorax to initiate inspiration. They are not commonly used in the critical care environment. Positive-pressure ventilators use a mechanical drive mechanism to force oxygen into the patient's lungs through an endotracheal or tracheostomy tube to initiate respiration.[40] There are four classifications of positive pressure ventilators based on the cycle variable: volume-cycled, pressure-cycled, flow-cycled, and time-cycled.[40,41] Volume-cycled ventilators are designed to deliver a breath until a preset volume is delivered. Pressure-cycled ventilators deliver a breath until a preset pressure is reached within the patient's airway. Flow-cycled ventilators deliver a breath until a preset inspiratory flow rate is achieved. Time-cycled ventilators deliver a breath over a preset time interval. Most of the newer ventilators are capable of using a variety of cycling mechanisms.[40] Fig. 14-3 depicts three commonly used ventilators in critical care.

Modes of Ventilation

The term *ventilator mode* refers to how the machine will ventilate the patient. In other words, selection of a particular mode of ventilation determines how much the patient will participate in his or her own ventilatory pattern. The choice depends on the patient's situation and the goals of treatment.[28] A large variety of modes are available[39,40,43-45] (Table 14-4). Many of these modes may be used in conjunction with each other. Because brands of ventilators vary in their ability to perform certain functions, not all modes are available on all ventilators.[42]

Ventilator Settings

A variety of settings on the ventilator allow the ventilator parameters to be individualized to the patient and the mode of ventilation selected[39,46] (Table 14-5). In addition, each ventilator has a patient-monitoring system that allows all aspects of the patient's ventilatory pattern to be assessed, monitored, and displayed. These monitoring capabilities include exhaled minute volume, exhaled tidal volume, total respiratory rate, peak pressure, plateau pressure, PEEP, mean airway pressure, spontaneous minute volume, spontaneous respiratory rate, circuit temperature, FIO_2, inspired tidal volume, pressure waveform, flow waveform, auto-PEEP, and respiratory mechanics. Monitoring capabilities vary slightly from one brand of ventilator to another.[43]

Complications

Mechanical ventilation is often lifesaving, but, similar to other interventions, it is not without complications. Some complications are preventable, whereas others can be minimized but not eradicated. Physiologic complications associated with mechanical ventilation include barotrauma, cardiovascular compromise, gastrointestinal disturbances, patient-ventilator asynchrony, and nosocomial pneumonia.

Barotrauma

Barotrauma occurs in mechanically ventilated patients as a result of alveolar over-distention. This causes alveo-

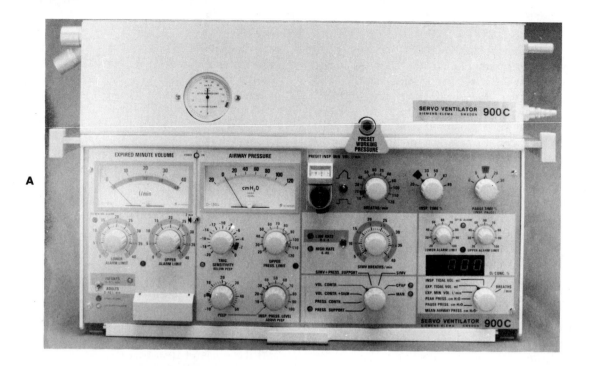

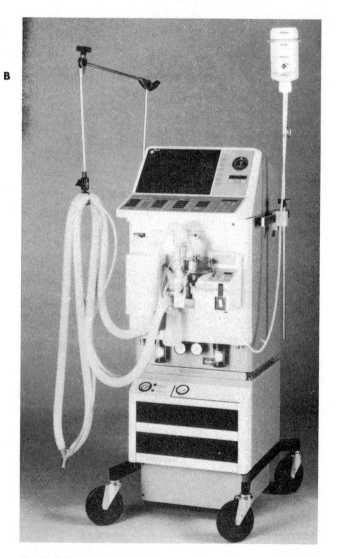

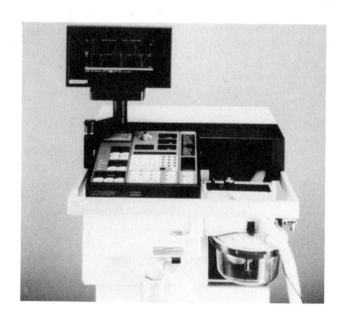

Fig. **14-3** Three types of volume-cycled ventilators. **A,** Servo 900C ventilator. **B,** BEAR 5 ventilator. **C,** Puritan-Bennett 7200 microprocessor ventilator. (From Dupuis YG: *Ventilators: theory and clinical application,* ed 2, St Louis, 1992, Mosby.)

TABLE 14-4

MODES OF MECHANICAL VENTILATION

MODE OF VENTILATION	CLINICAL APPLICATION	NURSING IMPLICATIONS
Control (volume or pressure) ventilation (CV): delivers gas at preset rate and tidal volume or pressure (depending on selected cycling variable), regardless of patient's inspiratory efforts	CV is used as the primary ventilatory mode in patients who are apneic	Used in patients unable to initiate a breath Spontaneously breathing patients must be sedated and/or paralyzed
Assist-control (volume or pressure) ventilation (A/C) or continuous mandatory ventilation (CMV): delivers gas at preset tidal volume or pressure (depending on selected cycling variable) in response to patient's inspiratory efforts and will initiate breath if patient fails to do so within preset time	A/C or CMV is used as the primary mode of ventilation in spontaneously breathing patients with weak respiratory muscles	Hyperventilation can occur in patients with increased respiratory rates Sedation may be necessary to limit the number of spontaneous breaths
Synchronous intermittent mandatory (volume or pressure) ventilation (SIMV): delivers gas at preset tidal volume or pressure (depending on selected cycling variable) and rate while allowing patient to breathe spontaneously; ventilator breaths are synchronized to patient's respiratory effort	SIMV is used both as a primary mode of ventilation in a wide variety of clinical situations and as a weaning mode	May increase the work of breathing and promote respiratory muscle fatigue
Positive end-expiratory pressure (PEEP): positive pressure applied at the end of expiration of ventilator breaths (used with CV, A/C, and SIMV) Constant positive airway pressure (CPAP): positive pressure applied during spontaneous breaths	PEEP and CPAP are used in patients with hypoxemia refractory to oxygen therapy; they increase functional residual capacity and improve oxygenation by opening collapsed alveoli at end expiration	Side effects include decreased cardiac output, barotrauma, and increased intracranial pressure No ventilator breaths are delivered in PEEP and CPAP mode unless used with CV, A/C, or SIMV
Pressure support ventilation (PSV): preset positive pressure used to augment patient's inspiratory efforts; patient controls rate, inspiratory flow, and tidal volume Volume-assured pressure support ventilation (VAPSV): tidal volume is set to ensure patient receives minimum tidal volume with each pressure support breath	PSV is used as the primary mode of ventilation in patients with stable respiratory drive, is used with SIMV to support spontaneous breaths, and is used as a weaning mode in patients who are difficult to wean	Advantages include increased patient comfort, decreased work of breathing and decreased respiratory muscle fatigue, and promotion of respiratory muscle conditioning
Independent lung ventilation (ILV): each lung is ventilated separately	ILV is used in patients with unilateral lung disease, bronchopleural fistulas, and bilateral asymmetric lung disease	Requires a double-lumen endotracheal tube, two ventilators, sedation, and/or pharmacologic paralysis
High frequency ventilation (HFV): delivers a small volume of gas at a rapid rate High-frequency positive-pressure ventilation (HFPPV): delivers 60-100 breaths/min High-frequency jet ventilation (HFJV): delivers 100-600 cycles/min High-frequency oscillation (HFO): delivers 900-3000 cycles/min	HFV is used in situations in which conventional mechanical ventilation compromises hemodynamic stability, with bronchopleural fistulas, during short-term procedures, and with diseases that create a risk of barotrauma	Patients require sedation and/or pharmacologic paralysis Inadequate humidification can compromise airway patency Assessment of breath sounds is difficult
Inverse ratio ventilation (IRV): proportion of inspiratory to expiratory time is greater than 1:1; can be initiated using pressure-controlled breaths (PC-IRV) or volume controlled breaths (VC-IRV)	IRV is used in patients with hypoxemia refractory to PEEP; the longer inspiratory time increases functional residual capacity and improves oxygenation by opening collapsed alveoli, and the shorter expiratory time induces auto-PEEP that prevents alveoli from recollapsing	Requires sedation and/or pharmacologic paralysis because of discomfort Increased intrathoracic pressure can result in excessive air trapping and decreased cardiac output

TABLE 14-5

VENTILATOR SETTINGS

PARAMETER	DESCRIPTION
Respiratory rate (f)	Number of breaths the ventilator delivers per minute; usual setting is 4-20 breaths/min
Tidal volume (V_T)	Volume of gas delivered to patient during each ventilator breath; usual volume is 5-15 ml/kg
Oxygen concentration (FIO_2)	Fraction of inspired oxygen delivered to patient; may be set between 21% and 100%; usually adjusted to maintain PaO_2 level greater than 60 mm Hg or SaO_2 level greater than 90%
I:E ratio	Duration of inspiration to duration of expiration; usual setting is 1:2 to 1:1.5 unless inverse ratio ventilation is desired
Flow rate	Speed with which the tidal volume is delivered; usual setting is 40-100 L/min
Sensitivity/ trigger	Determines the amount of effort the patient must generate to initiate a ventilator breath; it may be set for pressure-triggering or flow-triggering; usual setting for pressure-trigger is 0.5-1.5 cm H_2O below baseline pressure and for flow-trigger is 1-3 L/min below baseline flow
Pressure limit	Regulates the maximal pressure the ventilator can generate to deliver the tidal volume; when the pressure limit is reached, the ventilator terminates the breath and spills the undelivered volume into the atmosphere; usual setting is 10-20 cm H_2O above peak inspiratory pressure

lar rupture and air leakage into the pulmonary interstitial space. Once in the space, the air travels out through the hilum and into the mediastinum (pneumomediastinum), pleural space (pneumothorax), subcutaneous tissues (subcutaneous emphysema), pericardium (pneumopericardium), peritoneum (pneumoperitoneum), and retroperitoneum (pneumoretroperitoneum). The resultant disorders vary from the fairly benign to the potentially lethal. The most lethal include pneumothorax or pneumopericardium resulting in cardiac tamponade.[39,47,48]

Cardiovascular compromise

Positive-pressure ventilation increases intrathoracic pressure, which decreases venous return to the right side of the heart. Impaired venous return decreases preload, which results in a decrease in CO. As a secondary consequence, hepatic and renal dysfunction may occur. In addition, positive-pressure ventilation impairs cerebral venous return. In patients with impaired autoregulation, positive-pressure ventilation can result in increased intracranial pressure.[39,47,48]

Gastrointestinal disturbances

A number of gastrointestinal disturbances can also occur as a result of positive pressure ventilation. Gastric distention occurs when air leaks around the endotracheal or tracheostomy tube cuff and overcomes the resistance of the lower esophageal sphincter.[48] Vomiting can occur as a result of pharyngeal stimulation from the artificial airway.[39] These problems can be prevented by inserting a nasogastric tube and ensuring appropriate cuff inflation.[48] In addition, hypomotility and constipation may occur because of the administration of paralytic agents, analgesics, and sedatives, and because of immobility.[39]

Patient-ventilator asynchrony

As the normal ventilatory pattern is usually initiated by the establishment of negative pressure within the chest, the application of positive pressure can lead to patient difficulties in breathing on the ventilator. To achieve optimal ventilatory assistance, the patient should breath in synchrony with the machine. The selected mode of ventilation, the settings, and the type of ventilatory circuitry used can also increase the work of breathing and lead to the patient breathing out of synchrony with the ventilator. Patient-ventilatory asynchrony can result in a decrease in effectiveness of mechanical ventilation, the development of auto-PEEP, and psychologic distress for the patient. Patients who are not breathing in synchrony with the ventilator appear to be fighting or "bucking" the ventilator. To minimize this problem, the ventilator should be adjusted to accommodate the patient's spontaneous breathing pattern and to work with the patient. If this is not possible, the patient may need to be sedated and/or pharmacologically paralyzed.[39]

Nosocomial pneumonia

There is great potential for the development of nosocomial pneumonia after the placement of a artificial airway, as the tube bypasses or impairs many of the lung's normal defense mechanisms. Once an artificial airway is placed, contamination of the lower airway follows within 24 hours. This results from a number of factors that directly and indirectly promote airway colonization. The use of respiratory therapy devices (e.g., ventilators, nebulizers, and intermittent positive-pressure breathing machines) can also increase the risk of pneumonia. The severity of the patient's illness, acute lung injury, and/or malnutrition significantly increase the likelihood that an infection will occur. In addition, such therapeutic measures as nasogastric tubes, antacids, and histamine inhibitors facilitate the development of pneumonia. Nasogastric tubes promote aspiration by acting as a wick for stomach contents, and antacids and histamine inhibitors increase the pH level of the stomach, thus promoting the growth of bacteria that can then be aspirated.[20]

Weaning

Weaning is the gradual withdrawal of the mechanical ventilator and the reestablishment of spontaneous breathing.[39] Weaning should begin only after the original process requiring ventilator support for the patient has been corrected and patient stability has been achieved.[49]

Other factors to consider when weaning are length of time on ventilator, sleep deprivation, and nutritional status. Major factors that affect the patient's ability to wean include the ability of the lungs to participate in ventilation and respiration, cardiovascular performance, and psychologic readiness.[39] This discussion will focus on weaning the patient from short-term (3 days or less) mechanical ventilation. Weaning the patient from long-term mechanical ventilation is discussed in Chapter 13.

Readiness to wean

Once the decision is made to wean the patient, an assessment of the patient's readiness to wean should take place. Two strong predictors for weaning readiness are vital capacity (VC)/kg greater than or equal to 15 ml and negative inspiratory pressure (NIP) of -30 cm H_2O or less.[50]

Once readiness to wean has been established, the patient should be prepared for a weaning trial. The patient should be positioned upright to facilitate breathing and suctioned to ensure airway patency. In addition, the process should be explained to the patient and the patient offered reassurance and diversional activities. The patient should be assessed immediately before the start of the trial and frequently during the weaning period for signs of weaning intolerance, including SpO_2 less than 90%, greater than 20% change in heart rate from baseline, respiratory rate greater than 30%, and serious changes in cardiac rhythm.[51]

Weaning methods

A number of methods can be used to wean a patient from the ventilator. The method selected depends on the patient, pulmonary status, and the length of time on the ventilator. The three main methods for weaning are T-tube (T-piece) trials, SIMV, and PSV.[39]

T-tube. T-tube trials consist of alternating periods of ventilatory support (usually on A/C or CMV) with periods of spontaneous breathing. The trial is initiated by removing the patient from the ventilator and having the patient breathe spontaneously on a T-tube. After a length of time, the patient is placed back on the ventilator. The goal is to progressively increase the duration of time spent off the ventilator. During the weaning process, the patient should be observed closely for respiratory muscle fatigue.[39,49] CPAP may be added to prevent atelectasis and improve oxygenation.[49]

SIMV. The goal of SIMV weaning is the gradual transition from ventilatory support to spontaneous breathing. It is initiated by placing the ventilator in the SIMV mode and slowly decreasing the rate until zero (or close) is reached. The rate is usually decreased one to three breaths at a time, and an ABG analysis is usually obtained 30 minutes afterward. This method of weaning can increase the work of breathing, and thus the patient

should be closely monitored for signs of respiratory muscle fatigue.[39,49]

PSV. PSV weaning consists of placing the patient on the pressure support mode and setting the pressure support at a level that facilitates the patient's achieving a spontaneous tidal volume of 10 to 12 ml/kg. PSV augments the patient's spontaneous breaths with a positive-pressure "boost" during inspiration. During the weaning process, the level of pressure support is gradually decreased in increments of 3 to 6 cm H_2O while maintaining a tidal volume of 10 to 15 ml/kg until a level of 5 cm H_2O is achieved. If the patient is able to maintain adequate spontaneous respirations at this level, extubation is considered. PSV can also be used with SIMV weaning to help overcome the resistance in the ventilator system.[49]

Nursing Management

Nursing priorities for the patient with invasive mechanical ventilation include monitoring the patient for both patient-related and ventilator-related complications. Monitoring should include a routine total assessment, with particular emphasis on the pulmonary system, placement of the endotracheal tube, and observation for subcutaneous emphysema and synchrony with the ventilator. Assessment of the ventilator should include a review of all the ventilator settings and alarms.

Bedside evaluation of vital capacity, minute ventilation, arterial blood gas (ABG) values, and other pulmonary function tests may be warranted, according to the patient's condition. The use of pulse oximetry can facilitate continuous, noninvasive assessment of oxygenation. Static and dynamic compliance should also be monitored to assess for changes in lung compliance (Appendix B).

Some additional measures are required to maintain a trouble-free ventilator system. These include maintaining a functional MRB connected to oxygen at the bedside, ensuring that the ventilator tubing is free of water, positioning the ventilator tubing to avoid kinking, maintaining the patency of ventilator tubing and connections, changing ventilator tubing per hospital policy, and monitoring the temperature of the inspired air. In addition, a clear understanding of the alarms and their related problems is important (Table 14-6). **In the event that the ventilator malfunctions, the patient should be removed from the ventilator and ventilated manually with an MRB.**

NONINVASIVE MECHANICAL VENTILATION

Noninvasive mechanical ventilation is a relatively new method of ventilation that uses a mask to administer positive pressure instead of a endotracheal tube. Advantages to this type of ventilation include decreased frequency of nosocomial pneumonia, increased comfort, and the noninvasive nature of the procedure, which allows easy application and removal. It is indicated in variety of situations, including acute hypercapnia respiratory failure, acute hypoxemic respiratory failure, and when intubation is not

TABLE 14-6

TROUBLESHOOTING VENTILATOR ALARMS

PROBLEM	CAUSES	INTERVENTIONS
Low exhaled V_T	Altered settings; any condition that triggers high or low pressure alarm; patient stops spontaneous respirations; leak in system preventing V_T from being delivered; cuff insufficiently inflated; leak through chest tube; airway secretions; decreased lung compliance; spirometer disconnected or malfunctioning	Check settings; evaluate patient, check respiratory rate; check all connections for leaks; suction patient's airway; check cuff pressure; calibrate spirometer
Low inspiratory pressure	Altered settings; unattached tubing or leak around ET tube; ET tube displaced into pharynx or esophagus; poor cuff inflation or leak; tracheal-esophageal fistula; peak flows that are too low; low V_Ts; decreased airway resistance resulting from decreased secretions or relief of bronchospasm; increased lung compliance resulting from decreased atelectasis; reduction in pulmonary edema; resolution of ARDS; change in position	Reset alarm; reconnect tubing; modify cuff pressures; tighten humidifier; check chest tube; adjust peak flow to meet or exceed patient demand and correct for the patient's V_T reposition or change ET tube
Low exhaled minute volume	Altered settings; leak in system; airway secretions; decreased lung compliance; malfunctioning spirometer; decreased patient-triggered respiratory rate resulting from drugs; sleep; hypocapnia; alkalosis; fatigue; change in neurologic status	Check settings; assess patient's respiratory rate, mental status, and work of breathing; evaluate system for leaks; suction airway; assess patient for changes in disease state; calibrate spirometer
Low PEEP/CPAP pressure	Altered settings; increased patient inspiratory flows; leak; decreased expiratory flows from ventilator	Check settings and correct; observe for leaks in system; if unable to correct problem, increase PEEP setting
High respiratory rate	Increased metabolic demand; drug administration; hypoxia; hypercapnia; acidosis; shock; pain; fear; anxiety	Evaluate ABGs; assess patient; calm and reassure patient
High pressure limit	Improper alarm setting; airway obstruction resulting from patient fighting ventilator (holding breath as ventilator delivers V_T); patient circuit collapse; tubing kinked; ET tube in right mainstem bronchus or against carina; cuff herniation; increased airway resistance resulting from bronchospasm, airway secretions, plugs, and coughing; water from humidifier in ventilator tubing; decreased lung compliance resulting from tension pneumothorax; change in patient position; ARDS; pulmonary edema; atelectasis; pneumonia; or abdominal distention.	Reset alarms; clear obstruction from tubing; unkink and reposition patient off of tubing; empty water from tubing; check breath sounds; reassure patient and sedate if necessary; check ABGs for hypoxemia; observe for abdominal distention that would put pressure on the diaphragm; check cuff pressures; obtain chest x-ray and evaluate for ET tube position, pneumothorax, and pneumonia; reposition ET tube; give bronchodilator therapy
Low pressure oxygen inlet	Improper oxygen alarm setting; oxygen not connected to ventilator; dirty oxygen intake filter	Correct alarm setting; reconnect or connect oxygen line to a 50 psi source; clean or replace oxygen filter
I:E ratio	Inspiratory time longer than expiratory time; use of an inspiratory phase that is too long with a fast rate; peak flow setting too low while rate too high; machine too sensitive	Change inspiratory time or adjust peak flow; check inspiratory phase, or hold; check machine sensitivity
Temperature	Sensor malfunction; overheating resulting from too low or no gas flow; sensor picking up outside airflow (from heaters, open doors or windows, air conditioners); improper water levels	Test or replace sensor; check gas flow; protect sensor from outside source that would interfere with readings; check water levels

Modified from Flynn JBM, Bruce NP: *Introduction to critical care nursing skills,* St Louis, 1993, Mosby.

an option. Contraindications to noninvasive mechanical ventilation include hemodynamic instability, dysrhythmias, apnea, uncooperativeness, intolerance of the mask, and inability to maintain a patent airway, to clear secretions, and to properly fit the mask.[52,53]

Noninvasive mechanical ventilation can be applied using a nasal or facial mask and ventilator or a BiPAP (trademark of Respironics) machine (Fig. 14-4). This mode of therapy uses a combination of PSV (ventilator) or inspiratory positive airway pressure (IPAP) (BiPAP

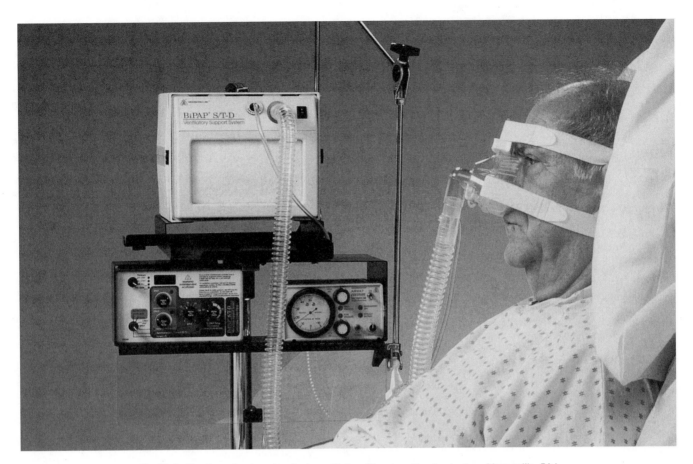

Fig. 14-4 Noninvasive mechanical ventilator. (Courtesy Respironics Inc., Murrysville, PA.)

machine) and PEEP (ventilator) or expiratory positive airway pressure (EPAP) (BiPAP machine) to assist the spontaneously breathing patient with ventilation. On inspiration, the patient receives PSV or IPAP to increase tidal volume and minute ventilation, which results in increased alveolar ventilation, decreased $PaCO_2$, relief of dyspnea, and reduced accessory muscle use. On expiration, the patient receives PEEP or EPAP to increase functional residual capacity, which results in increased PaO_2. Humidified supplemental oxygen is administered to maintain a clinically acceptable PaO_2 and timed breaths may be added if necessary.[52,53]

Nursing Management

Nursing priorities for patient with noninvasive mechanical ventilation include monitoring the patient for both patient-related and ventilator-related complications. As with invasive mechanical ventilation, the patient must be closely monitored while receiving noninvasive mechanical ventilation. Respiratory rate, accessory muscle use, and oxygenation status should be continually assessed to ensure the patient is tolerating this method of ventilation. Continued pulse oximetry with a set alarm parameter should be initiated.[52,53]

The key to ensuring adequate ventilatory support is a properly fitted mask. Either a nasal mask or a full face mask may be used, depending on the patient. A properly fitted mask minimizes discomfort for the patient and air leakage. Transparent dressings placed over the pressure points of the face help minimize air leakage and prevent facial skin necrosis from the mask. The BiPAP machine is able to compensate for airleaks.[52,53]

The patient should be positioned with the head of the bed elevated to 45 degrees to minimize the risk of aspiration and facilitate breathing. Insufflation of the stomach is a complication of this mode of therapy and places the patient at risk for aspiration. In addition, the patient should be closely monitored for gastric distention. Often patients are very anxious with high levels of dyspnea before initiation of noninvasive mechanical ventilation. Once adequate ventilation has been established, anxiety and dyspnea are usually sufficiently relieved. Heavy sedation should be avoided and, if needed, would constitute the need for intubation and invasive mechanical ventilation. Spending 30 minutes with the patient after the initiation of noninvasive ventilation is important because the patient needs reassurance and must learn how to breathe on the machine.[52,53]

References

1. O'Connor BS, Vender JS: Oxygen therapy, *Crit Care Clin* 11:67, 1995.
2. Carlton TJ, Anthonisen NR: A guide for judicious use of oxygen in critical illness, *J Crit Ill* 7:1744, 1992.
3. Scanlan CL, Thalken FR: Medical gas therapy. In Scanlan CL, Spearman CB, Sheldon RL, editors: *Egan's fundamentals of respiratory care*, ed 6, St Louis, 1995, Mosby.
4. Branson RD: The nuts and bolts of increasing arterial oxygenation: devices and techniques, *Respir Care* 38:672, 1993.
5. Durbin CG, Wallace KK: Oxygen toxicity in the critically ill patient, *Respir Care* 38:739, 1993.
6. Hanson CW, Marshall BE, Frasch HF, Marshall C: Causes of hypercarbia with oxygen therapy in patients with chronic obstructive pulmonary disease, *Crit Care Med* 24:23, 1996.
7. Kharasch M, Graff J: Emergency management of the airway, *Crit Care Clin* 11:53, 1995.
8. Somerson SJ, Sicilia MR: Emergency oxygen administration and airway management, *Crit Care Nurs* 12(4):23, 1992.
9. Stauffer JL: Medical management of the airway, *Clin Chest Med* 12:449, 1991.
10. Einarsson O, Rochester CL, Rosenbaum S: Airway management in respiratory emergencies, *Clin Chest Med* 15:13, 1994.
11. Stone DJ, Bogdonoff DL: Airway considerations in the management of patients requiring long-term endotracheal intubation, *Anesth Anal* 74:276, 1992.
12. Colice GL: Technical standards for tracheal tubes, *Clin Chest Med* 12:433, 1991.
13. Zarshenas Z, Sparschu RA: Catheter placement and misplacement, *Crit Care Clin* 10:417, 1994.
14. McCulloch TM, Bishop MJ: Complications of translaryngeal intubation, *Clin Chest Med* 12:507, 1991.
15. Wenig BL, Applebaum EL: Indications for and techniques of tracheotomy, *Clin Chest Med* 12:545, 1991.
16. Weilitz PB, Dettenmeier PA: Back to basics: test your knowledge of tracheostomy tubes, *Am J Nurs* 94(2):46, 1994.
17. Myers EN, Carrau RL: Early complications of tracheotomy: incidence and management, *Clin Chest Med* 12:589, 1991.
18. Wood DE, Mathisen DJ: Late complications of tracheotomy, *Clin Chest Med* 12:597, 1991.
19. Fink J: Humidity and aerosol therapy. In Scanlan CL, Spearman CB, Sheldon RL, editors: *Egan's fundamentals of respiratory care*, ed 6, St Louis, 1995, Mosby.
20. Chang VM: Protocol for prevention of complications of endotracheal intubation, *Crit Care Nurs* 15(5):19, 1995.
21. Goodnough SKC: Reducing tracheal injury and aspiration, *Dimens Crit Care Nurs* 7:324, 1988.
22. Tyler DO, Clark AP, Ogburn-Russell L: Developing a standard for endotracheal tube cuff care, *Dimens Crit Care Nurs* 10:54, 1991.
23. Bivona: *Fome-Cuf users' manual*, Gary, 1991, Bivona.
24. Glass CA, Grap MJ: Ten tips for safer suctioning, *Am J Nurs* 95(5):51, 1995.
25. Stone KS: Endotracheal suctioning in the critically ill, *Crit Care Nurs Curr* 7:5, 1989.
26. Gunderson LP, Stone KS, Hamlin RL: Endotracheal suctioning–induced heart rate alterations, *Nurs Res* 40:139, 1991.
27. Stone KS, et al: The effect of lung hyperinflation and endotracheal suctioning on cardiopulmonary hemodynamics, *Nurs Res* 40:76, 1991.
28. Grap MJ, Glass C, Corley M, Parks T: Endotracheal suctioning: ventilator vs manual delivery of hyperoxygenation breaths, *Am J Crit Care* 1(3):62, 1992.
29. Mancinelli-Van Atta J, Beck SL: Preventing hypoxemia and hemodynamic compromise related to endotracheal suctioning, *Am J Crit Care* 1(3):62, 1992.
30. Stone KS: Ventilator versus manual resuscitation bag as the method of delivering hyperoxygenation before endotracheal suctioning, *AACN Clin Iss Crit Care Nurs* 1:289, 1990.
31. Czarnik RE, et al: Deferential effects of continuous versus intermittent suction on tracheal tissue, *Heart Lung* 20:144, 1991.
32. Raymond SJ: Normal saline instillation before suctioning: helpful or harmful? A review of the literature, *Am J Crit Care* 4:267, 1995.
33. Hagler DA, Traver GA: Endotracheal saline and suction catheters: sources of lower airway contamination, *Am J Crit Care* 3:444, 1994.
34. Johnson KL, et al: Closed versus open endotracheal suctioning: costs and physiologic consequences, *Crit Care Med* 22:658, 1994.
35. Jablonski RS: The experience of being mechanically ventilated, *Qual Health Res* 4:186, 1994.
36. Williams ML: An algorithm for selecting a communication technique with intubated patients, *Dimens Crit Care Nurs* 11:222, 1992.
37. Bell SD: Use of Passy-Muir tracheostomy speaking valve in mechanically ventilated neurological patients, *Crit Care Nurs* 16(1):63, 1996.
38. Godwin JE, Heffner JE: Special critical care considerations in tracheostomy management, *Clin Chest Med* 12:573, 1991.
39. American College of Chest Physicians: ACCP consensus conference: mechanical ventilation, *Chest* 194:1833, 1993.
40. Scanlan CL, Blazer C: Physics and physiology of ventilatory support. In Scanlan CL, Spearman CB, Sheldon RL, editors: *Egan's fundamentals of respiratory care*, ed 6, St Louis, 1995, Mosby.
41. Kacmarek RM, Meklaus GJ: The new generation of mechanical ventilators, *Crit Care Clin* 6:551, 1990.
42. Dupuis YG: *Ventilators: theory and clinical application*, ed 2, St Louis, 1992, Mosby.
43. Bone RC, Eubanks DH: Second- and third-generation ventilators: sorting through available options, *J Crit Ill* 7:399, 1992.
44. Herridge MS, Slutsky AS: High frequency ventilation: a ventilatory technique that merits revisiting, *Respir Care* 41:385, 1996.
45. Brochard L: Pressure-limited ventilation, *Respir Care* 41:447, 1996.
46. Scanlan CL: Initiating and adjusting ventilatory support. In Scanlan CL, Spearman CB, Sheldon RL, editors: *Egan's fundamentals of respiratory care*, ed 6, St Louis, 1995, Mosby.
47. Dreyfuss D, Saumon G: Ventilator-induced lung injury, *Am J Respir Crit Care Med* 157:294, 1998.
48. Keith RL, Pierson DJ: Complications of mechanical ventilation, *Clin Chest Med* 17:439, 1996.
49. Weilitz PB: Weaning a patient from mechanical ventilation, *Crit Care Nurs* 13(4):33, 1993.
50. Hanneman SK, et al: Weaning from short-term mechanical ventilation: a review, *Am J Crit Care* 3:421, 1994.
51. Hannemann, SK: *Weaning from short-term mechanical ventilation*, Aliso Viejo, CA, 1998, American Association of Critical Care Nurses.
52. Abou-Shola N, Meduri GU: Noninvasive mechanical ventilation in patients with acute respiratory failure, *Crit Care Med* 24:705, 1996.
53. Meduri, GU: Noninvasive positive-pressure ventilation in patients with acute respiratory failure, *Clin Chest Med* 17:513, 1996.

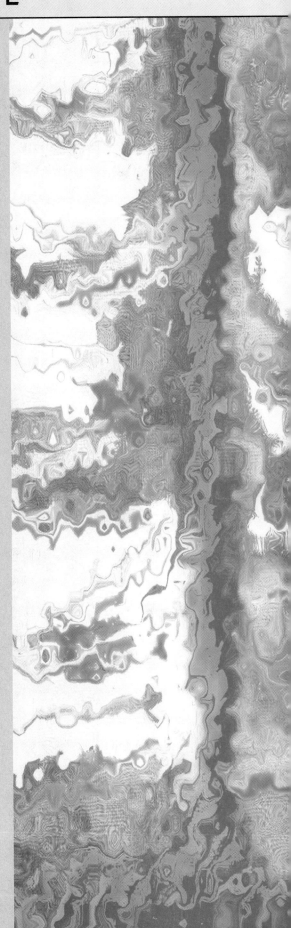

NEUROLOGIC
ALTERATIONS

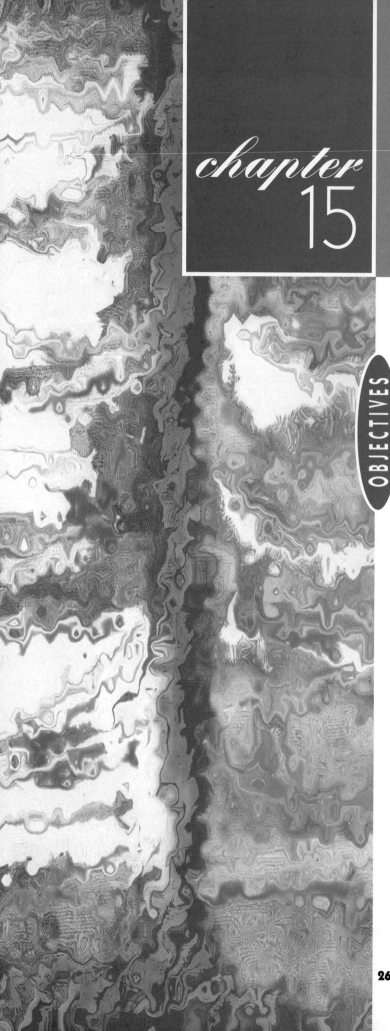

chapter 15

Neurologic Assessment and Diagnostic Procedures

Beverly Means Carlson

OBJECTIVES

- Identify the components of a neurologic history.
- Describe the five components of the neurologic assessment.
- Discuss the neurologic changes associated with intracranial hypertension.
- Identify key diagnostic procedures used in assessment of the patient with neurologic dysfunction.
- Discuss the nursing management of a patient undergoing a neurologic diagnostic procedure.

Assessment of the critically ill patient with neurologic dysfunction includes a review of the patient's health history, a thorough physical examination, and an analysis of the patient's laboratory data. Numerous invasive and noninvasive diagnostic procedures may also be performed to assist in the identification of the patient's disorder. This chapter focuses on priority clinical assessments, laboratory studies, and diagnostic procedures for the critically ill patient with a neurologic dysfunction.

CLINICAL ASSESSMENT

A thorough clinical assessment of the patient with neurologic dysfunction is imperative for the early identification and treatment of neurologic disorders. Once completed, the assessment serves as the foundation for developing the management plan for the patient. The assessment process can be brief or can involve a detailed history and examination, depending on the nature and immediacy of the patient's situation.

HISTORY

Neurologic assessment encompasses a wide variety of applications and a multitude of techniques. This chapter focuses on the type of assessment performed in a critical care environment. The one factor common to all neurologic assessments is the need to obtain a comprehensive history of events preceding hospitalization. An adequate neurologic history includes information about clinical manifestations, associated complaints, precipitating factors, progression, and familial occurrences. If the patient is incapable of providing this information, family members or significant others should be contacted as soon as possible. When someone other than the patient is the source of the history, it should be an individual who was in contact with the patient on a daily basis. Frequently, valuable information is gained, which directs the caregiver to focus on certain aspects of the patient's clinical assessment.

PHYSICAL EXAMINATION

Five major components make up the neurologic examination of the critically ill patient. **These assessment priorities are evaluation of (1) level of consciousness, (2) motor function, (3) pupillary function, (4) respiratory function, and (5) vital signs.** Until all five components have been assessed, a complete neurologic examination has not been performed.

Level of Consciousness

Assessment of the level of consciousness is the most important aspect of the neurologic examination. In most situations, a patient's level of consciousness deteriorates before any other neurologic changes are noted. These deteriorations often are subtle and must be monitored carefully. **Assessment of level of consciousness focuses on two priorities: (1) evaluation of arousal or alertness and (2) appraisal of content of consciousness or awareness.**[1] Universally accepted definitions for various levels of consciousness do not exist. The categories outlined in Box 15-1, although vague, are often used to describe the patient's level of consciousness.[1-3]

Evaluation of arousal

Assessment of the arousal component of consciousness is an evaluation of the reticular activating system and its connection with the thalamus and the cerebral cortex. Arousal is the lowest level of consciousness, and observation centers on the patient's ability to respond to verbal or noxious stimuli in an appropriate manner. To stimulate the patient, the nurse should begin with verbal stimuli in a normal tone. If the patient does not respond, the nurse should increase the stimuli by shouting at the patient. If the patient still does not respond, the nurse should further increase the stimuli by shaking the patient. Noxious stimuli should

---

BOX 15-1

CATEGORIES OF CONSCIOUSNESS

Alert—responds immediately to minimal external stimuli.
Lethargic—state of drowsiness or inaction in which the patient needs an increased stimulus to be awakened but is still easily arousable. Verbal, mental, and motor responses are slow and sluggish.
Obtunded—very drowsy when not stimulated. Follows simple commands when stimulated. A duller indifference to external stimuli exists, and response is minimally maintained.
Stuporous—minimal spontaneous movement. Arousable only by vigorous and continuous external stimuli. Motor responses to tactile stimuli are appropriate. Verbal responses are minimal and incomprehensible.
Comatose—vigorous stimulation fails to produce any voluntary neural response. Both arousal and awareness are absent. No verbal responses. Motor responses may be purposeful withdrawal to pain (light coma), nonpurposeful, or absent (deep coma).

BOX 15-2

NOXIOUS STIMULI

CENTRAL STIMULATION TECHNIQUES
- Trapezius pinch: performed by squeezing the trapezius muscle between the thumb and first two fingers.
- Sternal rub: performed by applying firm pressure to the sternum with the knuckles, using a rubbing motion.

PERIPHERAL STIMULATION TECHNIQUES
- Nail bed pressure: performed by applying firm pressure, using an object such as a pen, to the nailbed.
- Pinching of the inner aspect of the arm or leg: performed by firmly pinching a small portion of the patient's tissue on the sensitive inner aspect of the arm or leg.

---

follow if previous attempts to arouse the patient are unsuccessful. To assess arousal, central stimulation should be used (Box 15-2).

Appraisal of awareness

Content of consciousness is a higher level function and is concerned with assessment of the patient's orientation to person, place, and time. Assessment of content of consciousness requires the patient to give appropriate answers to a variety of questions. Changes in the patient's answers that indicate increasing degrees of confusion and disorientation may be the first sign of neurologic deterioration.[1]

Glasgow Coma Scale

The most widely recognized level of consciousness assessment tool is the Glasgow Coma Scale (GCS).[4] This scored scale is based on evaluation of three categories: eye opening, verbal response, and best motor response (Table 15-1). The best possible score on the GCS is 15, and the lowest score is 3. Generally a score of 7 or less on the GCS indicates coma. Originally the scoring system was developed to assist in general communication concerning the severity of neurologic injury. Recent testing of the GCS revealed a moderate to high agreement rating among both physicians and nurses.[5] Several points should be kept in mind when the GCS is used for serial assessment. It provides data about level of consciousness only and never should be considered a complete neurologic examination. It is not a sensitive tool for evaluation of an altered sensorium, nor does it account for possible aphasia. The GCS is also a poor indicator of lateralization of neurologic deterioration.[6] Lateralization involves decreasing motor response on one side or unilateral changes in pupillary reaction.

Motor Function

Assessment of motor function focuses on two priorities: (1) evaluation of muscle size and tone and (2) estimation of muscle strength. Each side should be assessed individually and then compared together.

Evaluation of muscle size and tone

Initially the muscles should be inspected for size and shape. The presence of atrophy or hypertrophy is noted. Muscle tone is assessed by evaluating the opposition to passive movement. The patient is instructed to relax the extremity while the nurse performs passive range of motion and evaluates the degree of resistance. Muscle tone is appraised for signs of flaccidity (no resistance), hypotonia (little resistance), hypertonia (increased resistance), spasticity, or rigidity.[7]

Estimation of muscle strength

Muscle strength is assessed by having the patient perform a number of movements against resistance. The strength of the movement is then graded on a six-point scale (Box 15-3). The upper extremities are tested by asking the patient to grasp, squeeze, and release the nurse's index and middle fingers. If weakness or asymmetry is suspected, the patient is instructed to extend both arms with the palms turned upward and hold that position with the eyes closed. If the patient has a weaker side, the arm will drift downward and pronate. The lower extremities are tested by asking the patient to push and pull the feet against resistance.[8]

Abnormal motor responses

If the patient is incapable of comprehending and following a simple command, noxious stimuli is required to determine motor responses. The stimuli is applied to each extremity separately to allow evaluation of individual extremity function. Peripheral stimulation is used to assess motor function.[9] Motor responses elicited by noxious stimuli are interpreted differently than those elicited by

TABLE 15-1

GLASGOW COMA SCALE

CATEGORY	SCORE	RESPONSE
Eye opening	4	Spontaneous: eyes open spontaneously without stimulation
	3	To speech: eyes open with verbal stimulation but not necessarily to command
	2	To pain: eyes open with noxious stimuli
	1	None: no eye opening regardless of stimulation
Verbal response	5	Oriented: accurate information about person, place, time, reason for hospitalization, and personal data
	4	Confused: answers not appropriate to question, but use of language is correct
	3	Inappropriate words: disorganized, random speech, no sustained conversation
	2	Incomprehensible sounds: moans, groans, and incomprehensible mumbles
	1	None: no verbalization despite stimulation
Best motor response	6	Obeys commands: performs simple tasks on command; able to repeat performance
	5	Localizes to pain: organized attempt to localize and remove painful stimuli
	4	Withdraws from pain: withdraws extremity from source of painful stimuli
	3	Abnormal flexion: decorticate posturing spontaneously or in response to noxious stimuli
	2	Extension: decerebrate posturing spontaneously or in response to noxious stimuli
	1	None: no response to noxious stimuli; flaccid

BOX 15-3

MUSCLE STRENGTH GRADING SCALE

0—No movement or muscle contraction
1—Trace contraction
2—Active movement with gravity eliminated
3—Active movement against gravity
4—Active movement with some resistance
5—Active movement with full resistance

voluntary demonstration. These responses may be classified into four categories as listed in Box 15-4.[8]

Pupillary Function

Assessment of pupillary function focuses on three priorities: (1) estimation of pupil size and shape, (2) evaluation of pupillary reaction to light, and (3) assessment of eye movements. Pupillary function is an extension of the autonomic nervous system. Parasympathetic control of the pupil occurs through innervation of the oculomotor nerve (CN III), which exits from the brainstem in the midbrain area. When the parasympathetic fibers are stimulated, the pupil constricts. Sympathetic control originates in the hypothalamus and travels down the entire length of the brainstem. When the sympathetic fibers are stimulated, the pupil dilates. Pupillary changes provide a valuable tool to assessment because of pathway location. The oculomotor nerve lies at the junction of the midbrain and the tentorial notch. Any increase of pressure that exerts force down through the tentorial notch compresses the oculomotor nerve. Oculomotor nerve compression results in a dilated, nonreactive pupil. Sympathetic pathway disruption occurs with involvement in the brainstem. Loss of sympathetic control leads to pinpoint, nonreactive pupils. Control of eye movements occurs with interaction of three cranial nerves: oculomotor (CN III), trochlear (CN IV), and abducens (CN VI). The pathways for these cranial nerves provide integrated function through the internuclear pathway of the medial longitudinal fasciculus (MLF) located in the brainstem. The MLF provides coordination of eye movements with the vestibular (CN VIII) nerve and the reticular formation.[7]

Estimation of pupil size and shape

Pupil size should be documented in millimeters with the use of a pupil gauge to reduce the subjectivity of

description. Although most people have pupils of equal size, a discrepancy up to 1 mm between the two pupils is normal. Inequality of pupils is known as anisocoria and occurs in 15% to 17% of the human population.[10] Change or inequality in pupil size, especially in patients who previously have not shown this discrepancy, is a significant neurologic sign. It may indicate impending danger of herniation and should be reported immediately. With the location of the oculomotor nerve (CN III) at the notch of the tentorium, pupil size and reactivity play a key role in the physical assessment of intracranial pressure changes and herniation syndromes. In addition to CN III compression, changes in pupil size occur for other reasons. Large pupils can result from the instillation of cycloplegic agents, such as atropine or scopolamine, or can indicate extreme stress. Extremely small pupils can indicate narcotic overdose, lower brainstem compression, or bilateral damage to the pons.[10]

Pupil shape also is noted in the assessment of pupils. Although the pupil is normally round, an irregularly shaped or oval pupil may be noted in patients with elevated intracranial pressure. An oval pupil can indicate the initial stages of CN III compression.[2] It has been observed that an oval pupil almost always is associated with an elevated intracranial pressure (ICP) between 18 and 35 mm Hg.[11]

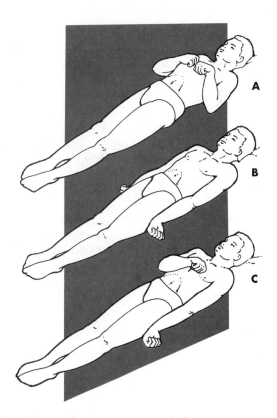

Fig. **15-1** Abnormal motor responses. **A,** Decorticate posturing. **B,** Decerebrate posturing. **C,** Decorticate posturing on right side and decerebrate posturing on left side of body.

BOX **15-4**

CLASSIFICATION OF ABNORMAL MOTOR FUNCTION

Spontaneous: Occurs without regard to external stimuli and may not occur by request.

Withdrawal: Occurs when the extremity receiving the painful stimulus flexes normally in an attempt to avoid the noxious stimulus.

Localization: Occurs when the extremity opposite to the extremity receiving pain crosses the midline of the body in an attempt to remove the noxious stimulus from the affected limb.

Decortication: An abnormal flexion response that may occur spontaneously or in response to a noxious stimuli (Fig. 15-1, *A*).

Decerebration: An abnormal extension response that may occur spontaneously or in response to noxious stimuli (Fig. 15-1, *B*).

Flaccid: Response to painful stimuli.

Evaluation of pupillary reaction to light

The pupillary light reflex depends on both optic nerve (CN II) and oculomotor nerve (CN III) function. The technique for evaluation of the pupillary light response involves use of a narrow-beamed bright light shone into the pupil from the outer canthus of the eye. If the light is shone directly onto the pupil, glare or reflection of the light may prevent the assessor's proper visualization. Pupillary reaction to light is identified as either brisk, sluggish, or nonreactive or fixed. Each pupil should be evaluated both for direct light response and for consensual response. The consensual pupillary response is constriction in response to a light shone into the opposite eye. This reflex occurs as a result of crossing of nerve fibers at the optic chiasm. Evaluation of consensual response is necessary to rule out optic nerve dysfunction as a cause for lack of a direct light reflex. Because the optic nerve is the afferent pathway for the light reflex, shining a light into a blind eye will produce neither a direct light response in that eye nor a consensual response in the opposite eye. A consensual response in the blind eye produced by shining a light into the opposite eye demonstrates an intact oculomotor nerve. Oculomotor compression associated with transtentorial herniation will affect both the direct light response and the consensual response in the affected pupil.[10,12]

Assessment of eye movement

In the conscious patient, the function of the three cranial nerves of the eye and their MLF innervation can be assessed by asking the patient to follow a finger through the full range of eye motion. If the eyes move together into all six fields, extraocular movements are intact.[7]

In the unconscious patient, assessment of ocular function and innervation of the MLF is performed by eliciting the doll's eyes reflex. If the patient is unconscious as a result of trauma, the nurse must ascertain the absence of cervical injury before performing this examination. To assess the oculocephalic reflex, the nurse holds the patient's eyelids open and briskly turns the head to one side while observing the eye movements, then briskly turns the head to the other side and observes. If the eyes deviate to the opposite direction in which the head is turned, doll's eyes are present and the oculocephalic reflex arc is intact (Fig. 15-2, *A*). If the oculocephalic reflex arc is not intact, the reflex is absent. This lack of response, in which the eyes remain midline and move with the head, indicates significant brainstem injury (Fig. 15-2, *B*). The reflex may also be absent in severe metabolic coma. An abnormal oculocephalic reflex is present when the eyes rove or move in opposite directions from each other (Fig. 15-2, *C*). Abnormal oculocephalic reflex indicates some degree of brainstem injury.[3,7]

Respiratory Function

Assessment of respiratory function focuses on two priorities: (1) observation of respiratory pattern and

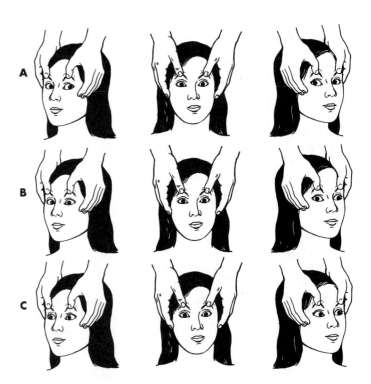

Fig. **15-2** Oculocephalic reflex (doll's eyes). **A,** Normal. **B,** Abnormal. **C,** Absent.

(2) evaluation of airway status. The activity of respiration is a highly integrated function that receives input from the cerebrum, brainstem, and metabolic mechanisms. A close correlation exists in clinical assessment among altered levels of consciousness, the level of brain or brainstem injury, and the respiratory pattern noted.[9] Under the influence of the cerebral cortex and the diencephalon, three brainstem centers control respirations. The lowest center, the medullary respiratory center, sends impulses through the vagus nerve to innervate muscles of inspiration and expiration. The apneustic and pneumotaxic centers of the pons are responsible for the length of inspiration and expiration and the underlying respiratory rate.[3]

Observation of respiratory pattern

Changes in respiratory patterns assist in identifying the level of brainstem dysfunction or injury (Table 15-2). Evaluation of respiratory pattern must also include evaluation of the effectiveness of gas exchange in maintaining adequate oxygen and carbon dioxide levels. Hypoventilation is not uncommon in the patient with an altered level of consciousness. Alterations in oxygenation or carbon dioxide levels can result in further neurologic dysfunction. ICP increases with hypoxemia or hypercapnia.[7]

Evaluation of airway status

Finally, assessment of the respiratory function in a patient with neurologic deficit must include assessment of airway maintenance and secretion control. Cough, gag,

TABLE **15-2**

RESPIRATORY PATTERNS

PATTERN OF RESPIRATION	DESCRIPTION OF PATTERN	SIGNIFICANCE
Cheyne-Stokes	Rhythmic crescendo and decrescendo of rate and depth of respiration; includes brief periods of apnea	Usually seen with bilateral deep cerebral lesions or some cerebellar lesions
Central neurogenic hyperventilation	Very deep, very rapid respirations with no apneic periods	Usually seen with lesions of the midbrain and upper pons
Apneustic	Prolonged inspiratory and/or expiratory pause of 2-3 sec	Usually seen in lesions of the mid to lower pons
Cluster breathing	Clusters of irregular, gasping respirations separated by long periods of apnea	Usually seen in lesions of the lower pons or upper medulla
Ataxic respirations	Irregular, random pattern of deep and shallow respirations with irregular apneic periods	Usually seen in lesions of the medulla

and swallow reflexes responsible for protection of the airway may be absent or diminished.[7]

Vital Signs

Assessment of vital signs focuses on two priorities: (1) evaluation of blood pressure and (2) observation of heart rate and rhythm. As a result of the brain and brainstem influences on cardiac, respiratory, and body temperature functions, changes in vital signs can indicate deterioration in neurologic status.

Evaluation of blood pressure

A common manifestation of intracranial injury is systemic hypertension. Cerebral autoregulation, responsible for the control of cerebral blood flow, frequently is lost with any type of intracranial injury. After cerebral injury, the body often is in a hyperdynamic state (increased heart rate, blood pressure, and cardiac output) as part of a compensatory response. With the loss of autoregulation as blood pressure increases, cerebral blood flow and cerebral blood volume increase and, therefore, ICP increases. Control of systemic hypertension is necessary to stop this cycle. However, caution must be exercised. The mean arterial pressure must be maintained at a level sufficient to produce adequate cerebral blood flow in the presence of elevated ICP. Attention must also be paid to the pulse pressure because widening of this value may occur in the late stages of intracranial hypertension.

Observation of heart rate and rhythm

The medulla and the vagus nerve provide parasympathetic control to the heart. When stimulated, this lower brainstem system produces bradycardia. Sympathetic stimulation increases the rate and contractility. Various intracranial pathologies and abrupt ICP changes can produce cardiac dysrhythmias, such as bradycardia, premature ventricular contractions (PVCs), atrioventricular (AV) block, or ventricular fibrillation and myocardial damage.[13]

Cushing's triad

Cushing's triad is a set of three clinical manifestations (bradycardia, systolic hypertension, and widening pulse pressure) related to pressure on the medullary area of the brainstem. These signs often occur in response to intracranial hypertension or a herniation syndrome. The appearance of Cushing's triad is a late finding that may be absent in neurologic deterioration. Attention should be paid to alteration in each component of the triad and intervention initiated accordingly.

NEUROLOGIC CHANGES ASSOCIATED WITH INTRACRANIAL HYPERTENSION

Assessment of the patient for signs of increasing intracranial pressure is an important responsibility of the critical care nurse. Increasing ICP can be identified by changes in level of consciousness, pupillary reaction, motor response, vital signs, and respiratory patterns (Figure 15-3).

LABORATORY STUDIES

The major laboratory study performed in the patient with neurologic dysfunction is cerebrospinal fluid (CSF) analysis obtained via a lumbar puncture or a ventriculostomy. A complete analysis of CSF is described in Table 15-3.

DIAGNOSTIC PROCEDURES

Table 15-4 presents an overview of the various diagnostic procedures used to evaluate the patient with neurologic dysfunction.[14-20]

Nursing Management

The nursing management of a patient undergoing a diagnostic procedure involves a variety of interventions. **Priorities are directed toward preparing the patient psychologically and physically for the procedure, monitoring the patient's responses to the procedure,**

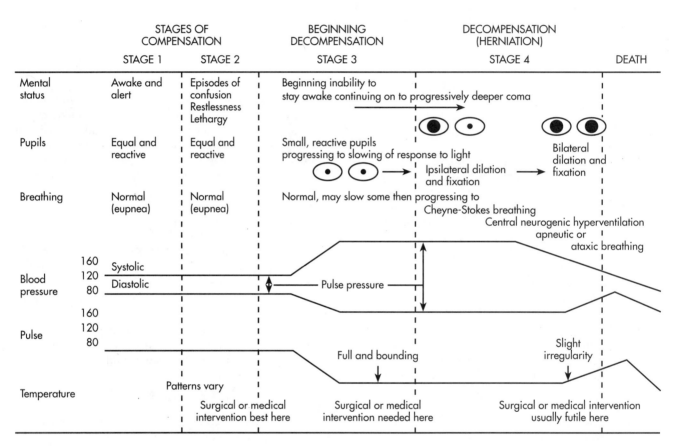

Fig. **15-3** Clinical correlates of compensated and decompensated phases of intracranial hypertension. (From Beare PG, Myers JL: *Principles and practice of adult health nursing,* ed 2, St Louis, 1994, Mosby.)

TABLE 15-3

CEREBROSPINAL FLUID ANALYSIS

PARAMETERS	NORMAL	ABNORMAL	POSSIBLE CAUSE
Pressure (initial readings)	75-180 mm H$_2$O (5-15 mm Hg)	<60 mm	Faulty needle placement Dehydration Spinal block along subarachnoid space Block of foramen magnum
		>200 mm	Muscle tension Abdominal compression Brain tumor Subdural hematoma Brain abscess Brain cyst Cerebral edema (any cause) Hydrocephalus
Color	Clear, colorless	Cloudy	Increased cell count Increased microorganisms
		Yellow	Xanthochromic (RBC pigments) High protein content
		Smoky	Presence of RBCs
Red blood cells	None	Blood-tinged Grossly bloody	Traumatic tap Traumatic tap Subarachnoid hemorrhage
White blood cells	0-6 mm^3	>10 mm^3 (cell counts range from below 100 to many thousands depending on causative factor; all are abnormal findings)	Occurs in many conditions: 　Bacterial infections of meninges 　Viral infections of meninges 　Neurosyphilis 　Tuberculous meningitis 　Metastatic neoplastic lesions 　Parasitic infections 　Acute demyelinating diseases 　Following introduction of air or blood into subarachnoid space
Protein*	15-45 mg/100 ml (1% of serum protein)	<10 mg/100 ml >60 mg/100 ml	Little clinical significance Occurs in many conditions: 　Complete spinal block 　Guillain-Barré syndrome 　Carcinomatosis of meninges 　Tumors close to pial or ependymal surfaces, or in cerebello-positive angle 　Acute and chronic meningitis 　Meningeal hemorrhage 　Demyelinating disorders 　Degenerative diseases
Glucose	50-75 mg/100 ml (approximately 60% of blood glucose level)	<40 mg/100 ml >100 mg/100 ml	Acute bacterial meningitis Tuberculous meningitis Meningeal carcinomatosis Diabetes
Chloride	700-750 mg/100 ml; 125 mM	<625 mg/100 ml >800 mg/100 ml	Hypochloremia Tuberculous meningitis Not of neurologic significance; correlated with blood levels of chloride

From Rudy E: *Advanced neurological and neurosurgical nursing*, ed 4, St. Louis, 1984, Mosby.
*Note: If CSF contains blood, this will raise the protein level.

and assessing the patient after the procedure. Preparing the patient includes teaching the patient about the procedure, answering any questions, and transporting and/or positioning the patient for the procedure. Monitoring the patient's responses to the procedure includes observing the patient for signs of pain, anxiety, or hemorrhage and monitoring vital signs. Assessing the patient after the procedure includes observing for complications of the procedure and medicating the patient for any postprocedure discomfort. **Any evidence of increasing intracranial pressure should be immediately reported to the physician, and emergency measures to maintain circulation must be initiated.**

NEUROLOGIC DIAGNOSTIC PROCEDURES

PROCEDURE	PURPOSES	COMMENTS

Arteriography (angiography)	• Visualizes extracranial and intracranial vasculature
	• Identifies aneurysm, AV malformation, vasospasm, vascular tumors
		• Contraindicated if patient has bleeding disorder or is receiving anticoagulants
		• May cause local hematoma, vasospasm, vessel occlusion, allergic reaction to contrast media, transient or permanent neurologic dysfunction
		• Before test:
		  • Patient usually NPO for 4 hours and sedated
		  • Allergy to iodine checked
		• After test:
		  • Contrast medium used, hydration ensured postprocedure
		  • Bed rest maintained for 8-12 hours
		  • Arterial puncture point monitored for hemorrhage or hematoma
		  • Neurovascular assessment of affected limb
		  • Necessary to monitor for indications of systemic emboli

Cisternogram	• Views CSF flow • Identifies hydrocephalus • Evaluates CSF leakage through a dural tear • Evaluates abnormality of structures at the base of the brain and upper cervical cord region	• Contraindicated in intracranial hypertension

Computed tomography (CT); computed axial tomography (CAT)	• Views intracranial structures: size, shape, location
	• Differentiates between tumors, hemorrhage, infarction
	• Identifies hydrocephalus, cerebral edema, infectious processes, trauma, aneurysm, hematoma, AV malformation, cerebral atrophy
		• Necessitates a cooperative patient
		• Possible use of contrast media
		  • Check for allergy to iodine and seafood before the study
		  • Patient will be NPO for 4-8 hours before the study
		  • Monitor for signs of allergic reaction
		  • Force fluids

Digital subtraction angiography (DSA)	• Visualizes vasculature, especially carotid and larger cerebral arteries
	• Evaluates occlusive vascular disease
	• Identifies tumors, aneurysms, AV malformation, vascular abnormalities
		• May be done intravenously or intraarterially
		  • IV: this method is less invasive and has fewer complications than cerebral angiography
		  • Intraarterial: care as for arteriogram
		• Use of contrast media
		  • Check for allergy to iodine and seafood before study
		  • Patient will be NPO for 4-8 hours before the study
		  • Monitor for signs of allergic reaction
		  • Force fluids

Electroencephalography (EEG)	• Differentiates epilepsy from mass lesion • Detects midline shift • Evaluates drug intoxication • Evaluates cerebral blood flow • May be used in designation of brain death	• May be asked to withhold stimulants, anticonvulsants, tranquilizers, antidepressants 24-48 hours before the study • Hair washed before and after procedure
Electromyography (EMG); nerve conduction velocity studies	• Detects muscle disease • Identifies peripheral neuropathies, nerve compression • Identifies nerve regeneration and muscle recovery	• Necessitates a cooperative patient • Contraindicated in patients on anticoagulants, with bleeding disorders, or with skin infection • May be uncomfortable for patient
Electronystagmography (ENG)	• Detects nystagmus, which may aid in identification of cerebellar or vestibular problem	

From Dennison RD: *Pass CCRN!*, St Louis, 1996, Mosby.

TABLE **15-4**

NEUROLOGIC DIAGNOSTIC PROCEDURES—cont'd

PROCEDURE	PURPOSES	COMMENTS
Evoked potentials	• Identifies neuromuscular disease, cerebrovascular disease, spinal cord injury, head injury, peripheral nerve disease, tumors • Determines prognosis in severe head injury • Is useful in diagnosis of multiple sclerosis, brainstem injury	• Hair washed before and after procedure
Isotope ventriculography	• Visualizes CSF circulation system	• No CSF withdrawn • May cause meningeal irritation, aseptic meningitis
Lumbar puncture or cisternal puncture	• Obtains CSF for analysis • Measures CSF pressure	• May be necessary to use cisternal puncture (higher risk) if scar tissue prevents lumbar puncture • Necessitates a cooperative patient • Contraindicated in patients with intracranial hypertension because herniation may occur • Contraindicated in bleeding disorders and in patients receiving anticoagulants • Patient kept flat for 4-8 hours to prevent headache • May cause headache, low back pain, meningitis, abscess, CSF leak, puncture of spinal cord
Magnetic resonance imaging (MRI)	• As for CT except better visualization of vasculature • Identifies vascular lesions, tissue abnormalities, cerebral hemorrhage, cerebral infarction, epileptic foci, multiple sclerosis • Identifies brainstem abnormalities	• More sensitive than CT scan, especially for posterior fossa • Necessitates a cooperative patient • Cannot be performed on a patient receiving mechanical ventilation • Contraindicated in patients with any implanted metallic device, including pacemakers

Myelography	• Visualization of spinal subarachnoid space
	• Detects spinal cord lesions, cord or nerve root compression
	• Detects pressure on spinal nerve roots
		• If done with oil-based iophendylate (Pantopaque)
		  • Patient must lie flat for 4-8 hours after study
		  • This substance may cause headache, nerve root irritation, allergic reaction, adhesive arachnoiditis
		• If done with water-soluble metrizamide (Amipaque)
		  • Patient should have head of bed elevated
		  • This substance may cause headache, nausea, vomiting, back and neck ache, chest pain, seizures, hallucinations, speech disorders, dysrhythmias, allergic reaction
		• Force fluids with either type of dye

Oculoplethysmography (OPG)	• Indirectly measures blood flow in the ophthalmic artery	• Contraindicated in patients who have undergone eye surgery within the last 6 months, who have had lens implants or cataracts, or who have had retinal detachment • May cause conjunctival hemorrhage, corneal abrasions, transient photophobia
Pneumoencephalography	• Visualizes ventricular system and subarachnoid space • Identifies intracranial tumors • Identifies cerebral atrophy	• Care as for LP • Contraindicated in patients with intracranial hypertension • May cause headache, nausea, vomiting, autonomic dysfunction, herniation, subdural hematoma, air embolus, seizures • Patient kept flat for 12-24 hours after study

Continued

TABLE 15-4

NEUROLOGIC DIAGNOSTIC PROCEDURES—cont'd

PROCEDURE	PURPOSES	COMMENTS
Positron emission tomography (PET) Single proton emission computed tomography (SPECT)	• Evaluates oxygen and glucose metabolism • Evaluates cerebral blood flow • Identifies cerebral ischemia, injuries, epilepsy, Alzheimer's disease	• Necessitates a cooperative patient • Contraindicated in pregnant patients
Radioisotope brain scan	• Identifies tumors, cerebrovascular disease, cerebral infarction, trauma, infectious processes, seizures	• Generally replaced by CT scan • Patient assured that amount of radioactive material is minimal • Necessitates a cooperative patient • Contraindicated in pregnant patients
Regional cerebral blood flow (xenon [^{133}Xe] inhalation)	• Evaluates blood flow to the cerebral cortex • Identifies cerebrovascular disease • Detects regions of increased or decreased perfusion • Determines presence of collateral blood flow • Evaluates cerebral vasospasm	• Patient assured that amount of radioactive material is minimal • Contraindicated in pregnant patients
Skull x-rays	• Detects skull fracture, facial fracture, tumor, bone erosion, cranial anomalies	• Linear and basilar fractures frequently missed by routine x-rays
Spinal cord arteriography	• Differentiates between spinal AV malformation, angioma, tumor, and ischemia	• As for arteriography • May cause thrombosis of spinal vessels, allergy to contrast agent
Spine x-rays	• Detects vertebral dislocation or fracture, degenerative disease, tumor, bone erosion, calcification	• Necessary to use caution to prevent fracture displacement and spinal cord injury • C1-C2 view best obtained via open mouth; C6-C7 best obtained with arms pulled down
Suboccipital puncture	• Obtains CSF for analysis • Measures CSF pressure • Is useful when lumbar puncture is contraindicated	• May cause trauma to the medulla
Ventriculography	• Obtains CSF for analysis • Measures CSF pressure • Is used especially when intracranial hypertension contraindicates LP	• May cause meningeal irritation, seizures, herniation, intracerebral or intraventricular hemorrhage

From Dennison RD: *Pass CCRN!*, St Louis, 1996, Mosby.

References

1. Plum F, Posner JB: *The diagnosis of stupor and coma*, ed 3, Philadelphia, 1980, FA Davis.
2. Hickey JV: *The clinical practice of neurological and neurosurgical nursing*, ed 3, Philadelphia, 1992, JB Lippincott.
3. Topel JL, Lewis SL: Examination of the comatose patient. In Weiner WJ, Goetz CG, editors: *Neurology for the non-neurologist*, ed 3, Philadelphia, 1994, JB Lippincott.
4. Teasdale G, Jennett W: Assessment of coma and impaired consciousness: a practical scale, *Lancet* 2:81, 1974.
5. Juarez VJ, Lyons M: Interrater reliability of the Glasgow Coma Scale, *J Neurosci Nurs* 27:283, 1995.
6. Segatore M, Way C: The Glasgow Coma Scale: time for change, *Heart Lung* 21:548, 1992.
7. Barker E: *Neuroscience nursing*, St Louis, 1994, Mosby.
8. Sullivan J: Neurologic assessment, *Nurs Clin North Am* 25:795, 1990.
9. Lower J: Rapid neuro assessment, *Am J Nurs* 92(6):38, 1992.
10. Bishop BS: Pathologic pupillary signs: self-learning module, part 1, *Crit Care Nurs* 11(6):59, 1991.
11. Marshall LF, et al: The oval pupil: clinical significance and relationship to intracranial hypertension, *J Neurosurg* 58:566, 1983.
12. Goodwin JA: Eye signs in neurologic diagnosis. In Weiner WJ, Goetz CG, editors: *Neurology for the non-neurologist*, ed 3, Philadelphia, 1994, JB Lippincott.
13. Keller C, Williams A: Cardiac dysrhythmias associated with central nervous system dysfunction, *J Neurosci Nurs* 25:349, 1993.
14. Mason PJB: Neurodiagnostic testing in critically injured adults, *Crit Care Nurs* 12(4):64, 1992.
15. Barnwell SL: Interventional neuroradiology, *West J Med* 158:162, 1993.
16. Fearon M, Rusy KL: Transcranial Doppler: advanced technology for assessing cerebral hemodynamics, *DCCN* 13:241, 1994.
17. Lucke KT, Kerr ME, Chovanes GI: Continuous bedside cerebral blood flow monitoring, *J Neurosci Nurs* 27:164, 1995.
18. Martin NA, Doberstein C: Cerebral blood flow measurement in neurosurgical intensive care, *Neurosurg Clin North Am* 5:607, 1994.
19. Buzea CE: Understanding computerized EEG monitoring in the intensive care unit, *J Neurosci Nurs* 27:292, 1995.
20. Nuwer MR: Electroencephalograms and evoked potentials: monitoring cerebral function in the neurosurgical intensive care unit, *Neurosurg Inten Care* 5:647, 1994.

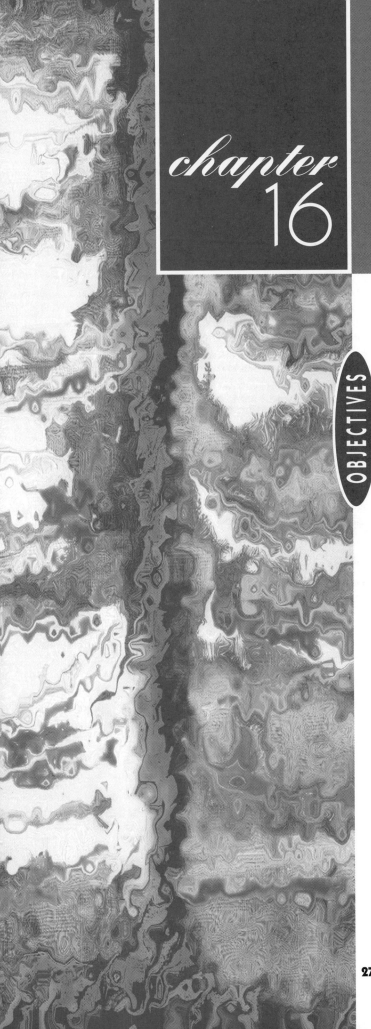

Beverly Means Carlson

chapter 16

Neurologic Disorders

- Describe the etiology and pathophysiology of selected neurologic disorders.
- Identify the clinical manifestations of selected neurologic disorders.
- Explain the treatment of selected neurologic disorders.
- Discuss the nursing priorities for managing a patient with selected neurologic disorders.

An understanding of the pathology of a disease or condition, the areas of assessment on which to focus, and the usual medical management allows the critical care nurse to more accurately anticipate and plan nursing interventions. Although a wide array of neurologic disorders exists, only a few routinely require care in the critical care environment.

COMA

Description and Etiology

Coma is a state of unconsciousness in which both wakefulness and awareness are lacking.[1] The patient cannot be aroused and demonstrates no voluntary movement.[2] Like consciousness, the state of coma comprises a continuum of many levels. The patient in a light coma demonstrates purposeful withdrawal in response to noxious stimuli. The patient in deep coma lacks any response, even to noxious stimuli. Between these two extremes, levels of coma are difficult to clearly differentiate.

The state of coma is actually a symptom, rather than a disease. It occurs as a result of some underlying process. And yet like any other life-threatening condition, coma requires identification and therapeutic management even

BOX 16-1

CAUSES OF COMA

STRUCTURAL LESIONS

Subarachnoid hemorrhage
Intracerebral hemorrhage
Subdural hematoma
Epidural hematoma
Thrombotic or embolic brain infarction
Brain tumor
Brain abscess
Trauma

METABOLIC OR TOXIC CONDITIONS

Meningitis
Encephalitis
Alcohol
Hepatic failure
Renal failure (uremia)
Cardiac failure
Ischemia, hypoxemia, anoxia
Hypercapnia
Hypoglycemia or hyperglycemia
Electrolyte imbalance (sodium, calcium, magnesium, phosphorus)
Water imbalance
Acidosis or alkalosis
Hypothyroidism (myxedema)
Addisonian crisis
Thiamine deficiency (Wernicke's encephalopathy)
Sepsis
Poisoning (lead, mushroom, cyanide, methanol, carbon monoxide)
Drug overdose
Lactic acidosis
Hypertensive encephalopathy
Hypothermia or hyperthermia
Postictal state

when the cause cannot be determined or treated. Although any number of diagnosis-related groups (DRGs) may apply to the patient in a coma, depending on the underlying cause and subsequent treatment, usually DRG 27 (Traumatic stupor and coma, coma greater than 1 hour) or DRG 23 (Nontraumatic stupor and coma) are used, with anticipated lengths of stay of 5.5 days and 4.6 days, respectively.[3]

The causes of coma can be divided into three general categories: structural neurologic lesions, metabolic or toxic conditions (Box 16-1), or psychiatric disorders (which are not discussed in this chapter). Structural lesions that can result in coma include vascular lesions, trauma, brain tumors, and brain abscesses. Metabolic or toxic conditions that can result in coma include cardiopulmonary decompensation, poisoning, alcohol, hypertensive encephalopathy, meningitis, encephalitis, postconvulsive states, and other metabolic conditions.

Pathophysiology

Consciousness involves both arousal, or wakefulness, and awareness. Neither of these functions is present in the patient in coma. Ascending fibers of the reticular activating system in the pons, hypothalamus, and thalamus maintain arousal as an autonomic function. Neurons in the cerebral cortex are responsible for awareness. Diffuse dysfunction of both cerebral hemispheres and/or diffuse or focal dysfunction of the reticular activating system is necessary to produce coma.[5] Small focal lesions in the posterior hypothalamic and midbrain regions can also produce coma, whereas unilateral cerebral lesions usually do not, unless they increase intracranial pressure (ICP). Alterations in cerebral function that can also produce coma include ischemia, hypoxia, infection, metabolic imbalance, toxic exposure, and structural disruption.

The pathophysiologic continuum of coma is comparable with the stages of anesthesia. Slight or moderate cortical depression produces clouding of consciousness, impairment of contact with the environment, loss of discrimination, and euphoria. In complete cortical suppression, motor and reflex functions are controlled solely by subcortical structures. Midbrain depression produces a loss of reflex response and a loss of several visceral functions. Finally, brainstem depression results in gradual abolition of respiratory and circulatory control.[2]

Assessment and Diagnosis

Diagnosis of the coma state is a clinical one, readily established by assessment of the level of consciousness. Determining the full nature and cause of coma, however, requires a thorough history and physical examination. A past medical history is essential because events immediately preceding the change in level of consciousness can often provide valuable clues as to the origin of the coma. When limited information is available and the coma is profound, the response of the patient to emergency treatment may provide clues to the underlying diagnosis, such as the patient who becomes responsive with the administration of naloxone can be presumed to have ingested some type of opiate.

Detailed serial neurologic examinations are essential for all patients in coma. Assessment of motor function, pupil responses, and respiratory pattern provides valuable diagnostic information.[4,6] Pupillary light responses are often the key to differentiating between structural and metabolic causes of coma because they are usually intact in metabolic-induced coma, with the exceptions of anoxic encephalopathy, barbiturate intoxication, and hypothermia. Focal or asymmetric motor deficits usually indicate structural lesions. Table 16-1 lists the clinical manifestations of metabolic and structural causes of coma.

Structural causes of coma are usually readily apparent with computed tomography (CT) scanning or magnetic resonance imaging (MRI). Lumbar puncture, unless contraindicated by signs of increased ICP, facilitates the analysis of CSF pressure and content. Laboratory studies are also used to identify metabolic or endocrine abnormalities. Occasionally, the cause of coma is never clearly determined.

TABLE 16-1

CLINICAL MANIFESTATIONS OF METABOLICALLY AND STRUCTURALLY INDUCED COMAS

MANIFESTATION	METABOLICALLY INDUCED COMA	STRUCTURALLY INDUCED COMA
Blink to threat (cranial nerves II, VII)	Equal	Asymmetric
Discs (cranial nerve II)	Flat, good pulsation	Papilledema
Extraocular movement (cranial nerves III, IV, VI)	Roving eye movements; normal doll's eyes and calorics	Gaze paresis, nerve III palsy, medial longitudinal fasciculus (MLF) syndrome (internuclear ophthalmoplegia)
Pupils (cranial nerves II, III)	Equal and reactive, may be large (e.g., atropine), pinpoint (e.g., opiates), or midposition and fixed (e.g., glutethimide [Doriden])	Asymmetric and/or nonreactive; may be midposition (midbrain injury), pinpoint (pons injury), large (tectal injury)
Corneal reflex (cranial nerve V, VII)	Symmetric response	Asymmetric response
Grimace to pain (cranial nerve VII)	Symmetric response	Asymmetric response
Motor function movement	Symmetric	Asymmetric
Tone	Symmetric	Paratonic, spastic, flaccid, especially if asymmetric
Posture	Symmetric	Decorticate, especially if symmetric; decerebrate, especially if asymmetric
Deep tendon reflexes	Symmetric	Asymmetric
Babinski sign	Absent or symmetric response	Present
Sensation	Symmetric	Asymmetric

From McCance KL, Huether SE: *Pathophysiology: the biologic basis for disease in adults and children,* ed 3, St Louis, 1998, Mosby.

Medical Management

The goal of medical management of the patient in a coma is identification and treatment of the underlying cause of the condition. Initial medical management includes emergency measures to support vital functions and prevent further neurologic deterioration. Protection of the airway and ventilatory assistance are frequently needed. Administration of thiamine (100 mg), glucose, and a narcotic antagonist is suggested whenever the cause of coma is not immediately known.[2,4,6] Thiamine is administered before glucose because the coma produced by thiamine deficiency, Wernicke's encephalopathy, can be precipitated by a glucose load.[2] The cervical neck is stabilized until traumatic injury is ruled out.

The patient who remains in coma after emergency treatment requires supportive measures to maintain physiologic body functions and prevent complications. Continued airway protection and nutritional support are essential. Fluid and electrolyte management is often complex because of alterations in the neurohormonal system. Anticonvulsant therapy may be necessary to prevent further ischemic damage to the brain.

Nursing Management

Nursing management of the patient in a coma incorporates a variety of nursing diagnoses (Box 16-2). Nursing management is directed by the specific etiology of the coma although some common interventions are used. One of the most important things to remember is that the patient in a coma is totally dependent on the health care team. **Nursing priorities are directed toward assessing** for changes in neurologic status and clues to the origin of the coma, supporting all bodily functions, preventing complications such as corneal damage, providing psychosocial and informational support to the family, and initiating rehabilitation measures such as coma stimulation therapy. Because a complete description of the nursing management of the comatose patient is beyond the scope of this text, only two key nursing measures are addressed: eye care and coma stimulation therapy.

Eye care

The blink reflex is often diminished or absent in the comatose patient. The eyelids may be flaccid and dependent on body positioning to remain in a closed position,

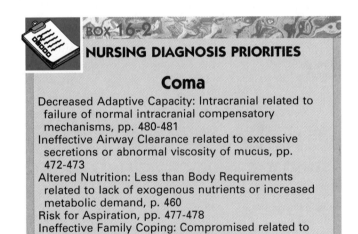

BOX 16-2

NURSING DIAGNOSIS PRIORITIES

Coma

Decreased Adaptive Capacity: Intracranial related to failure of normal intracranial compensatory mechanisms, pp. 480-481

Ineffective Airway Clearance related to excessive secretions or abnormal viscosity of mucus, pp. 472-473

Altered Nutrition: Less than Body Requirements related to lack of exogenous nutrients or increased metabolic demand, p. 460

Risk for Aspiration, pp. 477-478

Ineffective Family Coping: Compromised related to critically ill family member, pp. 452-453

and edema may prevent complete closure. Loss of these protective mechanisms results in drying and ulceration of the cornea, which can lead to permanent scarring and blindness.

Two interventions that are commonly used to protect the eyes are instilling saline or methyl cellulose lubricating drops and taping the eyelids in the shut position. Recent evidence suggests that an alternative technique may be more effective in preventing corneal epithelial breakdown.

In addition to instilling saline drops every 2 hours, a polyethylene film is taped over the eyes, extending beyond the orbits and eyebrows. The film creates a moisture chamber around the cornea and assists in keeping the eyes moist and in the closed position.[7] This technique also prevents damage to the eyes that results from tape or gauze being placed directly on the delicate skin of the eyelids.

Coma stimulation therapy

The purpose of coma stimulation is to stimulate the reticular activating system and increase the patient's level of alertness. This therapy is based on the belief that structured brain stimulation fosters brain recovery. Based on the belief that maximal reorganization of the brain takes place in the early weeks after an insult, coma stimulation therapy must begin in the critical care unit to increase the possibility for maximal recovery.[8-10]

The methods of stimuli used in coma stimulation therapy and the anticipated neurologic responses are listed in Boxes 16-3 and 16-4, respectively. Simple auditory and tactile stimulation are most often used in the critical care environment. Stimuli must be meaningful rather than random. Taped voices of family and friends talking to the patient have been found to be particularly effective.[10]

Some experts advocate bombarding the patient with stimuli up to 16 hours a day, whereas others support providing stimulation every hour. In the critical care unit, a program consisting of a single stimulation activity lasting no more than 10 to 30 minutes per session two to four times a day allows time for necessary patient care activities and rest periods.[9] Family visits and nursing activities will naturally augment this program with additional auditory and tactile stimulation.

Medical stability, including normal ICP and hemodynamic values, is required before initiation of coma stimulation, and the therapy is usually not started until the second week after neurologic insult. Any increase in ICP; sustained increase in blood pressure, heart rate, or respiratory rate; or development of seizure activity is considered unfavorable and reason to terminate or revise the stimulation program.[8]

CEREBROVASCULAR ACCIDENT

Cerebrovascular accident, commonly known as stroke, is a descriptive term for the onset of neurologic symptoms caused by the interruption of blood flow to the brain. Stroke is the third leading cause of death in the United States, preceded by heart disease and cancer. The number of survivors of stroke in the United States is estimated at

---

BOX 16-3

SENSORY STIMULATION USED IN COMA STIMULATION THERAPY

AUDITORY	VISUAL	OLFACTORY	GUSTATORY	TACTILE	KINESTHETIC
Verbal orientation	Photographs	Vinegar	Mouthwash swabs	Hand holding	Turning
Music	Penlight	Spices	Lemon juice	Rubbing lotion	Range of motion
Bells	Familiar objects	Perfume	Sweet or salty	Heat/cold	Chair
Clapping	Faces	Potpourri	solutions	Cotton balls	Tilt table
Tuning fork	Flashcards	Orange/lemon peel		Rough surfaces	
				Familiar objects	

From Sosnowski C, Ustik M: Early intervention: coma stimulation in the intensive care unit, *J Neurosci Nurs* 26:336, 1994.

BOX 16-4

RESPONSES TO STIMULATION

AUDITORY	VISUAL	OLFACTORY	GUSTATORY	TACTILE	KINESTHETIC
Startle reaction	Eye blink	Grimacing	Grimacing	Localization	Spasticity of joints
Visual tracking toward sound	Visual tracking	Tearing	Spitting	Withdrawal	Assisted ROM
Follows commands		Head turning	Swallowing	Posturing	Follows commands

From Sosnowski C, Ustik M: Early intervention: coma stimulation in the intensive care unit, *J Neurosci Nurs* 26:336, 1994.

3 million people. The morbidity associated with stroke is the leading cause of adult disability.[11] The annual cost for care and loss of productivity is nearly $20 billion.[12]

There are two basic types of stroke: ischemic and hemorrhagic. Hemorrhagic strokes are divided into subarachnoid hemorrhage and intracerebral hemorrhage. Cerebrovascular accident falls under DRG 14 (Specific Cerebrovascular Disorders, Except Transient Ischemic Attack) with an average length of stay of 6.8 days. If the patient has surgery to correct the underlying cause of the hemorrhage, then DRG 1 (Craniotomy, Age Greater than 17 Years Except for Trauma) or DRG 2 (Craniotomy, Age 0 to 17 Years) is used, with average lengths of stay of 10.3 and 10.6 days, respectively.[3]

Ischemic Stroke

Description and etiology

Ischemic stroke is a stroke that results from low cerebral flow, usually because of occlusion of a blood vessel. The occlusion can be either thrombotic or embolic in nature. Eighty percent of the 500,000 Americans that suffered a stroke in 1991 suffered an ischemic stroke.[12] The 30-day survival rate after ischemic stroke is approximately 67% to 85%.

Most thrombotic strokes are the result of the accumulation of atherosclerotic plaque in the vessel lumen, especially at bifurcations, or curves, of the vessel. The pathogenesis of cerebrovascular disease is identical to that of coronary vasculature. The greatest risk factor for ischemic stroke is hypertension. Other risk factors are diabetes, elevated blood lipids, obesity, smoking, stress, and family history. Common sites of atherosclerotic plaque are the bifurcation of the common carotid artery, the origins of the middle and anterior cerebral arteries, and the origins of the vertebral arteries.[13] Elderly women are at greater risk for cardioembolic stroke.[14]

An embolic stroke occurs when a small embolus from the heart or lower cerebral circulation travels distally and lodges in a small vessel, resulting in loss of blood supply. Up to one third of ischemic strokes are attributed to a cardioembolic phenomenon.[14,15] Risk factors include atrial fibrillation, coronary artery disease, and an enlarged heart. Aspirin and warfarin therapy are currently under investigation as preventive measures to guard against this complication in patients with chronic atrial fibrillation.

Pathophysiology

Ischemic stroke is a cerebral hemodynamic insult. When cerebral blood flow is reduced to a level insufficient to maintain neuronal viability, ischemic injury occurs. In focal stroke, an area of marginally perfused tissue surrounds a core of ischemic cells. Five minutes of anoxic insult initiates a chain of events producing brain infarction. Irreversible neuronal injury soon follows.[13] If infarction occurs, the affected brain tissue eventually softens and liquefies.

The phenomenon of a focal ischemic stroke is identical to that associated with myocardial infarction. Cerebral blood flow is diminished by either atherosclerotic vascular disease or embolus. Often a history of transient ischemic attacks (TIAs), brief episodes of neurologic symptoms, offers clues to the progressive severity of cerebrovascular disease. Sudden onset indicates embolism as the final insult to flow.[13] The size of the stroke depends on the size and location of the occluded vessel and the availability of collateral blood flow. Global ischemia results when severe hypotension or cardiopulmonary arrest produces a transient drop in blood flow to all areas of the brain.

Cerebral edema sufficient to produce clinical deterioration develops in 10% to 20% of patients with ischemic stroke and can result in intracranial hypertension. The edema results from a loss of normal metabolic function of the cells and peaks at 3 to 5 days. This process is commonly the cause of death during the first week after a stroke.[13] Secondary hemorrhage at the site of the stroke lesion, known as hemorrhagic conversion, and seizures are the two other major acute neurologic complications of ischemic stroke. Mortality rates in the first 20 days after ischemic stroke range from 8% to 30%.[13]

Assessment and diagnosis

The characteristic sign of an ischemic stroke is the sudden onset of focal neurologic signs.[12] These signs usually occur in combination. Box 16-5 lists common patterns of neurologic symptoms associated with an ischemic stroke. Hemiparesis, aphasia, and hemianopsia are common. Changes in level of consciousness usually only occur with brainstem or cerebellar involvement, seizure, hypoxia, hemorrhage, or elevated ICP. These changes may be exhibited as stupor, coma, confusion, and agitation. The reported frequency of seizures in patients with ischemic stroke is variable, ranging from 4% to 43%. If seizures occur, they are usually seen within 24 hours of insult.[13]

Confirmation of the diagnosis of ischemic stroke is the first step in the emergent evaluation of these patients. Differentiation from intracranial hemorrhage is vital. Noncontrast CT scanning is the method of choice for this purpose and is considered the most important initial diagnostic study. In addition to excluding intracranial hemorrhage, CT can also assist in identifying early neurologic complications and the etiology of the insult. An MRI will demonstrate actual infarction of cerebral tissue earlier than a CT but is less useful in the emergent differential diagnosis. Because of the strong correlation between acute ischemic stroke and heart disease, electrocardiography, chest x-ray, and cardiac monitoring are suggested to detect a cardiac etiology or co-existing condition. Echocardiography is also valuable in identifying a cardioembolic phenomenon when a sufficient index of suspicion warrants.[14] Laboratory evaluation of hematologic function, electrolyte and glucose levels, and renal and hepatic function is also recommended. Arterial blood gas analysis is performed if hypoxia is suspected, and an electro-

COMMON PATTERNS OF NEUROLOGIC ABNORMALITIES IN PATIENTS WITH ACUTE ISCHEMIC STROKES

LEFT (DOMINANT) HEMISPHERE

Aphasia; right hemiparesis; right-sided sensory loss; right visual field defect; poor right conjugate gaze; dysarthria; difficulty in reading, writing, or calculating

RIGHT (NONDOMINANT) HEMISPHERE

Neglect of the left visual space, left visual field defect, left hemiparesis, left-sided sensory loss, poor left conjugate gaze, extinction of left-sided stimuli, dysarthria, spatial disorientation

BRAINSTEM/CEREBELLUM/POSTERIOR HEMISPHERE

Motor or sensory loss in all four limbs, crossed signs, limb or gait ataxia, dysarthria, dysconjugate gaze, nystagmus, amnesia, bilateral visual field defects

SMALL SUBCORTICAL HEMISPHERE OR BRAINSTEM (PURE MOTOR STROKE)

Weakness of face and limbs on one side of the body without abnormalities of higher brain function, sensation, or vision

SMALL SUBCORTICAL HEMISPHERE OR BRAINSTEM (PURE SENSORY STROKE)

Decreases sensation of face and limbs on one side of the body without abnormalities of higher brain function, motor function, or vision

From Adams HP, et al: Guidelines for the management of patients with ischemic stroke: a statement for health care professionals from a special writing group of the Stroke Council, American Heart Association, *Circulation* 90:1589, 1994.

encephalogram is obtained if seizures are suspected. Lumbar puncture is only performed if subarachnoid hemorrhage is suspected and the CT is negative.[12]

Medical management

Emergent care must include airway protection and ventilatory assistance to maintain adequate tissue oxygenation. Hypertension is often present in the early period as a compensatory response and in most cases must not be lowered. Antihypertensive therapy is considered only if the mean blood pressure (BP) is greater than 130 mm Hg or the systolic BP is greater than 220 mm Hg.[12] Body temperature and glucose levels must also be normalized.

Medical management must also include the identification and treatment of acute complications, such as cerebral edema or seizure activity. Prophylaxis for these complications is not recommended. Surgical decompression is recommended if a large cerebellar infarction compresses the brainstem.

There is much conflicting evidence regarding a variety of interventions for the patient with acute ischemic stroke.[12] Heparin therapy has been used for years to prevent recurrent embolism; however, recent scientific studies have demonstrated conflicting results. The Stroke Council of the American Heart Association (AHA) has determined that evidence regarding the role of heparin in the patient with ischemic stroke is insufficient to make any recommendation regarding its use.[12]

Thrombolytic therapy for strokes has been approved for use in selected patients. It must be given within 3 hours of the onset of symptoms and the patient's CT scan must be negative for signs of hemorrhage. The recommended dose is 0.9 mg/kg (maximum 90 mg) of t-PA with the first 10% of the dose given as an intravenous bolus over 1 minute and the rest infused over 1 hour.[16] The following is a list of additional therapies that are currently under investigation: emergent carotid endarterectomy, embolectomy or angioplasty, hemodilution of the blood, or the administration of steroids, barbiturates, calcium channel blockers, nimodipine, naloxone, glutamate antagonists, or amphetamines.[12,15] The immediacy of treatment is a major factor in the documented effectiveness of several of these therapies.

Subarachnoid Hemorrhage

Description and etiology

Subarachnoid hemorrhage (SAH) is bleeding into the subarachnoid space, usually caused by rupture of a cerebral aneurysm or arteriovenous malformation (AVM). Subarachnoid hemorrhage accounts for 6% to 7% of all strokes—with nontraumatic SAH affecting more than 30,000 Americans each year. The incidence of SAH is greater in women and increases with age. The overall mortality rate is 25%, with most patients dying on the first day after insult. The rate of significant morbidity approximates 50% of all survivors.[17] The known risk factors for SAH include hypertension, smoking, alcohol use, and stimulant use.[17] As in ischemic stroke, the single most important risk factor is hypertension. Causes of SAH include cerebral aneurysms, AVMs, hypertensive intracerebral hemorrhages, and bleeding from a cerebral tumor.

Cerebral aneurysm. Cerebral aneurysm rupture accounts for more than 50% of all cases of spontaneous SAH.[18] An aneurysm is an outpouching of the wall of a blood vessel that results from weakening of the wall of the vessel. Ninety percent of aneurysms are congenital—the cause of which is unknown. The other 10% can be a result of traumatic injury (that stretches and tears the muscular middle layer of the arterial vessel), infectious material (most often from infectious vegetation on valves of the left side of the heart after bacterial endocarditis) that lodges against a vessel wall and erodes the muscular layer, or of undetermined cause. Multiple aneurysms occur in 20% to 25% of the cases and often are bilateral, occurring in the same location on both sides of the cerebral vascular system. It is possible for an individual to live a full life span with an unruptured cerebral aneurysm. Aneurysm rup-

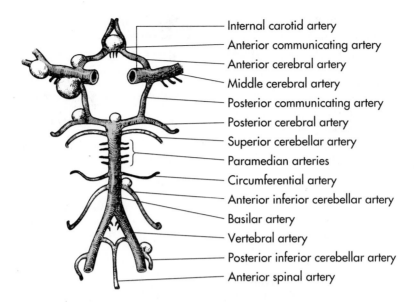

Fig. **16-1** The common sites of berry aneurysms. The size of the aneurysm in the drawing is proportional to the frequency of occurrence at the various sites. (From Wyngaarden JB, Smith LH, editors: *Cecil's textbook of medicine*, ed 16, Philadelphia, 1982, WB Saunders.)

ture usually occurs between 30 and 60 years of age, with peak incidence during the fifth decade of life.[18]

Arteriovenous malformation. Arteriovenous malformation rupture is responsible for less than 10% of all SAHs.[6] An AVM is a tangled mass of arterial and venous blood vessels that shunt blood directly from the arterial side into the venous side, bypassing the capillary system. They may be small, focal lesions or large diffuse lesions that occupy almost an entire hemisphere. AVMs are always congenital, though the exact embryonic cause for these malformations is unknown. They also occur in the spinal cord and renal, gastrointestinal, and integumentary systems. Small superficial AVMs are seen as port-wine stains of the skin. In contrast to the middle-aged population with SAH from aneurysm, SAH from an AVM usually occurs before the third decade of life.[6]

Pathophysiology

The pathophysiology of the two most common causes of SAH are distinctly different.

Cerebral aneurysm. As the individual with a congenital cerebral aneurysm matures, blood pressure rises and more stress is placed on the poorly developed and thin vessel wall. Ballooning out of the vessel occurs, giving the aneurysm a berry-like appearance. Most cerebral aneurysms are saccular or berry-like with a stem or neck. Aneurysms are usually small, 2 to 7 mm in diameter, and frequently occur at the base of the brain on the circle of Willis at the bifurcation of the blood vessels (Fig. 16-1).

The aneurysm becomes clinically significant when the vessel wall becomes so thin that it ruptures, sending arterial blood at a high pressure into the subarachnoid space. For a brief moment after the aneurysm ruptures, intracranial pressure is believed to approach mean arterial pres-

sure and cerebral perfusion falls. In other situations, the unruptured aneurysm expands and places pressure on surrounding structures. This is particularly true with posterior communicating artery aneurysms, as they put pressure on the oculomotor nerve (CN III) causing ipsilateral pupil dilation and ptosis.

Arteriovenous malformation. The pathophysiologic features of an AVM are related to the size and location of the malformation. An AVM is fed by one or more cerebral arteries, also known as feeders. These feeder arteries tend to enlarge over time and increase the volume of blood shunted through the malformation as well as increase the overall mass effect. Large, dilated, tortuous draining veins also develop as a result of increasing arterial blood flow being delivered at a higher than normal pressure. Normal vascular flow has a mean arterial pressure of 70 to 80 mm Hg, a mean arteriole pressure of 35 to 45 mm Hg, and a mean capillary pressure that drops from 35 to 10 mm Hg as it connects with the venous side. Lack of this capillary bridge allows blood with a mean pressure of 35 to 45 mm Hg to flow into the venous system. Because there is no muscular layer in a vein as there is in an artery, the veins become extremely engorged and rupture easily. Cerebral atrophy is also sometimes present in the patient with an AVM. It is the result of chronic ischemia because of the shunting of blood through the AVM and away from normal cerebral circulation.

Assessment and diagnosis

The patient with an SAH characteristically has an abrupt onset of pain, described as the "worst headache of my life." A brief loss of consciousness, nausea, vomiting, focal neurologic deficits, and a stiff neck may accompany the headache. The SAH may result in coma or death.

Patient history may reveal one or more incidences of sudden onset of headache with vomiting in the weeks preceding a major SAH. These are "warning leaks" of an aneurysm in which small amounts of blood ooze from the aneurysm into the subarachnoid space. The presence of blood is an irritant to the meninges, particularly the arachnoid membrane. This irritation causes headache, stiff neck, and photophobia. These small "warning leaks" seldom are detected because the condition is not severe enough for the patient to seek medical attention. If a neurologic deficit, such as third cranial nerve palsy, develops before aneurysm rupture, medical intervention is sought and the aneurysm may be surgically secured before the devastation of a rupture can occur. Symptoms of unruptured AVM—headaches with dizziness or syncope or fleeting neurologic deficits—may also be found in the history.

Diagnosis of SAH is based on clinical presentation, CT scan, and lumbar puncture. Noncontrast CT is the cornerstone of definitive SAH diagnosis.[17] In 92% of the cases, CT scan can demonstrate a clot in the subarachnoid space if performed within 24 hours of the onset of the hemorrhage. On the basis of the appearance and the location of the SAH, diagnosis of cause—aneurysm or AVM—may be made from the CT scan. MRI is relatively insensitive for detecting blood in the subarachnoid space.

If the initial CT scan is negative, an LP is performed to obtain CSF for analysis. CSF after SAH is bloody in appearance with a red blood cell count greater than 1000/mm.[3] If the lumbar puncture is performed more than 5 days after the SAH, CSF fluid is xanthochromic (dark amber), because the blood products have broken down. Cloudy CSF usually indicates some type of infectious process, such as bacterial meningitis, not a subarachnoid hemorrhage.

Once the SAH has been documented, a cerebral angiogram is necessary to identify the exact cause of the SAH. If a cerebral aneurysm rupture is the cause, an angiogram is also essential for identifying the exact location of the aneurysm in preparation for surgery. Once the aneurysm has been located, it is graded using the Hunt and Hess classification scale. This scale categorizes the patient based on the severity of the neurologic deficits associated with the hemorrhage (Box 16-6).[19] If AVM rupture is the cause, an angiogram is necessary to identify the feeding arteries and draining veins of the malformation.

Medical management

SAH is a medical emergency, and time is of the essence. Preservation of neurologic function is the goal. Initial treatment must always support vital functions. Airway management and ventilatory assistance may be necessary. Early diagnosis is also essential. A ventriculostomy is performed to control ICP if the patient's level of consciousness is depressed.[17]

Evidence suggests that only 19% of the deaths attributable to aneurysmal SAH are related to the direct effects

---

BOX 16-6

HUNT AND HESS CLASSIFICATION OF SUBARACHNOID HEMORRHAGE

Grade I	Asymptomatic or minimal headache and slight nuchal rigidity
Grade II	Moderate to severe headache, nuchal rigidity, no neurologic deficit other than cranial nerve palsy
Grade III	Drowsiness, confusion, or mild focal deficit
Grade IV	Stupor, moderate-to-severe hemiparesis, possible early decerebrate rigidity, and vegetative disturbances
Grade V	Deep coma, decerebrate rigidity, moribund appearance

---

of the initial hemorrhage.[20] In a recent major multicenter study, rebleeding accounted for 22% of deaths from aneurysmal SAH, cerebral vasospasm accounted for 23%, and nonneurologic medical complications accounted for 23%.[20] Therefore, once initial intervention has provided necessary support for vital physiologic functions, medical management of acute SAH is primarily aimed toward the prevention and treatment of the complications of SAH that can produce further neurologic damage and death.

Rebleeding. Rebleeding is the occurrence of a second SAH in an unsecured aneurysm or, less commonly, an AVM.[4] The incidence of rebleeding with conservative therapy is 20% to 30% in the first month, with the highest occurrence on the first day after initial hemorrhage.[22] Mortality with aneurysmal rebleeding is 48% to 78%.[23]

Historically, conservative measures to prevent rebleeding have included BP control and SAH precautions. An elevation in BP is a normal compensatory response to maintain adequate cerebral perfusion after a neurologic insult. In the belief that hypertension contributes to rebleeding, nitroprusside, propranolol, or hydralazine have been commonly used to maintain a systolic BP no greater than 150 mm Hg.[21] Recent evidence suggests that rebleeding has more to do with variations in BP rather than absolute values and that BP control does not lower the incidence of rebleeding.[17] Prophylactic anticonvulsant therapy is recommended to prevent seizures.[17]

Surgical aneurysm clipping. Definitive treatment for the prevention of rebleeding is surgical clipping with complete obliteration of the aneurysm. Timing of the surgery is a key medical management issue. Since the introduction of microsurgery and improved surgical techniques, patients commonly are taken to the operating room within the first 48 hours after rupture. This early surgical intervention to secure the aneurysm eliminates the risk of rebleeding and allows more aggressive therapy to be used in the postoperative period for the treatment of vasospasm. Early surgery also allows the neurosurgeon to flush out the excess blood and clots from the basal cisterns (reservoir of CSF around the base of the brain and circle of Willis) to reduce the risk of vasospasm. Early surgery is recommended for patients with a Grade I or Grade II SAH and for some patients with Grade III. In patients with a Grade III SAH, the initial hemorrhage did not produce significant neurologic deficit, but the risk of rebleeding with a tragically high incidence of mortality is present until the aneurysm is secured. Because of the patient's clinical condition and the technical difficulty of the surgery, early surgical repair of the aneurysm is not always possible. Early surgery continues to be controversial for patients with Grade IV or V SAH and those demonstrating vasospasm. However, recent studies have not supported the fear of worse ischemic sequelae with early surgery in these patients.[18] Careful consideration of the patient's clinical situation is necessary in determining the optimal time for surgery.

The surgical procedure involves a craniotomy to expose and isolate the area of aneurysm. A clip is placed over the neck of the aneurysm to eliminate the area of weakness. This is a technically difficult procedure that requires the skill of an experienced neurosurgeon. It is not uncommon, particularly in early surgery, for the clot to break away from the aneurysm as it is surgically exposed. Extensive hemorrhage into the craniotomy site results, and cessation of the hemorrhage often causes increased neurologic deficits. Deficits may also occur as a result of surgical manipulation to gain access to the site of the aneurysm.

Surgical AVM excision. Medical management of AVM traditionally has involved surgical excision or conservative management of such symptoms as seizures and headache. The decision for surgical excision depends on the location and size of the AVM. Some malformations are located so deep in the cerebral structures (the thalamus or midbrain) that attempts to remove the AVM would cause severe neurologic deficits. History of a previous hemorrhage and the patient's age and overall condition are also taken into account when making the decision regarding surgical intervention.

Surgical excision of large AVMs includes the risk of reperfusion bleeding. As feeding arteries of the AVM are clamped off, the arterial blood that usually flowed into the AVM is now diverted into the surrounding circulation. In many cases the surrounding tissue has been in a state of chronic ischemia and the arterial vessels feeding these areas are maximally dilated. As arterial blood begins to flow at a higher volume and pressure into these dilated arteries, seeping of blood from the vessels may occur. Evidence of reperfusion bleeding in the operating room is an indication that no more arterial blood can be diverted from the AVM without risk of serious intracerebral hemorrhage. In the postoperative phase, a low blood pressure is maintained to prevent further reperfusion bleeding. In large AVMs, two to four stages of surgery may be required over 6 to 12 months.

Embolization. Embolization is used to secure a cerebral aneurysm or AVM that is surgically inaccessible because of size, location, or medical instability of the patient. Embolization involves several new interventional neuroradiology techniques. All of the techniques use a percutaneous transfemoral approach in a manner similar to an angiogram. Under fluoroscopy, the catheter is threaded up to the internal carotid artery. Specially developed microcatheters are then manipulated into the area of the vascular anomaly and embolic materials are placed endovascularly. Three different embolization techniques are used, depending on the underlying pathologic derangement.

The first type of embolization is used to embolize an AVM. Small silastic beads or glue are slowly introduced into the vessels feeding the AVM. Blood flow then carries the material to the site and embolization is achieved. This procedure may be used in combination with surgery. One to three sessions of embolization of the feeding vessels are performed to reduce the size of the lesion before a craniotomy is performed for total excision. The primary risk of this procedure is lodging of the embolic substance in a vessel that feeds normal tissue. This occurrence creates an embolic stroke with the immediate onset of neurologic symptoms.

The second type of embolization involves placement of one or more detachable balloons into an aneurysmal sac or AVM. A liquid polymerizing agent is used to inflate the balloon. The material then solidifies within approximately 45 minutes.[21] The third techniques involves placement of one or more detachable platinum coils into an aneurysm to produce an endovascular thrombus. The advantage of this technique is that an electrical current creates positive charging of the coil, which induces electrothrombosis.[22,23] The most common complication of these two techniques is the development of distal ischemia resulting from emboli. Again, the onset of neurologic symptoms is immediate. Other risks include subtotal occlusion and intraprocedural rupture of the vasculature and death.

Pharmacologic therapy. For years the use of antifibrinolytic agents (aminocaproic acid) has been suggested in situations in which early surgery is not an option. Antifibrinolytic agents prevent the production of fibrin, which is responsible for the eventual dissolution of the clot at the tip of the aneurysm. Controversy continues to surround the use of these agents. Results of studies reporting a reduced incidence of rebleeding have been minimally positive. The main issue with the use of antifibrinolytic agents is the tendency of these drugs to increase the incidence and severity of the other common SAH complication—vasospasm. Clinical trials continue to evaluate the efficacy of this treatment.[17]

Cerebral vasospasm. The presence or absence of cerebral vasospasm significantly affects the outcome of aneurysmal SAH. This complication does not occur with SAH resulting from AVM rupture. Cerebral vasospasm is a narrowing of the lumen of the cerebral arteries. It is believed to be a response to subarachnoid blood clots coating the outer surface of the blood vessels.[24] Inasmuch as aneurysms occur at the circle of Willis, the major vessels responsible for feeding the cerebral circulation are affected by vasospasm. Depending on the arterial vessels involved in the vasospasm reaction, decreased arterial flow occurs in large areas of the cerebral hemispheres.

It is estimated that 50% of all SAH patients develop vasospasm, which is demonstrable by angiography. Thirty-two percent of these patients develop symptomatic vasospasm, resulting in ischemic stroke and/or death for 15% to 20% of them despite the use of maximal therapy.[17] The onset of vasospasm is usually 3 to 5 days after the initial hemorrhage, with maximal narrowing occurring at 5 to 14 days.[17] Vasospasm can last for 3 to 4 weeks.

A variety of therapies have been evaluated in an attempt to reverse or overcome cerebral vasospasm. To date, three treatments seem to have potential benefit: induced hypertensive, hypervolemic, hemodilution therapy; oral nimodipine; and transluminal cerebral angioplasty.

Hypertensive, hypervolemic, hemodilution therapy. Hypertensive, hypervolemic, hemodilution (HHH) therapy involves increasing the patient's blood pressure and cardiac output with vasoactive medications and diluting the patient's blood with fluid and volume expanders. Systolic BP is maintained between 150 and 160 mm Hg. The increase in volume and pressure forces blood through the vasospastic area at higher pressures. Hemodilution facilitates flow through the area by reducing blood viscosity. Many anecdotal reports exist of patients' neurologic deficits improving as systolic pressure increases from 130 mm Hg to between 150 and 160 mm Hg. The Stroke Council of the AHA has recommended this therapy for prevention and treatment of vasospasm.[17]

The obvious deterrent to use of induced hypertension is the risk of rebleeding in an unsecured aneurysm. Surgical clipping of the aneurysm before HHH therapy is preferred. Cerebral edema, elevated intracranial pressure, cardiac failure, and electrolyte imbalance are also risks of HHH therapy. Careful monitoring of the patient's neurologic status, hemodynamic parameters, ICP, and serum electrolytes is necessary.[17]

Oral nimodipine. Oral nimodipine is strongly recommended to reduce the poor outcomes associated with vasospasm. The exact nature of the effect of nimodipine is not clear, but use of the drug has demonstrated consistently positive effects on outcome without any demonstrable effect on the incidence or severity of vasospasm. Nimodipine is administered by mouth or nasogastric tube prophylactically in all patients with SAH. Nimodipine may produce hypotension, especially when administered concurrently with other antihypertensive agents. The drug is not effective if administered sublingually.[25] Intravenous administration of other calcium channel blockers is under investigation.[17]

Transluminal cerebral angioplasty. Transluminal cerebral angioplasty is used when pharmacologic management of cerebral vasospasm has failed.[26] It is only performed when CT or MRI provides evidence that infarction has not yet occurred. The procedure is performed by an interventional neuroradiologist, and the patient is under either local, general, or neuroleptic analgesia. The technique of cerebral angioplasty is very similar to that used in the coronary vasculature. Risks include intimal perforation or rupture cerebral artery thrombosis or embolism, recurrence of stenosis, and severe diffuse vasospasm unresponsive to therapy. Hemorrhage at the femoral site may also occur. Early evidence is promising, and this procedure is recommended when conventional therapy is unsuccessful.[17]

Hyponatremia. Hyponatremia develops in 10% to 43% of patients with SAH. It usually occurs around the same timeframe as vasospasm, several days after initial hemorrhage. There is strong evidence that the use of fluid restriction to treat hyponatremia is associated with poor outcome in the SAH patient. The AHA Stroke Council has strongly recommended that fluid restriction not be used in this instance and instead recommends sodium replenishment with isotonic fluids.[17]

Hydrocephalus. The development of hydrocephalus is a late complication that commonly occurs after SAH. Blood that has circulated in the subarachnoid space and has been absorbed by the arachnoid villi may obstruct the villi and reduce the rate of CSF absorption. Over time, increasing volumes of CSF in the intracranial space produce communicating hydrocephalus. Treatment consists of placing a drain to remove CSF. This can be accomplished temporarily by inserting a ventriculostomy or permanently by placing a ventriculoperitoneal shunt.

Intracerebral Hemorrhage

Description and etiology

Intracerebral hemorrhage (ICH) is bleeding directly into cerebral tissue, usually from a small artery. Causes of intracerebral hemorrhage are aneurysm or AVM rupture, trauma, or hypertensive hemorrhage. This section concentrates on hypertensive hemorrhage. Intracerebral hemorrhage destroys cerebral tissue, causes cerebral edema, and increases ICP. The incidence of hypertensive hemorrhage accounts for 2% of all deaths in the United States and is responsible for about 10% to 15% of all strokes annually.[14] ICH usually occurs in patients between 55 and 75 years old.

Intracerebral hemorrhage is most often caused by hypertensive rupture of a cerebral vessel. The cause of a hypertensive stroke is largely a longstanding history of hypertension. Blood dyscrasia (leukemia, hemophilia, sickle cell disease), anticoagulation therapy, and hemorrhage into brain tumors are other possible causes of intracerebral hemorrhage. Many patients develop headache and neurologic symptoms after straining to have a bowel movement. Often on questioning, the patient with a hypertensive hemorrhage admits to having discontinued antihypertensive medication 2 to 3 weeks before the hemorrhage.

Pathophysiology

The pathophysiology of intracerebral hemorrhage is caused by continued elevated blood pressure exerting force against smaller arterial vessels that have become damaged from arteriosclerotic changes. Eventually, these arteries break, and blood bursts from the vessels into the surrounding cerebral tissue, creating a hematoma. ICP rises precipitously in response to the increase in overall intracranial volume.

Assessment and diagnosis

Initial assessment usually reveals a critically ill patient who often is unconscious and requires ventilatory support. History from a relative or significant other describes a sudden onset of severe headache with rapid neurologic deterioration. Diagnosis is established easily with CT.

Vital signs usually reveal a severely elevated blood pressure (200/100 to 250/150 mm Hg), slow pulse, and deep, labored respirations. The patient arrives in the emergency room with many of the signs of increased ICP. Airway, breathing, and circulation must be addressed first to make sure that the airway is adequate, breathing patterns are acceptable, and circulation is present.

An antihypertensive medication usually is administered immediately to reduce the blood pressure to a relatively normal reading. If the hemorrhage is significant enough to cause increased ICP, the blood pressure must not be allowed to drop too rapidly or too low. If the blood pressure drops below 140 mm Hg systolic and ICP remains high, cerebral perfusion may be compromised.

Medical management

Medical management of a hypertensive hemorrhage is similar to that for a traumatic hemorrhage. Surgical removal of the clot depends on the size and location of the hematoma, the patient's ICP, and other neurologic symptoms. If the hematoma is large and causes a shift in cerebral structures or if ICP is elevated despite routine methods to lower it, a craniotomy for removal of the hematoma is performed. Nonsurgical management includes measures to maintain the ICP within normal limits and to support all other vital functions until the patient regains consciousness. The case fatality rate for intracerebral hemorrhagic strokes is approximately 50%.[14]

Nursing Management of Cerebrovascular Accident

Nursing management of the patient with a cerebrovascular accident incorporates a variety of nursing diagnoses (Box 16-7). **Nursing priorities are directed toward performing frequent neurologic and hemodynamic assess-**

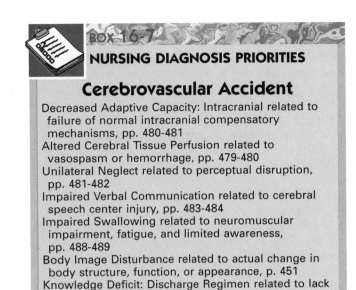

BOX 16-7

NURSING DIAGNOSIS PRIORITIES

Cerebrovascular Accident

Decreased Adaptive Capacity: Intracranial related to failure of normal intracranial compensatory mechanisms, pp. 480-481
Altered Cerebral Tissue Perfusion related to vasospasm or hemorrhage, pp. 479-480
Unilateral Neglect related to perceptual disruption, pp. 481-482
Impaired Verbal Communication related to cerebral speech center injury, pp. 483-484
Impaired Swallowing related to neuromuscular impairment, fatigue, and limited awareness, pp. 488-489
Body Image Disturbance related to actual change in body structure, function, or appearance, p. 451
Knowledge Deficit: Discharge Regimen related to lack of previous exposure to information, p. 443

ments, monitoring for complications, and educating the patient and family.

Performing frequent assessments

The goal of frequent assessments is early recognition of neurologic and/or hemodynamic deterioration. Close monitoring of the patient's neurologic signs and vital signs is essential and requires almost continuous observation. Automatic noninvasive devices, such as a blood pressure cuff and a pulse oximeter, are helpful. Seizure activity must be identified and treated immediately. It is essential that all personnel working with the patient be aware of the desired hemodynamic and neurologic parameters set by the physician and that the physician be notified at the first sign of any changes.

Monitoring for complications

The patient with a cerebrovascular accident should be monitored closely for signs of bleeding, vasospasm, and increased intracranial pressure. Other complications of stroke include aspiration, malnutrition, pneumonia, deep vein thrombosis, pulmonary embolism, decubitus ulcers, contractures, and joint abnormalities.[12] Nursing measures to prevent these complications are well-known.

Bleeding and vasospasm. In the patient with a cerebral aneurysm, sudden onset of or an increase in headache, nausea and vomiting, increased BP, and changes in respiration herald the onset of rebleeding. The first indication of vasospasm is usually the appearance of new focal or global neurologic deficits. SAH precautions must be implemented to prevent any stress or straining that could potentially precipitate rebleeding. Precautions include bedrest; a dark, quiet environment, and stool softeners. Short-acting analgesics and sedatives are used to relieve pain and anxiety. The patient must be kept calm. Limb restraints cause straining and must be avoided. If restraint is necessary, only a vest or jacket type of restraint is used. The head of the bed should be elevated to 35 to 45 degrees at all times. The patient is taught to avoid any activities that create the Valsalva maneuver, such as pushing with the legs to move up in bed, straining for a bowel movement, or holding his or her breath during procedures or discomfort. Deep vein thrombosis precautions are routinely implemented. Historically, family visitation has been limited, but with the vast research available documenting the benefit of family visitation, the nurse must develop an individualized visitation plan to meet the needs of each patient. Often, family members at the bedside can assist the patient to remain calm.

Increased intracranial pressure. There are numerous signs and symptoms of increased ICP. These include decreased level of consciousness, Cushing's triad (bradycardia, systolic hypertension, and bradypnea), diminished brainstem reflexes, papilledema, decerebrate posturing (abnormal extension), decorticate posturing (abnormal flexion), unequal pupil size, projectile vomiting, decreased pupillary response to light, altered breathing patterns, and headache.[27]

Additional complications that may be seen in the patient with a cerebrovascular accident are related to the area of the brain that has been damaged. Damage to the temporoparietal area can create a variety of disturbances that affect the patient's ability to interpret sensory information.[28] Damage to the dominant hemisphere (usually left) produces problems with speech and language and abstract and analytic skills. Damage to the nondominant hemisphere (usually right) produces problems with spatial relationships. The resulting deficits include agnosia, apraxia, and visual field defects. Perceptual deficits are not as readily noticeable as are motor deficits, but they may be more debilitating and can lead to the inability to perform skilled or purposeful tasks.[29]

The patient with cerebrovascular accident may also develop impaired swallowing.[30] Normal swallowing occurs in four phases that are controlled by the cranial nerves. Damage to the brain, brainstem, or cranial nerves can result in a variety of swallowing deficits that can place the patient at risk for aspiration. The stroke patient is observed for signs of dysphagia, including drooling; difficulty handling oral secretions; absence of gag, cough, or swallowing reflexes; moist, gurgly voice quality; decreased mouth and tongue movements; and the presence of dysarthria. A speech therapy consult is initiated if any of these signs are present, and the patient must not be orally fed. In the absence of these warning signs, the patient may be fed, as ordered by the physician, although he or she must be continually monitored for signs of aspiration.[31]

Educating the patient and family

Rehabilitation starts in the critical care area, with a multidisciplinary team designing and implementing an individualized plan for maximizing the patient's potential for neurologic rehabilitation. Early in the patient's hospital stay, the patient and family must be taught about cerebrovascular accident, its etiologies, and its treatment. As the patient moves toward discharge, teaching focuses on the interventions necessary for preventing the reoccurrence of the event and on maximizing the patient's rehabilitation potential. The patient's family must be encouraged to participate in the patient's care; learn how to feed, dress, and bathe the patient; and learn some basic rehabilitation techniques. In addition, the importance of participating in a neurologic rehabilitation program and/or a support group must be stressed.

GUILLAIN-BARRÉ SYNDROME

Description and Etiology

Guillain-Barré syndrome (GBS) is an inflammatory peripheral polyneuritis characterized by a rapidly progressive, ascending peripheral nerve dysfunction leading to paralysis. It is 90% to 100% reversible and is one of the most common peripheral nervous system diseases. Because of the need for ventilatory support, GBS is one of the few peripheral neurologic diseases that necessitates a critical care environment. The annual incidence of GBS is 1.6 to 1.9 per 100,000 persons. It occurs equally in males and females and is the most commonly acquired demyelinating neuropathy.[32] The incidence of GBS increased slightly for a period after the 1977 swine flu vaccinations.[33] The cause of GBS is unknown, but more than 60% of patients report a viral infection 2 to 4 weeks before the onset of clinical manifestations. The result is a possible autoimmune response of the peripheral nervous system.[34]

GBS falls under a variety of different DRGs, depending on whether the patient develops comorbid conditions (CC) or the need for continuous ventilatory support. DRG 18 (Cranial and Peripheral Nerve Disorders with CC) or DRG 19 (Cranial and Peripheral Nerve Disorders Without CC) are usually used and have average lengths of stay of 5.9 days and 4.1 days, respectively. If the patient requires mechanical ventilation or a tracheostomy, DRG 475 (Respiratory System Diagnosis with Ventilator Support) or DRG 483 (Tracheostomy Except for Face, Mouth, and Neck Diagnoses) are used, with anticipated lengths of stay of 11.6 days and 43.5 days, respectively.[3]

Pathophysiology

This disease affects the motor and sensory pathways of the peripheral nervous system as well as the autonomic nervous system functions of the cranial nerves. The major finding in GBS is a segmental demyelination process of the peripheral nerves. GBS is believed to be an autoimmune response to antibodies formed against a recent viral illness, usually upper respiratory or gastrointestinal. T-cells migrate to the peripheral nerves, resulting in edema and inflammation. Macrophages then invade the area and break down the myelin.[35] Inflammation around this demyelinated area causes further dysfunction.[34]

The myelin sheath of the peripheral nerves is generated by Schwann's cells and acts as an insulator for the peripheral nerve. Myelin promotes rapid conduction of nerve impulses by allowing the impulses to jump along the nerve via nodes of Ranvier. Disruption of the myelin fiber slows and may eventually stop the conduction of impulses along the peripheral nerves. In GBS, the more thickly myelinated fibers of motor pathways and the cranial nerves are more severely affected than are the thinly myelinated sensory fibers of cutaneous pain, touch, and temperature.[35]

Once the temporary inflammatory reaction stops, myelin-producing cells begin the process of reinsulating the demyelinated portions of the peripheral nervous system. When remyelination occurs, normal neurologic function should return. In some instances, the axon may be damaged during the inflammatory process. The degree of axonal damage is responsible for the degree of neurologic dysfunction that persists after recovery.[34]

Assessment and Diagnosis

Symptoms of GBS include motor weakness, paresthesias and other sensory changes, cranial nerve dysfunction (especially oculomotor, facial, glossopharyngeal, vagal, spinal accessory, and hypoglossal), and some autonomic dysfunction. The usual course of GBS begins with an abrupt onset of lower extremity weakness that progresses to flaccidity and ascends over a period of hours to days. Motor loss usually is symmetric, bilateral, and ascending. In the most severe cases, complete flaccidity of all peripheral nerves, including spinal and cranial nerves, occurs.[35]

Admission to the hospital occurs when lower extremity weakness prevents mobility. Admission to the critical care unit occurs when progression of the weakness threatens respiratory muscles. As the patient's weakness progresses, close observation is essential. Frequent assessment of the respiratory system, including ventilatory parameters such as inspiratory force and tidal volume, is necessary. The most common cause of death in patients with GBS is from respiratory arrest. As the disease progresses and respiratory effort weakens, intubation and mechanical ventilation are necessary. Continued, frequent assessment of neurologic deterioration is required until the patient reaches the peak of the disease and plateau occurs.[34]

The diagnosis of GBS is based on clinical findings plus CSF analysis and nerve conduction studies. CSF analysis demonstrates a normal protein initially, which elevates in the fourth to sixth week. No other changes in CSF occur. Nerve conduction studies that test the velocity at which nerve impulses are conducted show significant reduction as the demyelinating process of the disease suggests.[34]

Medical Management

With no curative treatment available, the medical management of GBS is limited. The disease simply must run

its course, which is characterized by ascending paralysis that advances over 1 to 3 weeks and then remains at a plateau for several weeks. The plateau stage is followed by descending paralysis and return to normal or near-normal function. The main focus of medical management is the support of bodily functions and the prevention of complications.[34]

Plasmapheresis is often used in an attempt to limit the severity and duration of the syndrome. Plasmapheresis involves plasma exchanges or washes that remove the antibodies that cause GBS. Exchanges are given over 10 to 15 days.[36] Controversy exists over the benefit of plasmapheresis. It is contraindicated in patients with hemodynamic instability. In a recently published study of 220 patients in a multicenter clinical trial, the long-term benefit of plasmapheresis demonstrated that 71% of the treatment group versus 52% of the control group had full muscular strength recovery at 1 year.[37] Research suggests that intravenous immunoglobulin may have beneficial effects in treating GBS. A recent large multicenter randomized trial has demonstrated promising results.[38] Immunoglobulin is a blood product; close monitoring during its administration and during plasmapheresis is necessary. Some physicians support the use of steroids for their antiinflammatory effect, although their effectiveness remains unclear.

Nursing Management

The nursing management of the patient with GBS incorporates a variety of nursing diagnoses and interventions (Box 16-8). The goal of nursing management is to support all normal body functions until the patient can do so on his or her own. Although the condition is reversible, the patient with GBS requires extensive long-term care because recovery can be a long process. **Nursing priorities are directed toward initiating rehabilitation, facilitating**

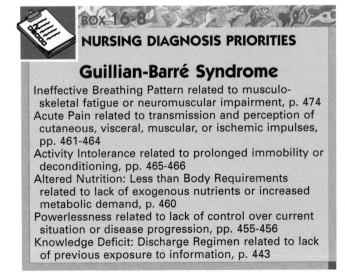

BOX 16-8

NURSING DIAGNOSIS PRIORITIES

Guillian-Barré Syndrome

Ineffective Breathing Pattern related to musculoskeletal fatigue or neuromuscular impairment, p. 474
Acute Pain related to transmission and perception of cutaneous, visceral, muscular, or ischemic impulses, pp. 461-464
Activity Intolerance related to prolonged immobility or deconditioning, pp. 465-466
Altered Nutrition: Less than Body Requirements related to lack of exogenous nutrients or increased metabolic demand, p. 460
Powerlessness related to lack of control over current situation or disease progression, pp. 455-456
Knowledge Deficit: Discharge Regimen related to lack of previous exposure to information, p. 443

nutritional support, providing comfort and emotional support, and educating patients and families.

Initiating rehabilitation

In patients with GBS, immobility may last for months. The usual course of GBS involves an average of 10 days of symptom progression and 10 days of maximum level of dysfunction, followed by 2 to 48 weeks of recovery. Although GBS is usually completely reversible, the patient will require physical and occupational rehabilitation because of the problems of long-term immobility. Rehabilitation starts in the critical care area, with a multidisciplinary team designing and implementing an individualized plan for maximizing the patient's potential for rehabilitation.

Facilitating nutritional support

Nutritional support is implemented early in the course of the disease. Because GBS recovery is a long process, adequate nutritional support will be a problem for an extended period. Nutritional support usually is accomplished through the use of enteral feeding, which is preferable to the use of total parenteral nutrition because it is less invasive and reduces the risk of infection in a patient who is highly vulnerable.

Providing comfort and emotional support

Pain control is another important component in the care of the patient with GBS. Although patients may have minimal to no motor function, most sensory functions remain, causing patients considerable muscle ache and pain. Because of the length of this illness, a safe, effective, long-term solution to pain management must be identified. These patients also require extensive psychologic support. Although the illness is almost 100% reversible, lack of control over the situation, constant pain or discomfort, and the long-term nature of the disorder create coping difficulties for the patient. GBS does not affect the level of consciousness or cerebral function. Patient interaction and communication are essential elements of the nursing management plan.

Educating the patient and family

Early in the patient's hospital stay, the patient and family must be taught about GBS and its different treatments. As the patient moves toward discharge, teaching focuses on the interventions to maximize the patient's rehabilitation potential. The patient's family must be encouraged to participate in the patient's care and to learn some basic rehabilitation techniques. In addition, the importance of participating in a neurologic rehabilitation program (if necessary) must be stressed.

CRANIOTOMY

Types of Surgery

A craniotomy is performed to gain access to portions of the CNS inside the cranium, usually to allow removal of a space-occupying lesion. Common procedures include

---

BOX 16-9

OPERATIVE TERMS

Burr hole	Hole made into the cranium using a special drill
Craniotomy	Surgical opening of the skull
Craniectomy	Removal of a portion of the skull without replacing it
Cranioplasty	Plastic repair of the skull
Supratentorial	Above the tentorium, separating the cerebrum from the cerebellum
Infratentorial	Below the tentorium; includes the brainstem and the cerebellum; an infratentorial surgical approach may be used for temporal or occipital lesions

---

tumor resection or removal, cerebral decompression, evacuation of hematoma or abscess, and clipping or removal of an aneurysm or arteriovenous malformation. Box 16-9 provides definitions of common neurosurgical terms. This section provides a generalized discussion of craniotomy care.

Most patients who undergo craniotomy for tumor resection or removal do not require care in a critical care unit. Those who do usually need intensive monitoring or are at greater risk of complications because of underlying cardiopulmonary dysfunction or the surgical approach used. One common procedure requiring routine postoperative care in the critical care unit is hypophysectomy or pituitary adenomectomy using either a transcranial or transsphenoidal approach.

Preoperative Care

Protection of the integrity of the CNS is a major priority of care for the patient awaiting a craniotomy. Optimal arterial oxygenation, hemodynamic stability, and cerebral perfusion are essential to maintaining adequate cerebral oxygenation. Management of seizure activity is essential to controlling metabolic needs.

Detailed assessment and documentation of the patient's preoperative neurologic status are imperative for accurate postoperative evaluation. Specific attention is placed on identifying and describing the nature and extent of any preoperative neurologic deficits.

Preoperative teaching is necessary to prepare both the patient and family for what to expect in the postoperative period. A description of the intravascular lines and intracranial catheters used during the postoperative period allows the family to focus on the patient, rather than be overwhelmed by masses of tubing. Some or all of the patient's hair is shaved off in the operating room and a large, bulky, turban-like craniotomy dressing is applied. Most patients experience some degree of postoperative eye or facial swelling and periorbital ecchymosis. An explanation of these temporary changes in appearance helps alleviate the shock and fear many patients and families experience in the immediate postoperative period.

All craniotomy patients require instruction to avoid activities known to produce sudden changes in intracranial pressure. These activities include bending, lifting, straining, and avoiding the Valsalva maneuver. Patients commonly elicit the Valsalva maneuver during repositioning in bed by holding their breath and straining with a closed epiglottis. Teaching the patient to continue to breathe deeply through the mouth during all position changes is an effective deterrent.

The patient undergoing transsphenoidal surgery requires preparation for the sensations associated with nasal packing. The patient often awakens with alarm because of the inability to breathe through the nose. Preoperative instruction in mouth breathing and avoidance of coughing, sneezing, or blowing of the nose facilitates postoperative cooperation.[39]

The psychosocial issues associated with the prospect of neurosurgery cannot be overemphasized. Few procedures are as threatening as those involving the brain or spinal cord. For some patients the fear of permanent neurologic impairment may be as or more ominous than the fear of death. Steps to meet the needs of the patient, as well as the family, include collaboration with clergy and social services personnel, patient-controlled visitation, and provision of as much privacy as the patient's condition permits. Both the patient and the family must be provided with the opportunity to express their fears and concerns apart from each other as well as jointly.

Surgical Considerations

While the emphasis in surgical approach for most other types of surgery is to gain adequate exposure of the surgical site, the neurosurgeon must select a route that also produces the least amount of disruption to the intracranial contents. Neural tissue is unforgiving. A significant portion of neurologic trauma and postoperative deficits is related to the surgical pathway through the brain tissue, rather than to the procedure performed at the site of pathology. Depending on the location of the lesion and the surgical route decided on, either a transcranial or a transsphenoidal approach is used to open the skull.

In the transcranial approach, a scalp incision is made and a series of burr holes are drilled into the skull to form an outline of the area to be opened. A special saw is then used to cut between the holes. In most cases the bone flap is left attached to the muscle to create a hinge effect. In some cases the bone flap is removed completely and either placed in the abdomen for later retrieval and implantation or discarded and replaced with synthetic material. Next the dura is opened and retracted. After the intracranial procedure, the dura and the bone flap are closed, the muscles and scalp are sutured, and a turban-like dressing is applied.[21]

The transsphenoidal approach is the technique of choice for removal of a pituitary tumor without extension into the intracranial vault.[39] This approach involves making a microsurgical entrance into the cranial vault via the nasal cavity. An otorhinolaryngologist performs the necessary steps to enter the sphenoid sinus and reach the anterior wall of the sella turcica. A neurosurgeon then opens the sphenoid bone and the dura to gain intracranial access. After removal of the tumor, the surgical bed is packed with a small section of adipose tissue grafted from the patient's abdomen or thigh. After closure of the intranasal structures, the otorhinolaryngologist places nasal splints and soft packing or nasal tampons impregnated with antibiotic ointment in the nasal cavities. Occasionally, epistaxis balloons are used instead. A nasal drip pad or mustache-type dressing is placed at the base of the nose to catch surgical drainage.[39]

The patient may be placed in a supine, prone, or even sitting position for a craniotomy procedure. A skull clamp connected to skull pins is used to position and secure the patient's head throughout the surgery. During a transsphenoidal approach or a transcranial approach into the infratentorial area, the patient's head is elevated during the surgery. This position places the patient at risk for an air embolism. Air can enter the vascular system either through the edges of the dura or a venous opening. Continuous monitoring of the patient's heart sounds by Doppler signal allows immediate recognition of this complication. If it occurs, an attempt may be made to withdraw the embolus from the right atrium through a central line. An immediate barrier to any further air entrance is created by flooding the surgical field with irrigation fluid and placing a moistened sterile surgical sponge over the surgical site.[21,39]

Several other procedures are used intraoperatively during a craniotomy to either facilitate the surgery or to prevent surgical complications. Hypothermia is used to decrease the metabolic needs of the brain. Controlled hypotension lessens blood loss during resection of an AVM or cerebral aneurysm. Hyperventilation is used to reduce the size or bulk of the brain through reduction in cerebral blood flow.[21]

Complications and Medical Management

Complications associated with a craniotomy include intracranial hypertension, surgical hemorrhage, fluid imbalance, CSF leak, deep vein thrombosis, gastric stress ulceration, and pulmonary infection.

Intracranial hypertension

Postoperative cerebral edema may be expected to peak 48 to 72 hours after surgery. If the bone flap is not replaced at the time of surgery, intracranial hypertension will produce bulging at the surgical site. Close monitoring of the surgical site is important so that integrity of the incision can be maintained. Postcraniotomy management of intracranial hypertension is usually accomplished through CSF drainage, hyperventilation, patient positioning, and steroid administration.

Surgical hemorrhage

Surgical hemorrhage after a transcranial procedure can occur in the intracranial vault and is manifested by signs and symptoms of increasing ICP. Hemorrhage after a transsphenoidal craniotomy may be evident from external drainage, patient complaint of persistent postnasal drip, or excessive swallowing. Postoperative hemorrhage requires surgical reexploration.

Fluid imbalance

Fluid imbalance in the postcraniotomy patient usually results from a disturbance in production or secretion of antidiuretic hormone (ADH). ADH is secreted by the posterior pituitary (neurohypophysis) gland. It stimulates the renal tubules and collecting ducts to retain water in response to low circulating blood volume or increased serum osmolality. Inoperative trauma or postoperative edema of the pituitary gland or hypothalamus can result in insufficient ADH secretion. The outcome is unabated renal water loss even when blood volume is low and serum osmolality is high. This condition is known as diabetes insipidus (DI). The polyuria associated with DI is often greater than 200 ml/hour. Urine specific gravity of 1.005 or less and elevated serum osmolality provide evidence of insufficient ADH. The loss of volume may produce hypotension and inadequate cerebral perfusion. DI is usually self-limiting, with fluid replacement being the only necessary therapy. In some cases, however, it may be necessary to administer vasopressin intravenously once or twice a day to control the loss of fluid.[40]

The syndrome of inappropriate antidiuretic hormone (SIADH) commonly occurs with neurologic insult and results from excessive ADH secretion.[40] SIADH is manifested by inappropriate water retention with hyponatremia in the presence of normal renal function. Urine specific gravity is elevated, and urine osmolality is greater than serum osmolality. The dangers associated with SIADH include circulating volume overload and electrolyte imbalance, both of which may impair neurologic functioning. SIADH is usually self-limiting, with the mainstay of treatment being fluid restriction.[40]

CSF leak

Leakage of CSF fluid results from an opening in the subarachnoid space, as evidenced by clear fluid draining from the surgical site. When this complication occurs after transsphenoidal surgery, it is evidenced by excessive, clear drainage from the nose or persistent postnasal drip. To differentiate CSF drainage from postoperative serous drainage, a specimen is tested for glucose content. A CSF leak is confirmed by glucose values of 30 mg/dL or greater. Management of the patient with a CSF leak includes bedrest and head elevation. Lumbar puncture or placement of a lumbar subarachnoid catheter may be used to reduce CSF pressure until the dura heals. Rarely, surgical reexploration is necessary.

Deep vein thrombosis

Deep vein thrombosis (DVT) has been reported to occur in 29% to 46% of all neurosurgical patients, as compared with a 25% incidence in general surgical patients. The risk is greater after removal of a supratentorial tumor and is increased twofold for patients whose surgery lasts for more than 4 hours.[41] Clinical manifestations of DVT include leg or calf pain, edema, localized tenderness, and pain with dorsiflexion or plantar flexion (Homan's sign). Unfortunately the patient with a DVT is often asymptomatic, and the diagnosis is not made until the patient experiences a pulmonary embolus.

The primary treatment for DVT is prophylaxis. Graduated elastic stockings and sequential pneumatic compression boots or stockings have been demonstrated to be effective in reducing the incidence of DVT. These devices are commonly used in the care of the neurosurgical patient, either alone or in combination. Effectiveness is enhanced when these devices are initiated in the preoperative period.[41,42] Low-dose heparin may also be used prophylactically in high risk patients. Recent evidence suggests that a combination of pneumatic compression therapy applied in the operating room and postoperative low-dose heparin is both safe and effective in preventing DVT in the neurosurgical patient.[43]

If a DVT develops in the postcraniotomy patient, the physician must weigh the risk of therapeutic heparinization versus the risk of pulmonary embolus (PE). There is evidence that a DVT in the distal circulation below the knee carries a much lower risk of PE than a DVT in the proximal circulation.[40] Even when a PE occurs, the use of therapeutic heparin doses in the neurosurgical patient is controversial.[42]

Stress ulcers

Historically, stress ulcers have been a common complication in neurosurgical patients, especially in those requiring long-term mechanical ventilation. Effective prophylactic measures for this complication include intravenous histamine$_2$ antagonists and early enteral feeding.

Pneumonia

The risk of pneumonia in the postoperative craniotomy patient is significantly increased if the patient remains in the critical care unit for more than 5 days because of prolonged intubation.[40] Adequate pulmonary hygiene and strict infection control measures are helpful to prevent this complication. Treatment consists of antibiotics and appropriate pulmonary management. Acute respiratory distress syndrome and neurogenic pulmonary edema may also occur in the postcraniotomy patient, possibly related to intracranial hypertension.

Numerous other complications may also occur after a craniotomy. Focal or grand mal seizure activity is common and is managed prophylactically with anticonvulsant therapy. Postoperative meningitis may result from surgical infection or CSF leak and is treated with antibiotics.[40] Cranial nerve dysfunction may occur either transiently or permanently as a result of surgical manipulation, edema, or anatomic disruption.[44] Compression of the optic chiasm with complete or partial visual loss may result from migration of the adipose tissue packing placed in a pituitary tumor bed and requires surgical reexploration.[39]

Postoperative Nursing Management

The nursing management of the neurosurgery patient incorporates a variety of nursing diagnoses and interventions (Box 16-10). As in preoperative care, the primary goal of postcraniotomy nursing management is protection of the integrity of the CNS. **Nursing priorities are directed toward preserving adequate cerebral perfusion, promoting arterial oxygenation, facilitating pain management, and maintaining surveillance for complications.** Frequent neurologic assessment is necessary to evaluate accomplishment of this objective and to identify and quickly intervene if complications do arise. Often a ventriculostomy is placed to facilitate ICP monitoring and/or CSF drainage.

Preserving adequate cerebral perfusion

Nursing interventions to preserve cerebral perfusion include patient positioning, fluid management, and avoidance of postoperative vomiting and fever.

Patient positioning is an important component of care for the craniotomy patient. The head of the bed should be elevated 30 to 45 degrees at all times to reduce the incidence of hemorrhage, facilitate venous drainage, and control ICP. Other positioning measures to control ICP include maintaining the patient's head in a neutral position at all times and avoiding neck or hip flexion. It is vital to adhere to these rules of positioning throughout all nursing activities, including linen changes and transporting the patient for diagnostic evaluation. Most craniotomy patients can still be turned from side to side within these restrictions, using pillows for support, except in some cases of extensive tumor removal, cranioplasty, and when the bone flap is not replaced. Specific orders from the surgeon must be obtained in these instances. The patient with an infratentorial incision may be restricted to only a very small pillow under the head to prevent strain on the incision. Avoidance of anterior or lateral neck flexion also protects the integrity of this type of incision.

Fluid management is another important component of postcraniotomy care. Hourly monitoring of fluid intake and output facilitates early identification of fluid imbalance. Urine specific gravity must be measured if DI is suspected. Fluid restriction may be ordered as a routine measure to lessen the severity of cerebral edema or as treatment for the fluid and electrolyte imbalances associated with SIADH.

Postoperative vomiting must be avoided to prevent sharp spikes in ICP and possibly surgical hemorrhage. Antiemetics are administered as soon as nausea is apparent. The patient is usually given nothing by mouth for at least 24 hours; then the diet is progressed as tolerated. Postoperative fever may also adversely affect ICP and increase the metabolic needs of the brain. Acetaminophen is administered either orally, rectally, or via a feeding tube. External cooling measures, such as a hypothermia blanket, may also be necessary.

Promoting arterial oxygenation

Routine pulmonary care is used to maintain airway clearance and prevent pulmonary complications. To prevent dangerous elevations in ICP, this care must be performed using proper technique and at time intervals that are adequately spaced from other patient care activities. If pulmonary complications do arise, consideration must be given to maintaining adequate oxygenation during repositioning. It may be necessary to restrict turning to only the side that places the good lung down.

Facilitating pain management

Pain management in the postcraniotomy patient primarily involves control of headache. Small doses of intravenous morphine may be used in the intensive care setting. As soon as oral analgesics can be tolerated, acetaminophen with codeine is used. Both of these analgesics cause constipation. Administration of stool softeners and initiation of a bowel program are important components of postcraniotomy care. Constipation is hazardous because straining to have a bowel movement can create significant elevations in blood pressure and ICP.

Maintaining surveillance for complications

The postoperative neurosurgery patient is at risk for infection, corneal abrasions, and injury from falls or seizures.

Care of the incision and surgical dressings is institution- and physician-specific. The rule of thumb for

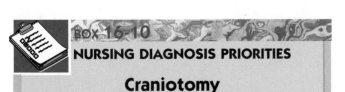

BOX 16-10

NURSING DIAGNOSIS PRIORITIES

Craniotomy

Decreased Adaptive Capacity: Intracranial related to failure of normal intracranial compensatory mechanisms, pp. 480-481

Altered Cerebral Tissue Perfusion related to vasospasm or hemorrhage, pp. 479-480

Acute Pain related to transmission and perception of cutaneous, visceral, muscular, or ischemic impulses, pp. 461-464

Body Image Disturbance related to actual change in body structure, function, or appearance, p. 451

Knowledge Deficit: Discharge Regimen related to lack of previous exposure to information, p. 443

a craniotomy dressing is to reinforce it as needed and change it only with a physician's order. Often times a drain is left in place to facilitate decompression of the surgical site. If a ventriculostomy is present, it is treated as a component of the surgical site. All drainage devices must be secured to the dressing to prevent unintentional displacement with patient movement. Sterile technique is required to prevent infection and resultant meningitis.

Routine eye care may be necessary to prevent corneal drying and ulceration. Periorbital edema interferes with normal blinking and eyelid closure, which are essential to adequate corneal lubrication. Saline drops are instilled every 2 hours. If the patient remains in a coma state, the eyes must also be covered with a polyethylene film extending over the orbits and eyebrows.[7]

The postcraniotomy patient may also experience periods of altered mentation. Protection from injury may require use of restraint devices. The side rails of the bed must also be padded to protect the patient from injury. Having a family member stay at the bedside and/or use of music therapy is often helpful to keep the patient calm during periods of restlessness. In rare circumstances, neuromuscular blockade and sedation may be necessary to control patient activity and metabolic needs on a short-term basis.

Increased patient activity, including ambulation, is begun as soon as tolerated in the postoperative period. Rehabilitation measures and discharge planning may begin in the critical care unit but are beyond the scope of this text. Transfer to a general care or rehabilitation unit is usually accomplished as soon as the patient is considered to be stable and without complication.

References

1. Multi-Society Task Force on PVS: Medical aspects of the persistent vegetative state (first of two parts), *N Engl J Med* 330:1499, 1994.
2. Haerer AF: *DeJong's the neurologic examination,* ed 5, Philadelphia, 1992, JB Lippincott.
3. *St Anthony's DRG guidebook* 1998, Reston, Va, 1997, St Anthony Publishing.
4. Berger JR: Clinical approach to stupor and coma. In Bradley WG, et al, editors: *Neurology in clinical practice: principles of diagnosis and management,* vol 1, ed 2, Boston, 1996, Butterworth-Heinemann.
5. Topel JL, Lewis SL: Examination of the comatose patient. In Weiner WE, Goetz CG, editors: *Neurology for the non-neurologist,* ed 3, Philadelphia, 1994, JB Lippincott.
6. Brust JCM: Coma. In Rowland LP, editor: *Merritt's textbook of neurology,* ed 9, Baltimore, 1995, Williams & Wilkins.
7. Cortese D, Capp L, McKinley S: Moisture chamber versus lubrication for the prevention of corneal epithelial breakdown, *Am J Crit Care* 4:425, 1995.
8. Sosnowski C, Ustik M: Early intervention: coma stimulation in the intensive care unit, *J Neurosci Nurs* 26:336, 1994.
9. Helwick LD: Stimulation programs for coma patients, *Crit Care Nurs* 14(4):47, 1994.
10. Jones R, et al: Auditory stimulation effect on a comatose survivor of traumatic brain injury, *Arch Phys Med Rehabil* 75:164, 1994.
11. Gwynn M: tPA in acute stroke—risk or reprieve? *J Neurosci Nurs* 25:180, 1993.
12. Adams HP, et al: Guidelines for the management of patients with acute ischemic stroke: a statement for healthcare professionals from a special writing group of the Stroke Council, American Heart Association, *Circulation* 90:1588, 1994.
13. Sacco RL: Pathogenesis, classification, and epidemiology of cerebrovascular disease. In Rowland LP, editor: *Merritt's textbook of neurology,* ed 9, Baltimore, 1995, Williams & Wilkins.
14. Hart RG: Cardiogenic embolism to the brain, *Lancet* 339:589, 1992.
15. Camarata PJ, Heros RC, Latchaw RE: "Brain attack": the rationale for treating stroke as a medical emergency, *Neurosurgery* 34:144, 1994.
16. McDowell FH, et al: *Stroke: the first hours—emergency evaluation and treatment,* Englewood, 1997, National Stroke Association.
17. Mayberg MR, et al: Guidelines for the management of aneurysmal subarachnoid hemorrhage: a statement for healthcare professionals from a special writing group of the Stroke Council, American Heart Association, *Circulation* 25:2315, 1994.
18. Rusy KL: Rebleeding and vasospasm after subarachnoid hemorrhage: a critical care challenge, *Crit Care Nurs* 16(1):41, 1996.
19. Hunt WE, Hess RM: Surgical risks as related to time of intervention in the repair of intracranial aneurysms, *J Neurosurg* 28:14, 1968.
20. Solenski NJ, et al: Medical complications of aneurysmal subarachnoid hemorrhage: a report of the multicenter, cooperative aneurysm study, *Crit Care Med* 23:1007, 1995.
21. Hickey JV: *The clinical practice of neurological and neurosurgical nursing,* ed 3, Philadelphia, 1992, JB Lippincott.
22. Coleman R, Sifri-Steele P: Treatment of posterior circulation aneurysms using platinum coils, *J Neurosci Nurs* 26:367, 1994.
23. Guglielmi G, et al: Carotid-cavernous fistula caused by a ruptured intracavernous aneurysm: endovascular treatment by electrothrombosis with detachable coils, *Neurosurgery* 31:591, 1992.
24. Findlay JM, Macdonald RL, Weir BK: Current concepts of pathophysiology and management of cerebral vasospasm following aneurysmal subarachnoid hemorrhage, *Cerebrovasc Brain Metab Rev* 3:336, 1991.
25. Counsell C, Gilbert M, Snively C: Nimodipine: a drug therapy for treatment of vasospasm, *J Neurosci Nurs* 27:54, 1995.
26. Grimes CM: Cerebral balloon angioplasty for treatment of vasospasm after subarachnoid hemorrhage, *Heart Lung* 20:431, 1991.
27. Wall BM, Philips JP, Howard JC: Validation of increased intracranial pressure and high risk of increased intracranial pressure, *Nurs Diagnosis* 5:74, 1994.
28. Olson E: Perceptual deficits affecting the stroke patient, *Rehabil Nurs* 16:213, 1991.
29. Baggerly J: Sensory perceptual problems following stroke: the "invisible" deficits, *Nurs Clin North Am* 26:997, 1991.
30. Phipps MA: Assessment of neurologic deficits in stroke: acute and rehabilitation implications, *Nurs Clin North Am* 26:957, 1991.
31. Baker DM: Assessment and management of impairments in swallowing, *Nurs Clin North Am* 28:793, 1993.
32. Lange DJ, Latov N, Trojaborg C: Acquired neuropathies. In Rowland LP, editor: *Merritt's textbook of neurology,* ed 9, Baltimore, 1995, Williams & Wilkins.
33. Keenlyside R, Brezman D: Fatal Guillain-Barré syndrome after the national influenza immunization program, *Neurology* 30:929, 1980.
34. Hund EF, et al: Intensive management and treatment of severe Guillain-Barré syndrome, *Crit Care Med* 21:433, 1993.

35. Ross AP: Nursing interventions for persons receiving immunosuppressive therapies for demyelinating pathology, *Nurs Clin North Am* 28:829, 1993.

36. Murray DP: Impaired mobility: Guillain-Barré syndrome, *J Neurosci Nurs* 25:100, 1993.

37. French Cooperative Group on Plasma Exchange: Plasma exchange in Guillain-Barré syndrome: one year follow-up, *Ann Neurol* 32:94, 1992.

38. Chipps E, Skinner C: Intravenous immunoglobulin: implications for use in the neurological patient, *J Neurosci Nurs* 26:8, 1994.

39. McEwen DR: Transsphenoidal adenomectomy, *AORN J* 61:321, 1995.

40. Levin AB: Intensive care. In Wilkins RH, Rengachary SS, editors: *Neurosurgery,* ed 2, vol 1, New York, 1996, McGraw-Hill.

41. Powers SK, Maliner LI: Prevention and treatment of thromboembolic complications in neurosurgical patients. In Wilkins RH, Rengachary SS, editors: *Neurosurgery,* ed 2, vol 1, New York, 1996, McGraw-Hill.

42. Fowler SB: Deep vein thrombosis and pulmonary emboli in neuroscience patients, *J Neurosci Nurs* 27:224, 1995.

43. Frim DM, et al: Postoperative low-dose heparin decreases thromboembolic complications in neurosurgical patients, *Neurosurgery* 30:830, 1992.

44. Geary SM: Nursing management of cranial nerve dysfunction, *J Neurosci Nurs* 27:102, 1995.

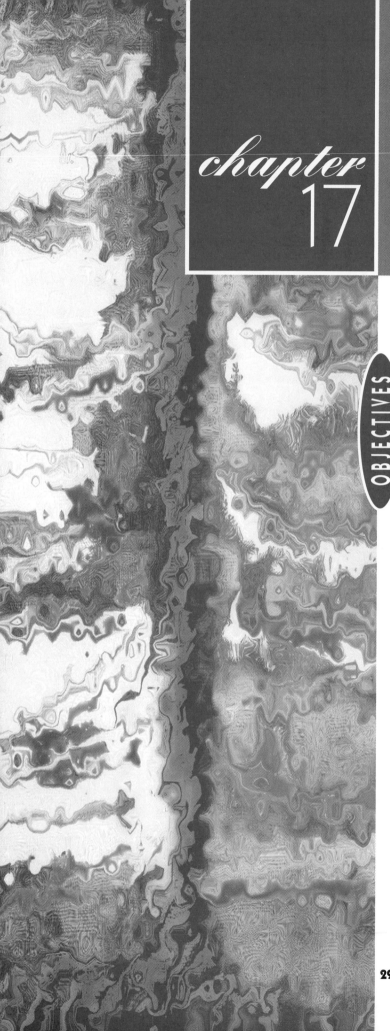

chapter 17

Neurologic Therapeutic Management

Kathleen A. Mendez

OBJECTIVES

- Discuss the concept of cerebral autoregulation.
- Calculate cerebral perfusion pressure.
- Describe the therapies commonly used to treat intracranial hypertension.
- Identify the different types of intracranial pressure monitoring devices.
- List the four supratentorial herniation syndromes.

Despite the diversity of neurologic abnormalities, one aspect of the critical care management of patients with neurologic disorders is common to a wide variety of these pathologic conditions. This chapter focuses on the priority interventions used to manage the critically ill patient with intracranial hypertension.

ASSESSMENT OF INTRACRANIAL PRESSURE

Monro-Kellie Hypothesis

The intracranial space comprises three components: brain substance (80%), cerebrospinal fluid (CSF) (10%), and blood (10%).[1] Under normal physiologic conditions, the ICP is maintained below 15 mm Hg mean pressure.[2] Essential to the understanding of the pathophysiology of ICP, the Monro-Kellie hypothesis proposes that an increase in volume of one intracranial component must be compensated by a decrease in one or more of the other components, so total volume remains fixed. This compensation, although limited, includes displacing CSF from the intracranial vault to the lumbar cistern, increasing CSF absorption, and compressing the low-pressure

TABLE **17-1**		

MECHANISMS OF ICP ELEVATION

PATHOPHYSIOLOGY	EXAMPLE	TREATMENT
DISORDERS OF CSF SPACE		
Overproduction of CSF	Choroid plexus papilloma	Diuretics, surgical removal
Communicating hydrocephalus from obstructed arachnoid	Old subarachnoid hemorrhage	Surgical drainage from lumbar intrathecal site
Noncommunicative hydrocephalus	Posterior fossa tumor obstructing aqueduct	Surgical drainage by ventricular drainage
Interstitial edema	Any of above	Surgical drainage of CSF
DISORDERS OF INTRACRANIAL BLOOD		
Intracranial hemorrhage causing increased ICP	Epidural hematoma	Surgical drainage
Vasospasm	Subarachnoid hemorrhage	Hypervolemia and hypertensive therapy
		Calcium channel antagonists
Vasodilation	Elevated $Paco_2$	Hyperventilation and adequate oxygenation
Increasing cerebral blood volume and ICP	Hypoxia	
DISORDERS OF BRAIN SUBSTANCE		
Expanding mass lesion with local vasogenic edema causing increased ICP	Brain tumor	Steroids Surgical removal
Ischemic brain injury with cytotoxic edema increasing ICP	Anoxic brain injury from cardiac or respiratory arrest	Resistant to therapy
Increased cerebral metabolic rate increasing cerebral blood flow and ICP	Seizures, hyperthermia	Anticonvulsant medications, especially barbiturates; control fever

From Helfaer MA, Kirsch JR: *Crit Care Rep* 1:12, 1989.

venous system. Pathophysiologic alterations that can elevate ICP are outlined in Table 17-1.

Volume-Pressure Curve

When capable of compliance, the brain can tolerate significant increases in intracranial volume without much increase in ICP. The amount of intracranial compliance, however, is limited. Once this limit has been reached, a state of decompensation with increased ICP results. As the ICP rises, the relationship between volume and pressure changes, and small increases in volume may cause major elevations in ICP (Fig. 17-1). The exact configuration of the volume-pressure curve and the point at which the steep rise in pressure occurs vary among patients. The configuration of this curve also is influenced by the cause and the rate of volume increases within the intracranial vault; for example, neurologic deterioration occurs more rapidly in a patient with an acute epidural hematoma than in a patient with a meningioma of the same size.[3]

Cerebral Blood Flow and Autoregulation

Cerebral blood flow (CBF) corresponds to the metabolic demands of the brain and is normally 50 ml/100 g of brain tissue/minute. Although the brain makes up only 2% of body weight, it requires 15% to 20% of the resting cardiac output and 15% of the body's oxygen

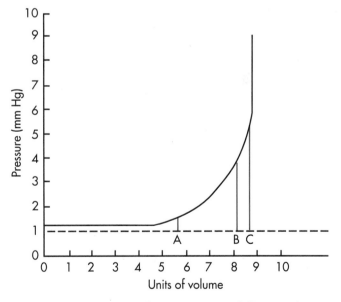

Fig. **17-1** Intracranial volume-pressure curve. *A,* Pressure is normal and increases in intracranial volume are tolerated without increases in intracranial pressure. *B,* Increases in volume may cause increases in pressure. *C,* Small increases in volume may cause larger increases in pressure.

demands. The normal brain has a complex capacity to maintain constant CBF despite wide ranges in arterial pressure—an effect known as *autoregulation*. Mean arterial pressure (MAP) of 50 to 150 mm Hg does not alter CBF when autoregulation is present. Outside the limits of autoregulation, CBF becomes passively dependent on the perfusion pressure.[3]

Factors other than arterial blood pressure that affect CBF are conditions that result in acidosis, alkalosis, and changes in metabolic rate. Conditions that cause acidosis (e.g., hypoxia, hypercapnia, and ischemia) result in cerebral vascular dilation. Conditions causing alkalosis (e.g., hypocapnia) result in cerebral vascular constriction. Normally, a reduction in metabolic rate (e.g., from hypothermia or barbiturates) decreases CBF, and increases in metabolic rate (e.g., from hyperthermia) increase CBF.[4]

Arterial blood gases exert a profound effect on CBF. Carbon dioxide, which affects the pH of the blood, is a potent vasoactive substance. Carbon dioxide retention (hypercapnia) leads to cerebral vasodilation, with increased cerebral blood volume, whereas hypocapnia leads to cerebral vasoconstriction and a reduction in cerebral blood volume.[3] Prolonged hypocapnia, however, especially at an arterial partial pressure of carbon dioxide ($PaCO_2$) less than 20 mm Hg, can produce cerebral ischemia.[5] Low arterial partial pressure of oxygen (PaO_2), especially below 40 mm Hg, leads to cerebral vasodilation, which increases the intracranial blood volume and can contribute to increased ICP. High PaO_2 has not been shown to affect CBF in either direction.

Metabolic activity in the brain significantly influences CBF. Normally, when cerebral metabolic activity increases, CBF also increases to meet the demand. Any pathologic process that decreases CBF could lead to a mismatch between metabolic demand and blood supply, resulting in cerebral ischemia.[5]

Cerebral Perfusion Pressure

Measuring CBF in the clinical setting is difficult. Cerebral perfusion pressure (CPP), an estimated pressure, is the blood pressure gradient across the brain and is calculated as the difference between the incoming MAP and the opposing ICP on the arteries (CPP = MAP − ICP). The CPP in the average adult is approximately 80 to 100 mm Hg, with a range of 60 to 150 mm Hg. The CPP should be maintained near 80 mm Hg to provide adequate blood supply to the brain. If the CPP drops below this point, ischemia may develop. A sustained CPP of 30 mm Hg or less usually will result in neuronal hypoxia and cell death. When the mean systemic arterial pressure equals the ICP, CBF may cease.[6]

Assessment Techniques

Signs and symptoms

The numerous signs and symptoms of increased ICP include decreased level of consciousness, Cushing's triad (bradycardia, systolic hypertension, and bradypnea), di-

minished brainstem reflexes, papilledema, decerebrate posturing (abnormal extension), decorticate posturing (abnormal flexion), unequal pupil size, projectile vomiting, decreased pupillary reaction to light, altered breathing patterns, and headache.[7] Patients may exhibit one or all of these symptoms, depending on the underlying cause of the elevation in ICP. **One of the earliest and most important signs of increased ICP is a decrease in level of consciousness. This change should be reported immediately to the physician.**

Monitoring the techniques

The common sites for monitoring ICP are the intraventricular space, the subarachnoid space, the epidural space, and the parenchyma. Each system has advantages and disadvantages for monitoring ICP (Table 17-2).[1,8] The type of monitor chosen depends on both the suspected pathologic condition and physician's preferences.

Ventriculostomy. The type of monitor placed in the ventricular system usually is a small catheter known as a ventriculostomy catheter. It is inserted through a burr hole with the patient under local anesthesia and usually is placed in the anterior horn of the lateral ventricle. If at all possible, the side chosen for placement of the ventriculostomy is the nondominant hemisphere[1,8,9] (Fig. 17-2, A).

Subarachnoid bolt. The second type of monitor frequently used is the subarachnoid bolt or screw. This small, hollow device is placed in a patient under local anesthesia through a burr hole, with the distal end lying in the subarachnoid or subdural space. Inserting this device (Fig. 17-2, B) is easier than the ventriculostomy catheter.[1,8]

Epidural monitor. Another type of device commonly used is the epidural monitor, also placed through a burr hole while the patient is under local anesthesia. The physician strips the dura away from the inner table of the skull before inserting the epidural monitor. The most common type of epidural monitor is the fiberoptic or pneumatic sensor although other implantable epidural transducers often are used for long-term monitoring[1,8] (Fig. 17-2, C).

Fiberoptic catheter. The fourth type of ICP monitoring system is the fiberoptic transducer-tipped catheter. This small (4 Fr) catheter can be placed intraventricularly, intraparenchymally (Fig. 17-2, D), in the subarachnoid space, or in the subdural space.[1,8]

Intracranial pressure waves

The ICP pulse waveform is observed on a continuous, real time pressure display, and corresponds to each heartbeat. The waveform arises primarily from pulsations of the major intracranial arteries, receiving retrograde venous pulsations as well.[3]

Normal ICP waveform. The normal ICP wave has three or more defined peaks (Fig. 17-3). The first peak, or P_1, is called the *percussion wave*. Originating from the pulsations of the choroid plexus, it has a sharp peak and is fairly consistent in its amplitude. The second peak, or P_2, is called the *tidal wave*. The tidal wave is more variable

TABLE 17-2

COMPARISON OF ICP MONITORING SYSTEMS

SYSTEM	ADVANTAGES	DISADVANTAGES
Ventricular catheter	Access for CSF drainage and sampling Access for determination of volume-pressure curve Direct measurement of pressure Access for medication instillation	Difficulty locating lateral ventricle Risk of intracerebral bleeding or edema at cannula track Risk of infection Need for transducer repositioning with head movement
Subarachnoid bolt/screw	Useful if ventricles are small No penetration of brain Decreased risk of infection Access for CSF sampling Direct measurement of pressure	Unable to drain CSF Unreliable pressure when high ICP herniates brain into bolt Requires intact skull Need for transducer repositioning with head movement
Epidural sensor	Ease of insertion No dural penetration Lower risk of infection No adjustment of transducer needed with head movement	Unable to drain CSF Unable to recalibrate or rezero after placement Questionable accuracy of sensing ICP through dura Separate large monitoring system required
Fiberoptic transducer-tipped catheter	Versatile system, which can be placed in ventricle, subarachnoid space, or brain tissue Able to monitor intraparenchymal pressure No adjustment of transducer needed with head movement	Catheter relatively fragile Unable to recalibrate or rezero after placement Separate monitoring system required

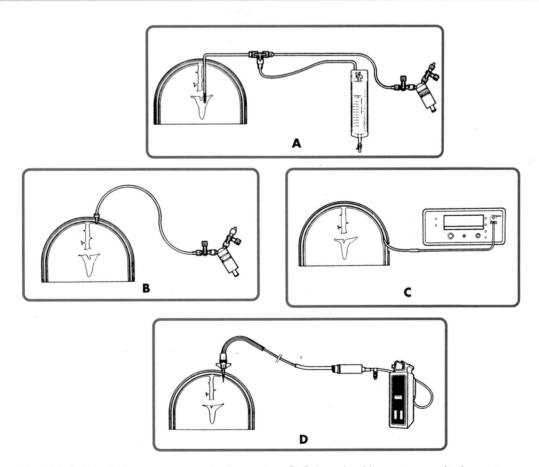

Fig. **17-2 A,** Ventricular pressure monitoring system. **B,** Subarachnoid pressure monitoring system. **C,** Epidural pressure monitoring system. **D,** Fiberoptic intraparenchymal pressure monitoring system. (Courtesy Camino NeuroCare, San Diego, CA.)

in shape and amplitude, ending on the dicrotic notch. The P_2 portion of the pulse waveform has been most directly linked to the state of decreased compliance. When the P_2 component is equal to or higher than P_1, decreased compliance occurs. Immediately after the dicrotic notch is the third wave, P_3, which is called the *dicrotic wave*. After the dicrotic wave, the pressure usually tapers down to the diastolic position unless retrograde venous pulsations add a few more peaks.[3]

A, B, and C pressure waves are not true waveforms (Fig. 17-4). Rather they are the graphically displayed trend data of ICP pressures over time. These waves reflect spontaneous alterations in ICP associated with respiration, systemic blood pressure, and deteriorating neurologic status.[8]

A waves. Also called *plateau waves* because of their distinctive shape, A waves are the most clinically significant of the three types. They usually occur in an already elevated baseline ICP (>20 mm Hg) and are characterized by sharp increases in ICP of 30 to 69 mm Hg, which plateau for 2 to 20 minutes and then return to baseline. The actual cause of A waves is unknown, but they may result from vasodilation and increased CBF, decreased venous outflow (and therefore increased cerebral blood volume), fluctuations in $PaCO_2$ (and therefore changes in cerebral blood volume), or decreased CSF absorption. B waves frequently precede A waves. Plateau waves are considered significant because of the reduced cerebral perfusion pressure associated with ICP in the 50 to 100 mm Hg range. Transient signs of intracranial hypertension such as a decreased level of consciousness, bradycardia, pupillary changes, or respiratory changes may accompany these waves. Some research suggests that prolonged increases in ICP associated with plateau waves could result in transient as well as permanent cell damage from ischemia.[1,8]

B waves. B waves are sharp, rhythmic oscillations with a sawtooth appearance that occur every 30 seconds to 2 minutes and can raise the ICP from 5 to 70 mm Hg. They are a normal physiologic phenomenon that can occur in any patient, but they are amplified in states of low intracranial compliance. B waves appear to reflect fluctuations in cerebral blood volume. Decompensation of normal intracranial volume compensatory capacity is indicated by B waves with a high amplitude (>15 mm Hg pressure change from peak to trough of wave).[1,8]

C waves. C waves are smaller rhythmic waves that occur every 4 to 8 minutes and at normal levels of ICP. They are related to normal fluctuations in respiration and systemic arterial pressure. C waves are considered clinically insignificant.[1,8]

MANAGEMENT OF INTRACRANIAL HYPERTENSION

Once intracranial hypertension is documented, therapy must be prompt to prevent secondary insults. Although the exact pressure level denoting intracranial hypertension remains uncertain, most current evidence suggests that ICP generally should be treated when it exceeds 20 mm Hg.[4] All therapies are directed toward reducing the volume of one or more of the components (blood, brain, CSF) that lie within the intracranial vault. A major goal of therapy is to determine the cause of the elevated pressure and, if possible, remove the cause.[10] In the absence of a surgically treatable mass lesion, intracranial hypertension is treated medically. Nurses play an important role in rapid assessment and implementation of appropriate therapies for reducing ICP.

Nursing priorities for the management of intracranial hypertension include keeping the patient's head

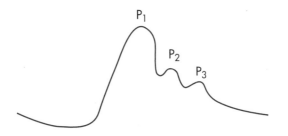

Fig. **17-3** Components of a normal intracranial pressure waveform. (From Barker E: Intracranial pressure and monitoring. In Barker E, editor: *Neuroscience nursing*, St Louis, 1994, Mosby.)

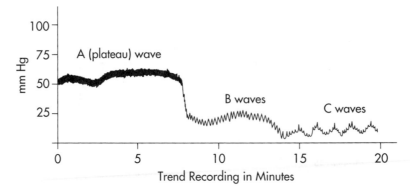

Fig. **17-4** Abnormal intracranial pressure waveforms. (From Barker E: Intracranial pressure and monitoring. In Barker E: *Neuroscience nursing*, St Louis, 1994, Mosby.)

elevated to maintain a cerebral perfusion pressure of at least 70 mm Hg and an intracranial pressure of 20 mm Hg or less, maintaining normothermia and controlled ventilation to ensure a $PaCO_2$ level of 25 to 30 mm Hg and PaO_2 level greater than 70 mm Hg; decreasing environmental stimuli, administering diuretic agents, anticonvulsants, and medications to ensure systolic blood pressure between 140 to 160 mm Hg; and performing ventricular drainage (if ventriculostomy catheter is present).

Patient Positioning

Positioning of the patient is a significant factor in the prevention and treatment of elevated ICP. Elevation of the head of the bed should be maintained to enhance venous drainage from the brain.[11,12] Positions that impede venous return from the brain cause elevations in ICP. Obstruction of jugular veins or an increase in intrathoracic or intraabdominal pressure is communicated as increased pressure throughout the open venous system, thereby impeding drainage from the brain and increasing ICP. Positions that decrease venous return from the head (e.g., Trendelenburg, prone, extreme flexion of the hips, angulation of the neck) should be avoided if possible. If changes to positions such as Trendelenburg are necessary to provide adequate pulmonary care, critical care nurses must closely monitor ICP and vital signs. Mechanisms to reduce intracranial pressure (e.g., sedation, ventricular drainage) also may be employed during the time the patient is in the Trendelenburg position.[13] Other impediments to cerebral venous drainage are positive end-expiratory pressure (PEEP) greater than 5 to 10 cm H_2O pressure, coughing, suctioning, tight tracheostomy tube ties, and the Valsalva maneuver.[3] The goal in positioning the patient is to maintain a cerebral perfusion pressure of at least 70 mm Hg and an intracranial pressure of 20 mm Hg or less. Carefully monitoring of intracranial pressure, cerebral perfusion pressure, systolic blood pressure is warranted with any change in the patient's position.[14]

Hyperventilation

Controlled hyperventilation has been an important adjunct of therapy for the patient with increased ICP. If the $PaCO_2$ can be reduced from its normal level of 35 to 40 mm Hg to a range of 25 to 30 mm Hg in the patient with intracranial hypertension, vasoconstriction of cerebral arteries, reduction of cerebral blood flow, and increased venous return will result. Reducing the intracranial blood volume results in a general reduction in ICP.[4] The use of controlled hyperventilation is currently under investigation. Research indicates that in certain situations of increased ICP, vasoconstriction of the cerebral vessels already has occurred. In these cases further application of controlled hyperventilation could cause vasoconstriction to such an extent that cerebral ischemia occurs.[15] Documentation shows that high levels of $PaCO_2$ cause cerebral

vasodilation and contribute to elevated ICP. For this reason $PaCO_2$ levels greater than 40 mm Hg are considered dangerous.[2]

Although hypoxemia should obviously be avoided, excessively high levels of oxygen offer no benefits.[3] In fact, increasing inspired oxygen concentrations (FIO_2) above 60% may lead to toxic changes in lung tissue. The increasing use of devices that monitor oxygen saturation (e.g., pulse oximetery) has led to greater awareness of circumstances such as suctioning and restlessness that can cause oxygen desaturation and therefore elevate ICP.

Environmental Control

Any treatment modality that increases the incidence of noxious stimulation to the patient carries with it the potential for increasing ICP. Such noxious stimuli include pain as a result of injuries sustained with the initial trauma, the presence of an endotracheal tube, coughing, suctioning, repositioning, bathing, and many routine nursing care procedures. In patients with poor intracranial compliance, stimuli can increase ICP. Only essential interventions should be done, and they should be spread out over time so as to limit any cumulative effects. Gentle touch can be used to help patients relax. Gentle stroking of the face, hands, and back or foot massage may be beneficial as shown by ICP and vital signs.[11,16]

To ensure adequate ventilation ($PaCO_2$ level of 25 to 30 and PaO_2 level greater than 70) and in anticipation of the deleterious effects of noxious stimuli on ICP, nurses may use sedatives alone or in combination with neuromuscular blocking agents. Use of these medications is recommended only in patients who have an ICP monitor in place, because sedation and neuromuscular blocking agents affect the reliability of neurologic assessment. Although sedation of the unconscious patient can obscure portions of the neurologic examination, its benefit may outweigh the risks.[16,17]

Temperature Control

Directly proportional to body temperature, cerebral metabolic rate increases 5% to 7% per degree centigrade of increase in body temperature.[5] This fact is significant because as the cerebral metabolic rate increases, blood flow to the brain must increase to meet the tissue demands. To avoid the increase in blood volume associated with an increased cerebral metabolic rate, nurses must prevent hyperthermia in the patient with a brain injury. Antipyretics and cooling devices should be used when appropriate while the source of the fever is being determined.[11,17]

Conversely, hypothermia reduces cerebral metabolic rate. Research done in severely head-injured patients who were unresponsive to barbiturate therapy for control of intractable intracranial hypertension demonstrated a significant decrease in ICP when subjected to mild hypothermia between 33.5° C and 34.5° C.[18]

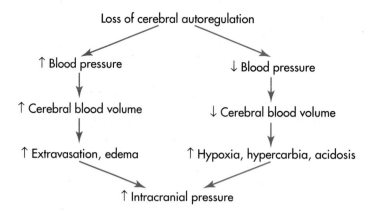

Fig. **17-5** Loss of pressure autoregulation.

Blood Pressure Control

Sustained systolic arterial hypertension (>160 mm Hg) in conjunction with elevated ICP should be vigorously treated. Control of systemic arterial hypertension may require nothing more than the administration of a sedative agent. Small, frequent doses may be sufficient to blunt noxious stimuli and prevent them from triggering rises in blood pressure. When sedation proves inadequate in controlling systemic arterial hypertension, primary antihypertensive agents are used. Care must be taken in choosing these agents because many of the peripheral vasodilators are also cerebral vasodilators (e.g., nitroprusside and nitroglycerin). However, all antihypertensives are believed to cause some degree of cerebral vasodilation. To reduce this vasodilating effect, cotreatment with beta blockers (e.g., propranolol and labetalol) may be beneficial.[17] Fig. 17-5 shows the relationship to blood pressure and ICP.

Seizure Control

The incidence of posttraumatic seizures in the head-injured population has been estimated at 5%. Because of the risk of a secondary ischemic insult associated with seizures, many physicians prescribe anticonvulsant medications prophylactically. Seizures cause metabolic requirements to increase, which results in elevation of cerebral blood flow, cerebral blood volume, and ICP even in paralyzed patients. If blood flow cannot match demand, ischemia will develop, cerebral energy stores will be depleted, and irreversible neuronal destruction will occur. The usual anticonvulsant regimen for seizure control includes phenytoin or phenobarbital, or both, in therapeutic doses.[16,17]

Lidocaine

Various forms of sensory stimulation (including tracheal intubation, laryngoscopy, and endotracheal suctioning) may provoke marked increases in ICP and MAP. One therapy used to prevent cerebral ischemia and acute in-

tracranial hypertension has been the administration of lidocaine through an endotracheal tube or through intravenous infusion before nasotracheal suctioning.[4] Lidocaine is believed to be effective in blunting ICP spikes secondary to tracheal stimulation. Studies have found that peak lidocaine concentrations are linearly related to the administered dose and that the rate of absorption depends on the vascularity of the site of administration.[4] It also has been documented that lidocaine is initially distributed to the lungs, then to the heart and kidneys, and then to muscle and adipose tissue.[19]

Cerebrospinal Fluid Drainage

Cerebrospinal fluid drainage for intracranial hypertension may be used with other treatment modalities. CSF drainage is accomplished by the insertion of a pliable catheter into the anterior horn of the lateral ventricle (ventriculostomy), preferably on the nondominant side. Such drainage can help support the patient through periods of cerebral edema by controlling spikes in ICP. One of the major advantages of the ventriculostomy is its dual role as both a monitoring device and a treatment modality. Because CSF provides a favorable medium for the development of infection, flawless aseptic technique must be followed during insertion and maintenance of the system. The ventricular system is connected to a drainage bag and is then maintained as a closed system for the period of time the ventriculostomy remains in place—usually 3 to 5 days[8] (Figs. 17-6 and 17-7).

Diuretics

Osmotic agents

Clinicians have known for decades that osmotic agents effectively reduce ICP. The mechanism by which these diuretics reduce ICP continues as a subject of investigational interest. One theory is that these agents act by remaining relatively impermeable to the blood-brain barrier, thereby drawing water from normal brain tissue to plasma. The direction of flow is from the hypoconcen-

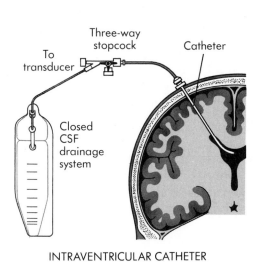

INTRAVENTRICULAR CATHETER

Fig. **17-6** Intermittent drainage system. Intermittent drainage involves draining CSF via a ventriculostomy when ICP exceeds the upper pressure parameter set by the physician. Intermittent drainage involves opening the three-way stopcock to allow CSF to flow into the drainage bag for brief periods (30 to 120 seconds) until the pressure is below the upper pressure parameter. (From Barker E: Intracranial pressure and monitoring. In Barker E: *Neuroscience nursing,* St Louis, 1994, Mosby.)

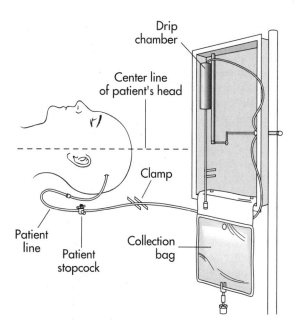

Fig. **17-7** Continuous drainage system. Continuous drainage involves placing the drip chamber of the drainage system at a specified level above the foramen of Monro (usually 15 cm). The system is left open to allow continuous drainage of CSF into the chamber (which drains into a collection bag) against a pressure gradient that prevents excessive drainage and ventricular collapse. (Courtesy Codman/Johnson & Johnson Professional Inc., Raynham, MA.)

trated cerebral tissue to the hyperconcentrated cerebral vasculature. If the situation becomes reversed and the tissue becomes hyperconcentrated in relation to the cerebral vasculature, a rebound phenomenon could occur. These agents have little direct effect on edematous cerebral tissue situated in an area of defective blood-brain barrier; instead, they require an intact blood-brain barrier for osmosis to occur.[20]

The most widely used osmotic diuretic is mannitol, a large molecule that is retained almost entirely in the extracellular compartment and has little to no rebound effect noted with other osmotic diuretics. Mannitol may improve perfusion to ischemic areas of the brain, producing cerebral vasoconstriction and resulting in a reduction of ICP.[20]

Perhaps the most frequent difficulty associated with the use of osmotic agents is the production of electrolyte disturbances. Careful attention should be paid to body weight and fluid and electrolyte stability. Serum osmolality should be kept between 300 and 320 mOsm/L. Hypernatremia and hypokalemia are frequently associated with repeated administration of osmotic agents. Central venous pressure readings should be monitored to prevent hypovolemia.[20]

Nonosmotic agents

Loop diuretics have also been used to decrease ICP. Furosemide, a nonosmotic diuretic, may act differently from osmotic agents by pulling sodium and water from

edematous areas and, perhaps, by decreasing CSF production. One advantage of furosemide administration over the use of osmotic diuretics is that its effect is not generally associated with increases in serum osmolality. Therefore electrolyte imbalances may not be as severe with the use of nonosmotic diuretics.[17]

High-Dose Barbiturate Therapy

Barbiturate therapy is a treatment protocol developed for the management of uncontrolled intracranial hypertension that has not responded to the conventional treatments previously described. Uncontrolled ICP is defined as ICP greater than 20 mm Hg for 30 minutes or ICP greater than 40 mm Hg for 15 minutes or more or CPP lower than 50 mm Hg that does not respond to aggressive use of conventional therapies.[5]

Although the specific action of barbiturates in the reduction of ICP is unclear, several theories explain their effect on the central nervous system (CNS) and the subsequent cerebral protection they provide. Barbiturates increase the cerebral vascular resistance in the undamaged portions of the brain, resulting in a decrease cerebral blood flow and shunting of blood to the damaged portions of the brain. Systemic blood pressure also is lowered, reducing hydrostatic pressure in the damaged cerebral tissue and helping arrest edema formation. Barbiturates also slow cerebral metabolism by reducing the functional electrical generation of the neurons. This decreases cerebral metabolism and thus lessens the glucose and oxygen demands of the brain. Barbiturates are also effective anticonvulsants and may suppress subclinical seizure activities. Finally, some researchers postulate that barbiturates are scavengers of free radicals and thereby prevent cell membrane damage and destruction.[17]

The two most commonly used drugs in high-dose barbiturate therapy are pentobarbital and thiopental. The goal with either of these drugs is a reduction of ICP to 15 to 20 mm Hg while a MAP of 70 to 80 mm Hg is maintained. Patients are maintained on high-dose barbiturate therapy until ICP has been controlled within the normal range for 24 hours. Barbiturates should never be stopped abruptly but should be tapered slowly over approximately 4 days.[5]

Complications of high-dose barbiturate therapy can be disastrous without a specific and organized approach. The most frequent complications are hypotension, hypothermia, and myocardial depression. If any complications occur and are allowed to persist unchecked, they may cause secondary insults to an already damaged brain. Hypotension, the most common complication, results from peripheral vasodilation and can be compounded in an already dehydrated patient who has received large doses of an osmotic diuretic in an attempt to control ICP. Careful monitoring of fluid status by central venous pressure or a pulmonary artery catheter can help to prevent this complication. Myocardial depression results from cardiac muscle suppression and can be avoided by frequent monitoring of fluid status, cardiac output, and serum drug levels. If an adequate cardiac output cannot be maintained in the presence of normothermia, barbiturates must be reduced, regardless of serum levels.[17]

HERNIATION SYNDROMES

The goal of neurologic evaluation, ICP monitoring, and treatment of increased ICP is to prevent herniation. Herniation of intracerebral contents results in the shifting of tissue from one compartment of the brain to another and places pressure on cerebral vessels and vital function centers of the brain. If unchecked, herniation rapidly causes death as a result of the cessation of cerebral blood flow and respirations.

Supratentorial Herniation

There are four types of supratentorial herniation syndrome: central or transtentorial, uncal, cingulate, or transcalvarial (Fig. 17-8).

Uncal herniation

Uncal herniation is most frequently noted herniation syndrome. In uncal herniation, a unilateral, expanding mass lesion, usually of the temporal lobe, increases ICP, causing lateral displacement of the tip of the temporal lobe (uncus). Lateral displacement pushes the uncus over

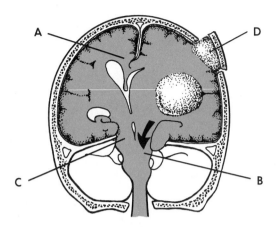

Fig. **17-8** Supratentorial herniation. *A*, Cingulate. *B*, Uncal. *C*, Central. *D*, Transcalvarial.

the edge of the tentorium, puts pressure on the oculomotor nerve (cranial nerve III) and posterior cerebral artery ipsilateral to the lesion, and flattens the midbrain against the opposite side.[3,21]

Clinical manifestations of uncal herniation include ipsilateral pupil dilation, decreased level of consciousness, respiratory pattern changes leading to respiratory arrest, and contralateral hemiplegia leading to decorticate or decerebrate posturing. If no intervention occurs, uncal herniation results in fixed and dilated pupils, flaccidity, and respiratory arrest.[3,21]

Central or transtentorial herniation

In central herniation, an expanding mass lesion of the midline, frontal, parietal, or occipital lobes results in downward displacement of the hemispheres, basal ganglia, and diencephalon through the tentorial notch. Central herniation often is preceded by uncal and cingulate herniation.[3,21]

Clinical manifestations of central or transtentorial herniation include loss of consciousness; small, reactive pupils progressing to fixed, dilated pupils; respiratory changes leading to respiratory arrest; and decorticate posturing progressing to flaccidity. In the late stages, uncal and central herniation syndromes affect the brainstem similarly.[3,21]

Cingulate herniation

Cingulate herniation occurs when an expanding lesion of one hemisphere shifts laterally and forces the cingulate gyrus under the falx cerebri. Cingulate herniation occurs frequently. Whenever a lateral shift is noted on a CT scan, cingulate herniation has occurred. Little is known about the effects of cingulate herniation, and there are no clinical manifestations that assist in its diagnosis. Cingulate herniation is not in itself life-threatening, but if the expanding mass lesion that caused cingulate herniation is not controlled, uncal or central herniation follows.[3,20]

Transcalvarial herniation

Transcalvarial herniation is the extrusion of cerebral tissue through the cranium. In the presence of severe cerebral edema, transcalvarial herniation occurs through an opening from a skull fracture or craniotomy site.[3]

Infratentorial herniation

There are two infratentorial herniation syndromes: upward transtentorial herniation and downward cerebellar herniation.

Upward transtentorial herniation. Upward transtentorial herniation occurs when an expanding mass lesion of the cerebellum causes protrusion of the vermis (central area) of the cerebellum and the midbrain upward through the tentorial notch. Compression of the third cranial nerve and diencephalon occur. Blockage of the central aqueduct and distortion of the third ventricle obstruct CSF flow. Deterioration progresses rapidly.[3,21]

Downward cerebellar herniation. Downward cerebellar herniation occurs when an expanding lesion of the cerebellum exerts pressure downward, sending the cerebellar tonsils through the foramen magnum. Compression and displacement of the medulla oblongata occur, rapidly resulting in respiratory and cardiac arrest.[3,21]

References

1. Richmond TS: Intracranial pressure monitoring, *AACN Clin Iss Crit Care Nurs* 4:148, 1993.
2. Boss BJ: Concepts of neurologic dysfunction. In McCance K, Huether S, editors: *Pathophysiology: the biologic basis for disease in adults and children,* ed 2, St Louis, 1994, Mosby.
3. Barker E: Intracranial pressure and monitoring. In Barker E, editor: *Neuroscience nursing,* St Louis, 1994, Mosby.
4. Chestnut RM, Marshall LF: Management of head injury: treatment of abnormal intracranial pressure, *Neurosurg Clin North Am* 2:267, 1991.
5. Hickey JV: *The clinical practice of neurological and neurosurgical nursing,* ed 3, Philadelphia, 1991, JB Lippincott.
6. Vos HR: Making headway with intracranial hypertension, *Am J Nurs* 93 (2):28, 1993.
7. Wall BM, Philips JP, Howard JC: Validation of increased intracranial pressure and high risk for increased intracranial pressure, *Nurs Diag* 5:74, 1994.
8. McQuillan KA: Intracranial pressure monitoring: technical imperatives, *AACN Clin Iss Crit Care* 2:623, 1991.
9. Cummings R: Understanding external ventricular drainage, *J Neurosci Nurs* 24:84, 1992.
10. Wrobel CJ, Marshall LF: Closed head injury management dilemmas. In Long DM, editor: *Current therapy in neurological surgery,* ed 3, St Louis, 1992, Mosby.
11. Andrus C: Intracranial pressure: dynamics and nursing management, *J Neurosci Nurs* 23:85, 1991.
12. Feldman Z, et al: Effect of head elevation on intracranial pressure, cerebral perfusion, and cerebral blood flow in head-injured patients, *J Neurosurg* 76:207, 1992.
13. Fontaine DK, McQuillan K: Positioning as a nursing therapy in trauma care, *Crit Care Nurs Clin North Am* 1:105, 1990.
14. March K, et al: Effect of backrest position on intracranial and cerebral perfusion pressures, *J Neurosci Nurs* 22:375, 1990.
15. Yundt KD, Diringer MN: The use of hyperventilation and its impact on cerebral ischemia in the treatment of traumatic brain injury, *Crit Care Clin* 13:163, 1997.
16. Arbour R: Aggressive management of intracranial dynamics, *Crit Care Nurs* 18(3):30, 1998.
17. Frank JI: Management of intracranial hypertension, *Med Clin North Am* 77:61, 1993.
18. Nikas DL: Commentary on the effect of mild hypothermia on uncontrolled hypertension after severe head injury and the use of moderate therapeutic hypothermia for patients with severe head injuries: a preliminary report, *AACN Nurs Scan Crit Care* 4(1):14, 1994.
19. Brucia JJ, Owen DC, Rudy EB: The effects of lidocaine on intracranial hypertension, *J Neurosci Nurs* 24:205, 1992.
20. Paczynski RP: Osmotherapy: basic concepts and controversies, *Crit Care Clin* 13:105, 1997.
21. Morrison CAM: Brain herniation syndromes, *Crit Care Nurs* 7(5):34, 1987.

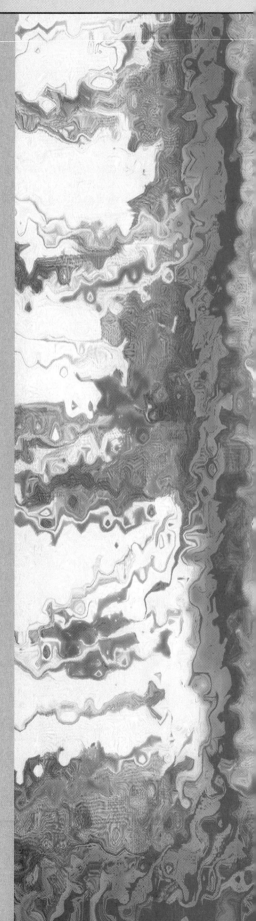

UNIT SIX

RENAL ALTERATIONS

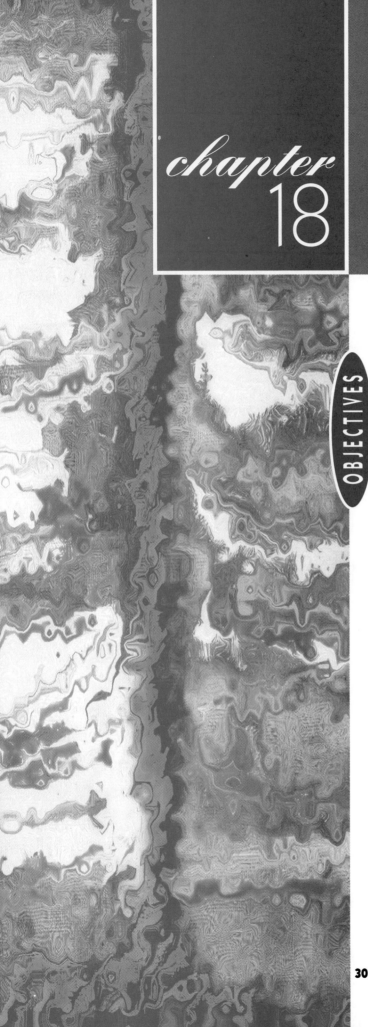

chapter 18

Renal Assessment and Diagnostic Procedures

Mary Schira

OBJECTIVES

● Describe the priorities of the renal nursing assessment.

● Identify ways in which alterations of hemoglobin and hematocrit levels can signal fluid volume deficit or excess.

● Explain the reason elevations of blood urea nitrogen and creatinine signal renal dysfunction.

HISTORY

A renal history begins with a description of the chief symptom, stated in the patient's own words. A description of the chief complaint includes the onset, location, duration, and factors that lessen or aggravate the problem.[1] Descriptions of any treatment sought by the individual, medications taken to alleviate symptoms (both prescription and nonprescription), or procedures performed to improve the problem often are helpful in determining the extent and potentially the nature of the current complaint.

Predisposing factors for acute renal dysfunction are elicited during the history, including the use of over-the-counter medicines, herbs, and/or vitamins; recent infections requiring antibiotic therapy; and any diagnostic procedures performed using radioopaque contrast media.[2] Nonsteroidal antiinflammatory drugs (such as ibuprofen), antibiotics (especially aminoglycosides), and iodine-based dyes are potentially nephrotoxic, and it is important to assess for them when an individual has renal-related symptoms. In addition, the individual is questioned about any recent strenuous physical exercise. Exercise-induced rhabdomyolysis and resulting acute renal failure symptoms are much more likely in an individual who is unconditioned or poorly conditioned for strenuous physical activity.[3] A history of recent onset of

307

nausea and vomiting or appetite loss caused by taste changes (uremia causes a metallic taste) may also provide clues to the rapid onset of renal problems.[2] Finally, symptoms that indicate rapid fluid volume gains are also sought. For example, rapid weight gains of more than 2 pounds per day or sleeping on additional pillows or sitting in a chair to sleep are signals of volume overload and potential kidney dysfunction.

PHYSICAL EXAMINATION

Inspection

Inspection of patients is focused on three priorities: bleeding, volume, and edema.

Bleeding

Visual inspection related to the kidneys generally focuses on the flank and abdomen. Renal trauma is suspected if a purplish discoloration is present on the flank (Turner's sign) or near the posterior eleventh or twelfth ribs.[4] Bruising, abdominal distention, and abdominal guarding may also signal renal trauma or a hematoma around a kidney.

Volume

Inspection is especially helpful in looking for signs of volume depletion or overload that might signal kidney problems. Fluid volume assessment begins with an inspection of the patient's neck veins. The supine position facilitates normal venous distention. An absence of distention (or flat neck veins) indicates hypovolemia. Assessment continues with the head of the bed elevated 45 to 90 degrees.[1] If the neck veins remain distended more than 2 cm above the sternal notch with the head of the bed at 45 degrees, fluid overload may be present.[5]

Hand vein inspection is also helpful in assessing volume status and is performed by observing for venous distention when the hand is held in the dependent position. Venous filling that takes longer than 5 seconds suggests hypovolemia. When the hand is elevated, the distention should disappear within 5 seconds. If distention does not disappear within 5 seconds after the hand is elevated, fluid overload is suspected.

Assessment of skin turgor provides additional data for identifying fluid-related problems. As the skin over the forearm is picked up and released, the rapidity of its return to its normal position is observed. Normal elasticity and fluid status allow an almost immediate return to shape once the skin is released. In hypovolemia, however, the skin remains raised and does not return to its normal position for several seconds. Because of the loss of skin elasticity in elderly persons, skin turgor assessment in the forearm is not accurate for fluid assessment of this age group. Rather, skin turgor may be more reliable in the shoulder or anterior chest area.

Finally, inspection of the oral cavity provides clues to fluid volume status. When hypovolemia exists, the mucous membranes of the mouth become dry. However, mouth breathing can also dry the mucous membranes temporarily. Therefore a more accurate way to assess the oral cavity is to inspect the mouth with the use of a tongue blade. Dryness of the oral cavity is more indicative of hypovolemia than are complaints of a dry mouth.[5]

Edema

Edema is the presence of excess fluid in the interstitial space and can be a sign of volume overload. In the presence of volume excess, edema may be present in dependent areas of the body such as the feet and legs. The presence of edema, however, does not always indicate fluid volume overload. A loss of albumin from the vascular space and peripheral vascular disease can cause edema in the presence of hypovolemia or normal fluid volume states.

Edema can be assessed by applying fingertip pressure on the skin over a bony prominence, such as the ankles, pretibial areas (shins), and sacrum. If the indentation made by the fingertip does not disappear within 30 seconds, "pitting" edema is present. Pitting edema indicates increased interstitial volume and is not evident until a fluid weight gain of approximately 10% has occurred.[6] Edema may also appear in the hands, around the eyes, and in the cheeks. Dependent areas, such as the feet and sacrum, are the most likely to demonstrate edema in patients confined to a wheelchair or bed. One way of measuring the extent of edema is by a subjective scale of 1 to 4, with 1 indicating only minimal pitting with fingertip pressure and 4 indicating severe pitting.

Auscultation

Auscultation of patients is focused on three priorities: heart, blood pressure, and lungs.

Heart

Auscultation of the heart requires not only assessing rate and rhythm but also listening for extra sounds. Fluid overload is often accompanied by a third or fourth heart sound, which may be heard with the bell of the stethoscope. Increased heart rate alone offers little data about fluid volume, but combined with a low blood pressure may indicate hypovolemia.

The heart is also auscultated for the presence of a pericardial friction rub. A rub can best be heard at the third intercostal space to the left of the sternal border, with the individual leaning slightly forward. The presence of a pericardial friction rub indicates pericarditis and may result from uremia or pericardial infection in a patient with renal failure.

Blood pressure

Blood pressure and heart rate changes are very useful in assessing fluid volume deficit. In stable critically ill patients or in patients on a telemetry unit, orthostatic vital sign measurements provide clues to blood loss, dehydration, unexplained syncope, and the effects of some antihypertensive medications.[7] A drop in blood pressure of more than 20 mm Hg or a rise in pulse rate of more than 20 beats per minute from the lying to sitting or from sitting to standing positions represents orthostatic hypotension. The drop in blood pressure occurs because the venous circulation is so volume depleted that a sufficient preload is not immediately available after the position change. The heart rate increases in an attempt to maintain cardiac output and circulation. Orthostatic hypotension often produces subjective feelings of weakness, dizziness, or faintness. Although orthostatic hypertension is often a sign of hypovolemia, peripheral vascular disease may also be responsible. Peripheral vascular disease often damages the venous circulation of the lower extremities and decreases blood return to the heart, leading to a blood pressure drop in a normovolemic individual.

Lungs

Lung assessment is also extremely important in gauging fluid status. Crackles indicate fluid overload. Dyspnea with mild exertion or dyspnea at night that prevents sleeping in a supine position or that awakens the person may indicate pooling of fluid in the lungs. Shallow, gasping breaths with periods of apnea reflect severe acid-base imbalances.

Palpation

Palpation of patients is focused on one priority: determining the size and shape of the kidneys. Palpation of the kidneys is accomplished by using the bimanual capturing approach. Capturing is done by placing one hand posteriorly under the flank of the supine patient with fingers pointing to the midline, while placing the opposite hand just below the ribcage anteriorly. The patient is asked to inhale deeply while pressure is exerted to bring the hands together. As the patient exhales, the examiner should feel the kidney between the hands. After each kidney is palpated in this manner, the two should be compared for size and shape. Each kidney should be firm and smooth and be of equal size.[8] The examiner is usually unable to palpate a normal left kidney. The right kidney is more easily palpated because of its lower position, as it is displaced downward by the liver. However, it is not uncommon to be unable to palpate normal kidneys in obese patients.

Percussion

Percussion of patients is focused on two priorities: kidneys and the abdomen.

Kidneys

Percussion of a kidney is performed with the patient in a side-lying or sitting position, with the examiner's hand placed over the costovertebral angle (lower border of the ribcage on the flank). Striking the back of the hand with the opposite fist produces a painless, dull thud, which is normal. Pain may indicate infection or injury resulting from trauma.

Abdomen

Observation and percussion of the abdomen are of value in assessing fluid status. Percussing the abdomen (using the same procedure as for the kidneys but placing the patient supine) can result in a dull sound (solid bowel contents or fluid) or a hollow sound (gaseous bowel).[1,10]

Ascites, severe fluid distention of the abdominal cavity, is an important observation in determining fluid imbalances. Differentiating ascites from distortion caused by solid bowel contents is accomplished by producing a fluid wave. A fluid wave is elicited by exerting pressure to the abdominal midline while one hand is placed on the right or left flank. Tapping the opposite flank produces a wave in the accumulated fluid that can be felt under the hands. Other signs of ascites include a protuberant, rounded abdomen and abdominal striae.[10]

Individuals with renal failure may have ascites caused by volume overload, which forces fluid into the abdomen because of increased capillary hydrostatic pressures. However, ascites may or may not represent fluid volume excess. Severe ascites in persons with compromised hepatic function may result from hypovolemia. The ascites occurs because the increased vascular pressure associated with hepatic dysfunction forces fluid and plasma proteins from the vascular space into the interstitial space and abdominal cavity.

FLUID BALANCE ASSESSMENT

Fluid balance assessment in patients is focused on three priorities: weight, intake and output, and hemodynamic monitoring.

Weight

One of the most important assessments of renal and fluid status is the patient's weight. In the critical care unit, weight is monitored on every patient and is an important vital sign measurement. Significant fluctuations in body weight over a 1- to 2-day period indicate fluid gains and losses. Rapid weight gains or losses of greater than 2 pounds per day generally indicate fluid rather than nutritional factors. One liter of fluid equals 1 kg or approximately 2.2 pounds.

Intake and output

Like patient weight, intake and output are monitored on all patients in the critical care unit. Intake and output can be compared with the patient's weight to evaluate accurately the gain or loss of fluid. Urinary output plus insensible fluid losses (perspiration, stool, and water vapor from the lungs) can range widely from 750 to 2400 ml/day. When intake exceeds output (excessive intravenous fluid, decreased renal output), a positive fluid balance exists. In impaired renal function, the positive fluid balance results in fluid volume overload. Conversely, if

TABLE 18-1

HEMODYNAMIC ASSESSMENT OF FLUID STATUS

MEASUREMENT	VOLUME DEPLETION	VOLUME OVERLOAD
CVP	<2 mm Hg	>6 mm Hg
PAWP	<8 mm Hg	>12 mm Hg
CI	<2.2 L/min/m²	>4.4 L/min/m²
MAP	Decreased	Increased

BOX 18-1

IMPORTANT ASPECTS OF FLUID AND ELECTROLYTE ASSESSMENT

FLUID STATUS
Skin turgor
Mucous membranes
Intake and output
Presence of edema/ascites
Diaphoresis
Fever
Neck and hand vein engorgement
Lung sounds—crackles
Dyspnea, orthopnea
CVP <2 mm Hg, >6 mm Hg
PAWP <8 mm Hg, >12 mm Hg
Tachycardia
Hypertension, hypotension
Orthostasis
CI <2.2 L/min/m², >4.4
S_3, S_4 heart sounds
Headache
Blurred vision
Papilledema
Mental changes

ELECTROLYTE STATUS
Serum osmolality
Complete blood count (CBC)
Serum electrolyte level
Electrocardiogram tracings (potassium, calcium, magnesium changes)
Behavioral and/or mental changes
Chvostek's, Trousseau's signs (calcium levels)
Changes in peripheral sensation (numbness, tremor)
Muscle strength
Gastrointestinal changes (nausea and vomiting)
Therapies that alter electrolyte status (gastrointestinal suction, diuretics, antihypertensives, calcium channel blockers)

output exceeds intake (fever, increased respiration, profuse sweating, vomiting, diarrhea, gastric suction, diuretic therapy), a negative fluid balance exists and volume deficit results. During a 24-hour period, fever can increase skin and respiratory losses by as much as 75 ml/degree of Fahrenheit temperature rise.

In many cases, individuals with acute renal failure (ARF) will exhibit a decrease in urine output, or oliguria (less than 400 ml/day). However, in most patients with ARF, as in those with early intrarenal ARF, there may be a fairly normal or only slightly decreased urine output that reflects water removal without solute removal. Therefore renal function cannot be accurately determined by urine output alone.[11]

Hemodynamic monitoring

Body fluid status is accurately reflected in the measurement of cardiovascular hemodynamics. Measurements such as central venous pressure (CVP), pulmonary artery wedge pressure (PAWP), cardiac index (CI), and mean arterial pressure (MAP) provide a clear picture of the increases or decreases in vascular volume returning to and being ejected from the heart. Indeed, both volume depletion and overload are easily detected by use of central venous or arterial catheters from which pressure measurements can be obtained (Table 18-1).

Other observations

Renal system dysfunction often leads to electrolyte as well as fluid imbalances. Some of the disturbances in fluid and electrolyte levels are accompanied by clinical manifestations less measurable than those previously mentioned but that, nonetheless, indicate a change from normal function. Box 18-1 summarizes the important aspects to consider during fluid and electrolyte assessment.

Sudden or slowly developing changes in mental status must be investigated. For example, acidosis often results in disorientation. Lethargy, coma, and confusion may result from sodium, calcium, or magnesium excess or deficit. Apprehension or anxiety may be secondary to sodium deficit, a shift of fluid from the plasma to the interstitium, or respiratory changes caused by fluid volume overload.[10]

Finally, apathy and withdrawal often accompany hypovolemic states.[10] Patients with renal failure with systemic increases in electrolytes, fluids, and nitrogenous waste products can also exhibit apathy, restlessness, confusion, and withdrawal.[2] The speed of onset will vary according to how rapidly (or slowly) the renal failure progresses and alters homeostasis.

LABORATORY ASSESSMENT

Serum

Blood urea nitrogen

Blood urea nitrogen (BUN) is a by-product of protein metabolism. The normal value for BUN is 9 to 20 mg/dL and is increased when renal function deteriorates.[13] With renal dysfunction, the BUN is elevated because of a decrease in the glomerular filtration rate (GFR) and, therefore, a fall in urea excretion. Numerous other factors may also affect the BUN and creatinine in the critically ill patient (malnutrition, volume status, bleeding). Therefore the BUN must be evaluated along with creatinine.

Creatinine

Creatinine is also a by-product of protein and normal cell metabolism and appears in serum in amounts proportional to the body muscle mass. Although slightly higher in males than females, the normal serum creatinine level is about 0.7 to 1.5 mg/dL.[13] Creatinine is easily excreted by the renal tubules and is not reabsorbed or secreted in the tubules. Measuring the amount of creatinine in the excreted urine and the amount of creatinine in the blood over 24 hours provides accurate information about kidney function (creatinine clearance).[2,9] Creatinine levels are fairly constant and are affected by fewer factors than BUN. As a result, the serum creatinine level is a better indicator of renal function than BUN. In addition, the ratio of BUN to creatinine (normally 10-20:1) is a useful indicator in identifying a specific type of renal dysfunction.

Osmolality

The serum osmolality reflects the concentration or dilution of vascular fluid. The normal serum osmolality is 275 to 295 mOsm/L.[13] When the serum osmolality level increases (e.g., with insufficient fluid intake or excessive losses), antidiuretic hormone (ADH) is released from the pituitary gland and stimulates increased water reabsorption. This expands the vascular space, brings the serum osmolality back to normal, and results in a more concentrated urine (and thus an elevated urine osmolality). The opposite occurs with a decreased serum osmolality level, which inhibits the production of ADH. The decreased ADH results in increased excretion of water through the kidneys, producing dilute urine with a low osmolality, and brings the serum osmolality back to normal. Measurement of serum osmolality is a useful parameter in determining fluid balance and fluid replacement therapy in critically ill patients.

Anion gap

The anion gap is a calculation of the difference between the measurable cations (sodium and potassium) and the measurable anions (chloride and bicarbonate).[5] The value represents the remaining unmeasurable anions present in the ECF (phosphates, sulfates, ketones, lactate). The formula generally used in the calculation of the anion gap is as follows:

$$Na^+ - (Cl^- + HCO_3^-)$$

A normal anion gap is 1 to 12 mEq/L and should not exceed 14 mEq/L. An increased anion gap level reflects overproduction or decreased excretion of acid products and correlates with serum pH measurement.

Hemoglobin and hematocrit

The hemoglobin (Hgb) and hematocrit (Hct) levels can indicate increases or decreases in intravascular fluid volume. Both Hgb and Hct vary between genders, with the Hgb in males normally 13.5 to 17.5 g/dL and in females 12 to 16 g/dL. The Hct ranges from 40% to 54% in males and 37% to 47% in females. Hgb transports oxygen and carbon dioxide and is important in maintaining cellular metabolism and acid-base balance.[13]

The Hct is the percentage of red blood cells (RBCs) in a volume of whole blood. An increase in the Hct often indicates a fluid volume deficit, which results in hemoconcentration. Conversely, a decreased Hct can indicate fluid volume excess because of the dilutional effect of the extra fluid load. Decreases, however, can also result from anemias, blood loss, liver damage, or hemolytic reactions.[13]

In individuals with acute renal failure, anemia may occur early in the disease, so that a decreased Hct may either indicate the anemia of renal failure or reflect fluid volume overload. If the Hct is dropping but the Hgb remains constant, then the cause is fluid volume overload. If both the Hct and the Hgb are decreased, this indicates a true loss of RBCs.

Albumin

Slightly more than 50% of the total plasma protein is serum albumin. It is manufactured in the liver, with a normal blood level of 3.5 to 5.5 g/dL.[13] Albumin is primarily responsible for the maintenance of colloid osmotic pressure, which functions to hold fluid in the vascular space. The blood vessel walls, because of their impermeability to plasma proteins, prevent albumin from leaving the vascular space. However, in some disease states such as third-degree burns (cell membrane destruction) or ARF resulting from the nephrotic syndrome (increased glomerular capillary permeability to protein), albumin escapes from the vascular space and enters the interstitial space. The result is peripheral edema.

A decreased albumin level can occur as a result of protein-calorie malnutrition, which occurs in many critically ill patients in whom available stores of albumin are depleted. A decrease in the plasma oncotic pressure results, and fluid shifts from the vascular space to the interstitial space. Liver disease or severe injury to the liver also causes a fall in albumin levels as the diseased liver fails to synthesize sufficient albumin. Furthermore, severe portal hypertension can force albumin and other plasma proteins into the abdominal cavity, resulting in ascites.

Increased albumin levels are rare. The body uses a fixed amount of protein for energy and body cell replacement and converts excess protein into stored fat. If all plasma protein levels are elevated, fluid volume deficit (hemoconcentration) is suspected.

Urine Analysis

Analysis of the urine provides excellent information about the patient's renal function and condition relative to fluids and electrolytes. Specific tests and abnormal indications are presented in Table 18-2.[4,8,9,11,15]

pH

Urine pH indicates the acidity or alkalinity of the urine. The normal urinary pH level is 6.0, which is acidic, but may range from 4.5 to 8.0. The kidney regulates acid-base balance; therefore, more hydrogen ions are excreted than bicarbonate ions, creating the acidity of the urine. Changes in renal function produce changes in urinary pH.

An increase in urinary acidity (decreased pH) indicates retention of sodium and acids by the body, which would be present in intrarenal ARF. Conversely, a decrease in urinary acidity (increased pH or more alkaline) means the body is retaining bicarbonate.

TABLE 18-2

URINALYSIS RESULTS

TEST	NORMAL	INCREASED	DECREASED
pH	4.5-8.0	Alkalosis	Acidosis
			Intrarenal ARF
Specific gravity	1.003-1.030	Volume deficit	Volume overload
		Glycosuria	
		Proteinuria	
		Prerenal ARF (>1.020)	
Osmolality	300-1200 mOsm/kg	Volume deficit	Volume excess
		Prerenal ARF (urine osmolality > serum osmolality)	Intrarenal ARF (urine osmolality < serum osmolality)
Protein	30-150 mg/24 hr	Trauma	
		Infection	
		Intrarenal ARF	
		Transient with exercise	
		Glomerulonephritis	
Sodium	27-287 mEq/24 hr	High sodium diet	Prerenal ARF
		Intrarenal ARF	
Creatinine	1-2 g/24 hr		Intrarenal ARF
			Chronic renal failure
Urea	6-17 g/24 hr		Intrarenal ARF
			Chronic renal failure
Myoglobin	Absent	Crush injury	
		Rhabdomyolysis	
RBCs	0-5	Trauma	
		Intrarenal ARF	
		Infection	
		Strenuous exercise	
		Renal artery thrombus	
WBCs	0-5	Infection	
Bacteria	None-few	Infection	
Casts	None-few	RBC: Glomerular disease	
		WBC: Pyelonephritis	
		Glomerular disease	
		Nephrotic syndrome	
		Epithelial: Glomerular disease	

Specific gravity

Specific gravity measures the density or weight of urine compared with that of distilled water. The normal urinary specific gravity is 1.003 to 1.030 as compared to the normal specific gravity of distilled water at 1.000.

The specific gravity indicates the ability of the kidneys to dilute or concentrate the urine. Decreases in specific gravity reflect the inability of the kidneys to excrete the usual solute load into the urine (less dense with fewer solutes). Increases in specific gravity (a more concentrated urine) occur with fluid volume deficit as the result of fever, vomiting, or diarrhea. An increased specific gravity can also occur with diabetes or glomerular membrane disease, both of which allow glucose and protein to pass into the urine, thereby increasing urine density.

Osmolality

The urinary osmolality more accurately pinpoints fluid balance than does the serum osmolality value. The serum osmolality largely reflects serum sodium concentration and therefore is subject to more influences than

the urinary osmolality. The simultaneous measurement of both the serum and urinary osmolality levels provides an accurate assessment of fluid status. Normal urinary osmolality is 300 to 1200 mOsm/kg and depends on reabsorption or excretion of water in the kidney tubules. The urinary osmolality level increases (and urine output decreases) during fluid volume deficit because of the retention of fluid by the body. Conversely, the urinary osmolality level decreases (and urine output increases) during volume excess because fluid is excreted by the kidneys.

Protein

Protein is normally absent from urine because the large protein molecule cannot pass across the normal glomerular capillary membrane. Consistent appearance of protein in urine suggests compromise of the glomerular membrane and possible intrarenal acute renal failure or the chronic effects of diabetes mellitus. The amount of protein in the urine is often directly correlated to the severity of the damage and may exceed 4.0 g/day.

TABLE 18-3

RENAL DIAGNOSTIC STUDIES

STUDY	PURPOSES	COMMENTS
Kidneys, ureters, and bladder (KUB)	• Outlines kidneys, ureters, bladder • Evaluates size, shape, and position of kidneys • Identifies location of calculi	• Also called flat plate of abdomen • Bowel preparation such as cathartics: may be prescribed if to be followed by IVP

Intravenous pyelogram (IVP)	• Evaluates position, size, shape, and location of kidneys
	• Provides visualization of internal kidney (parenchyma, calices, pelvis)
	• Evaluates filling of renal pelvis
	• Outlines ureters and bladder
	• Identifies presence of cysts and tumors
	• Identifies obstructions, congenital abnormality
		• Also called excretory urogram
		• Contraindicated in renal insufficiency, multiple myeloma, pregnancy, congestive heart failure, sickle cell disease
		• Bowel preparation such as cathartics as prescribed
		• NPO for 8 hours before the test
		• Contrast media used
		  • Check for allergy to iodine before the study
		  • Monitor for allergic reaction postprocedure
		  • Ensure hydration postprocedure

Retrograde pyelogram	• Evaluates position, size, shape, and location of kidneys
	• Outlines ureters and bladder
	• Identifies presence of cysts and tumors
	• Identifies obstructions
		• Does not require the kidney to excrete the dye so may be used in patients with renal insufficiency
		• Bowel preparation such as cathartics as prescribed
		• NPO for 8 hours before the test
		• Contrast media used
		  • Check for allergy to iodine before the study
		  • Monitor for allergic reaction postprocedure
		  • Ensure hydration postprocedure
		• Urinary tract infection or sepsis possible
		  • Monitor patient for clinical indications

Nephrotomogram	• Evaluates segments of the kidney at different levels
	• Differentiates cysts from solid masses
		• Bowel preparation such as cathartics as prescribed
		• NPO for 8 hours before the test
		• Contrast media used
		  • Check for allergy to iodine prior to the study
		  • Monitor for allergic reaction postprocedure
		  • Ensure hydration postprocedure

Modified with permission from Dennison R: *Pass CCRN!*, St Louis, 1996, Mosby.

Continued

Electrolytes

Levels of electrolytes in the urine are not as frequently measured as are levels in serum but can also yield information about kidney function. To measure urinary electrolyte levels, a 24-hour urine sample is often required. Urine electrolyte levels are highly variable, and the electrolytes depend on the kidneys for adequate excretion. Consequently, changes in urinary electrolyte levels are highly suggestive of renal impairment. Urinary sodium is especially useful in clarifying the causes of acute renal failure (ARF). Lower than normal levels (<20 mEq/L) generally indicate prerenal ARF, while normal and increased levels (>20 mEq/L) indicate intrarenal ARF.

Sediment

The presence of sediment, such as epithelial cells and casts, aids in identifying problems related to the kidneys. In addition, the presence or absence of urine sediment can be helpful in identifying the etiology of ARF.[9,15] In prerenal ARF, the kidneys are not damaged and urinary sediment is normal. However, in intrarenal ARF, the kidney tubules are damaged and urine sediment is abnormal, with the presence of casts and epithelial cells. Casts are shells or clumps of cellular breakdown or protein materials that form in the renal tubular system and are washed out in the urinary flow.

Hematuria

Both obvious and microscopic hematuria may signal renal damage. Although a few RBCs in the urine are normal, apparently bloody urine indicates bleeding within the urinary tract or renal trauma.[4,9] Microscopic hematuria may occur normally after strenuous exercise or the insertion of a retention catheter but should disappear within 48 hours.

DIAGNOSTIC PROCEDURES

Table 18-3 presents an overview of the various diagnostic procedures[16] used to evaluate the patient with renal dysfunction.

TABLE **18-3**

RENAL DIAGNOSTIC STUDIES—cont'd

STUDY	PURPOSES	COMMENTS
Ultrasonography	• Evaluates fluid vs solid mass • Identifies obstructions • Identifies cysts, abscesses, tumors, polycystic kidney disease • Identifies hemorrhage • Identifies urinary tract obstruction and leaks	• No special preparation • Can be safely done in patients with renal failure • Contrast media sometimes used
Renal radionu-clide scan (reno-gram)	• Evaluates position, size, shape, and location of kidneys • Identifies abscesses, cysts, tumors • Evaluates renal perfusion • Evaluates glomerular filtration, tubular function, and excretion • Assesses status of renal transplant	• Amount of radioactive material minimal • Not scheduled within 24 hours after IVP • Patient required to void before scan • Fluids encouraged postprocedure

Computed to-mography (CT) scan	• Provides a view of kidneys, retroperitoneal space, bladder, prostate
	• Evaluates kidney size
	• Evaluates the kidney for tumors, abscesses, and obstructions
		• No special preparation
		• Can be safely used in patients with renal failure
		• Contrast medium sometimes used
		  • Check for allergy to iodine before the study
		  • Monitor for allergic reaction postprocedure
		  • Ensure hydration postprocedure

Magnetic reso-nance imaging (MRI)	• Differentiation between cyst and solid mass • Identifies infarction, trauma, obstructions	• More specific than renal ultrasonography or CT scan because it shows subtle density changes • Cannot be used in patients with any implanted metallic device, including pacemakers • No special preparation required

Renal arteriogra-phy	• Evaluates renal vasculature
	• Identifies renal artery stenosis
	• Identifies cysts, tumors, infarction, trauma
		• Bowel preparation cathartics as prescribed
		• NPO for 8 hours before the test
		• Sedative usually prescribed before the procedure
		• Contrast media used
		  • Check for allergy to iodine before the study
		  • Monitor for allergic reaction postprocedure
		  • Ensure hydration postprocedure
		• Postprocedure
		  • Keep extremity in which catheter was placed immobilized in a straight position for 6 to 12 hours
		  • Monitor arterial puncture point for hemorrhage or hematoma
		  • Monitor neurovascular status of affected limb
		  • Monitor for indications of systemic emboli

Renal biopsy	• Obtains tissue specimen for microscopic evaluation	• May be performed open or closed
		• Clotting profile is evaluated preprocedure
		• Type and crossmatch for 2 units of blood preprocedure
		• Usually not performed if patient has only one functioning kidney (unless being done to evaluate possible transplant rejection)
		• Closed biopsy contraindicated in bleeding abnormalities, polycystic disease, hydronephrosis, neoplasm, urinary tract infection, and uncooperative patient
		• Postprocedure
		  • Maintain pressure dressing and bed rest for 24 hours
		  • Observe for hematuria, flank pain, or hypotension

Nursing Management

The nursing management of a patient undergoing a diagnostic procedure involves a variety of interventions. **Priorities are directed toward the patient psychologically and physically for the procedure, monitoring the patient's responses to the procedure, and assessing the patient after the procedure.** Preparing the patient includes assessing the patient for dye allergies, teaching the patient about the procedure, answering any questions, and transporting and/or positioning the patient. Monitoring the patient's response to the procedure includes observing for signs of pain, anxiety, or hemorrhage and monitoring vital signs. Assessing the patient after the procedure includes observing for complications of the procedure and medicating the patient for any postprocedural discomfort. **Any evidence of bleeding or decompensation in vital signs must be reported to the physician immediately.**

References

1. Bates B: *A guide to physical examination and history taking,* ed 6, Philadelphia, 1995, JB Lippincott.
2. Richard C: Assessment of renal structure and function. In Lancaster L, editor: *Core curriculum for nephrology nursing,* ed 3, Pitman, NJ, 1995, American Nephrology Nurses Association.
3. Fishbane S: Exercise-induced renal and electrolyte changes, *Phys Sportsmed* 23(8):39, 1996.
4. Talbot L, Meyers-Marquardt M: *Critical care assessment,* ed 2, St Louis, 1993, Mosby.
5. Metheny NM: *Fluid and electrolyte balance—nursing considerations,* Philadelphia, 1987, JB Lippincott.
6. Grimes J, Burns E: *Health assessment in nursing practice,* ed 3, Boston, 1992, Jones & Bartlett.
7. Roper M: Back to basics. Assessing orthostatic vital signs, *Am J Nurs* 96(8):43, 1996.
8. Brundage D: *Renal disorders,* St Louis, 1992, Mosby.
9. Weems J: *Quick reference to renal critical care nursing,* Gaithersburg, Md, 1991, Aspen.
10. Malasanos L, Barkauskas V, Stoltenberg-Allen K: *Health assessment,* ed 4, St Louis, 1990, Mosby.
11. Anderson R: Prevention and management of acute renal failure, *Hosp Pract* 27(8):61, 1993.
12. Chulay M, Guzzetta C, Dossey B: *AACN handbook of critical care nursing,* 1997, Appleton & Lange.
13. Fischbach F: *A manual of laboratory diagnostic tests,* ed 5, Philadelphia, 1996, JB Lippincott.
14. Stark J: Interpreting BUN/creatinine levels. It's not as simple as you think, *Nurs 94* 24(9):58, 1994.
15. Waite L, Krumberger J: *Noncardiac critical care nursing,* Albany, NY, 1994, Delmar.
16. Dennison RD: *Pass CCRN!,* St Louis, 1996, Mosby.

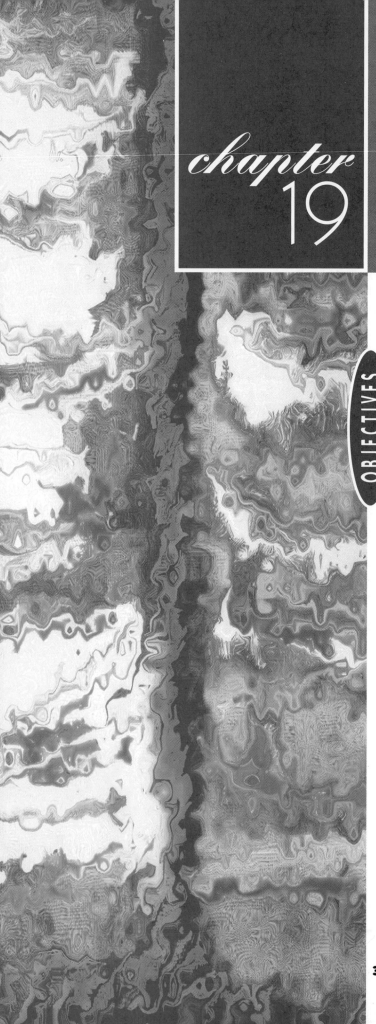

chapter 19

Renal Disorders and Therapeutic Management

Judith R. Glann

OBJECTIVES

- Describe the etiologies of acute renal failure.
- Describe the stages of acute tubular necrosis.
- Identify the priorities of nursing management in acute renal failure.
- Identify the differences among hemodialysis, peritoneal dialysis, and continuous renal displacement therapy.

ACUTE RENAL FAILURE

Description and Etiology

Acute renal failure (ARF) is a clinical syndrome that is characterized by an abrupt decline in glomerular filtration rate (GFR) with subsequent retention of metabolic waste products from protein catabolism (azotemia) and an inability to maintain electrolyte and acid-base homeostasis.[1,2] This change in renal function also disturbs the regulation of fluid volume. Oliguria, or a urine output less than 400 ml/day, is a classic finding in ARF[3] and occurs in about half of the patients admitted to critical care units.[1,4] ARF is usually reversible if the appropriate treatment is initiated promptly.

However, if the condition goes untreated or if the patient does not respond to treatment, the acute condition may lead to chronic renal failure, with significant morbidity and mortality. ARF is a serious complication in the critically ill patient and mortality remains high, ranging from 50% to 80%, even with advanced critical care and dialysis techniques.[5] Insults from gastrointestinal (GI) bleeding, sepsis, burns, trauma injuries (rhabdomyolysis), multisystem organ dysfunction syndrome (MODS), and central nervous system (CNS) changes often are implicated in deaths related to ARF.[2,4] ARF is

BOX 19-1

ETIOLOGY OF ACUTE RENAL FAILURE

PRERENAL

Hemorrhage
Severe gastrointestinal losses
Burns
Shock
Cirrhosis
Renal trauma
Volume depletion (actual loss or "third-spacing")
Heart failure
Renal losses (diuretics, diabetes insipidus, osmotic
    diuresis)
Severe dehydration
Hypotension
Sepsis
Embolism, thrombosis (bilateral renal vascular
    obstruction)
Anesthesia, surgery (increased renal vascular
    resistance)

INTRARENAL

Thrombus
Stenosis
Hypertensive sclerosis
Glomerulonephritis
Pyelonephritis
Acute tubular necrosis
Diabetic sclerosis
Toxic damage
Acute aortic necrosis

POSTRENAL

Obstructions (stenosis, calculi)
Prostatic disease
Tumors
Bladder obstruction, inflection
Neurogenic bladder
Ureteral obstruction

covered under DRG 316, with an anticipated length of stay of 7.1 days.[6]

Prerenal azotemia is a physiologic response to an insult that occurs before blood reaches the kidney. The primary characteristic is that the kidney and the functioning unit, the nephron, are intact but an alteration in renal perfusion interferes with the production of normal volume of urine. The hypotension leads to oliguria.[5] The hypoperfusion decreases the GFR, leading to oliguria. The nephrons remain normal, and a return to normal renal function is possible with prompt treatment of the underlying cause of the prerenal condition (i.e., dehydration, hypotension, cardiac failure, anesthesia, surgery, embolism, thrombosis, sepsis[5]). About 70% of critical care patients suffer from a sequela of events that can precipitate prerenal azotemia.[7] The term *azotemia* is used to describe an acute rise in blood urea nitrogen (BUN).

Intrarenal azotemia, also known as *intrinsic, primary,* or *parenchymal damage,* is the physiologic response to an insult that occurs at the site of the nephrons. It may involve both the glomeruli and the tubular epithelium. This is more commonly known as acute tubular necrosis (ATN). About 25% of patients admitted to critical care units suffer from this ischemic/toxic condition. It usually results in temporary renal damage and can present with different degrees of alteration in renal function.[5]

Postrenal azotemia is the physiologic response caused by the disruption of the normal flow of urine or urinary obstruction by any source from the kidney to the urethra.[5] The blockage results in retention of fluid, electrolytes and waste products and fewer than 5% of patients suffer from this.[7] Anuria or urine output less than 400 ml over 24 hours[3] occurs more commonly in postrenal obstruction[6] (Box 19-1). As with prerenal conditions, prompt treatment aimed at alleviating the obstruction will restore normal kidney function and prevent permanent kidney damage.[4,7]

ACUTE TUBULAR NECROSIS

Description and Etiology

ATN results from either nephrotoxic or ischemic injury that damages the renal tubular epithelium and, in severe cases, extends to the basement membrane.[1,3,7] Injury that is limited to the epithelial layer recovers sooner than injury that also involves the basement membrane. ATN is the most common form of intrarenal failure, making up approximately 75% of cases, and accounts for the vast majority of cases of hospital-acquired ARF.[1,7] Damage to the cellular structures in this area prevents normal concentration of urine, filtration of wastes, and regulation of acid-base, electrolyte, and water balance. A number of disorders can result in ATN, and several contributing factors may work together to bring about tubular damage.[1] Common causes of ATN are shown in Box 19-2. Causes are usually divided into two categories: ischemic and toxic.

Ischemic acute tubular necrosis

Ischemic damage occurs irregularly along the tubular membranes, causing areas of tubular cell damage and cast formation. Perfusion to the kidneys is obliterated or severely reduced, which causes the autoregulation properties of the afferent and efferent arterioles, which regulate GFR, to be lost.[8] Ischemia results if the ischemic episode is prolonged.

Toxic acute tubular necrosis

Toxic damage results from nephrotoxins, usually drugs, chemical agents, or bacterial endotoxins, which cause uniform, widespread damage. The renal tubular cells are constantly at risk for damage because of their normally high blood flows, high oxygen requirements, and the constant reabsorption and secretion of metabolites.

ETIOLOGY OF ACUTE TUBULAR NECROSIS

ISCHEMIC
Hemorrhage
Excessive diuretic use
Burns
Peritonitis
Sepsis
Heart failure
Myocardial ischemia
Pulmonary emboli
Transfusion reactions
Obstetric complications (severe toxemia, abruptio placentae, placenta previa, uterine rupture)
Severe dehydration
Severe, prolonged hypotension
Shock: cardiogenic, hypovolemic, septic
Major trauma; crush injuries

TOXIC
Rhabdomyolysis
Hypercalcemia
Gram-negative sepsis
Nephrotoxic medications (aminoglycosides, cephalosporins, antimicrobials, antineoplastic agents, analgesics containing phenacetin)
Heavy metals
Radiocontrast media
Insecticides, pesticides, fungicides
Carbon tetrachloride
Methanol
Street drugs such as phencyclidine (PCP)

Pathophysiology

The mechanisms responsible for tubular dysfunction in ischemic ATN are multifactorial and explain the pathophysiology behind ATN. Accumulation of "cellular debris" in the tubular lumen (tubular obstruction) from interstitial edema or from an accumulation of casts and sloughing tissue can create an obstruction. Filtration ceases when tubular hydrostatic pressure reaches that of glomerular filtration pressure. This decreases the formation of urine because of the nonavailability of filtrate to process.[9,10] The result of tubular cell swelling causes an obstruction that decreases capillary blood flow, leading to further ischemia and cell injury.[9] Adenosine triphosphate (ATP) decreases, causing cellular dysfunction. This results in an accumulation of intracellular calcium and the production of oxygen-free radicals that can cause tubular cell injury.[9]

Phases of Acute Tubular Necrosis

Onset phase

The onset (initiating) phase is the period of time from which an insult occurs until cell injury. Ischemic injury is evolving during this time. The GFR is decreased because of impaired renal blood flow and decreased glomerular ultrafiltration pressure. This disrupts the integrity of the tubular epithelium, which backleaks the glomerular filtrate.[7] The phase lasts from hours to days, depending on the cause, with toxic factors lasting longer. If treatment is initiated during this time, irreversible damage can be alleviated. A longer course of recovery reflects the presence of more extensive tubular injury.[5]

Oliguric/anuric phase

The oliguric/anuric phase, characterized by the presence of urine output <360 ml/24 hours,[5] is the second phase of ATN, and lasts 5 to 8 days in the nonoliguric patient and 10 to 16 days in the oliguric patient.[10] This phase is also referred to as the maintenance phase because total support of renal function is often required during this period. Oliguria is a sign that the damage to the tubule is probably extensive and severe.[5] ATN is often reversible and may last from a few hours to several weeks, depending on the cause and severity of renal tubular cell injury.[10] During the oliguric/anuric phase, the GFR is greatly reduced, which leads to increased levels of BUN, elevated creatinine levels, electrolyte abnormalities (hyperkalemia, hyperphosphatemia, hypocalcemia), and metabolic acidosis.[1,4,11]

Diuretic phase

The third phase, the diuretic phase, lasts 7 to 14 days and is characterized by an increase in GFR and sometimes polyuria with a urine output as high as 2 to 4 L/day.[1,4] If the patient is receiving hemodialysis during this phase, the polyuria will not be evident because excess volume will be removed by dialysis. During the diuretic phase, tubular function returns slowly and tubular reabsorption may not increase as quickly as GFR. The kidneys can clear volume but not solutes, which, with a large diuresis, can lead to volume depletion.[1]

Recovery phase

The last phase of ATN is the recovery or convalescent phase. Both oliguric and nonoliguric patients will increase their urine output.[10] During this stage, renal function slowly returns to normal or near normal. If significant renal parenchymal damage has occurred, BUN and creatinine levels may never return to normal.[1,4]

Assessment and Diagnosis

Laboratory assessment

Electrolyte imbalances in ARF are discussed in Table 19-1. Normal and abnormal urinalysis findings and significance are summarized in Table 18-2 in the previous chapter. Laboratory assessments always include a test of BUN and serum creatinine levels. BUN is neither the sole indicator of ARF nor the most reliable indicator of renal damage because, although it reflects cellular damage, the BUN level is easily changed by protein intake, blood in the GI tract, or cell catabolism.[2,9]

Creatinine, on the other hand, is an accurate reflection of renal damage because it is almost totally excreted by

TABLE 19-1

SERUM ELECTROLYTE DISTURBANCES IN ACUTE RENAL FAILURE

ELECTROLYTE DISTURBANCE	SERUM VALUE	FINDINGS
POTASSIUM		
Hypokalemia	Less than 3.5 mEq/L (rare)	Muscular weakness Cardiac irregularities on ECG Abdominal distention and flatulence Paresthesia Decreased reflexes Anorexia Dizziness Confusion Increased sensitivity to digitalis
Hyperkalemia	Greater than 5.0 mEq/L	Irritability and restlessness Anxiety Nausea and vomiting Abdominal cramps Weakness Numbness and tingling (fingertips and circumoral) Cardiac irregularities on ECG
SODIUM		
Hyponatremia	Less than 135 mEq/L	Disorientation Muscle twitching Nausea and vomiting Abdominal cramps Headaches Seizures Dizziness Postural hypotension Cold, clammy skin Decreased skin turgor Tachycardia Oliguria
Hypernatremia	Greater than 145 mEq/L	Extreme thirst Dry, sticky mucous membranes Altered mentation Seizures (later stages)
CALCIUM		
Hypocalcemia	Less than 8.5 mg/dL or 4.5 mEq/L	Irritability Muscular tetany Muscle cramps Decreased cardiac output (decreased contractions) Bleeding (decreased ability to coagulate) ECG changes Positive Chvostek's sign Positive Trousseau's sign
Hypercalcemia	Greater than 10.5 mg/dL or 5.8 mEq/L	Deep bone pain Excessive thirst Anorexia Lethargy Weakened muscles
MAGNESIUM		
Hypomagnesemia	Less than 1.4 mEq/L	Choroid and athetoid muscle activity Facial tics Spasticity Cardiac dysrhythmias
Hypermagnesemia	Greater than 2.5 mEq/L	CNS depression Respiratory depression Lethargy Coma Bradycardia ECG changes

Continued

TABLE **19-1**		

SERUM ELECTROLYTE DISTURBANCES IN ACUTE RENAL FAILURE—cont'd

ELECTROLYTE DISTURBANCE	SERUM VALUE	FINDINGS
PHOSPHATE		
Hypophosphatemia	Less than 3.0 mg/dL	Hemolytic anemias Depressed white cell function Bleeding (decreased platelet aggregation) Nausea, vomiting, and anorexia
Hyperphosphatemia	Greater than 4.5 mg/dL	Tachycardia Nausea Diarrhea Abdominal cramps Muscle weakness Flaccid paralysis Increased reflexes
CHLORIDE		
Hypochloremia	Less than 98 mEq/L	Hyperirritability Tetany or muscular excitability Slow respirations
Hyperchloremia	Greater than 108 mEq/L	Weakness Lethargy Deep, rapid breathing Possible unconsciousness (later stages)
ALBUMIN		
Hypoalbuminemia	Less than 3.8 g/dL	Muscle wasting Peripheral edema (fluid shift) Decreased resistance to infection Poorly healing wounds

the renal tubules. Elevated levels of serum creatinine can reflect damage to 50% of the nephrons or more.[9] If the patient is making sufficient urine, the creatinine clearance can be measured from the urine. A normal urine creatinine clearance is 120 ml/minute. It decreases in renal failure. However, many critical care patients in ARF do not make urine; therefore, the health care team must depend on the serum creatinine level instead.

Radiologic findings

Sonography, tomography, and angiography can help pinpoint the causal mechanism and even help differentiate between acute diseases and chronic renal failure. Radiologic contrast media have been implicated in the development and worsening of renal disorders. For example, patients with a history of coronary artery disease, diabetes, or renal disease can suffer from acute renal problems when contrast medium is not adequately cleared because of an already compromised circulatory or renal system.[12]

Hemodynamic monitoring and fluid balance

Because hypovolemia is the usual precursor of ischemic tubular damage, careful assessment of fluid losses from all potential sources is important. Taking frequent blood pressure measurements and monitoring hemodynamic values are other means of evaluating fluid status.

Changes in CO and PAWP values will indicate decreases or increases in intravascular volume.

Medical Management

Treatment goals for patients experiencing ARF focus on compensating for the deterioration of renal function. Medical interventions for ARF are directed toward three basic goals: (1) prevention, (2) correcting the causative mechanism, and (3) promoting regeneration of the remaining functional capacity. Medical management is based on the three categories or causes of ARF.[2]

Acute renal failure prevention

The only truly effective remedy for ARF is prevention. For effective prevention, the patient's risk for ARF must be known. Principles of prevention include avoiding the use of nephrotoxic drugs in the elderly and in those with chronic renal failure as well as avoiding the use of nonsteroidal antiinflammatory drugs for pain relief in patients taking antibiotics or recovering from major surgery. Delaying the use of intravascular x-ray contrast medium until the patient is rehydrated and antibiotics have been discontinued can help preserve kidney function in the high-risk patient. If this is not possible, low-dose dopamine can be infused to improve diuresis or dobutamine given to help increase creatinine clearance.[2] Dopamine

TABLE 19-2

FREQUENTLY USED INTRAVENOUS SOLUTIONS

NAME	ELECTROLYTES		INDICATIONS
CRYSTALLOIDS*			
Dextrose in water (D₅W)— isotonic	None		To maintain volume To replace mild loss To provide minimal calories
Normal saline solution (0.9% NaCl)	Sodium Chloride Osmolality	154 mEq/L 154 mEq/L 308 mEq/L	To maintain volume To replace mild loss To correct mild hyponatremia
Half-strength saline solution (0.45% NaCl)	Sodium Chloride	77 mEq/L 77 mEq/L	For free water replacement To correct mild hyponatremia For free water and electrolyte replacement (used in fluid- and electrolyte-restricted conditions)
Lactated Ringer's solution	Sodium Potassium Calcium Chloride Lactate pH	130 mEq/L 4 mEq/L 2.7 mEq/L 107 mEq/L 27 mEq/L 6.5	For fluid and electrolyte replacement (contraindicated for patients with renal or liver disease or in lactic acidosis)
COLLOIDS			
5% Albumin (Albumisol)	Albumin Sodium Osmolality Osmotic pressure pH	50 g/L 130 to 160 mEq/L 300 mOsm/L 20 mm Hg 6.4 to 7.4	For volume expansion For moderate protein replacement For achievement of hemodynamic stability in shock states
25% Albumin (salt-poor)	Albumin Globulins Sodium Osmolality pH	240 g/L 10 g/L 130 to 160 mEq/L 1500 mOsm/L 6.4 to 7.4	Concentrated form of albumin sometimes used with diuretics to move fluid from tissues into the vascular space for diuresis
Hetastarch	Sodium Chloride Osmolality Colloid osmotic pressure	154 mEq/L 154 mEq/L 310 mOsm/L 30-35 mm Hg	Synthetic polymer (6% solution) used for volume expansion For hemodynamic volume replacement after cardiac surgery, burns, sepsis
Low molecular weight dextran (LMWD)	Glucose polysaccharide molecules with an average molecular weight of 40,000, no electrolytes		For volume expansion and support (contraindicated for patients with bleeding disorders)
High molecular weight dextran (HMWD)	Glucose polysaccharide molecules with an average molecular weight of 70,000, no electrolytes		Used prophylactically in some cases to prevent platelet aggregation, available in either saline or glucose solutions

*For the crystalloid solutions that contain electrolytes, specific concentrations of electrolytes and pH will vary according to manufacturers.

has been associated with maintaining renal blood flow (RBF) and improving the glomerular filtration rate. Furosemide, used in pre-ATN, encourages passage of tubular cellular debris and augments the effect of RBF in conjunction with dopamine.[5]

Fluid balance

Prerenal failure is caused by decreased perfusion and is often associated with trauma, hemorrhage, or other fluid losses. Prerenal failure requires two specific methods of management: fluid and electrolyte restoration and stimulation of urinary output with diuretics.[2]

The objectives of fluid replacement are to replace losses of fluids and electrolytes and to prevent fluid im-

balance in the face of ongoing loss.[12] Maintenance fluid therapy is initiated only when oral fluid intake is clinically inadvisable.[1] Maintenance fluids are calculated with consideration for individual body surface area. Adults require approximately 1500 ml/m²/24 hours.[12] Requirements may be altered by fever, burns, environmental temperature, humidity changes, and other injuries.[12] The rate of replacement depends on cardiopulmonary reserve, adequacy of renal mechanisms, ongoing loss, and type of fluid required.

Crystalloids and colloids. Crystalloids and colloids refer to two different types of intravenous fluids that are frequently used for volume management in the critically ill. Refer to Table 19-2 for frequently used intravenous solutions. Crystalloid solutions, which are balanced salt solutions, are in widespread use for both maintenance infusions and replacement therapy. The choice of fluid and the amount of fluid are based on the patient's general condition and ability to tolerate this intervention.[5]

Colloids are solutions containing oncotically active particles that are employed to expand intravascular volume to achieve and maintain hemodynamic stability. The effect from colloid volume expansion can last as long as 24 hours. The goal is to increase PAWP, mean arterial pressure (MAP), and CI to a therapeutic level.

Adequacy of IV fluid replacement depends on strict ongoing evaluation and frequent adjustment. Frequent monitoring of serum electrolyte levels is required, and strictly regulated intake and output are correlated with daily weight records. Finally, hemodynamic readings are frequent and ongoing. If, following a fluid challenge, the increase in CVP is only minimal, this indicates the need for fluid replacement. Continued decreases in CVP, PAWP, and CI indicate ongoing volume losses. Significant rises in CVP and PAWP, with a fall in CI, may indicate hypervolemia with underlying cardiac failure.

Fluid restriction. Fluid restriction constitutes a large part of the medical treatment for renal failure. Fluid restriction is used to prevent circulatory overload and interstitial edema when excess volume cannot be removed by the kidneys. The fluid requirements are calculated on the basis of daily urinary volumes and insensible losses. Obtaining daily weights and keeping accurate intake and output records are essential. Renal failure patients are usually restricted to 1 L of fluid if urinary output is 500 ml or less and insensible losses range from 500 to 750 ml/day.

Fluid removal. Intrarenal failure involves the introduction of increased amounts of water, solutes, and potential toxins into the circulation; thus prompt measures are needed to decrease their levels. Diuretics are used to stimulate the urinary output. However, hemodialysis or hemofiltration are the treatments of choice, particularly if volume overload creates pulmonary and cardiac compromise. Severe hyperkalemia almost always necessitates hemodialysis because of the life-threatening cardiac dysrhythmias resulting from hyperkalemia.[13] Hemodialysis may also be initiated for severe azotemia when other treatments are contraindicated.

Electrolyte balance
Potassium. Electrolyte levels require frequent observation, especially in the critical phases of renal failure. Potassium may quickly reach levels of 6.0 mEq/L and above. Specific ECG changes are associated with hyperkalemia, specifically peaked T waves, a widening of the QRS interval, and ultimately ventricular tachycardia or fibrillation.[13] If hyperkalemia is present, all potassium supplements are stopped.[14] If the patient is producing urine, IV diuretics can be administered. Acute hyperkalemia can be treated temporarily by an IV infusion of insulin and glucose. An infusion of 100 ml of 50% dextrose accompanied by 20 units of regular insulin forces potas-

sium out of the serum and into the cells. Sodium bicarbonate (40 to 160 mEq) may be infused to promote higher excretion of potassium in the urine, particularly if the serum pH is below 7.10. Finally, sodium polystyrene sulfonate (Kayexalate), a cation-exchange resin, is mixed in water and sorbitol and given orally, rectally, or through a nasogastric (NG) tube. The resin binds potassium in the bowel, which eliminates it in the feces. Kayexalate and dialysis are the only permanent methods of potassium removal.[13,14]

Sodium. Dilutional hyponatremia, associated with renal failure, can be corrected with fluid restriction.[15] If, however, sodium stores actually are depleted, hypertonic 3% saline solution is sometimes administered intravenously as a replacement. In addition, sodium levels may be raised during dialysis by changing the amount of sodium in the dialysate bath.[3]

Calcium and phosphorus. Calcium levels are reduced in renal failure. This reduction results from multiple factors, among which is hyperphosphatemia. Aluminum hydroxide preparations are administered orally or via an NG tube to bind phosphorus in the bowel and thus eliminate it from the body. This lowers the serum phosphorus level and increases the calcium blood level. Calcium may also be increased by use of calcium supplements, vitamin D preparations, and synthetic calcitrol.[16]

Nutrition
The nutritional aspects of renal failure involve increased energy expenditure, the extensive catabolic state, and the negative nitrogen balance.[5] If the patient is anorexic and malnourished, total parenteral nutrition (TPN) can be provided and the excess TPN fluid volume removed during hemodialysis or hemofiltration. The renal diet restricts protein, potassium, sodium, and phosphorus. Protein restriction may vary to limit azotemia (increased BUN). Carbohydrates are encouraged, primarily to provide needed energy for healing.[9]

Medications
Care must be taken in the use of diuretics to avoid creating secondary electrolyte abnormalities. Diuretic therapy is thought to increase renal blood flow, GFR, and intratubular pressure while decreasing the possibility of tubular obstruction and dysfunction. Both osmotic and loop diuretics may be effective in decreasing the initial insult to the renal system if given promptly at the onset of oliguria.[2]

Nursing Management
Nursing management of patients with acute renal failure incorporates a variety of nursing diagnoses (Box 19-3). **Nursing priorities are directed toward preventing infectious complications, optimizing fluid balance, preventing electrolyte imbalance, and addressing psychosocial issues with patients and families.**

The critical care patient with ARF is at risk for infectious complications. Signs of infection, such as increased

NURSING DIAGNOSIS PRIORITIES

Acute Renal Failure

- Fluid Volume Excess related to renal dysfunction, p. 487
- Altered Renal Tissue Perfusion related to decreased renal blood flow, p. 485
- Anxiety related to threat to biologic, psychologic, and/or social integrity, p. 448
- Decreased Cardiac Output related to alterations in preload, p. 467
- Risk for Infection risk factors: protein-calorie malnourishment, invasive monitoring devices, p. 494
- Body Image Disturbance related to functional dependence on life-sustaining technology, p. 450

BOX 19-4

INDICATIONS AND CONTRAINDICATIONS FOR HEMODIALYSIS

INDICATIONS

BUN >90 mg/dL
Serum creatinine >9 mg/dL
Hyperkalemia
Drug toxicity
Intravascular and extravascular fluid overload
Metabolic acidosis
Symptoms of uremia:
   Pericarditis
   GI bleeding
   Mental changes
Contraindications to other forms of dialysis

CONTRAINDICATIONS

Hemodynamic instability
Inability to anticoagulate
Lack of access to circulation

WBC count, redness at a wound or IV site, or increased temperature, are a cause for concern.

Frequent assessment of intake and output, particularly in response to diuretics, is a necessary part of nursing management for the patient in renal failure. Hemodynamic values and daily weights are correlated with the intake and output to confirm fluid overload. Urinary output is measured throughout all phases of ARF. During the diuretic phase, as urinary function returns, it may be necessary to replace the fluids and electrolytes that are lost during this phase.

Hyperkalemia, hypocalcemia, hyponatremia, hyperphosphatemia, and acid-base imbalances all occur during ARF.[2] Clinical manifestations of these electrolyte imbalances must be prevented and their associated side effects controlled. The imbalances with the most potential hazard are hyperkalemia and hypocalcemia, which can result in life-threatening cardiac dysrhythmias. Dilutional hyponatremia may develop as fluid overload worsens in the patient with oliguria. Monitoring the serum sodium level is important to prevent this complication. Hyperphosphatemia results in severe pruritus. Nursing care is directed at soothing the itching by performing frequent skin care with emollients, discouraging scratching, and administering phosphate-binding medications. The acid-base imbalances that occur with renal failure are monitored by arterial blood gas analysis.

DIALYSIS

A wide range of options is available for the treatment of ARF, including the following: hemodialysis, peritoneal dialysis, and continuous renal replacement therapy.[3,11]

Hemodialysis

Hemodialysis roughly translates as "separating from the blood."[17] Indications and contraindications for hemodialysis are listed in Box 19-4. As a treatment, hemodialysis literally separates and removes from the blood the excess

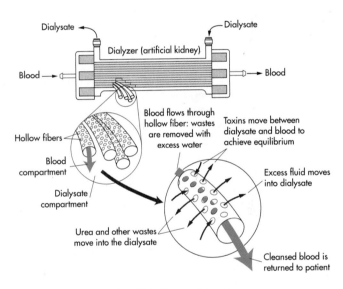

Fig. **19-1** Hemodialyzer.

electrolytes, fluids, and toxins by use of a dialyzer. Although efficient in removing chemicals, it does not remove all metabolites. Furthermore, electrolytes, toxins, and fluids increase between treatments, requiring hemodialysis on a regular basis. Each dialysis treatment takes 3 to 4 hours. In the acute phases of renal failure, dialysis is performed daily.

Hemodialyzer

Hemodialysis works by circulating blood outside the body through synthetic tubing to a *dialyzer*, which consists of hollow-fiber tubes as shown in Fig. 19-1. The components of a hemodialysis system are shown in Fig. 19-2. While the blood flows through the membranes, which are semipermeable, a fluid known as the dialysate

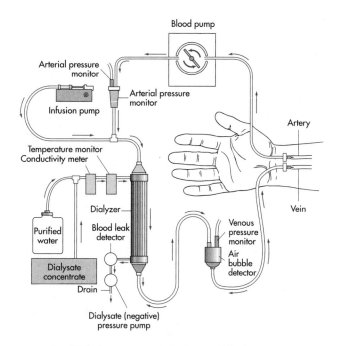

Fig. **19-2** Components of a hemodialysis system.

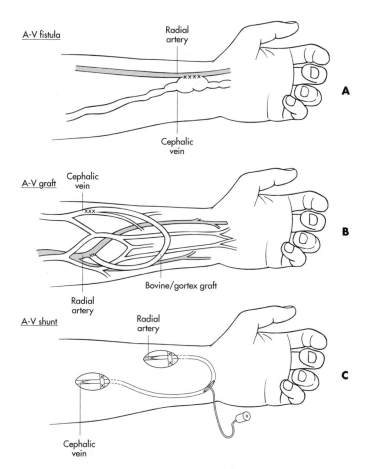

Fig. **19-3** Methods of vascular access for hemodialysis. **A,** Arteriovenous fistula between vein and artery. **B,** Internal synthetic graft corrects artery and vein. **C,** External synthetic cannula, or shunt, with T-connector.

bath bathes the membranes and, through osmosis and diffusion, performs exchanges of fluid, electrolytes, and toxins from the blood to the bath.[18] The blood and bath are shunted in opposite directions (countercurrent flow) through the dialyzer to maintain the osmotic and chemical gradients at their highest.

Ultrafiltration

To remove fluid, a positive hydrostatic pressure is applied to the blood and a negative hydrostatic pressure is applied to the dialysate bath. The two forces together, called *transmembrane pressure*, pull and squeeze the excess fluid from the blood. The difference between the two values (expressed in millimeters of mercury) represents the transmembrane pressure and results in fluid extraction, known as *ultrafiltration*, from the vascular space.[18]

Anticoagulation

Heparin is added to the system just before the blood enters the dialyzer. Without the heparin, the blood would clot because its presence outside the body and its passage through foreign substances initiate the clotting mechanism. Heparin can be administered by bolus injection or intermittent infusion.

Vascular access for hemodialysis

Hemodialysis requires access to the bloodstream. Various types of permanent arteriovenous (A-V) accesses have been created. The common denominator is access to the arterial circulation and return to the venous circulation. Femoral and subclavian catheters (used most frequently in acute care situations) permit access to the venous circulation only.

Subclavian and femoral vein catheters

A dual-lumen venous catheter is the most commonly used form of vascular access for acute hemodialysis. It has a central partition running the length of the catheter. The outflow catheter pulls the blood flow through openings that are proximal to the inflow openings on the opposite side. This design avoids dialyzing the same blood just returned to the area (recirculation), which can severely reduce the procedure's efficiency.[17,18] A silicone rubber, dual-lumen catheter with a Dacron cuff that is designed to decrease the incidence of catheter-related infections is also available.[17]

Subclavian and femoral veins are usually catheterized in cases of ARF when short-term access is required or when vascular access is nonfunctional in a patient requiring immediate hemodialysis. Both subclavian and femoral catheters can be inserted at the bedside. When the subclavian vein is not available, a shorter dialysis catheter is used for placement into the femoral vein.

Arteriovenous fistula

The arteriovenous (A-V) fistula is created by surgically visualizing a peripheral artery and vein, creating an opening in the artery and the vein, and anastomosing the two open areas. Anastomoses may be side-to-side, end-to-side, or end-to-end.[3,11,18] The high arterial flow creates swelling of the vein, or a *pseudoaneurysm,* at which point—when healed—a large-bore needle can be inserted to obtain outflow. Inflow is accomplished through a second large-bore needle inserted into a peripheral vein distal to the fistula (Fig. 19-3, *A*). If the patient's vessels are adequate, fistulas are the preferred mode of access because of the durability of blood vessels and the relatively few complications in comparison to the other accesses. Development of sufficient flow to the fistula, however, may require weeks to months. Attempting to obtain flow from underdeveloped fistulas often causes painful vascular spasm and reduced flow.

Arteriovenous grafts

Arteriovenous (A-V) grafts are the most frequently used access for treating chronic renal failure. The graft is a tube formed of Gortex, which is surgically implanted in the limb. The area is surgically opened, and an artery and a vein are located. A tunnel is created, either straight or U-shaped, in the tissue where the graft is placed. Anastomoses are made with the graft ends connected to the artery and vein. The blood is allowed to flow through the graft, and the surgical area is closed. The graft creates a raised area that looks like a large peripheral vein just under the skin and peripheral tissue layers (Fig. 19-3, *B*). Two large-bore needles are used for outflow and inflow to the graft. For both grafts and fistulas, after needle removal at the end of the hemodialysis treatment, firm pressure must be applied to stem bleeding.

Arteriovenous shunt

Because of the advent of subclavian and femoral catheters, arteriovenous (A-V) shunts are used infrequently today in critical care. If, however, long-term hemodialysis is required, a permanent vascular access is necessary to permit rapid blood access to be obtained through an external arteriovenous shunt (Fig. 19-3, *C*). The arteriovenous shunt requires a peripheral artery, usually radial or ulnar, and a peripheral vein, such as the cephalic or basilic. A cutdown is performed on each vessel. The vessel tips are sutured in place. When not being used for dialysis, a straight connector or a heparin T device connects the peripheral artery and vein. Blood flows in a U-shaped fashion from the higher arterial pressure to the lower venous system. Shunts may also be inserted in the thigh or ankle areas.

Medical management

Medical management involves the decision to place a vascular access device and the most appropriate type and location for each patient. Patients in the critical care setting require vascular access if they suffer from ARF or chronic renal failure and require hemodialysis.[12]

Some patients with chronic renal failure are admitted to the hospital to receive lytic therapy (streptokinase, or urokinase) to lyse a thrombus in the vascular access. In some cases, this may require invasive procedures such as angiography or surgery to remove clots.

Nursing management

Nursing management of patients with arteriovenous shunt, fistula, and grafts are delineated in Table 19-3. **Nursing priorities are directed toward preventing complications, detecting early signs of shunt malfunction, and preventing infection.**

Continuous Renal Replacement Therapy

Continuous renal replacement therapy (CRRT) is used as an alternative to hemodialysis in patients with hemodynamic instability.[19] It is a continuous therapy lasting 12 hours or longer in which blood is circulated from an artery to a vein—or from vein to vein—through a highly porous hemofilter.[11,16,20] The system allows for continuous fluid removal from the plasma, the amount ranging from 5 to 45 ml/minute, depending on the particular CRRT system used, plus removal of urea, creatinine, and electrolytes.[16,21] If large amounts of fluid are removed, replacement solutions are infused. If fluid removal is low, this is not required. Indications and contraindications for CRRT are listed in Box 19-5.

In an ideal situation, the hydrostatic pressure exerted by the patient's MAP forms the basis for the continuous flow of blood through the hemofilter. To maintain this flow of blood, a MAP greater than 70 mm Hg is desirable. The removed ultrafiltrate can be drained by gravity flow or by a suction-assisted collection system.[16] However, because many critically ill patients do not have a MAP greater than 70 mm Hg—sufficient to provide adequate flow through the system—in many critical care units a roller pump is added to the system to augment flow. The various CRRT systems are shown in Fig. 19-4.

Because controlled removal and replacement of fluid are possible with CRRT, hemodynamic stability is maintained. This makes CRRT highly advantageous for use in the patient with MODS.[3,20] The four most frequently seen forms of CRRT are:

1. Slow continuous ultrafiltration (SCUF)
2. Continuous arteriovenous hemofiltration (CAVH)
3. Continuous arteriovenous hemodialysis (CAVHD)
4. Continuous venovenous hemodialysis (CVVHD)

The first three types of CRRT require an arterial access (SCUF, CAVH, CAVHD)[20]; the last one requires only venous access (CVVHD).[22] The decision as to which type of therapy to initiate is based on myriad factors, including clinical assessment, metabolic status, severity of uremia, and whether a particular treatment modality is available at that institution. A comparison of CRRT approaches is found in Table 19-4, and a discussion of each of these methods follows.

Slow continuous ultrafiltration

SCUF, as the name implies, slowly removes fluid, 100 to 300 ml/hour, through a process of ultrafiltration.[20-23]

TABLE 19-3

COMPLICATIONS AND NURSING MANAGEMENT OF ARTERIOVENOUS SHUNT, FISTULA, AND GRAFT

TYPE	COMPLICATIONS	NURSING MANAGEMENT
Shunt	Clotting Dislodgment Skin erosion Infection Bleeding	Monitor for clinical manifestations of infection. Monitor for clinical manifestations of thrombosis (darkening of blood, separation of serum or cellular compartment blood in tubing, decreased temperature of tubing). Assess insertion site daily for erosion around insertion sites. Use strict aseptic technique during dressing changes at insertion sites. Teach patients to avoid sleeping on or prolonged bending of accessed limbs. Keep two shunt clamps attached to patients' clothing or access dressing at all times.
Fistula	Thrombosis Infection Pseudoaneurysm Vascular steal syndrome Venous hypertension Carpal tunnel syndrome Inadequate blood flow	Teach patients to avoid wearing constrictive clothing on limbs containing access. Teach patients to avoid sleeping on or prolonged bending of accessed limb. Use aseptic technique when cannulating access. Avoid repetitious cannulation of one segment of access. Offer comfort measures, such as warm compresses and ordered analgesics, to lessen pain of vascular steal. Teach patients to develop blood flow in the fistulas through exercises (squeezing a rubber ball) while applying mild impedance to flow just distal to the access (at least once per day for 10 to 15 minutes).
Graft	Bleeding Thrombosis False aneurysm formation Infection Arterial or venous stenosis Vascular steal syndrome	Avoid too early cannulation of new access. Teach patients to avoid wearing constrictive clothing on accessed limbs. Avoid repeated cannulation of one segment of access. Use aseptic technique when cannulating access. Monitor for changes in arterial or venous pressure while patients are on dialysis. Provide comfort measures to reduce pain of vascular steal (e.g., warm compresses, analgesics as ordered).

BOX 19-5

INDICATIONS AND CONTRAINDICATIONS FOR CONTINUOUS RENAL REPLACEMENT THERAPY

INDICATIONS

Need for large fluid volume removal in the hemodynamically unstable patient
Hypervolemic or edematous patients unresponsive to diuretic therapy
Patients with MODS
Ease of fluid management in patients requiring large daily fluid volume, such as replacement for oliguria, TPN administration
Contraindications to hemodialysis and peritoneal dialysis
Inability to anticoagulate
Uncontrolled electrolyte imbalances or uremia
Cardiogenic shock or cardiopulmonary edema
Removal of uremic toxins
Acute electrolyte imbalances

CONTRAINDICATIONS

Hematocrit >45%
Lack of arterial access (for SCUF, CAVH, CAVHD only)

This process consists of an exchange of fluid, solutes, and solvents across a semipermeable membrane.[20] Because small amounts of fluid are removed via this process, it is a treatment of choice for patients with acute heart failure and diminished renal perfusion who are unresponsive to diuretics.

Continuous arteriovenous hemofiltration

CAVH is indicated when the patient's clinical condition warrants removal of significant volumes of fluid and solutes. Fluid is removed by ultrafiltration in volumes of 5 to 20 ml/minute or 7 to 30 L in 24 hours.[24] Increased removal of solutes such as urea, creatinine, or other nonprotein-bound toxins is accomplished by increasing flow through the hemofilter via the addition of a prehemofilter replacement fluid (Fig. 19-4, B).

Continuous arteriovenous hemodialysis

CAVHD requires arterial access but is technically different from the two previously described methods because it contains a slow (15 to 30 ml/minute) countercurrent drainage flow on the membrane side of the hemofilter[24] (Fig. 19-3, C). The countercurrent flow is through the hemodialyzer. Countercurrent means the blood flows in one direction and the dialysate flows in the opposite direction. This increases its clearance of ure-

TABLE 19-4

COMPARISON OF CONTINUOUS RENAL REPLACEMENT THERAPY METHODS

TYPE	ULTRAFILTRATION RATE	FLUID REPLACEMENT	INDICATION
SCUF	100 to 300 ml/hr	None	Fluid removal
CAVH	500 to 800 ml/hr	Predilution or postdilution, calculating an hourly net loss	Fluid removal, moderate solute removal
CAVHD	500 to 800 ml/hr	Predilution or postdilution, subtracting the dialysate and then calculating an hourly net loss	Fluid removal, maximum solute removal
CVVHD		Same as CAVHD	Fluid removal and solute removal

SCUF, Slow continuous ultrafiltration; *CAVH,* continuous arteriovenous hemofiltration; *CAVHD,* continuous arteriovenous hemodialysis; *CVVHD,* continuous venovenous hemodialysis.

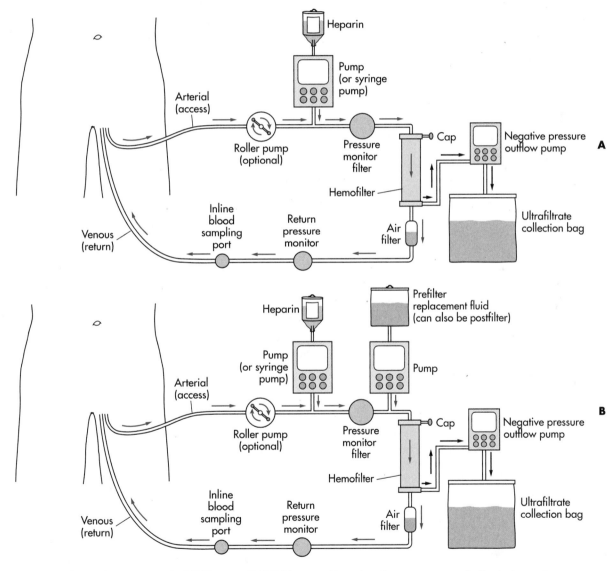

Fig. **19-4** CRRT systems. **A,** SCUF setup. **B,** CAVH setup. Note that the systems are similar but vary in complexity, depending on what function is to be performed. For example, the CVAH setup differs from the SCUF setup in that it contains prefilter replacement fluid and a pump so that significant blood volume can be removed. (The red arrows indicate blood flow, and the black arrows indicate ultrafiltrate flow.)

Continued

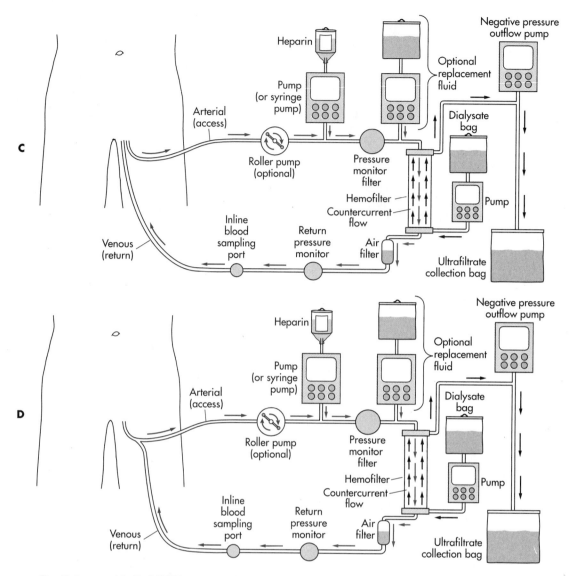

Fig. **19-4—cont'd. C,** CAVHD setup. **D,** CVVHD setup. The CAVHD setup and CVVHD setup differ from the SCUF setup and CAVH setup in that they have additional countercurrent flow. (The red arrows indicate blood flow, and the black arrows indicate ultrafiltrate flow.)

mic toxins and makes it more like traditional hemodialysis.[20] CAVHD is the most efficient form of CRRT.[16]

CAVHD is indicated in patients who require large-volume removal for severe uremia or critical acid-base imbalances or who are diuretic resistant. A MAP of at least 70 mm Hg is desirable for effective volume removal and dialysis, and it is most effective when used over days, not hours.

The circuit uses the same basic connection and hemofiltration concepts as CAVH but has the added benefit of a pump driver circuit. CVVH operations are independent of the mean systemic arterial pressure. It allows removal of solutes and modification of the volume and composition of the extracellular fluid to occur over time. If the goal of therapy is to remove fluid, the ultrafiltration rate may be lower than if the goal is solute removal. With solute removal, the ultrafiltration rate should be 2-4 ml/

minute. If the goal is fluid removal, the ultrafiltration rate is not as important as the net fluid balance for the patient.[25]

Continuous venovenous hemodialysis

CVVHD is a newer method of renal replacement therapy. The advantage of CVVHD is that arterial access is not required. The CVVHD system is set up in the same way as CAVHD and also includes a slow countercurrent drainage flow on the membrane side of the hemofilter (Fig. 19-4, *D*). The indications for CVVHD are the same as for CAVHD.

Vascular Access for CRRT

Single-lumen, large-bore catheters are placed into an artery and vein. Usually, the femoral site is selected because of its large size and accessibility.

Medical management

The choice of blood purification to use in ARF is a medical decision. Age, sex, and preexisting chronic conditions are of little help in determining the need for hemofiltration or hemodialysis, and often it is the acute clinical diagnosis that is the deciding factor.[2] In trauma the location of injury is important. For example, patients with head and abdominal injury have a poorer prognosis than those with chest and limb damage. Multisystem organ failure often involves the kidneys; however, the number of organ systems involved and the severity of their involvement have been shown to be of very limited prognostic importance, at least at the onset of ARF.[2] Infectious complications are associated with a grave prognosis. Dialysis is prescribed for almost anyone who develops severe ARF unless the patient is clearly dying.[2]

Intermittent hemodialysis or CRRT is usually begun before the BUN level exceeds 90 mg/dL or the creatinine exceeds 9 mg/dL. It is controversial whether daily treatment is more effective than treatment every other day.[2] The patient's serum creatinine, BUN, and fluid volume status are the deciding factors. CRRT is often prescribed when the BUN level is approximately 60 mg/dL. CRRT is more effective in the early stages of ARF. If severe electrolyte imbalance or fluid overload is present, even earlier intervention may be required.[2]

Nursing management

Nursing management of the patient receiving CRRT is vital for the maintenance of treatment equipment and for the detection of changes that may indicate dysfunction or deterioration in physical condition (refer to Table 19-5). **Nursing priorities are directed toward monitoring dialysis equipment and procedures for potential malfunction and monitoring the patient's hemodynamic, fluid and electrolyte status, and any indications of bleeding.**

Peritoneal Dialysis

Peritoneal dialysis (PD) involves the introduction of sterile dialyzing fluid through an implanted catheter into the abdominal cavity. The dialysate bathes the peritoneal membrane, which covers the abdominal organs and overlies the capillary beds that support the organs. By the processes of osmosis, diffusion, and active transport, excess fluid and solutes travel from the peritoneal capillary fluid through the capillary walls, through the peritoneal membrane, and into the dialyzing fluid. After a selected time period, the fluid is drained out of the abdomen by gravity (Fig. 19-5). The process is then repeated at regular prescribed intervals. Indications and contraindications for PD are listed in Box 19-6.

The volume of dialysate instilled into the abdomen affects the clearance. During acute PD, 3.5 L/hour provides a urea clearance of 26 ml/minute. During chronic, continuous PD, 2 L exchanges every 4 hours provide a clearance of 7 ml/minute. The dialysate should be instilled at body temperature to be comfortable, provide

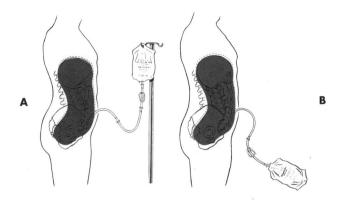

Fig. **19-5** Peritoneal dialysis. **A,** Inflow. **B,** Outflow (drains by gravity).

BOX 19-6

INDICATIONS AND CONTRAINDICATIONS FOR PERITONEAL DIALYSIS

INDICATIONS

Uremia
Volume overload
Electrolyte imbalances
Hemodynamic instability
Lack of access to circulation
Removal of high molecular weight toxins
Patients with nonrenal critical illness who are receiving PD for chronic renal failure
Severe cardiovascular disease
Inability to anticoagulate
Contraindication to hemodialysis

CONTRAINDICATIONS

Recent abdominal surgery
History of abdominal surgeries with adhesions and scarring
Significant pulmonary disease
Need for rapid fluid removal
Peritonitis

some vasodilation, and provide increased solute transport in the peritoneum. The length of time the solution remains in the peritoneal cavity (dwell time) and the solution composition affect the outcome. The dwell time affects the amount of fluid removed from the peritoneal capillaries, although a longer dwell time will not remove proportionately more fluid because of osmotic equilibration across the membranes. The various glucose concentrations of the dialysate provide for different rates of fluid removal.

Peritoneal dialysis catheter placement

Two types of catheters are used for PD: the rigid stylet and the silicone catheter. The single-use *rigid stylet catheter* can be inserted at the bedside for immediate initiation of dialysis. Patient mobility is limited when the rigid stylet is in place because of the possibility of perfora-

TABLE 19-5

PROBLEMS, ETIOLOGIES, CLINICAL MANIFESTATIONS, AND NURSING INTERVENTIONS RELATED TO CRRT

PROBLEM	ETIOLOGY	CLINICAL MANIFESTATIONS	NURSING MANAGEMENT
Decreased ultrafiltration rate	Hypotension Dehydration Kinked lines Bending of catheters Clotting of filter	Ultrafiltration rate decreased Minimal flow through blood lines	Observe filter and arteriovenous system. Control blood flow. Control coagulation time. Position patients on back. Lower height of collection container.
Filter clotting	Obstruction Insufficient heparinization Hypotension	Ultrafiltration rate decreased, despite height of collection container being lower	Control heparinization. Maintain continuous heparinization. Call physician. Remove system. Prime catheters with heparin. Prime a new system and connect it. Start predilution with 1000 ml saline 0.9% solution per hour. Do not use three-way stopcocks.
Hypotension, secondary to hypovolemia	Increased ultrafiltration rate Blood leak Disconnection of one of lines	Bleeding	Control amount of ultrafiltration. Control access sites. Clamp lines. Call physician.
Fluid and electrolyte changes	Too much/little removal of fluid Inappropriate replacement of electrolytes Inappropriate dialysate	Changes in mentation ↑ or ↓ CVP, PAWP ECG change ↑ or ↓ BP and heart rate Abnormal electrolyte levels	Observe for changes in central venous pressure or pulmonary capillary wedge pressure. Observe for changes in vital signs. Observe electrocardiogram for changes as a result of electrolyte abnormalities. Monitor output values every hour. Control ultrafiltration.
Bleeding	System disconnection ↑ Heparin dose	Oozing from catheter insertion site or connection	Monitor activated clotting time (ACT) no less than once every hour. Adjust heparin dose within specifications to maintain ACT. Observe dressing on vascular access for blood loss. Observe for blood in filtrate (filter leak).
Access dislodgment or infection	Catheter/connections not secured Break in sterile technique Excessive patient movement	Bleeding from catheter site or connections Inappropriate flow/infusion Fever Drainage at catheter site	Observe access site at least once every 2 hr. Ensure that clamps are available within easy reach at all times. Observe strict sterile technique when dressing vascular access.
Hypothermia	Extracorporeal nature of circuit	↓ Temperature Shivering	Warm filter, replacement fluids, and/or blood products
Air embolism	Air from circuit; lack of air detection alarm	↑ RR SOB Anxiety Chest pain	Position patient on left side and notify physician Discontinue therapy
Cardiac arrest			Clamp ultrafiltrate Initiate CPR/ACLS

tion.[26] The *silicone catheter* usually is inserted surgically, although it can be inserted at the bedside. This catheter is designed for multiple treatments over extended periods. Because the catheter is extremely flexible, the patient is able to move freely with minimal discomfort.[26]

Most catheters have an external segment, a tunnel segment that passes through subcutaneous tissue and muscle, a cuff for stabilization at the peritoneal membrane, and an external segment with numerous holes for fast delivery and drainage of dialysate.

Peritoneal dialysis complications

Complications of PD can be numerous. The complications, which range from annoying to severe, require careful observation and intervention to control or even prevent further problems.[27] However, with the exception of peritonitis, complications from PD are less severe than those associated with hemodialysis.

Medical management

PD is generally used for long-term chronic renal failure. One acute clinical situation that may have applica-

TABLE 19-6

COMPLICATIONS AND NURSING MANAGEMENT OF PERITONEAL DIALYSIS

COMPLICATIONS	NURSING MANAGEMENT
Peritonitis	Assess for signs and symptoms: cloudy effluent, abdominal pain, rebound tenderness, nausea and vomiting, and fever. Obtain effluent sample for culture. Administer antibiotics as ordered. Teach patient and family signs and symptoms of peritonitis and its prevention.
Exit site infection	Monitor site daily for signs and symptoms of infection: enduration, erythema, purulence, and hyperthermia. Increase daily cleaning of site. Apply topical antibiotics as ordered (controversial). Teach patient and family to avoid agents such as creams and lotions around exit site.
Catheter-tunnel infection	Assess for signs and symptoms of infection: pain along tunnel, enduration for several centimeters away from catheter, erythema leading away from the exit site, and drainage at exit site or as tunnel is "milked" toward exit site. Teach patient and family signs and symptoms of infection. Teach patient and family to avoid pulls or tugs on the catheter or trauma to the exit site. Emphasize the need to maintain cleansing regimen at exit site.
Fluid obstruction	Change position of patient (i.e., standing, lying, side-lying, knee chest). Relieve patient's constipation. Irrigate the catheter. Ensure that sufficient fluid is in abdomen (sometimes requires a residual reservoir of approximately 50 ml).
Rectal pain	Ensure a sufficient reservoir of fluid. Use slow infusion rate.
Shoulder pain	Ensure that all air is primed from infusion tubing. Attempt draining the effluent with the patient in the knee-chest position. Administer mild analgesics as ordered.
Hernias	Monitor for increase in size of or pain in area of hernia. Decrease volume of exchanges as ordered. Dialyze with patient in the supine position. Use abdominal binder or support for patient (as long as not binding on catheter exit site). Avoid initiation of PD until exit site healing has taken place (approximately 1 to 2 weeks) if possible.
Fluid overload	Increase use of hypertonic solutions. Decrease by-mouth (PO) fluid intake. Shorten dwell times. Weigh patient frequently. Monitor lung sounds and peripheral edema.
Dehydration	Assess patient for decreased skin turgor, muscle cramps, hypotension, tachycardia, and dizziness. Discontinue hypertonic solutions. Increase PO fluid intake. Lengthen dwell times.
Blood-tinged effluent	Monitor for change in effluent color (clear yellow to pink or rusty). Administer heparin, as ordered, to avoid fibrin formation. Obtain patient history about catheter trauma and patient activity before appearance of complication.

tion for PD is patients with a head injury. In this case, PD is advised because no anticoagulation is needed, the osmolality changes are not pronounced, and pressure changes in the CNS are avoided.[27]

Nursing management

Nursing management of the patient receiving PD is directed toward prevention and detection of complications related to PD (Table 19-6). **Nursing priorities for patients include observation for signs of infection, fluid volume status, and signs and symptoms related to PD catheter and dialysis complications.**

The critical care nurse is cognizant of those drugs that are eliminated by the kidney and that are dialyzed during hemodialysis. Some of the drugs more frequently encountered in critical care and that are affected by renal failure or hemodialysis are listed in Table 19-7. The molecular weight of medications, the higher water solubility of some medications that make them easily removed by dialysis, or the ability of the medications to bind with proteins and therefore not be removed by dialysis are factors that affect the blood level of the medication.

TABLE 19-7

IMPACT OF RENAL FAILURE AND HEMODIALYSIS ON SELECTED DRUGS

DRUG	NORMAL DRUG METABOLISM AND EXCRETION	PERCENT OF NORMAL DOSE ADJUSTMENT IN RENAL FAILURE CAUSED BY DECREASED CREATININE CLEARANCE (ml/minute)*	EFFECT OF HEMODIALYSIS
ANTIINFECTIVES **Antibiotics**			
Amikacin†	94%-99% renal excretion	—	Dialyzed
Ampicillin	73%-92% renal excretion 12%-24% hepatic metabolism	Creatinine clearance 10-50: 100% of normal dose every 6-12 hours Creatinine clearance <10: 50%-100% of normal dose every 12 hours	Moderately dialyzed
Clindamycin	10% renal excretion 85% hepatic metabolism (some active metabolites)	No change	Not dialyzed
Cefazolin	>95% renal excretion	Creatinine clearance 10-50: 50%-100% of normal dose every 12 hours Creatinine clearance <10: 50% of normal dose every 24 hours	Moderately dialyzed
Cefotaxime	40%-65% renal excretion 40%-60% hepatic metabolism (active metabolite has 25% activity of parent)	Creatinine clearance 10-50: 50%-100% of normal dose every 8-12 hours Creatinine clearance <10: 50% of normal dose every 8-12 hours	Moderately dialyzed
Ceftriaxone	40%-67% renal excretion 40% hepatic metabolism	Creatinine clearance 10-50: no change Creatinine clearance <10: decrease dose only with hepatic failure	Questionably dialyzed
Cefoxitin	78%-99% renal excretion	Creatinine clearance 10-50: 50%-100% of normal dose every 12-24 hours Creatinine clearance <10: 25% of normal dose every 24 hours	Moderately dialyzed
Ceftazidime	>85% renal excretion	Creatinine clearance 10-50: 50% of normal dose every 6-8 hours Creatinine clearance <10: 25% of normal dose every 12-24 hours	Dialyzed
Ciprofloxacin	62% renal excretion 38% hepatic metabolism	Creatinine clearance 10-50: 75% of normal dose every 12 hours Creatinine clearance <10: 50%-75% of normal dose every 24 hours	Slightly dialyzed
Cefotetan	50%-89% renal excretion 12% hepatic metabolism	Creatinine clearance 10-50: 50%-100% of normal dose every 12-24 hours Creatinine clearance <10: 25%-50% of normal dose every 24 hours	Moderately dialyzed
Erythromycin	5%-15% renal excretion 85%-95% hepatic metabolism	No change	Slightly dialyzed
Gentamycin†	90%-97% renal excretion		Dialyzed
Imipenem	60%-75% renal excretion 22% hepatic metabolism	Creatinine clearance 10-50: 50%-75% of normal dose every 8-12 hours Creatinine clearance <10: 25%-50% of normal dose every 12 hours	Moderately dialyzed
Mezlocillin	45%-65% renal excretion 35%-55% hepatic metabolism	Creatinine clearance 10-50: 100% of normal dose every 6-8 hours Creatinine clearance <10: 50% of normal dose every 8 hours	Slightly dialyzed

Modified from Bubp JL, Rodondi LC, Gamberloglio JG: Renal dialysis. In Koda-Kimble MA, Young LY, editors: *Applied therapeutics: the clinical use of drugs,* ed 5, Vancouver, Wash, 1992, Applied Therapeutics; and Aweeka FT: Drug dosing in renal failure. In Koda-Kimble MA, Young LY: *Applied therapeutics: the clinical use of drugs,* ed 5, Vancouver, Wash, 1992, Applied Therapeutics.

*The degree of renal failure is assessed by the creatinine clearance. Normal creatinine clearance is 120 ml/minute; it decreases in renal failure. In renal failure, drug dosages are reduced either by decreasing the amount of drug administered each dose, lengthening the time between doses, or both.

†Aminoglycosides (amikacin, gentamycin, and tobramycin): these drugs have a narrow therapeutic window, which means that the range between the therapeutic level and the toxic level is small, and they require close monitoring. In addition, drug clearance is affected by multiple factors. Refer to a pharmacist or pharmacokinetic text for recommendations.

TABLE 19-7

IMPACT OF RENAL FAILURE AND HEMODIALYSIS ON SELECTED DRUGS—cont'd

DRUG	NORMAL DRUG METABOLISM AND EXCRETION	PERCENT OF NORMAL DOSE ADJUSTMENT IN RENAL FAILURE CAUSED BY DECREASED CREATININE CLEARANCE (ml/minute)*	EFFECT OF HEMODIALYSIS
ANTIINFECTIVES—cont'd			
Antibiotics—cont'd			
Nafcillin	25%-30% renal excretion Up to 70% hepatic metabolism	No change	Not dialyzed
Penicillin‡	50% renal excretion 19% hepatic metabolism		Moderately dialyzed
Piperacillin	50%-60% renal excretion Up to 30%-40% hepatic metabolism	Creatinine clearance 10-50: 100% of normal dose every 6-8 hours Creatinine clearance <10: 50%-75% of normal dose every 8 hours	Moderately dialyzed
Sulfamethoxazole	10% renal excretion 65%-80% hepatic metabolism	Creatinine clearance 10-50: 100% of normal dose every 12-24 hours Creatinine clearance <10: 100% of normal dose every 24 hours	Slightly dialyzed
Tobramycin†	90%-97% renal excretion		Dialyzed
Trimethoprim	20%-35% renal excretion 53%-80% hepatic metabolism	Creatinine clearance 10-50: 100% of normal dose every 12-24 hours Creatinine clearance <10: 100% of normal dose every 24 hours	Slightly dialyzed
Vancomycin	80%-90% renal excretion 10%-20% hepatic metabolism	Requires individualized dosing regimens	Not dialyzed
Antifungals			
Amphotericin B	3%-5% renal excretion 95%-97% hepatic metabolism	Creatinine clearance 10-50: 100% of normal dose every 24 hours Creatinine clearance <10: 100% of normal dose every 24-48 hours	Not dialyzed
Fluconazole	70% renal excretion Some hepatic metabolism	Creatinine clearance 10-50: 50% of normal dose every 24 hours Creatinine clearance <10: 25% of normal dose every 24 hours	Moderately dialyzed
Ketoconazole	3% renal excretion 51% hepatic metabolism	No change	Not dialyzed
Antivirals			
Acyclovir	70%-80% renal excretion 14% hepatic metabolism	Creatinine clearance 10-50: 100% of normal dose every 12-24 hours Creatinine clearance <10: 50% of normal dose every 24 hours	Dialyzed
Gancyclovir	>90% renal excretion	Creatinine clearance 10-50: 1.25-2.5 mg/kg every 24 hours Creatinine clearance <10: 1.25 mg/kg every 24 hours	Dialyzed
CARDIOVASCULAR DRUGS			
Beta-blockers			
Atenolol	75% renal excretion 10% hepatic metabolism	Creatinine clearance <50: 50% dose reduction and titrate as needed	Moderately dialyzed
Labetalol	5% renal excretion 95% hepatic excretion	No change	Not dialyzed

‡Penicillin G: methods have been developed to calculate dosage based on changes in creatinine clearance. However, none of these methods have been subjected to careful clinical trials. Other factors can also affect patients' responses to therapy. Refer to a pharmacist or pharmacokinetic text for recommendations. *Continued*

TABLE 19-7

IMPACT OF RENAL FAILURE AND HEMODIALYSIS ON SELECTED DRUGS—cont'd

DRUG	NORMAL DRUG METABOLISM AND EXCRETION	PERCENT OF NORMAL DOSE ADJUSTMENT IN RENAL FAILURE CAUSED BY DECREASED CREATININE CLEARANCE (ml/minute)*	EFFECT OF HEMODIALYSIS
CARDIOVASCULAR DRUGS—cont'd			
Beta-blockers			
Metoprolol	10% renal excretion 90% hepatic metabolism	No change	Metabolites dialyzed
Nadolol	75% renal excretion 25% hepatic metabolism	Creatinine clearance <50: 50% dose reduction and titrate as needed	Moderately dialyzed
Propranolol	<1% renal excretion Primarily hepatic metabolism	No change	Not dialyzed
ACE inhibitors			
Captopril	36%-42% renal excretion 50% hepatic metabolism	Creatinine clearance 10-50: No change Creatinine clearance <10: 25% dose reduction and titrate as needed	Moderately dialyzed
Enalapril	61% renal excretion 33% hepatic metabolism	Creatinine clearance <50: 50% dose reduction and titrate as needed	Moderately dialyzed
Calcium channel blockers			
Nifedipine	100% hepatic metabolism	No change	Not known
Verapamil	100% hepatic metabolism	No change	Not dialyzed
Antidysrhythmics			
Digoxin	70% renal excretion	Creatinine clearance 10-50: 50% dose reduction and titrate as needed Creatinine clearance <10: 75% dose reduction and titrate as needed	Moderately dialyzed
Lidocaine	100% hepatic metabolism	No change	Not dialyzed
Procainamide	50%-60% renal excretion Hepatic metabolism to active NAPA metabolite	Creatinine clearance 10-50: 100% of normal dose every 6-12 hours Creatinine clearance <10: 100% of normal dose every 12-24 hours	Moderately dialyzed
ANALGESICS			
Codeine	Hepatic metabolism	Creatinine clearance 10-50: 25% of normal dose and titrate as needed Creatinine clearance <10: 50% of normal dose and titrate as needed	Not known
Ibuprofen	45%-60% excreted unchanged and as metabolites	No change	Not dialyzed
Meperidine	10% renal excretion Hepatic metabolism	Creatinine clearance 10-50: 75%-100% of normal dose every 6 hours Creatinine clearance <10: 50% of normal dose every 6-8 hours and use with caution	Not known
ANTICONVULSANTS/SEDATIVES			
Anticonvulsants			
Phenobarbital	10%-40% renal excretion Hepatic metabolism	Creatinine clearance 10-50: No change Creatinine clearance <10: Slight dosage decrease	Moderately dialyzed
Phenytoin	Hepatic metabolism	No change	Not dialyzed
Sedatives			
Diazepam	Renal excretion of active metabolites Hepatic metabolism	Reduction of dose and titration as needed Not known	Not dialyzed
Midazolam	Not known		
H₂ BLOCKERS			
Cimetidine	40%-80% renal excretion	Creatinine clearance 10-50: 25% dose reduction Creatinine clearance <10: 50% dose reduction	Slightly dialyzed
Famotidine	Significant renal excretion Small hepatic metabolism	Creatinine clearance <10: 100% of normal dose every 24-48 hours	
Ranitidine	70% renal excretion	Creatinine clearance 10-50: 25% dose reduction	Slightly dialyzed

Modified from Bubp JL, Rodondi LC, Gamberloglio JG: Renal dialysis. In Koda-Kimble MA, Young LY, editors: *Applied therapeutics: the clinical use of drugs*, ed 5, Vancouver, Wash, 1992, Applied Therapeutics; and Aweeka FT: Drug dosing in renal failure. In Koda-Kimble MA, Young LY: *Applied therapeutics: the clinical use of drugs*, ed 5, Vancouver, Wash, 1992, Applied Therapeutics.
NAPA, N-acetylprocainamide.

References

1. Douglas S: Acute tubular necrosis: diagnosis, treatment and nursing implications, *AACN Clin Issues Crit Care Nurs* 3(3):688, 1992.
2. Kjellstrand C, Barsoum R: Management of acute renal failure. In Jacobson H, Sinker G, Klohr S, editors: *The principles and practice of nephrology,* ed 2, St Louis, 1995, Mosby.
3. Baer C, Lancaster LE: Acute renal failure, *Crit Care Nurs Q* 14(4):1, 1992.
4. Lancaster LE: Renal response to shock, *Crit Care Nurs Clin North Am* 2(2):221, 1990.
5. Stark J: Acute renal failure: focus on advances in acute tubular necrosis, *Crit Care Clin N Am* 10(2):159-170, 1998.
6. *St. Anthony's DRG guidebook* 1996, Reston, Va, 1996, St. Anthony Hospital.
7. Brady H, Singer G: Acute renal failure, *Lancet* 346:1533, 1995.
8. Cheney P: Early management and physiologic changes in crush syndrome, *Crit Care Nurs Q* 17(2):62, 1994.
9. Toto K: Acute renal failure: a question of location, *Am J Nurs* 92(11):44, 1992.
10. Tisher C, Wilcox C, editors: *Nephrology for the house officer,* ed 2, Baltimore, 1993, Williams & Wilkins.
11. Stark JL: Acute tubular necrosis: differences between oliguria and nonoliguria, *Crit Care Nurs Q* 14(4):22, 1992.
12. Brundage D, editor: *Renal disorders,* St Louis, 1995, Mosby.
13. Braxmeyer DL, Keyes JL: The pathophysiology of potassium balance, *Crit Care Nurs* 16(5):59, 1995.
14. Innerarity SA: Electrolyte emergency in the critically ill renal patient, *Crit Care Nurs Clin North Am* 2(1):89, 1990.
15. Cluitman FH: Management of severe hypernatremia: rapid or slow corrections, *Am J Med* 88:161, 1990.
16. Price CA: Continuous renal replacement therapy: the treatment of choice for acute renal failure, *ANNA J* 18(3):239, 1992.
17. Gutch C, Stoner M, Corea A: *Review of hemodialysis for nurses and dialysis personnel,* ed 5, St Louis, 1993, Mosby.
18. Pechman P: Acute hemodialysis: issues in critical illness, *AACN Clin Issues Crit Care Nurs* 3(3):545, 1992.
19. Politoski G, et al: Continuous renal replacement: a natural perspective, *AACN/NKF Crit Care Clin North Am* 10(2):171-177, 1998.
20. Bosworth C: SCUF/CAVH/CAVHD. Critical differences, *Crit Care Nurs Q* 14(4):45-55, 1992.
21. Price CA: An update on continuous renal replacement therapies, *AACN Clin Issues Crit Care Nurs* 3(3):597, 1992.
22. Forni LG, Hilton PJ: Continuous hemofiltration in the treatment of acute renal failure, *N Engl J Med* 336(18):1303-1309, 1997.
23. Bonaventure J: Mechanisms of ischemic acute renal failure, *Kidney Int* 43:1160, 1993.
24. Higley RR: Continuous arteriovenous hemofiltration; a case study, *Crit Care Nurs* 16(5):37, 1996.
25. Headrick C: Adult/pediatric CVVH: the pump, the patient, the circuit, *Crit Care Clin North Am* 10(2):197-207, 1998.
26. Smith LJ: Peritoneal dialysis in the critically ill, *AACN Clin Issues Crit Care Nurs* 3(3):558, 1992.
27. Graham-Macaluso M: Complications of peritoneal dialysis: nursing care plans to document teaching, *ANNA J* 18(5):479, 1991.

GASTROINTESTINAL ALTERATIONS

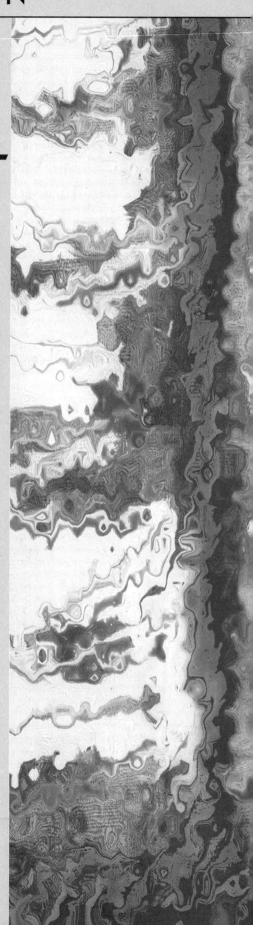

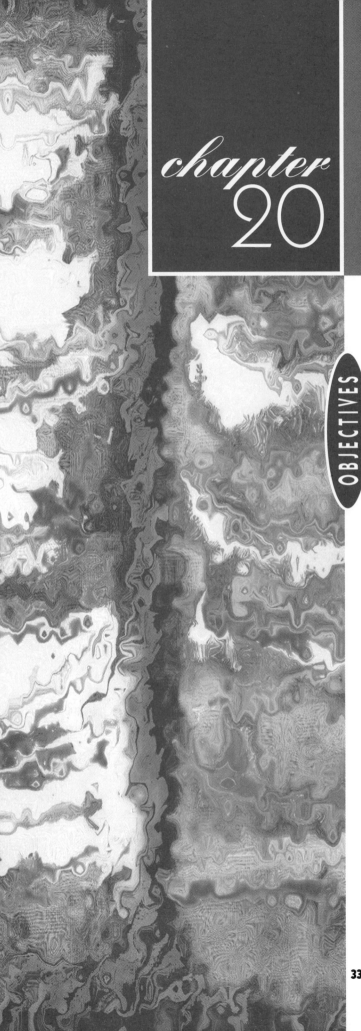

chapter 20

Gastrointestinal Assessment and Diagnostic Procedures

Nancy McLaughlin

OBJECTIVES

● Identify the components of a gastrointestinal history.

● Describe inspection, palpation, percussion, and auscultation of the patient with gastrointestinal dysfunction.

● Delineate the clinical significance of selected laboratory tests used in the assessment of gastrointestinal disorders.

● Identity key diagnostic procedures used in assessment of the patient with gastrointestinal dysfunction.

● Discuss the nursing management of a patient undergoing a gastrointestinal diagnostic procedure.

Assessment of the critically ill patient with gastrointestinal (GI) dysfunction includes a review of the patient's health history, a thorough physical examination, and an analysis of the patient's laboratory data. Numerous invasive and noninvasive diagnostic procedures may also be performed to assist in the identification of the patient's disorder. This chapter focuses on priority clinical assessments, laboratory studies, and diagnostic tests for the critically ill patient with gastrointestinal dysfunction.

CLINICAL ASSESSMENT

A thorough clinical assessment of the patient with GI dysfunction is imperative for the early identification and treatment of GI disorders. Once completed, the assessment serves as the foundation for developing the management plan for the patient. The assessment process can be brief or can involve a detailed history and examination, depending on the nature and immediacy of the patient's situation.[1]

HISTORY

Taking a thorough and accurate history is extremely important to the assessment process. The patient's history provides the foundation and direction for the rest of the assessment. The overall goal of the patient interview is to expose key clinical manifestations that will facilitate the identification of the underlying cause of the illness. This information will then assist in the development of an appropriate management plan.[2]

The initial presentation of the patient determines the rapidity and direction of the interview. For a patient in acute distress, the history should be curtailed to just a few questions about the patient's chief complaint and precipitating events. For a patient in no obvious distress, the history focuses on four different areas: (1) review of the patient's present illness, (2) overview of the patient's general gastrointestinal status including previous GI diagnostic studies or interventional procedures, (3) examination of the patient's personal and social history including dietary habits, nutritional status, bowel characteristics (stool descriptions), alcohol intake, and dependence on laxatives or enemas, and (4) survey of the patient's family history including metabolic disorders, malabsorption syndromes, and cancer of the GI tract.[3,4]

PHYSICAL EXAMINATION

The physical assessment helps establish baseline data about the physical dimensions of the patient's situation. The physical examination helps establish baseline data about the physical dimensions of the patient's situation.[3] The abdomen is divided into four quadrants (left upper, right upper, left lower, and right lower), with the umbilicus as the middle point, to facilitate the identification of the location of examination findings (Fig. 20-1 and Box 20-1). The assessment proceeds when the patient is as comfortable as possible and in the supine position; however, the position may need readjustment if it elicits pain. To prevent stimulation of GI activity, the order for the assessment should be changed to inspection, auscultation, percussion, and palpation.[4]

Inspection

Inspection should be performed in a warm, well-lighted environment with the patient in a comfortable position with the abdomen exposed. Although assessment of the GI system classically begins with inspection of the abdomen, the patient's oral cavity also must be inspected to determine any unusual findings. Abnormal findings of the mouth include joint tenderness, inflammation of the gums, missing teeth, dental caries, ill-fitting dentures, and mouth odor.[5]

The skin is observed for pigmentation, lesions, striae, scars, petechiae, signs of dehydration, and venous pat-

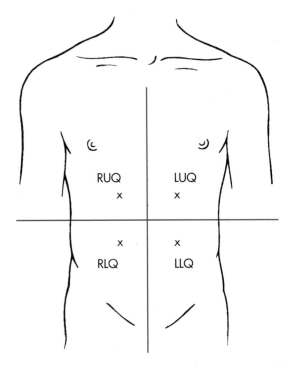

Fig. **20-1** Four quadrants of the abdomen. *RUQ,* right upper quadrant; *LUQ,* left upper quadrant; *RLQ,* right lower quadrant; *LLQ,* left upper quadrant. (From Barkauskas V, et al: *Health and physical assessment,* ed 2, St Louis, 1998, Mosby.)

BOX 20-1

ANATOMIC CORRELATES OF THE FOUR QUADRANTS OF THE ABDOMEN

RIGHT UPPER QUADRANT

Liver and gallbladder
Pylorus
Duodenum
Head of pancreas
Right adrenal gland
Portion of right kidney
Hepatic flexure of colon
Portions of ascending
 and transverse colon

LEFT UPPER QUADRANT

Left lobe of liver
Spleen
Stomach
Body of pancreas
Left adrenal gland
Portion of left kidney
Splenic flexure of colon
Portions of transverse
 and descending colon

RIGHT LOWER QUADRANT

Lower pole of right
 kidney
Cecum and appendix
Portion of ascending
 colon
Bladder (if distended)
Ovary and salpinx
Uterus (if enlarged)
Right spermatic cord
Right ureter

LEFT LOWER QUADRANT

Lower pole of left kidney
Sigmoid colon
Portion of descending
 colon
Bladder (if distended)
Ovary and salpinx
Uterus (if enlarged)
Left spermatic cord
Left ureter

From Malasanos L, Barkauskas V, Stoltenberg-Allen K: *Health assessment,* ed 4, St Louis, 1990, Mosby.

tern. Pigmentation may vary considerably within normal range because of race and ethnic background, although the abdomen is generally lighter in color than other, exposed areas of the skin. Abnormal findings include jaundice, skin lesions, and a tense and glistening appearance of the skin. Old striae (stretch marks) are generally silver in color, while pink purple striae may be indicative of Cushing's syndrome.[4] A bluish discoloration of the umbilicus (Cullen's sign) or of the flank (Turner's sign) is indicative of intraperitoneal bleeding.[1]

The abdomen is observed for contour (noting if it is flat, slightly concave, or slightly round), for symmetry, and for movement. Marked distention is an abnormal finding. In particular, ascites may cause generalized distention and bulging flanks. Asymmetric distention may be indicative of organ enlargement or a mass. Peristaltic waves should not be visible except in very thin patients. In the case of intestinal obstruction, hyperactive peristaltic waves may be noted. Pulsation in the epigastric area is frequently a normal finding, but increased pulsation may be indicative of an aortic aneurysm. Symmetric movement of the abdomen with respirations is usually seen in men.[4,5]

Auscultation

Auscultation of patients is focused on two priorities: bowel sounds and presence of bruits. Auscultation of the abdomen provides clinical data regarding the status of the motility of the bowel. Initially, the examiner must listen with the diaphragm of the stethoscope below and to the right of the umbilicus. Proceeding methodically through all four quadrants, the examiner lifts and places the diaphragm of the stethoscope lightly against the abdomen. Normal bowel sounds include high-pitched, gurgling sounds that occur approximately every 5 to 15 seconds or at a rate of 5 to 34 times each minute. Colonic sounds are low pitched and have a rumbling quality. A venous hum may also be audible at times.[6] See Table 20-1 for list of abnormal abdominal sounds.

Abnormal findings include the absence of bowel sounds throughout a 5-minute period, extremely soft and widely separated sounds, and increased sounds with a high-pitched, loud rushing sound (peristaltic rush). Absent bowel sounds may occur as a result of inflammation, ileus, electrolyte disturbances, and ischemia. Bowel sounds may be increased with diarrhea and early intestinal obstruction.[6] The abdomen should also be auscultated for the presence of bruits using the bell of the stethoscope. Bruits are created by turbulent flow over a partially obstructed artery and are always considered an abnormal finding. The aorta, right and left renal arteries, and iliac arteries should be auscultated.[5,6]

Percussion

Percussion of patients is focused on one priority: the abdomen. Percussion is used to elicit information about deep organs, such as the liver, spleen, and pancreas. As the abdomen is a sensitive area, muscle tension may interfere with this part of the assessment. Because percussion often helps relax tense muscles, it is performed before palpation. Percussion, in the absence of disease, is most helpful in delineating the position and size of the liver and spleen, and it also assists in the detection of fluid, gaseous distention, and masses in the abdomen.[5]

Percussion should proceed systemically and lightly in all four quadrants. Normal findings include tympany over the stomach when empty, tympany or hyperreso-

TABLE **20-1**	
ABNORMAL ABDOMINAL SOUNDS	
SOUND	**CAUSE**
Hyperactive bowel sounds (borborygmi) Loud and prolonged	Hunger, gastroenteritis, or early intestinal obstruction
High-pitched, tinkling sounds	Intestinal air and fluid under pressure; characteristic of early intestinal obstruction
Decreased (hypoactive) bowel sounds Infrequent and abnormally faint	Possible peritonitis or ileus
Absence of bowel sounds (confirmed only after auscultation of all four quadrants and continuous auscultation for 5 min)	Temporary loss of intestinal motility, as occurs with complete ileus
Friction rubs High-pitched sounds heard over liver and spleen (RUQ and LUQ), synchronous with respiration	Pathologic conditions such as tumors or infection that cause inflammation of organ's peritoneal covering
Bruits Audible swishing sounds that may be heard over aortic, iliac, renal, and femoral arteries	Abnormality of blood flow (requires additional evaluation to determine specific disorder)
Venous hum Low-pitched, continuous sound	Increased collateral circulation between portal and systemic venous systems

From Doughty DB, Jackson DB: *Gastrointestinal disorders*, St Louis, 1993, Mosby.

TABLE 20-2

SELECTED LABORATORY STUDIES OF GI FUNCTION

TEST	NORMAL FINDINGS	CLINICAL SIGNIFICANCE OF ABNORMAL FINDINGS
Stool studies	Resident microorganisms: clostridia, enterococci, *Pseudomonas*, a few yeasts	Detection of *Salmonella typhi* (typhoid fever), *Shigella* (dysentery), *Vibrio cholerae* (cholera), *Yersinia* (enterocolitis), *Escherichia coli* (gastroenteritis), *Staphylococcus aureus* (food poisoning), *Clostridium botulinum* (food poisoning), *Clostridium perfringens* (food poisoning), *Aeromonas* (gastroenteritis)
	Fat: 2-6 g/24 hr	Steatorrhea (increased values) can result from intestinal malabsorption or pancreatic insufficiency
	Pus: none	Large amounts of pus are associated with chronic ulcerative colitis, abscesses, and anal-rectal fistula
	Occult blood: none (Ortho-Tolidin or guaiac test)	Positive tests associated with bleeding
	Ova and parasites: none	Detection of *Entamoeba histolytica* (amebiasis), *Giardia lamblia* (giardiasis), and worms
D-Xylose absorption	5-hr urinary excretion: r4.5 g/L Peak blood level: >30 mg/dL	Differentiation of pancreatic steatorrhea (normal D-xylose absorption) from intestinal steatorrhea (impaired D-xylose absorption)
Gastric acid stimulation	11-20 mEq/hr after stimulation	Detection of duodenal ulcers, Zollinger-Ellison syndrome (increased values), gastric atrophy, gastric carcinoma (decreased values)
Manometry (use of water-filled catheters connected to pressure transducers passed into the esophagus, stomach, colon, or rectum to evaluate contractility)	Values vary at different levels of the intestine	Inadequate swallowing, motility, sphincter function
Culture and sensitivity of duodenal contents	No pathogens	Detection of *Salmonella typhi* (typhoid fever)

From McCance KL, Huether SE: *Pathophysiology: the biologic basis for disease in adults and children,* ed 3, St Louis, 1998, Mosby.

nance over the intestine, and dullness over the liver and spleen. Abnormal areas of dullness may indicate an underlying mass. Solid masses, enlarged organs, and a distended bladder also produce areas of dullness. Dullness over both flanks may be indicative of ascites and requires further assessment.[6]

Palpation

Palpation of patients is focused on two priorities: light and deep palpation of the abdominal area. Palpation is the assessment technique most useful in detecting abdominal pathologic conditions. Both light and deep palpation of each organ and quadrant should be completed. Light palpation assesses the depth of skin and fascia, which has a depth of palpation of approximately 1 cm. Deep palpation assesses the rectus abdominis muscle and is performed bimanually to a depth of 4 to 5 cm. Deep palpation is most helpful in detecting abdominal masses. Areas in which the patient complains of tenderness should be palpated last.[6]

Normal findings include no areas of tenderness or pain, no masses, and no hardened areas. Persistent invol-

untary guarding may indicate peritoneal inflammation, particularly if it continues even after relaxation techniques are used. Rebound tenderness, in which pain increases with quick release of palpated area, is indicative of an inflamed peritoneum.[4]

LABORATORY STUDIES

The value of various laboratory studies used to diagnose and treat diseases of the GI system has often been emphasized. No single study, however, provides an overall picture of the various organs' functional state. Also, no single value is predictive by itself. More than 100 laboratory studies have been proposed for the study of the GI system.[7] Laboratory studies used in the assessment of GI function, liver function, and pancreatic function are found in Tables 20-2, 20-3, and 20-4, respectively.

DIAGNOSTIC PROCEDURES

Table 20-5 presents an overview of the various diagnostic procedures used to evaluate the patient with GI dysfunction.[4,8-18]

TABLE 20-3

COMMON LABORATORY STUDIES OF LIVER FUNCTION

TEST	NORMAL VALUE	INTERPRETATION
SERUM ENZYMES		
Alkaline phosphatase	13-39 U/ml	Increases with biliary obstruction and cholestatic hepatitis
Aspartate amino transferase (AST; previously SGOT)	5-40 U/ml	Increases with hepatocellular injury
Alanine amino transferase (ALT; previously SGPT)	5-35 U/ml	Increases with hepatocellular injury
Lactate dehydrogenase (LDH)	200-500 U/ml	Isoenzyme LD_5 is elevated with hypoxic and primary liver injury
5'-Nucleotidase	2-11 U/ml	Increases with increase in alkaline phosphatase and cholestatic disorders
BILIRUBIN METABOLISM		
Serum bilirubin		
Indirect (unconjugated)	<0.8 mg/dL	Increases with hemolysis (lysis of red blood cells)
Direct (conjugated)	0.2-0.4 mg/dL	Increases with hepatocellular injury or obstruction
Total	<1.0 mg/dL	Increases with biliary obstruction
Urine bilirubin	0	Decreases with biliary obstruction
Urine urobilinogen	0-4 mg/24 hr	Increases with hemolysis or shunting of portal blood flow
SERUM PROTEINS		
Albumin	3.5-5.5 g/dL	Reduced with hepatocellular injury
Globulin	2.5-3.5 g/dL	Increases with hepatitis
Total	6-7 g/dL	
A/G ratio	1.5:1-2.5:1	Ratio reverses with chronic hepatitis or other chronic liver disease
Transferrin	250-300 µg/dL	Liver damage with decreased values, iron deficiency with increased values
Alpha-fetoprotein	6-20 ng/ml	Elevated values in primary hepatocellular carcinoma
BLOOD CLOTTING FUNCTIONS		
Prothrombin time	11.5-14 sec or 90%-100% of control	Increases with chronic liver disease (cirrhosis) or vitamin K deficiency
Partial thromboplastin time	25-40 sec	Increases with severe liver disease or heparin therapy
Bromsulphalein (BSP) excretion	<6% retention in 45 min	Increased retention with hepatocellular injury

From McCance KL, Huether SE: *Pathophysiology: the biologic basis for disease in adults and children,* ed 3, St Louis, 1998, Mosby.

TABLE 20-4

COMMON LABORATORY STUDIES OF PANCREATIC FUNCTION

TEST	NORMAL VALUE	CLINICAL SIGNIFICANCE
Serum amylase	60-180 Somogyi units/ml	Elevated levels with pancreatic inflammation
Serum lipase	1.5 Somogyi units/ml	Elevated levels with pancreatic inflammation (may be elevated with other conditions; differentiates with amylase, isoenzyme study)
Urine amylase	35-260 Somogyi units/hr	Elevated levels with pancreatic inflammation
Secretin test	Volume 2-5 g/24 hr; Bicarbonate concentration: >80 mEq/L; Bicarbonate output: >10 mEq/L/30 sec	Decreased volume with pancreatic disease as secretin stimulates pancreatic secretion
Stool fat	2-5 g/24 hr	Measures fatty acids; decreased pancreatic lipase increases stool fat

From McCance KL, Huether SE: *Pathophysiology: the biologic basis for disease in adults and children,* ed 3, St Louis, 1998, Mosby.

TABLE 20-5

GASTROINTESTINAL DIAGNOSTIC PROCEDURES

PROCEDURE	EVALUATES	COMMENTS
Barium enema (also called *lower GI series*) (Note: meglumine diatrizoate [Gastrografin] may be used, especially if bowel perforation is suspected)	• Visualizes the movement, position, and filling of various segments of the colon after instillation of barium by enema • Diagnoses colorectal lesions, diverticulitis, inflammatory bowel disease, strictures, fistulas • Evaluates colon size, length, and patency	• Low fiber diet for 1 to 3 days before procedure • Bowel preparation with bowel irrigation (e.g., GoLYTELY) and cathartics • NPO for 8 to 12 hours before procedure • Necessary for cathartics to be given after procedure • Contraindicated if bowel perforation or obstruction exists
Barium swallow, upper GI series, and small bowel follow-through (Note: ordered according to which area or areas need to be evaluated—e.g., upper GI with small bowel follow-through means stomach, pylorus, duodenum; barium swallow with upper GI means esophagus, stomach, pylorus) (Note: meglumine diatrizoate [Gastrografin] may be used especially if bowel perforation is suspected)	• Visualizes the position, shape, and activity of the esophagus, stomach, duodenum, and jejunum • Diagnoses esophageal lesions, varices, or esophageal motility disorders; hiatal hernia, gastric ulcers and tumors, small bowel obstruction, small bowel lesions, and Crohn's disease • Evaluates gastric and small bowel motility	• Bowel preparation with bowel irrigation (e.g., GoLYTELY) and cathartics • NPO for 8 to 12 hours before procedure • Necessary for cathartics to be given after procedure • Contraindicated if bowel perforation or obstruction exists
Celiac or mesenteric arteriography	• Evaluates portal vasculature • Diagnoses source of gastrointestinal bleeding • Evaluates cirrhosis, portal hypertension, vascular damage resulting from trauma, intestinal ischemia, tumors • May be used to treat GI bleeding using vasopressin	• Bowel preparation (e.g., cathartics) as prescribed • NPO for 8 hours before procedure • Sedative usually prescribed before procedure • Contrast media used • Check for allergy to iodine before procedure • Monitor for allergic reaction postprocedure • Ensure hydration postprocedure • Postprocedure • Keep extremity in which catheter was placed immobilized in a straight position for 6 to 12 hours • Monitor arterial puncture point for hemorrhage or hematoma • Monitor neurovascular status of affected limb • Monitor for indications of systemic emboli
Cholecystography (oral, intravenous, percutaneous transhepatic, or common bile duct)	• Assesses gallbladder function, patency of the biliary system, and presence of gallstones • Diagnoses extrahepatic or intrahepatic jaundice, biliary calculi, biliary obstruction, common bile duct injury	• Percutaneous transhepatic cholangiography contraindicated in patients with bleeding disorders • Fatty meal the day before procedure but fat-free evening meal • Enema given the evening before procedure • NPO 8 to 12 hours before procedure

From Dennison RD: *Pass CCRN!*, St Louis, 1996, Mosby.

TABLE 20-5

GASTROINTESTINAL DIAGNOSTIC PROCEDURES—cont'd

PROCEDURE	EVALUATES	COMMENTS

		• Contrast medium administered orally the evening before the procedure, administered intravenously immediately before the procedure, injected percutaneously into the bile duct or injected directly into the common bile duct during surgery
		  • Check for allergy to iodine before procedure
		  • Monitor for allergic reaction postprocedure
		  • Ensure hydration postprocedure
		• Necessary to monitor for clinical indications of bile leakage, hemorrhage, or peritonitis after percutaneous transhepatic cholangiography

Computed tomographic (CT) scan of abdomen	• Diagnoses tumors, pancreatic cancer or cysts, pancreatitis, biliary tract disorders, obstructive versus nonobstructive jaundice, cirrhosis, liver metastases, ascites, lymph node metastases, aneurysm
	• Evaluates vasculature and focal points found on nuclear scans
	• Used to direct biopsy of tumors or aspiration of abscess
		• No special preparation required
		• If contrast medium used:
		  • Check for allergy to iodine before procedure
		  • Monitor for allergic reaction postprocedure
		  • Ensure hydration postprocedure

Endoscopic retrograde cholangiopancreatography (ERCP)	• Diagnoses biliary stones, ductal stricture, ductal compression, neoplasms of the pancreas and biliary system • Evaluates patency of biliary and pancreatic ducts, jaundice, pancreatitis, cholecystitis, hepatitis	• Same as for esophagogastroduodenoscopy • Contraindicated if patient uncooperative or if bilirubin >3.5 mg/dl; acute pancreatitis • Necessary to monitor for clinical indications of pancreatitis (most common complication) after study • Necessary to monitor for clinical indications of sepsis
Endoscopy • Esophagogastroduodenoscopy • Colonoscopy • Proctosigmoidoscopy	• Directly visualizes mucosa of areas of the GI tract • Esophagogastroduodenoscopy extended to visualize the pancreas and gallbladder • Esophagogastroduodenoscopy used to diagnose esophagitis, esophageal ulcers, esophageal strictures, esophageal varices, hiatal hernia, gastritis, gastric ulcers, pyloric obstruction, pernicious anemia, foreign bodies, duodenal inflammation or ulcers and to evaluate esophageal or gastric motility, bleeding, lesions, status of surgical anastomoses • Esophagoscopy, gastroscopy also used therapeutically for sclerosis of varices • Proctosigmoidoscopy used to diagnose rectosigmoid cancer, strictures, polyps, inflammatory processes, hemorrhoids and evaluate bleeding from rectosigmoid, surgical anastomoses • Colonoscopy used to diagnose diverticular disease, obstruction, strictures, radiation injury, polyps, neoplasms, bleeding, ischemia • Colonoscopy or sigmoidoscopy used therapeutically for removal of polyps • Biopsies taken during any endoscopy	• Sedation sometimes prescribed, especially for colonoscopy • Bowel preparation with gastric irrigation (e.g., GoLYTELY) and cathartics required before lower GI endoscopy • NPO 4 to 8 hours before study • If sedation used, NPO maintained until gag reflex returns • Close monitoring after procedure for clinical indications of perforation, hemorrhage

Continued

TABLE 20-5		

GASTROINTESTINAL DIAGNOSTIC PROCEDURES—cont'd

PROCEDURE	EVALUATES	COMMENTS
Flat plate of abdomen	• Diagnoses perforated viscus, paralytic ileus, mechanical obstruction, intraabdominal mass • Evaluates the distribution of visceral gas (and identifies free air in the peritoneum indicative of bowel perforation) • Evaluates organ size	• No preparation required

Liver biopsy	• Obtains tissue specimen for microscopic evaluation
	• Diagnoses liver disease or malignancy
		• May be performed open or closed
		  • Open biopsy is done in surgery
		  • Closed biopsy may be done at bedside
		• Clotting profile evaluated preprocedure
		  • Closed biopsy is contraindicated if platelet count is <100,000/mm^3
		• Requires cooperative patient who will take a deep breath and hold for closed biopsy
		• Necessary to type and crossmatch for 2 units of blood preprocedure
		• NPO for 4 to 8 hours before procedure
		Postprocedure
		• Patient positioned on right side for 2 hours
		• Pressure dressing applied; patient on bed rest for 24 hours
		• Observe for
		  • Hemorrhage: hypotension, dyspnea (subphrenic hematoma)
		  • Pneumothorax: dyspnea, chest pain, diminished breath sounds on right, hypoxemia
		  • Sepsis: fever, leukocytosis

Liver scan	• Diagnoses cirrhosis, hepatitis, tumors, abscesses, cysts, tuberculosis	• No preparation required
Magnetic resonance imaging (MRI)	• Evaluates liver, biliary tree, pancreas, spleen • Differentiates between cyst and solid mass • Diagnoses hepatic metastasis • Evaluates abscesses, fistulas, source of GI bleeding • Used for staging of colorectal cancer	• Cannot be used in patients with any implanted metallic device, including pacemakers • No special preparation required • Cannot be done on a patient being mechanically ventilated
Paracentesis	• Analyzes fluid removed during peritoneal tap • Diagnoses intraperitoneal bleeding with diagnostic peritoneal lavage	• Necessary to monitor for peritoneal leakage after paracentesis • Necessary to monitor for clinical indications of infection or peritonitis after paracentesis
Percutaneous transhepatic portography	• Diagnoses esophageal varices and visualizes portal venous circulation	• As for arteriogram
Radionuclide imaging (hepatobiliary scintigraphy) • HIDA scan • PIPIDA scan	• Diagnoses hepatocellular disease, hepatic metastasis, biliary disease, lower GI bleeding, gastric reflux	• NPO 2 hours before procedure
Schilling's test	• Evaluates ileal absorption of vitamin B$_{12}$ • Diagnoses pernicious anemia caused by intrinsic factor deficiency and inadequate ileal absorption of intrinsic factor-vitamin B$_{12}$ complex	• IM vitamin B$_{12}$ and oral radioactive vitamin B$_{12}$ administered; 24-hour urine specimen collected
Ultrasound of abdomen	• Evaluates the pancreas, biliary ducts, gallbladder, liver • Diagnoses stage of rectal cancer, abdominal abscesses, hepatocellular disease, splenomegaly, pancreatic or splenic cysts • Differentiates obstructive from nonobstructive jaundice	• Necessary to clear all barium from the GI tract before ultrasonography • NPO for 8 hours before procedure • If for evaluation of gallbladder: fat-free meal the evening before procedure

From Dennison RD: *Pass CCRN!*, St Louis, 1996, Mosby.

Nursing Management

The nursing management of a patient undergoing a diagnostic procedure involves a variety of interventions. **Priorities are directed toward preparing the patient psychologically and physically for the procedure, monitoring the patient's responses to the procedure, and assessing the patient after the procedure.** Preparing the patient includes teaching the patient about the procedure, answering any questions, and transporting and/or positioning the patient for the procedure. Monitoring the patient's responses to the procedure includes observing the patient for signs of pain, anxiety, or hemorrhage and monitoring vital signs. Assessing the patient after the procedure includes observing for complications of the procedure and medicating the patient for any postprocedure discomfort. **Any evidence of gastrointestinal bleeding should be immediately reported to the physician and emergency measures to maintain circulation must be initiated.**

References

1. O'Toole MT: Advanced assessment of the abdomen and gastrointestinal problems, *Nurs Clin North Am* 24:771, 1990.
2. Gehring PE: Physical assessment begins with a history, *RN* 54(11):26, 1991.
3. Bates B: *A guide to physical examination,* ed 6, Philadelphia, 1995, JB Lippincott.
4. Barkauskas V, et al: *Health and physical assessment,* ed 2, St Louis, 1998, Mosby.
5. Thompson JM, et al: *Mosby's clinical nursing,* ed 4, St Louis, 1997, Mosby.
6. Holmgren C: Perfecting the art: abdominal assessment, *RN* 55(3):28, 1992.
7. Normal reference values, *N Engl J Med* 327(10):718, 1992.
8. Doughty DB, Jackson DB: *Gastrointestinal disorders,* St Louis, 1993, Mosby.
9. Kovacs TOG, Jensen DM: Therapeutic endoscopy for upper gastrointestinal bleeding. In Taylor MB, editor: *Gastrointestinal emergencies,* Baltimore, 1992, Williams & Wilkins.
10. Porter DH, Kim D: Angiographic intervention in upper gastrointestinal bleeding. In Taylor MB, editor: *Gastrointestinal emergencies,* Baltimore, 1992, Williams & Wilkins.
11. Elta GH: Approach to the patient with gross gastrointestinal bleeding. In Yamada T, editor: *Textbook of gastroenterology,* vol 1, Philadelphia, 1991, JB Lippincott.
12. Roszler MH: Plain film radiologic examination of the abdomen, *Crit Care Clin* 10:277, 1994.
13. Ramano WM, Platt JF: Ultrasound of the abdomen, *Crit Care Clin* 10:297, 1994.
14. Dobranowski J, et al: *Procedures in gastrointestinal radiology,* New York, 1990, Springer-Verlag.
15. Eisenberg RL: *Gastrointestinal radiology,* ed 2, Philadelphia, 1990, JB Lippincott.
16. Zingas AP: Computed tomography of the abdomen in the critically ill, *Crit Care Clin* 10:321, 1994.
17. Davis LR, Fink-Bennet D: Nuclear medicine in the acutely ill patient. I. *Crit Care Clin* 10:265, 1994.
18. Niedzwick L, Stringer C: Liver biopsy and nursing intervention, *Gastroenterol Nurs* 17(1):17, 1994.

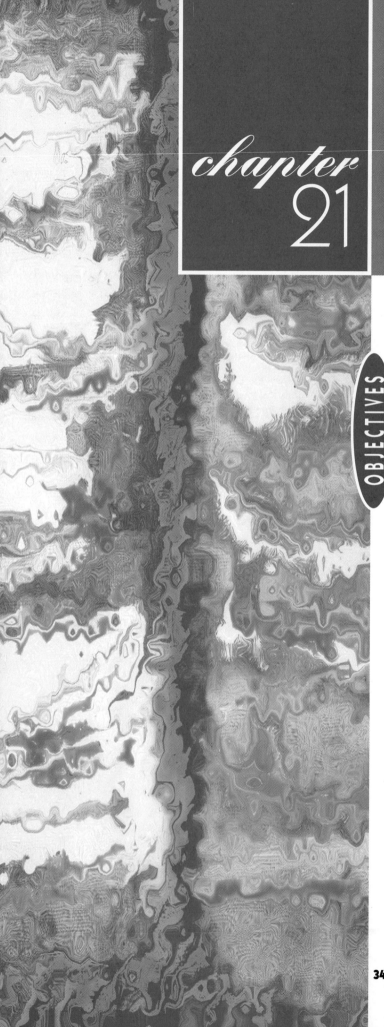

chapter 21

Gastrointestinal Disorders and Therapeutic Management

Nancy McLaughlin

OBJECTIVES

● **Describe the etiology and pathophysiology of selected gastrointestinal disorders.**

● **Identify the clinical manifestations of selected gastrointestinal disorders.**

● **Explain the treatments of selected gastrointestinal disorders.**

● **Discuss the nursing priorities for managing a patient with selected gastrointestinal disorders.**

● **Outline the use and care of gastrointestinal tubes.**

Understanding the pathology of the a disease, the areas of assessment on which to focus, and the usual medical management allows the critical care nurse to more accurately anticipate and plan nursing interventions. This chapter focuses on gastrointestinal disorders commonly seen in the critical care environment.

ACUTE GASTROINTESTINAL HEMORRHAGE

Description and Etiology

Gastrointestinal (GI) hemorrhage is a medical emergency that remains a very common complication of critical illness[1] and results in almost 300,000 hospital admissions yearly.[2] Despite advances in medical knowledge and nursing care, the mortality for acute GI bleeding has not changed in more than 50 years;[2] it remains approximately 10%.[3]

GI hemorrhage falls under two different DRGs depending on whether the patient develops complications or comorbid conditions (CC). DRG 174 (GI Hemorrhage With CC) and DRG 175 (GI Hemorrhage Without CC) have average lengths of the stay of 5.2 days and 3.2 days respectively.[4]

GI hemorrhage can occur from bleeding in the lower or upper GI tract. Causes for acute lower GI hemorrhage include ulcerative colitis, diverticulosis, angiodysplasias, and trauma.[2,5] Most cases of GI hemorrhage, however, result from bleeding in the upper GI tract due to a variety of disorders, including peptic ulcers, stress ulcers, and esophagogastric varices.[2,3,6]

Peptic ulcers

Peptic ulcers (gastric and duodenal ulcers), resulting from the breakdown of the gastroduodenal mucosal lining, are the leading cause of upper GI hemorrhage, accounting for approximately 50% of cases.[2,7] Normally, protection of the gastric mucosa from the digestive effects of gastric secretions is accomplished in several ways. First, the gastroduodenal mucosa is coated by a glycoprotein mucus. The mucus forms a gel that prevents the back diffusion of acid and pepsin and helps to maintain a mucosal-luminal pH gradient. Second, gastroduodenal epithelial cells secrete bicarbonate, which augments the actions of the glycoprotein mucus in maintaining this pH gradient. Finally, gastroduodenal epithelial cells are protected structurally against damage from acid and pepsin inasmuch as they are connected by tight junctions that help prevent acid penetration. Through these mechanisms, gastroduodenal mucosal pH is maintained above 6, even when the luminal pH is as low as 1.5.[7]

Peptic ulceration occurs when these protective mechanisms cease to function, thus allowing gastroduodenal mucosal breakdown. Once the mucosal lining is penetrated, gastric secretions autodigest the layers of the stomach resulting in damage the mucosal and submucosal layers of the stomach or duodenum. This results in damage to blood vessels and subsequent hemorrhage. There are number of factors that can disrupt gastroduodenal mucosal resistance, including the use of nonsteroidal anti-inflammatory drugs, the bacterial action of *Helicobacter pylori*, decreased mucosal bicarbonate secretion, and cigarette smoking.[8]

Stress ulcers

Stress ulcers, also known as hemorrhagic erosive gastritis, describes the gastric mucosal abnormalities often found in the critically ill patient. These abnormalities develop rapidly within hours of admission and range from superficial mucosal erosions to deep ulcers and are usually limited to the stomach.[1,9] GI hemorrhage is estimated to occur in 2% to 6% of patients who develop stress ulcers, with an associated mortality of 50% to 80%. Stress ulcers are the second leading cause of upper GI hemorrhage, accounting for approximately 20% of cases.[9]

Stress ulcers result from the same mechanisms as peptic ulcers but the contributing factor is thought to be decreased mucosal blood flow, which results in ischemia and degeneration of the mucosal lining.[9,10] Patients at risk include those in high physiologic stress situations, such as occur with thermal injury, head trauma, extensive surgery, shock, or acute neurologic disease.[1] In the burn patient, stress ulcers are often referred to as Curling's ulcers and in the brain-injured patient, they are often called Cushing's ulcers. In addition to decreased mucosal blood flow, excessive acid secretion resulting from overstimulation of the parasympathetic nervous system contributes to the development of Cushing's ulcers.[1,10]

Esophagogastric varices

Esophagogastric varices develop as a result of portal hypertension secondary to hepatic cirrhosis. Rupture and hemorrhage occurs in 19% to 40% of the patients with varices and has an associated mortality of 40% to 70%.[11] Variceal bleeding is the third leading cause of GI hemorrhage, accounting for approximately 15% of cases.[3]

Engorged and distended blood vessels of the esophagus and proximal stomach are referred to as esophagogastric varices. Varices are the result of hepatic cirrhosis, a chronic disease of the liver that results in damage to the liver sinusoids. Without adequate sinusoid function, resistance to portal blood flow is increased and pressures within the liver are elevated. This leads to a rise in portal venous pressure (portal hypertension), causing collateral circulation to divert portal blood from areas of high pressure within the liver to adjacent areas of low pressure outside the liver, such as into the veins of the esophagus, spleen, intestines, and stomach. The tiny thin-walled vessels of the esophagus and proximal stomach that receive this diverted blood lack sturdy mucosal protection. The vessels become engorged and dilated, forming esophagogastric varices that are vulnerable to damage from gastric secretions, resulting in subsequent rupture and hemorrhage.[11,12]

Pathophysiology

GI hemorrhage is a life-threatening disorder that is characterized by acute, massive GI bleeding. Regardless of the etiology, acute GI hemorrhage results in hypovolemic shock, initiation of the shock response, and the development of multiple organ dysfunction syndrome if left untreated[10] (Fig. 21-1). The most common cause of death in GI hemorrhage though is exacerbation of the underlying disease not intractable hypovolemic shock.[2]

Assessment and Diagnosis

The initial clinical presentation of the patient with acute GI hemorrhage will be hypovolemic shock, which varies depending of the amount of blood lost[13] (Table 21-1). Hematemesis (bright red or brown/coffee ground emesis), hematochezia (bright red stools), and melena (black, tarry, or dark red stools) are the hallmarks of GI hemorrhage.[10]

The patient who is vomiting blood is usually bleeding from a source above the duodenojejunal junction as re-

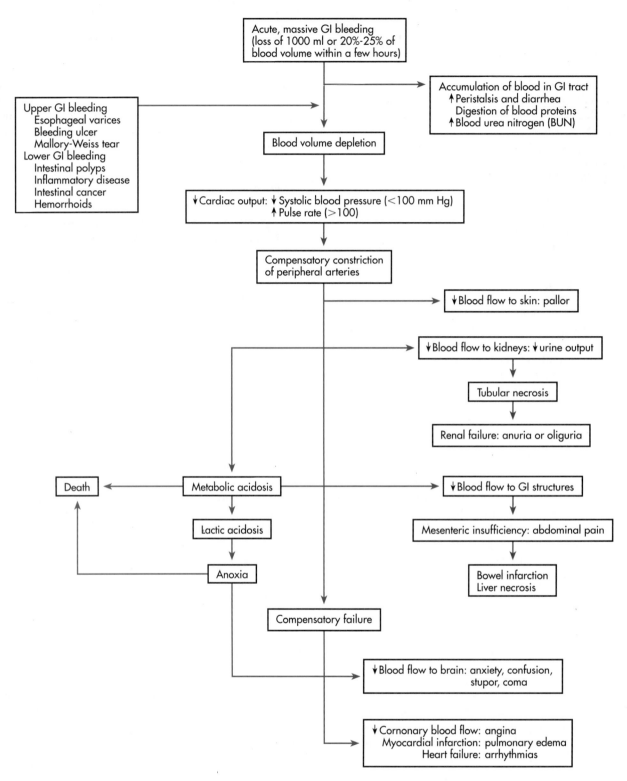

Fig. **21-1** Pathophysiology of acute gastrointestinal hemorrhage. (From McCance KL, Huether SE: *Pathophysiology: the biological basis for disease in adults and children*, ed 3, St Louis, 1998, Mosby.)

verse peristalsis is seldom sufficient to cause hematemesis if the bleeding point is below this area. The emesis may be bright red or coffee-ground in appearance, depending on the amount of gastric contents at the time of the bleeding and the length of time the blood has been in contact with gastric secretions. Gastric acid converts bright red hemoglobin to brown hematin, accounting for the coffee-ground appearance of the emesis. Bright red emesis results from profuse bleeding with little contact with gastric secretions.[2]

TABLE 21-1

SEVERITY OF BLOOD LOSS

BLOOD VOLUME LOSS	CLINICAL SIGNS AND SYMPTOMS
<15% total blood volume (<1000 ml)	HR normal or <100 bpm supine Capillary refill WNL Urine output >30 ml/hr Anxiety may be present
15%-30% total blood volume (1000 ml)	Systolic BP >90 mm Hg Decreased pulse (pressure) HR 100-120 bpm Capillary refill >3 sec Increased respiratory rate Urine output 25-30 ml/hr Weakness May have mental status changes
31%-40% total blood volume (1500-2000 ml)	HR >120 bpm Systolic blood pressure 70-90 mm Hg Cool, pale skin Increased respiratory rate Urine output 1-15 ml/hr Mental status changes
>40% total blood volume (>2000 ml)	HR >140 bpm Mean arterial pressure <50 mm Hg Confused/lethargic Cold, clammy skin Urine output minimal

From Kinney MR, et al: *AACN's clinical reference for critical care nursing*, ed 4, St Louis, 1998, Mosby.

The presence of blood in the GI tract results in increased peristalsis and diarrhea. Hematochezia occurs from massive lower GI hemorrhage and, if rapid enough, upper GI hemorrhage. Melena occurs from digestion of blood from an upper GI hemorrhage and may take several days after the bleeding has stopped to clear.[2,10]

Laboratory tests can help determine the extent of bleeding, although it is important to realize that the patient's hemoglobin and hematocrit are poor indicators of the severity or rapidity of blood loss. As whole blood is lost, plasma and red blood cells are lost in the same proportion; thus if the patient's hematocrit is 45% before a bleeding episode, it will still be 45% several hours later.[1,6,10] It may take as long as 48 hours for the patient's hemoglobin and hematocrit to equilibrate after an episode of blood loss.[10]

To isolate the source of bleeding, an urgent fiberoptic endoscopy is usually undertaken. If performed within 12 hours of the bleeding event, endoscopy has a 90% accuracy rate. Before initiating the endoscopy, the patient must be hemodynamically stabilized and the area to be visualized cleared of blood. Angiography is done when the endoscopy fails to identify the source of bleeding or it is impossible to get a clear view the GI tract because of continued active bleeding.[13]

Medical Management

In order to reduce mortality related to GI hemorrhage, patients at risk should be identified early and interventions to reduce gastric acidity and to support the gastric mucosal defense mechanisms should be implemented. Management of the patient at risk for GI hemorrhage should include prophylactic administration of pharmacologic agents for gastric acid neutralization. These agents include antacids, histamine blockers, cytoprotective agents, and gastric proton pump inhibitors.[1,9]

The goals of medical management of the patient with GI hemorrhage are fluid resuscitation to achieve hemodynamic stability, therapeutic procedures to control and/or stop bleeding, and diagnostic procedures to determine the exact etiology of the bleeding.

Fluid resuscitation

The initial treatment priority is the restoration of adequate circulating blood volume to treat or prevent shock. This is accomplished with the administration of intravenous infusions of crystalloids, blood and blood products. A pulmonary artery catheter should be placed to provide a more decisive guide to fluid replacement therapy. A large NG tube should be inserted and lavaged till clear with water or normal saline. Lavaging is used to confirm the diagnosis of active bleeding, slow the bleeding, and prepare the esophagus, stomach, and proximal duodenum for endoscopic evaluation.[13]

Control of bleeding

In the patient with GI hemorrhage related to peptic ulcer disease, bleeding hemostasis may be accomplished via endoscopic thermal therapy or endoscopic injection therapy. Endoscopic thermal therapy uses heat to cauterize the bleeding vessel while endoscopic injection therapy uses a variety of agents, such as hypertonic saline, epinephrine, and dehydrated alcohol, to induced localized vasoconstriction of the bleeding vessel.[14] Intra-arterial infusion of vasopressin into the gastric artery or intra-arterial injection of an embolizing agent (Gelfoam pledgets, stainless steel coils, platinum microcoils, and polyvinyl alcohol particles) can also be performed during arteriography to control bleeding once the site has been identified.[15] Intra-arterial administration of vasopressin is less effective for duodenal lesions because of the dual blood supply of duodenum. GI hemorrhage resulting from stress ulcers is managed in a similar fashion.[1]

In acute variceal hemorrhage, control of bleeding may be initially accomplished by endoscopic sclerotherapy, endoscopic variceal band ligation, and/or intravenous vasopressin administration. If these therapies fail, esophagogastric balloon tamponade and/or transjugular intrahepatic portosystemic shunting (TIPS) may become necessary. Endoscopic sclerotherapy controls bleeding via the injection of a sclerosing agent in or around the varices. This creates an inflammatory reaction that induces vasoconstriction and results in the formation of a venous thrombosis. During endoscopic variceal band ligation, latex bands are placed around the varices to create an obstruction to stop the bleeding. Intravenous administration of vasopressin reduces portal venous pressure and slows blood flow by constricting the splanchnic arteriolar bed. Balloon tamponade tubes (Sengstaken-Blakemore, Linton, and Minnesota tubes) halt hemorrhaging by applying direct pressure against bleeding vessels while decompressing the stomach. During a TIPS procedure, a channel between the systemic and portal venous systems is created to redirect portal blood, thereby reducing portal hypertension and decompressing the varices to control bleeding.[12,16]

The patient who remains hemodynamically unstable despite volume replacement needs urgent surgery. Indications for surgery include poor prognosis, loss of 30% of estimated blood volume within 24 hours, administration of greater than 1500 ml blood transfusions within 24 hours, massive hemorrhage to the point of shock, and rebleeding despite medical and endoscopic interventions.[13] Operative procedures to control bleeding from gastric or duodenal ulcers include vagotomy, pyloroplasty, partial gastrectomy, subtotal gastrectomy, and Billroth I and II procedures.[10] Operative procedures to control bleeding esophagogastric varices include portacaval shunt, mesocaval shunt, splenorenal shunt, and liver transplantation.[12] Operative procedures to control bleeding from stress ulcers include total gastrectomy (bleeding generalized) and oversew of the ulcers (bleeding localized).[13]

Nursing Management

All critically ill patients should be considered at risk for stress ulcers and thus GI hemorrhage. Routine assessments should include gastric fluid pH monitoring every 2 to 4 hours, with a goal of keeping the pH greater than 5. Gastric pH measurements, either via litmus paper or direct nasogastric tube probes, may be used to assess gastric fluid pH and the need for or effectiveness of prophylactic agents. In addition, patients at risk should be assessed for the presence of bright red or coffee-ground emesis, bloody nasogastric aspirate, and bright red, black, or dark-red stools. Any signs of bleeding should be promptly reported to the physician.[1]

Nursing management of a patient experiencing acute GI hemorrhage incorporates a variety of nursing diagnoses (Box 21-1). **Nursing priorities are directed towards administering volume replacement, controlling the bleeding, monitoring for complications, and educating the patient and family.**

Administering volume replacement

Measures to facilitate volume replacement include obtaining intravenous access and administering prescribed fluids and blood products. Two large-diameter peripheral intravenous catheters should be started to facilitate the rapid administration of prescribed fluids.

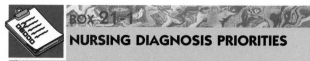

NURSING DIAGNOSIS PRIORITIES

Acute Gastrointestinal Hemorrhage

- Fluid Volume Deficit related to absolute loss, p. 486
- Decreased Cardiac Output related to alterations in preload, pp. 467-468
- Altered Nutrition: Less than Body Requirements related to lack of exogenous nutrients and increased metabolic demand, p. 460
- Powerlessness related to health care environment or illness-related regimen, pp. 455-456
- Knowledge Deficit: Discharge Regimen related to lack of previous exposure to information, p. 443

Controlling the bleeding

One measure to control active bleeding is gastric lavage. It is used to decrease gastric mucosal blood flow and evacuate blood from the stomach. Gastric lavage is performed by inserting a large-bore nasogastric tube into the stomach and irrigating it with normal saline or water until the returned solution is clear. It is important to keep accurate records of the amount of fluid instilled and aspirated as to ascertain the true amount of bleeding. Historically, iced saline was favored as a lavage irrigant.[13] Research has shown, however, that low-temperature fluids shift the oxyhemoglobin dissociation curve to the left, decrease oxygen delivery to vital organs, and prolong bleeding time and prothrombin time. Iced saline may also further aggravate bleeding; therefore, room-temperature water or saline is the currently preferred irrigant for use in gastric lavage.[2]

Monitoring for complications

In addition to monitoring the patient's response to care, the patient should also be continuously observed for signs of gastric perforation. Although a rare complication, gastric perforation constitutes a surgical emergency. Signs and symptoms include sudden, severe, generalized abdominal pain, with significant rebound tenderness and rigidity. Perforation should be suspected when fever, leukocytosis, and tachycardia persist despite adequate volume replacement.[2]

Educating the patient and family

Early in the patient's hospital stay, the patient and family should be taught about acute GI hemorrhage, its etiologies and treatments. As the patient moves toward discharge, teaching should focus on the interventions necessary for preventing the reoccurrence of the precipitating disorder. If the patient is an alcohol abuser, the patient should be encouraged to stop drinking and should be referred to a alcohol cessation program.

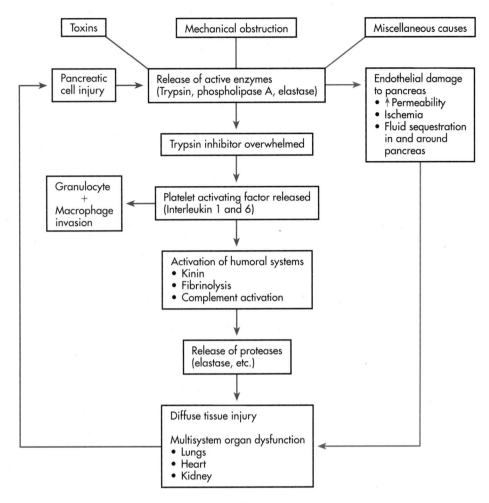

Fig. **21-2** Pathophysiology of acute pancreatitis. (From Kinney MR, et al: *AACN's clinical reference for critical care nursing,* ed 4, St Louis, 1998, Mosby.)

ACUTE PANCREATITIS

Description and Etiology

Pancreatitis is an inflammation of the pancreas that produces exocrine and endocrine dysfunction. It can be classified as acute or chronic. Acute pancreatitis is best described as an acute onset of mild or severe abdominal pain, accompanied by a rise in pancreatic enzymes indicating inflammation. No permanent damage to the pancreas occurs, and, once the primary cause is eliminated, complete resolution should occur.[17]

Acute pancreatitis falls under DRG 204 (Disorders of Pancreas Except Malignancy) with an average length of the stay of 6.4 days.[4]

The two most common causes of acute pancreatitis are biliary disease (gallstones) and alcoholism.[18,19] Other much less common causes include peptic ulcer disease, surgical trauma, hyperparathyroidism,[20] vascular disease, and the use of certain drugs.[21] In 10% to 25% of patients with acute pancreatitis, no etiologic factor can be determined.[22]

Pathophysiology

In acute pancreatitis, the normally inactive digestive enzymes become prematurely activated within the pancreas itself, creating the central pathophysiologic mechanism of acute pancreatitis, namely autodigestion.[20] The enzymes become activated through a variety of mechanisms, including obstruction or damage to the pancreatic duct system, alterations in the secretory processes of the acinar cells, infection, ischemia, and other idiopathic factors[23] (Fig. 21-2).

Trypsin is the enzyme that becomes activated first and initiates the autodigestion process by triggering the secretion of proteolytic enzymes phospholipase A, elastase, and kinin. Phospholipase A, in the presence of bile, digests the phospholipids of cell membranes. This causes severe pancreatic parenchymal and adipose tissue necrosis, with subsequent release of free fatty acids. Elastase activation causes dissolution of the elastic fibers of blood vessels and ducts, leading to hemorrhage. Kinin activation results in decreased peripheral vascular resistance, vasodilation, and increased vascular permeability.[20,23]

Together these proteases and phosopholipases cause pancreatic inflammation and swelling. Extravasation of plasma and red blood cells in the area surrounding the pancreas causes fluid to be redistributed from the intravascular space to the retroperitoneum and bowel. With large amounts of plasma volume sequestration, hypovolemia and hypotension occur and the patient goes into shock.[20,24]

Assessment and Diagnosis

The clinical manifestations of acute pancreatitis are from mild to severe and often mimic other disorders. Epigastric to midabdominal pain may vary from mild and tolerable to severe and incapacitating. Many patients report a twisting or knifelike sensation that radiates to the low dorsal region of the back. Nausea or vomiting, or both, may accompany the pain.[23] The patient may obtain some comfort by leaning forward or by lying down with knees drawn up. Other clinical findings include abdominal guarding, distention, hypertension, abdominal mass, jaundice, hematemesis, and melena.[23]

The results of GI auscultation vary according to the presence or absence of bowel sounds; abdominal palpitation reveals tenderness and guarding. Uncommon inspection findings, that could indicate pancreatic hemorrhage, include Turner's sign (gray-blue discoloration of the flank) and Cullen's sign (discoloration of the umbilical region).[23] Neuromuscular irritability may result from electrolyte deficiencies, but, although muscle weakness or tremors may appear, tetany rarely develops.[20]

Assessment of laboratory data usually demonstrates elevated levels of serum amylase and lipase. Serum lipase is more pancreas-specific than amylase and a more accurate marker for acute pancreatitis. Amylase present in other body tissues and other disorders, such as cerebral trauma, mumps, renal insufficiency, burns, and shock, may contribute to an elevated level. However, amylase is excreted in urine, unlike other serum enzymes, and this clearance increases with acute pancreatitis. Measurement of urinary vs. serum amylase should be considered in light of the patient's creatinine clearance. In addition, serum amylase may be elevated for only 2 days in mild cases. If the patient delays seeking treatment, and, the amylase level is not measured within 2 to 7 days after the onset of the symptoms, a normal level (false-negative) may be noted. Leukocytosis, hypocalcemia, hyperglycemia, hyperbilirubinemia, and hypoalbuminemia may also be present.[22]

Medical Management

The goals of medical management of the patient with acute pancreatitis are fluid resuscitation to achieve hemodynamic stability, minimization of pancreatic function, and correction of metabolic alterations.[23] In addition, the management of systemic and local complications is critical.

Fluid resuscitation

Intravenous crystalloids, typically Ringer's lactate, and colloids are administered immediately to prevent hypovolemic shock and to maintain hemodynamic stability. Assessment of fluid replacement therapy should include blood pressure, heart rate, capillary refill, and strict I&O. In severe forms of the disease, the use of a pulmonary artery catheter guides such fluid management.[24]

Minimization of pancreatic function

To minimize pancreatic function, the pancreas should be placed "at rest." Interventions to suppress pancreatic stimulation include insertion of a nasogastric tube and initiation of gastric suction, restricting all oral food and fluids, and bed rest.[23] In addition, antacids or histamine blockers should be administered to elevate the pH of gastric secretions.[17]

Correction of metabolic alterations

Electrolytes are monitored closely and abnormalities, such as hypocalcemia, hypokalemia, and hypomagnesemia, should be treated. If hyperglycemia develops, exogenous insulin is given. Supplemental oxygen is also needed.[23]

Nursing Management

Nursing management of the patient with pancreatitis incorporates a variety of nursing diagnoses (Box 21-2). **Nursing priorities are directed toward correcting fluid and electrolyte imbalances, facilitating pain manage-**

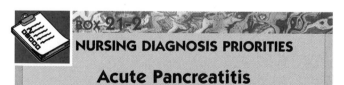

Box 21-2

NURSING DIAGNOSIS PRIORITIES

Acute Pancreatitis

- Acute Pain related to transmission and perception of cutaneous, visceral, muscular, ischemia impulses, pp. 461-464
- Fluid Volume Deficit related to relative fluid loss, pp. 486-487
- Altered Nutrition: Less Than Body Requirements related to lack of exogenous nutrients or increased metabolic demand, p. 460
- Anxiety related to threat to biologic, psychologic, and/or social integrity, pp. 448-450
- Knowledge Deficit: Discharge Regimen related to lack of previous exposure to information, p. 443

ment, promoting gas exchange, monitoring for complications, and educating the patient and family.

Correcting fluid and electrolyte imbalances

Assisting with insertion of a pulmonary artery catheter and/or central venous catheter to guide fluid replacement therapy is an important nursing function as is the continuous assessment of the patient's hemodynamic status once the catheter is in place. Monitoring for signs of hypovolemia, electrolyte imbalances (hypocalcemia, hypokalemia, and hypomagnesemia), hyperglycemia, and sepsis, as well as implementing aggressive measures, as ordered, to correct these problems are also key nursing measures.[23]

Facilitating pain management

Pain management is a major priority for the patient with acute pancreatitis as the patient may be in severe pain. The administration of analgesics to achieve pain relief is of critical importance. For years, meperidine (Demerol) had been thought to be the preferred agent in the patient with acute pancreatitis because morphine may produce spasms at the sphincter of Oddi. This belief is now being seriously questioned because morphine is the more effective analgesic, has been found to have minimal effects on the sphincter of Oddi,[23] and as long as pancreatic stimulation is controlled the issue is no longer important.[17] Positioning the patient in the knee-to-chest position and implementing measures to rest the pancreas (nothing by mouth and nasogastric suction) also assist in pain control. Relaxation techniques may augment analgesia.

Promoting gas exchange

Accurate pulmonary assessment is vital because abdominal pain often results in shallow, rapid breathing, which can precipitate respiratory insufficiency. Pulmonary crackles, shortness of breath, and hypoxemia indicate the development of atelectasis, pneumonia, and/or acute respiratory failure. Mediators released as part of the inflammatory-immune response can facilitate the development of acute respiratory distress syndrome. Measures to improve oxygenation and ventilation are of critical importance.

Monitoring for complications

Pancreatic complications include phlegmon, necrosis and abscess, and pseudocyst. A phlegmon is a space-occupying mass that is best described as an inflamed hardened area of the pancreas. Although it can spontaneously resolve, a phlegmon can cause damage to the surrounding organs, resulting in necrosis. The necrotic areas of the pancreas can lead to the development of a widespread pancreatic infection (infected pancreatic necrosis) or a localized infection (pancreatic abscess). An abscess is a collection of purulent inflammatory exudate either within or around the pancreas. It can perforate, resulting in hemorrhage or peritonitis.[24] A pseudocyst is a collection of pancreatic fluid enclosed in a fibrous capsule, resulting from an obstruction in the main pancreatic duct. A pancreatic pseudocyst can resolve spontaneously, rupture resulting in peritonitis, erode a major blood vessel resulting in hemorrhage, become infected resulting in sepsis, or invade surrounding structures resulting in obstruction. If the patient develops an infected necrotic pancreas, infected pseudocyst, or abscess, surgery is usually indicated. A variety of surgical procedures may be performed, including wide sump drainage and debridement and open packing and drainage.[25]

Educating the patient and family

Early in the patient's hospital stay, the patient and family should be taught about acute pancreatitis, its etiologies and its treatment. As the patient moves toward discharge, teaching should focus on the interventions necessary for preventing the reoccurrence of the precipitating disorder. If the patient has sustained permanent damage to the pancreas, the patient will require teaching specific to diet modification and supplemental pancreatic enzymes. Diabetes education may also be necessary. If the patient is an alcohol abuser, he or she should be encouraged to stop drinking and should be referred to a alcohol cessation program.

ACUTE INTESTINAL OBSTRUCTION

Description and Etiology

Acute intestinal obstruction occurs when bowel contents fail to move forward. It can be classified as either functional (non-mechanical) or mechanical. Functional obstruction, also known as a neurogenic obstruction or a paralytic ileus, results from the absence of peristalsis due either to ischemia or neuromuscular dysfunction.[26] A functional obstruction presents in a similar way to a mechanical obstruction except for the bowel sounds, which are decreased or absent.[27] Mechanical obstruction results from occlusion of the small or large bowel lumen[28] and can be further classified as strangulated or simple, depending on the presence or absence of blood flow to surrounding bowel wall.[26] Mechanical obstructions can also be classified as high small intestinal, low small intestinal, and colonic, depending on their location.

Acute intestinal obstruction falls under two different DRGs, depending on whether the patient develops complications or comorbid conditions (CC). DRG 180 (GI Obstruction With CC) and DRG 181 (GI Obstruction Without CC) have average lengths of the stay of 5.7 days and 3.7 days, respectively.[4]

Functional obstructions can be the result of an intraabdominal problem or an extraabdominal problem. Specific causes include the postoperative state, sepsis, electrolyte imbalances, trauma, and the use of opiates, chemotherapeutic agents, or cardiac drugs.[26] Mechanical obstructions can be the result of extrinsic lesions, intrinsic lesions, and objects blocking the intestinal lumen.[26] Most mechanical obstructions occur in the small intestine, with

ETIOLOGIES OF INTESTINAL OBSTRUCTIONS

FUNCTIONAL OBSTRUCTIONS
Intraabdominal

Peritonitis
Pancreatitis
Bowel ischemia
Abdominal surgery or trauma

Extraabdominal

Rib, spine, or pelvic trauma
Retroperitoneal surgery or trauma
Myocardial infarction
Pneumonia
Electrolyte abnormalities (hypokalemia, hypomagnesemia)
Metabolic disturbances
Sepsis
Drugs

MECHANICAL OBSTRUCTION
Extrinsic lesions

Adhesions
Hernias
Volvulus
Tumors

Intrinsic lesions

Tumors
Intussusception
Congenital atresia or stenosis
Bowel ischemia
Bowel inflammation (radiation enteritis, Crohn's disease)
Diverticulitis

Blockage of intestinal lumen

Gallstones
Impaction (fecal, barium, bezoars, worms)
Tumors

abdominal adhesions generally the causative factor.[27] Obstructions of the large intestine are generally due to malignant tumors.[28] Box 21-3 lists the etiologies of functional and mechanical obstructions.[26-28]

Pathophysiology

Regardless of the etiology, once a obstruction develops, fluid and gas accumulate in the bowel lumen proximal to the point of obstruction (Fig. 21-3). Trapped fluids cause bowel distention and bowel wall edema, which triggers the secretion of more fluid and electrolytes into the lumen, resulting in progressive distention. Typically, the fluid and electrolyte shifts are much more pronounced in mechanical obstructions, as opposed to functional obstructions. Large losses of sodium, potassium, and chloride occur as well as a loss of hydrogen ions from the stomach. As the obstruction continues, the vascular space becomes rapidly depleted, which results in dehydration, hypotension, and hypovolemic shock. If intestinal distention progresses, bowel wall edema will ultimately impede venous and arterial supply, causing ischemia (strangulation), bowel necrosis, and perforation. Once the bowel perforates, peritonitis and sepsis ensue.[29]

Assessment and Diagnosis

Patients with acute intestinal obstruction may initially present with vague warning symptoms, such as abdominal distention, nausea, vomiting, obstipation, constipation, cramping abdominal pain, and abnormal bowel sounds. In the patient with a mechanical obstruction, bowel sounds are high-pitched, tinkling, and hyperactive proximal to the obstruction site and hypoactive or absent distal to the obstruction as opposed to the patient with a functional obstruction where the bowel sounds are low-pitched and hypoactive or absent.[26-28] The patient may also exhibit signs of dehydration, such as dry mucous membranes, poor skin turgor, tachycardia, and hypotension.[29]

Small bowel obstructions, which comprise about two thirds of mechanical obstructions, usually present with rapid onset of cramplike abdominal pain, nausea, vomiting (may be projectile), and abdominal distention. The patient may continue to pass small amounts of stool or flatus. Abdominal pain is severe and frequent with short quiet periods between peristaltic rushes. The higher the obstruction is located in the intestine, the more intense the pain.[27]

Large bowel obstructions, about one third of mechanical obstructions, generally have an insidious onset of low grade, crampy pain, marked abdominal distention, and obstipation. Nausea and vomiting are rare, and the patient's history will frequently include a change in bowel habits and report of weight loss. Vomiting may occur late and contain fecal material, requiring immediate attention.[28]

Diagnosis of intestinal obstruction is aided by radiologic examination. A chest x-ray and serial abdominal flatplate films taken with the patient standing or sitting and supine reveal dilated loops of gas-filled bowel. Barium or meglumine diatrizoate (Gastrografin) enemas are used to locate the exact site and the degree of obstruction. Laboratory data may reveal an elevated serum amylase, an elevated white blood cell count (marked elevation with complete or necrotic obstructions), hyponatremia, and hypokalemia.[29]

Medical Management

The goals of medical management of the patient with a bowel obstruction are decompression of the intestine with a nasogastric suctioning and relief or removal of the obstruction. Antibiotic prophylaxis should also be initiated for patient with large bowel obstructions.[29]

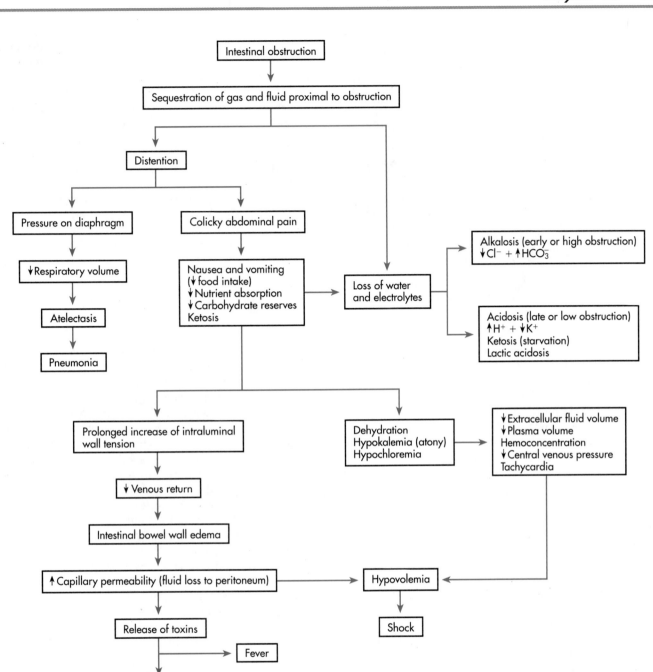

Fig. **21-3** Pathophysiology of intestinal obstruction. (From McCance KL, Huether SE: *Pathophysiology: the biological basis for disease in adults and children,* ed 3, St Louis, 1998, Mosby.)

Decompression of the intestine

Much controversy exists over whether a nasogastric tube or a nasointestinal tube should be placed for decompressing small bowel mechanical obstructions.[29] Nasointestinal tubes are contraindicated for large bowel mechanical obstructions.[26] Decompression of the upper GI tract of gas and fluids relieves abdominal distension and controls nausea and vomiting. In addition, the patient should receive nothing by mouth.

Removal or relief of the obstruction

Functional obstructions generally resolve within 24 to 72 hours with conservative therapy that includes placing the patient on nothing by mouth, decompressing the upper GI tract with nasogastric suction, stimulating motility pharmacologically, and eliminating underlying aggravating factors. Partial small bowel obstructions may also resolve with this conservative therapy.[27] Surgical intervention is required when the obstruction fails to resolve

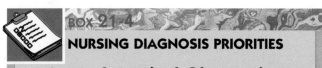

within a reasonable time or if there is evidence of a strangulation, bowel necrosis, and perforation. Complete mechanical obstructions also require surgical intervention.[26] When the patient is not acutely ill, surgical resection can be a one-stage procedure with reanastomosis of the bowel, therefore eliminating the need for a temporary colostomy. More often a two- or three-stage procedure is used and a temporary colostomy created.[29]

Nursing Management

Nursing management of the patient with an acute intestinal obstruction incorporates a variety of nursing diagnoses (Box 21-4). **Nursing priorities are directed toward ensuring the patency of the nasogastric tube, correcting fluid and electrolyte imbalances, monitoring for complications, and educating the patient and family.**

Ensuring patency of the nasogastric tube

Once a nasogastric tube is inserted, it should be checked regularly for placement and patency to ensure adequate decompression.

Correcting fluid and electrolyte imbalances

Outputs greater than 1000 ml/8 hours can occur; therefore, the patient should be monitored closely for electrolyte imbalances (hyponatremia and hypokalemia) and fluid volume deficit. Accurate intake and output must be maintained. Intravenous fluid and electrolyte solutions should be administered to prevent dehydration and replace lost electrolytes. Fluid and electrolyte balance is most often achieved with normal saline and potassium supplement administration.[26,29]

Monitoring for complications

Bowel necrosis and perforation are potential complications of colonic obstruction, and both can progress to sepsis. Bowel necrosis occurs as a result of impaired cir-

culation to the bowel wall (strangulation) and sustained excessive intraluminal pressure. Bowel perforation results from over-distention of the bowel lumen and is a sequelae to bowel necrosis. These complications carry a high mortality and can be avoided by astute clinical observations, followed by prompt surgical intervention.[26]

Educating the patient and family

Early in the patient's hospital stay, the patient and family should be taught about acute intestinal obstruction, its etiologies and treatments. As the patient moves toward discharge, teaching should focus on the interventions necessary for preventing the reoccurrence of the precipitating etiology. If the patient has either a temporary or permanent colostomy, he or she will also require ostomy teaching.

FULMINANT HEPATIC FAILURE

Description and Etiology

Fulminant hepatic failure (FHF) is a medical emergency that is best described as severe acute liver failure (hepatocellular necrosis) accompanied by hepatic encephalopathy. It has a mortality rate as high as 90% and generally occurs in patients without pre-existing liver disease, although it is occasionally seen in patients with compensated chronic liver disease. As liver transplantation is one of the few definitive treatments for FHF, the patient with FHF should be transferred to a critical care unit and strongly considered for referral to a major medical center where transplant services are available.[30,31]

Fulminant hepatic failure falls under two different DRGs, depending on whether the patient develops complications or comorbid conditions (CC). DRG 205 (Disorders of Liver Except Malignancy, Cirrhosis, and Alcoholic Hepatitis With CC) and DRG 206 (Disorders of Liver Except Malignancy, Cirrhosis, and Alcoholic Hepatitis Without CC) have average lengths of the stay of 6.8 days and 4.2 days, respectively.[4]

The etiologies of FHF include infections, drugs, toxins, hypoperfusion, metabolic disorders, and surgery (Box 21-5). Patients presenting with FHF are usually healthy before the onset of symptoms, as it tends to occur in patients with no known liver history. Therefore it is imperative that a thorough medication and health history is explored in order to determine a possible etiology. The patient should be questioned about exposure to environmental toxins, hepatitis, intravenous drug use, and sexual history. Viral hepatitis, drug toxicity, poisoning, and metabolic disorders, such as Reye's syndrome and Wilson's disease, should be considered.[30-32]

Pathophysiology

Fulminant hepatic failure is a syndrome characterized by the development of acute liver failure over 1 to 3 weeks, followed by the development of hepatic encephalopathy within 8 weeks, in a patient with a previously healthy

BOX 21-5

ETIOLOGIES OF FULMINANT HEPATIC FAILURE

INFECTIONS

Hepatitis A, B, C, D, E, non-A, non-B, non-C
Herpes simplex virus (types 1 and 2)
Epstein-Barr virus
Varicella zoster
Dengue fever virus
Rift Valley fever virus

DRUGS/TOXINS

Industrial substances (chlorinated hydrocarbons, phosphorus)
Amanita phalloides (mushrooms)
Aflatoxin (herb)
Medications (isoniazid, rifampin, halothane, methyldopa, tetracycline, valproic acid, monoamine oxidase inhibitors, phenytoin, nicotinic acid, tricyclic antidepressants, isoflurane, ketoconazole, co-trimethoprim, sulfasalazine, pyrimethamine, octreotide)
Acetaminophen toxicity
Cocaine

HYPOPERFUSION

Venous obstructions
Budd-Chiari syndrome
Veno-occlusive disease
Ischemia

METABOLIC DISORDERS

Wilson's disease
Tyrosinemia
Heat stroke
Galactosemia

SURGERY

Jejunoileal bypass
Partial hepatectomy
Liver transplant failure

OTHER

Reye's syndrome
Acute fatty liver of pregnancy
Massive malignant infiltration
Autoimmune hepatitis

BOX 21-6

STAGING OF HEPATIC ENCEPHALOPATHY

I Euphoria or depression, mild confusion, slurred speech, disordered sleep rhythm; slight asterixis and normal electroencephalogram (EEG)
II Lethargy, moderate confusion; marked asterixis and abnormal EEG
III Marked confusion, incoherent speech, sleeping but arousable; asterixis present and abnormal EEG
IV Coma; initially responsive to noxious stimuli, later unresponsive; asterixis absent and abnormal EEG

sion contribute to the development of ascites.[31,33] Hepatic encephalopathy is thought to be the result of failure of the liver to detoxify various substances in the blood stream and may be worsened by metabolic and electrolyte imbalances.[31]

The patient may also experience a variety of other complications including cerebral edema, cardiac dysrhythmias, acute respiratory failure, and acute renal failure. Cerebral edema develops as a result of breakdown of the blood-brain barrier and astrocyte swelling. Hypoxemia, acidosis, electrolyte imbalances, and/or cerebral edema can precipitate the development of cardiac dysrhythmias. Acute respiratory failure, progressing to ARDS, can result from pulmonary edema, aspiration pneumonia, and atelectasis. Acute renal failure caused by acute tubular necrosis, hypotension, or hemorrhage may also develop.[31]

Assessment and Diagnosis

Early recognition of FHF is extremely important. The diagnosis should include potentially reversible conditions, such as autoimmune hepatitis, as well as differentiate from decompensating chronic liver disease. Prognostic indicators, such as coma grade, serum bilirubin, prothrombin time, coagulation factors, pH, and investigation of potential etiologies, should be noted.

Signs and symptoms of FHF include headache, hyperventilation, jaundice, personality changes, palmar erythema, spider nevi, bruises, and edema. The patient should be evaluated for the presence of asterixis or "liver flaps," best described as the inability to voluntary sustain a fixed position of the extremities. Asterixis is best demonstrated by having the patient extend the arms and dorsiflex the wrists, resulting in downward flapping of the hands. Hepatic encephalopathy is assessed using a grading system that stages the encephalopathy according to the patient's clinical manifestations[32] (Box 21-6). Diagnostic findings include elevated serum bilirubin, AST, alkaline phosphatase, serum ammonia, and decreased serum albumin. Arterial blood gases reveal respiratory

liver. Generally the interval between the actual failure of the liver and the onset of hepatic encephalopathy is less than 2 weeks. The underlying cause is massive necrosis of the hepatocytes.[30-32]

Acute liver failure results in a number of derangements, including impaired bilirubin conjugation, decreased production of clotting factors, depressed glucose synthesis, and decreased lactate clearance. This results in jaundice, coagulopathies, hypoglycemia, and metabolic acidosis.[31] Other effects of acute liver failure include increased risk of infection and altered carbohydrate, protein, and glucose metabolism. Hypoalbuminemia, fluid and electrolyte imbalances, and acute portal hyperten-

alkalosis and/or metabolic acidosis. Hypoglycemia, hypokalemia, and hyponatremia may also be present.[31]

Factors I (fibrinogen), II (prothrombin), V, VII, IX, and X are produced by the liver exclusively. Of these, the prothrombin time may be the most useful test in the evaluation of acute FHF as levels may be 40 to 80 seconds above control values. Decreased levels of plasmin and plasminogen and increased levels of fibrin and fibrin split products are also noted. Platelet counts are often decreased, sometimes to <80,000/mm.[31]

Medical Management

The goals of medical management of the patient with FHF are decreased absorption of ammonia and treatment of complications. As treatment is primarily supportive, medical interventions are directed toward management of the multiple system impact of FHF.

Decreased absorption of ammonia

Neomycin or lactulose is administered to remove or decrease production of ammonia in the large intestine. Neomycin, which is given orally or rectally, reduces bacterial flora of the colon. This aids in decreasing ammonia formation by decreasing bacterial action on protein in the feces. Side effects include renal toxicity and hearing impairment. Lactulose is a synthetic ketoanalog of lactose and is split into lactic acid and acetic acid in the intestine. It is given orally, via nasogastric tube, or as a retention enema. The result is the creation of an acidic environment that decreases bacterial growth. Lactulose also traps ammonia and has a laxative effect that promotes expulsion.[33]

Treatment of complications

Bleeding is best controlled through prevention. As these patients are at risk for acute GI hemorrhage, stress ulcer prophylaxis is essential. If the patient develops active bleeding, Vitamin K, fresh frozen plasma (to maintain reasonable prothrombin time), and platelet transfusions are necessary. Metabolic disturbances, such as hypoglycemia, metabolic acidosis, hypokalemia and hyponatremia, should be monitored and treated appropriately. Prophylactic antibiotic administration may be initiated as the patient is at high risk for an infection. The development of cerebral edema necessitates the need for intracranial pressure (ICP) monitoring. Mannitol (although not suggested for patients experiencing associated renal failure), albumin, and hyperventilation may be used to decrease ICP. If renal failure develops, continuous renal replacement therapy should be initiated. Intubation and mechanical ventilation are necessary as hypoxemia develops. Hemodynamic instability is a common complication requiring fluid administration and vasoactive medications to avoid prolonged episodes of hypotension.[30-33]

If FHF continues and the patient shows no immediate signs of improvement or reversal, the patient should be considered for a liver transplant. Prompt referral to a transplant center should be a high priority for patients experiencing FHF.[31]

Nursing Management

Nursing management of the patient with FHF incorporates a variety of nursing diagnoses (Box 21-7). **Nursing priorities are directed toward monitoring and treating complications and educating the patient and family.**

Monitoring and treating complications

Nursing assessments include monitoring for signs of hypoxemia, increased ICP, hypoglycemia, bleeding, and infections. Continuous arterial saturation monitoring (pulse oximetry) as well as arterial blood gas analysis are helpful in assessing adequacy of respiratory efforts. Strict monitoring of intake and output and electrolyte balance is essential. As neurologic condition worsens, the nurse should be aware that respiratory depression and arrest can occur quickly. Use of benzodiazepines and other sedatives are discouraged in the FHF patient because of the "masking" of pertinent neurologic changes and further potentiating hepatic encephalopathy. This is often difficult for the nurse to understand because these patients may be extremely agitated and combative and require restraints for patient protection. A thorough neurologic assessment should be performed at least every hour.

Educating the patient and family

Early in the patient's hospital stay, the patient and family should be taught about FHF, its etiologies and treatment. As the patient moves toward discharge, teaching should focus on the interventions necessary for preventing the reoccurrence of the precipitating etiology. If the patient is considered a liver transplant candidate, the patient and family will need significant information regarding the procedure and care. Liver transplant evaluation may include screening for medical contraindications, HIV serology, anticipated compliance, and assessment of

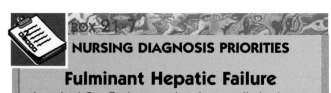

NURSING DIAGNOSIS PRIORITIES

Fulminant Hepatic Failure

- Impaired Gas Exchange related to ventilation/perfusion mismatching or intrapulmonary shunting, p. 476
- Decreased Cardiac Output related to alterations in preload, pp. 467-468
- Decreased Adaptive Capacity: Intracranial related to failure of normal compensatory mechanisms, pp. 480-481
- Risk for Infection, pp. 494-495
- Body Image Disturbance related to actual change in body structure, function, or appearance, p. 451
- Knowledge Deficit: Discharge Regimen related to lack of previous exposure to information, p. 443

the social support system. Psychiatric and other specialty team consults are necessary for a thorough evaluation of the patient's suitability for a transplant.

THERAPEUTIC MANAGEMENT

Gastrointestinal Intubation

Because GI intubation is so commonly used in critical care units, it is important for nurses to know the clinical indications and responsibilities inherent in its use. The four categories of GI tubes are based on function—nasogastric suction tubes, long intestinal tubes, esophagogastric balloon tamponade tubes, and feeding tubes.

Nasogastric suction tubes

Nasogastric suction tubes (Levin, Salem sump) remove fluid regurgitated into the stomach, prevent accumulation of swallowed air, may partially decompress the bowel, and reduce the patient's risk for aspiration. These tubes can also be used for collecting specimens and administering tube feedings. The tube is passed through the nose into the nasopharynx and then down through the pharynx into the esophagus and stomach. The length of time the nasogastric tube remains in place depends on its use. The tube is then placed to gravity, low-intermittent suction, low continuous suction, or, in rare instances, clamped.

Nursing management is focused on preventing complications common to this therapy, such as ulceration and necrosis of the nares, esophageal reflux, esophagitis, esophageal erosion and stricture, gastric erosion, and dry mouth and parotitis from mouth breathing. In addition, interference with ventilation and coughing, aspiration, and loss of fluid and electrolytes can also be critical problems. Interventions include irrigating the tube every 4 hours with normal saline, ensuring the blue air vent of the Salem sump is patent and maintained above the level of the patient's stomach, and providing frequent mouth and nares care.

Long intestinal tubes

Miller-Abbott, Cantor, Johnston, and Baker tubes are examples of long intestinal tubes that are placed either preoperatively or intraoperatively. The long length allows removal of contents from the intestine that cannot be accomplished by a nasogastric tube. These tubes can decompress the small bowel and can splint the small bowel intraoperatively or postoperatively. Because progression of the tubes depends on bowel peristalsis, their use is contraindicated in patients with paralytic ileus and severe mechanical bowel obstructions.

Interventions used in the care of the patient with a long intestinal tube are similar to those with a nasogastric tube. The patient should be observed for gaseous distention of the balloon section, which makes removal difficult; rupture of the balloon or spillage of mercury into the intestine; overinflation of the balloon, which can lead to intestinal rupture; and reverse intussusception if the tube is removed rapidly. Intestinal tubes should be removed slowly, usually 6 inches of the tube is withdrawn every hour.

Esophagogastric balloon tamponade tubes

Currently there are three different types of balloon tamponade tubes available: Sengstaken-Blakemore tube, the Linton tube, and the Minnesota tube. The Sengstaken-Blakemore tube has three lumens—one for the gastric balloon, one for esophageal balloon, and one for the gastric suction (Fig. 21-4, *A*). The Linton tube also has three lumens—one for the gastric balloon, one for gastric suction, and one for esophageal suction (Fig. 21-4, *B*). The Minnesota tube has four lumens—one for the gastric balloon, one for the esophageal balloon, one for gastric suction, and one for esophageal suction (Fig. 21-4, *C*). The Minnesota tube is preferable to the other tubes as it offers both a gastric and an esophageal balloon and allows suction to be applied both above and below the balloons (in the stomach and in the esophagus).[34]

Balloon tamponade tubes are inserted by the physician. Once the tube is passed into the stomach and placement assessed, the gastric balloon is inflated with 250 to 300 ml of air (or as specified by the tube manufacturer). The tube is then placed under tension so that the gastric balloon places pressure on the gastroesophageal junction. Two to three pounds of tension is usually applied using a helmet with a constant traction spring device. Once secured in place the esophageal balloon is inflated to a pressure of 25 to 45 mm Hg. Low intermittent suction is applied to both the gastric and esophageal ports. Once the patient's bleeding has stopped for 24 hours, the esophageal balloon is deflated, and, if rebleeding does not occur over the next 24 hours, the gastric balloon is deflated. If there is no further bleeding, the tube is discontinued 24 hours later.[34]

Nursing management of the patient with a balloon tamponade tube includes monitoring for rebleeding and observing for complications of the tube. The most common complication is pulmonary aspiration, which can be limited by emptying the stomach and placing an endotracheal tube before passing the balloon tamponade tube. Additional complications include esophageal erosion and rupture, balloon migration, and nasal necrosis. Balloon migration can be a potentially life-threatening complication. If the gastric balloon is allowed to slowly deflate or ruptures, the esophageal balloon migrates upward where it can occlude the patient's airway. If the patient develops respiratory distress, the gastric and esophageal balloon ports should be cut immediately.[34]

Transjugular Intrahepatic Portosystemic Shunt

A transjugular intrahepatic portosystemic shunt (TIPS) is an angiographic interventional procedure for decreasing portal hypertension. Recent data suggests that TIPS is advocated in patients with portal hypertension that are also

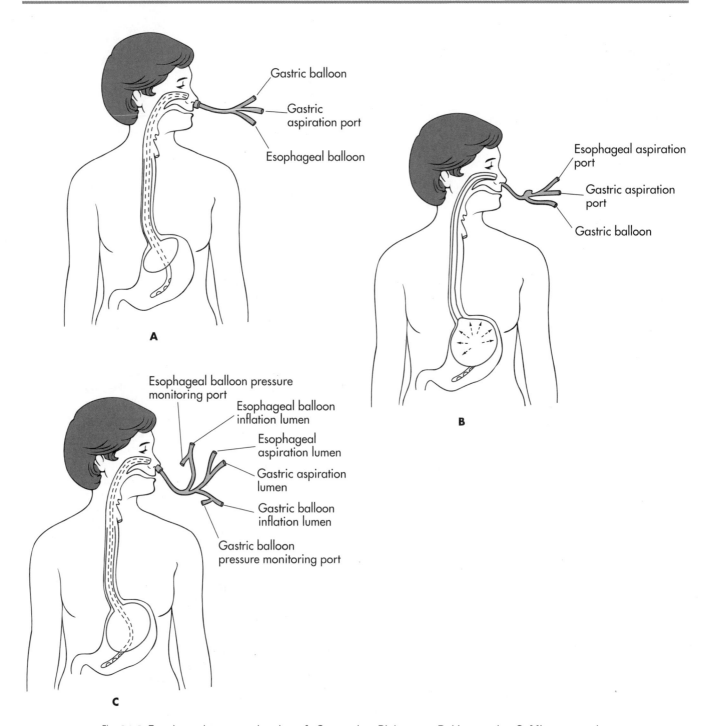

Fig. **21-4** Esophageal tamponade tubes. **A,** Sengstaken-Blakemore. **B,** Linton tube. **C,** Minnesota tube.

experiencing active bleeding, poor liver reserve, in transplant patients, or in patients with other operative risks.[35] The TIPS procedure is usually performed by a gastroenterologist, vascular surgeon, or interventional radiologist.

Portal hypertension is first confirmed via direct measurement of the pressure in the portal vein (gradient >10 mm Hg). Cannulation is achieved via the internal jugular vein and an angiographic catheter is advanced into the middle or right hepatic vein. The midhepatic vein is then catheterized and a new route is created connecting the portal and hepatic veins, using a needle and guidewire with a dilating balloon. A expandable stainless steel stent is then placed in the liver parenchyma to maintain that connection (Fig. 21-5). The increased resistance in the liver is therefore bypassed.[36]

TIPS may be performed on patients with bleeding varices, refractory bleeding varices, or as a "bridge" to liver transplant if the candidate becomes hemodynamically unstable. Post-procedure care should include observation for overt (cannulation site) or covert (intrahepatic site)

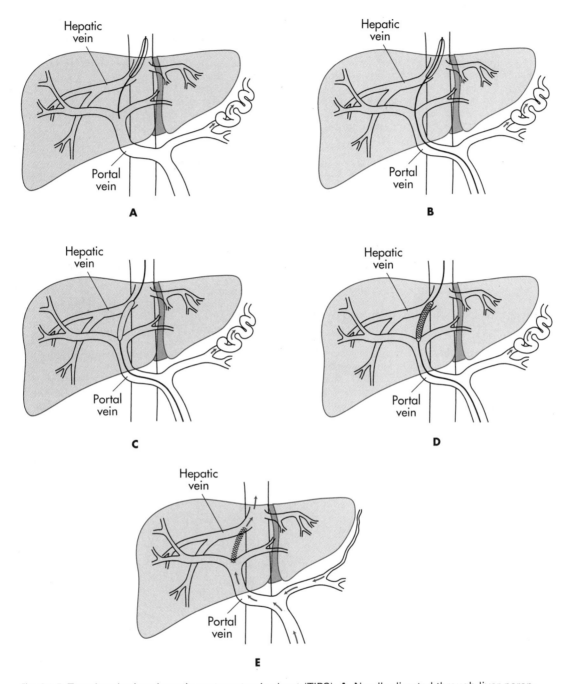

Fig. **21-5** Transjugular intrahepatic portosystemic shunt (TIPS). **A,** Needle directed through liver paren-chyma to portal vein. **B,** Needle and guidewire passed down to midportal vein. **C,** Balloon dilation. **D,** De-ployment of stent. **E,** Intrahepatic shunt from portal to hepatic vein. (Zemel G, et al: Percutaneous transjugular portosystemic shunt, *JAMA* 266:391, 1991.)

bleeding, hepatic or portal vein laceration (resulting in rapid loss of blood volume), and inadvertent puncture of surrounding organs. Other complications include bile duct trauma, stent migration and stent thrombosis. Loss of shunt patency occurs 5% to 75% of the time as a result of shunt thrombosis or stenosis. The 30-day mortality rate for this procedure is approximately 24% to 45%.[36]

References

1. Prevost SS, Oberle A: Stress ulceration in the critically ill pa-tient, *Crit Care Nurs Clin North Am* 5:163, 1993.
2. Zimmerman HM, Curfman KL: Acute gastrointestinal bleeding, *AACN Clin Issues Crit Care Nurs* 8:449, 1997.
3. Brewer TG: Treatment of acute gastroesophageal variceal hemorrhage, *Med Clin North Am* 77:993, 1993.
4. *St Anthony's DRG guidebook 1998*, Reston, VA, 1997, St An-thony Publishing.

5. DeMarkles MP, Murphy JR: Acute lower gastrointestinal bleeding, *Med Clin North Am* 77:1085, 1993.
6. Gupta PK, Fleischer DE: Nonvariceal upper gastrointestinal bleeding, *Med Clin North Am* 77:973,
7. Mertz HR, Walsh JH: Peptic ulcer pathophysiology, *Med Clin North Am* 75:799, 1991.
8. McQuaid KR, Isenberg JI: Medical therapy of peptic ulcer disease, *Surg Clin North Am* 72:885, 1992.
9. Fisher RL, Pipkin GA, Wood JR: Stress-related mucosal disease: pathophysiology, prevention, and treatment, *Crit Care Clin* 11:323, 1995.
10. Huether SE, McCance KL, Tarmina MS: Alterations of digestive function. In McCance KL, Huether SE, editors: *Pathophysiology: the biological basis for disease in adults and children*, ed 3, St Louis, 1998, Mosby.
11. Joff DL, Chung RT, Friedman LS: Management of portal hypertension and its complications, *Med Clin North Am* 80:1021, 1996.
12. McEwen DR: Management of alcoholic cirrhosis of the liver, *AORN J* 64:214, 1996.
13. Geier DL, Cooke AR: Upper GI bleeding: a five step approach to diagnosis and treatment, *J Crit Illness* 7:1676, 1992.
14. Sugawa C, Joseph AL: Endoscopic interventional management of bleeding duodenal and gastric ulcers, *Surg Clin North Am* 72:317, 1992.
15. Rosen RJ, Sanchez G: Angiographic diagnosis and management of gastrointestinal hemorrhage: current concepts, *Radiol Clin North Am* 32:951, 1994.
16. Jutabha R, Jensen DM: Management of upper gastrointestinal bleeding in the patient with chronic liver disease, *Med Clin North Am* 80:1035, 1996.
17. Smith SL, Butler RW: *Acute pancreatitis. Part I. An overview*, Aliso Viejo, CA, 1993, American Association of Critical Care Nurses.
18. Steer ML: Acute pancreatitis. In Taylor MB, editor: *Gastrointestinal emergencies*, Baltimore, 1992, Williams & Wilkins.
19. Singh M, Simsek H: Ethanol and the pancreas, *Gastroenterology* 98:1051, 1990.
20. Brown A: Acute pancreatitis: pathophysiology, nursing diagnoses, and collaborative problems, *Focus Crit Care* 18(2):121, 1991.
21. Ranson JHC: Complications of pancreatitis. In Taylor MB, editor: *Gastrointestinal emergencies*, Baltimore, 1992, Williams & Wilkins.
22. Ransom J: The current management of acute pancreatitis, *Adv Surg* 28:93, 1995.
23. Krumberger JM: Acute pancreatitis, *Crit Care Nurs Clin North Am* 5:185, 1993.
24. Forsmark CC, Toskes PP: Acute pancreatitis: medical management, *Crit Care Clin* 11:295, 1995.
25. Butler RW, Smith: *Acute pancreatitis. Part II. Complications and surgical management*, Aliso Viejo, CA, 1993, American Association of Critical Care Nurses.
26. McConnell EA: Loosening the grip of intestinal obstructions, *Nursing* 24(3):34, 1994.
27. Scovill WA: Small bowel obstruction. In Cameron JL, editor: *Current surgical therapy*, ed 5, St Louis, 1995, Mosby.
28. Choti MA: Obstruction of the large bowel. In Cameron JL, editor: *Current surgical therapy*, ed 5, St Louis, 1995, Mosby.
29. Steinhagen RM, Aufses AH: Acute abdominal obstruction: when to consider nonoperative therapy, *J Crit Illness* 8:209, 1993.
30. Ganger D, et al: Hepatic failure. In Parrillo JE, Bone RC, editors: *Critical care medicine: principles of diagnosis and management*, St Louis, 1994, Mosby.
31. Bernstein D, Tripodi J: Fulminant hepatic failure, *Crit Care Clin* 14:181, 1998.
32. Kucharski SA: Fulminant hepatic failure, *Crit Care Nurs Clin North Am* 5:141, 1993.
33. Elrod R: Problems of the liver, biliary tract, and pancreas. In Lewis SM, Collier IC, Heitkemper MM, editors: *Medical-surgical nursing: assessment and management of clinical problems*, ed 4, St Louis, 1996, Mosby.
34. Amato EJ: A nursing reference: gastrointestinal tubes and drains. Part II: esophageal tubes, *Crit Care Nurs* 3(1):46, 1983.
35. Becker YT, et al: The role of elective operation in the treatment of portal hypertension, *Ann Surg* 62:171, 1996.
36. Bouley G, et al: Transjugular intrahepatic portosystemic shunt: an alternative, *Crit Care Nurs* 16(1):26, 1996.

ENDOCRINE
ALTERATIONS

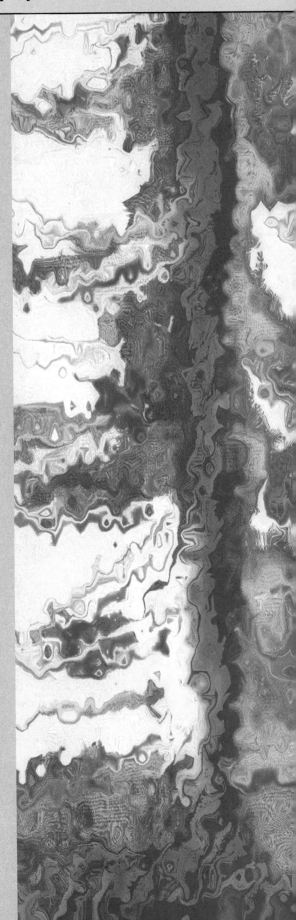

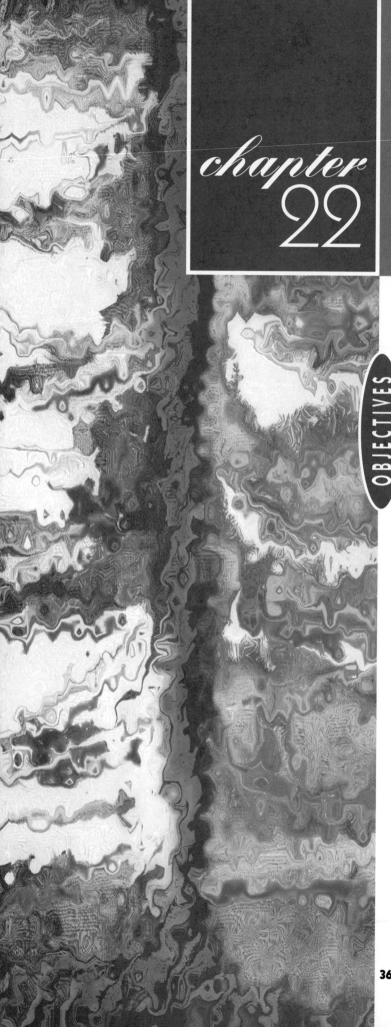

Endocrine Assessment and Diagnostic Procedures

JoAnn M. Clark

- **Identify the components of an endocrine history.**

- **Describe clinical findings of a patient with pancreatic, posterior pituitary, and thyroid dysfunction.**

- **Delineate the clinical significance of selected laboratory tests used in the assessment of endocrine disorders.**

- **Outline important diagnostic procedures for detection of selected endocrine disorders.**

Assessment of the patient with endocrine dysfunction is a systematic process that incorporates both a history and a physical examination. Most of the endocrine glands, except for the gonads and thyroid, are deeply encased in the human body. Although the placement of the glands provides security for the glandular functions, their resulting inaccessibility prevents them from being examined in the usual fashion. Nevertheless, the endocrine glands can be assessed in an indirect manner. The nurse who understands the metabolic actions of the hormones produced by those glands assesses the physiology of the gland by monitoring that gland's target tissue (Fig. 22-1). This chapter focuses on priority clinical assessments, laboratory studies, and diagnostic tests for the critically ill patient with endocrine dysfunction.

HISTORY

The initial presentation of the patient determines the rapidity and direction of the interview. For a patient in acute distress, the history is curtailed to just a few questions about the patient's chief complaint and precipitating events. For a patient in no obvious distress, the his-

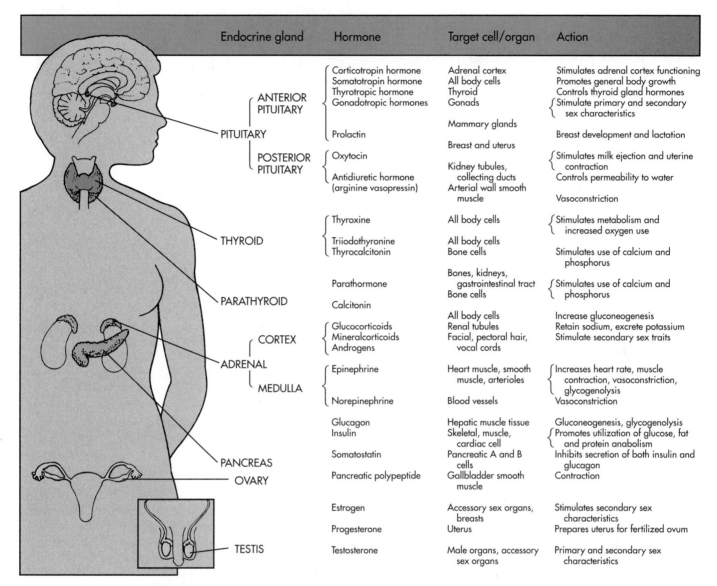

Endocrine gland	Hormone	Target cell/organ	Action
ANTERIOR PITUITARY	Corticotropin hormone	Adrenal cortex	Stimulates adrenal cortex functioning
	Somatotropin hormone	All body cells	Promotes general body growth
	Thyrotropic hormone	Thyroid	Controls thyroid gland hormones
	Gonadotropic hormones	Gonads	Stimulate primary and secondary sex characteristics
PITUITARY	Prolactin	Mammary glands	Breast development and lactation
		Breast and uterus	
POSTERIOR PITUITARY	Oxytocin	Kidney tubules, collecting ducts	Stimulates milk ejection and uterine contraction
	Antidiuretic hormone (arginine vasopressin)	Arterial wall smooth muscle	Controls permeability to water
			Vasoconstriction
THYROID	Thyroxine	All body cells	Stimulates metabolism and increased oxygen use
	Triiodothyronine	All body cells	
	Thyrocalcitonin	Bone cells	Stimulates use of calcium and phosphorus
PARATHYROID	Parathormone	Bones, kidneys, gastrointestinal tract	Stimulates use of calcium and phosphorus
	Calcitonin	Bone cells	
ADRENAL CORTEX	Glucocorticoids	All body cells	Increase gluconeogenesis
	Mineralcorticoids	Renal tubules	Retain sodium, excrete potassium
	Androgens	Facial, pectoral hair, vocal cords	Stimulate secondary sex traits
ADRENAL MEDULLA	Epinephrine	Heart muscle, smooth muscle, arterioles	Increases heart rate, muscle contraction, vasoconstriction, glycogenolysis
	Norepinephrine	Blood vessels	Vasoconstriction
PANCREAS	Glucagon	Hepatic muscle tissue	Gluconeogenesis, glycogenolysis
	Insulin	Skeletal, muscle, cardiac cell	Promotes utilization of glucose, fat and protein anabolism
	Somatostatin	Pancreatic A and B cells	Inhibits secretion of both insulin and glucagon
	Pancreatic polypeptide	Gallbladder smooth muscle	Contraction
OVARY	Estrogen	Accessory sex organs, breasts	Stimulates secondary sex characteristics
	Progesterone	Uterus	Prepares uterus for fertilized ovum
TESTIS	Testosterone	Male organs, accessory sex organs	Primary and secondary sex characteristics

Fig. **22-1** Location of endocrine glands with hormones, target cell/organ, and hormone action.

tory focuses on four different areas: (1) review of the patient's present illness, (2) overview of the patient's general endocrine status, (3) examination of the patient's general health status, and (4) survey of the patient's lifestyle. Areas to be included in the interview are outlined in Box 22-1.[1]

PANCREAS

Physical Assessment

Insulin, which is produced by the pancreas, is responsible for glucose metabolism. Acute dysfunction of the pancreas can result in insufficient insulin production. Conversely, adequate insulin production may exist with a receptor side resistance to circulating insulin, resulting in decreased levels of the insulin hormone. Thus the signs and symptoms of pancreatic dysfunction often manifest as hyperglycemia. **Assessment priorities for the patient with pancreatic dysfunction focus on observation for signs and symptoms of hyperglycemia.**

Observation for signs of hyperglycemia

The consequences of hyperglycemia affect a variety of body systems; therefore, all systems must be assessed for signs and symptoms. The patient may complain of blurred vision, headache, weakness, fatigue, drowsiness, anorexia, nausea, and abdominal pain. Upon inspection, the patient has flushed skin, polyuria, polydipsia, and vomiting. Excessively high blood glucose causes the patient's level of consciousness to be anywhere from lethargic to comatose. In addition, the patient's breathing is deep and rapid (Kussmaul's respirations) with a fruity odor to the breath. Auscultation of the abdomen reveals hypoactive bowel sounds and palpation elicits tender-

ENDOCRINE NURSING HISTORY

HISTORY
Chief complaint
History of present problem
  Onset
  Duration
  Signs/symptoms
  Treatments
History of pancreatic problems, surgery, diabetes, carbohydrate imbalances, thyroid disease, or kidney problems
Head or neurologic disorders
Recent severe infection or surgical trauma
Past or current treatments using hyperalimentation, peritoneal dialysis, or hemodialysis
Recent, unexplained changes in weight, thirst, hunger, or urination patterns
Changes in mental abilities (i.e., memory loss, momentary disorientation, difficulty concentrating, lethargy)
Recent changes in daily levels of activities, (e.g., decreased endurance level, fatigue, weakness)
Usage of prescription or over-the-counter drugs
Presence of acute stress
Family history of present illness (e.g., carbohydrate imbalance)

ness. Percussion reveals diminished deep tendon reflexes. Because hyperglycemia results in osmotic diuresis, the patient's fluid volume status is also assessed. Signs of dehydration include tachycardia, orthostatic hypotension, and poor skin turgor.

Laboratory Studies

Pertinent laboratory tests for the pancreas measure the amount of insulin produced by the pancreatic β cells and the effectiveness of insulin in transporting glucose from the blood stream into the cell. The test, while not a routine laboratory test for the individual with diabetes, reveals whether insulin can maintain a constant serum glucose level as well as contribute to the metabolism of fats and protein. When adequate insulin is unavailable to permit glucose to be used for fuel, the body is forced to break down noncarbohydrate sources, such as fat and protein, as alternate energy sources (gluconeogenesis). The liver, which normally contributes to protein and fat metabolism, is unable to complete gluconeogenesis as rapidly as the body requires fuel sources. The end result is accumulation of "waste products" from incomplete protein and fat gluconeogenesis. Tests to determine the osmolality, glucose level, and ketone level identify the residual effects of incomplete glucose uptake and use by the cells.

Insulin

The normal value of serum insulin is 5 to 20 mU/ml. This measurement of insulin levels, obtained by a sensi-tive radioimmunoassay test, indicates the amount of insulin circulating in the bloodstream during a period of fasting. The release of insulin depends on the concentration of blood glucose; in the healthy person, when glucose levels rise, insulin levels also rise. Conversely, when serum glucose levels are low, insulin secretion is inhibited. A fasting blood sample is preferred for evaluation of serum insulin levels, although insulin levels are not typically measured to determine diabetes mellitus.

Glucose

The normal fasting serum or plasma value of glucose, when measured by a blood test, is 70 to 110 mg/dL. The fasting whole blood value is 60 to 100 mg/dL. The nonfasting value is 85 to 125 mg/dL. A fasting blood sample is read as a simple, numeric value, but it actually measures many complex, interrelated processes. The circulating blood glucose level is derived from three sources—exogenous intake of glucose, release of glycogen stores (glycogenolysis), and breakdown of noncarbohydrate sources (gluconeogenesis). The glucose reading measures the ability of the pancreatic A cells to balance the release of glucagon with the β-cell release of insulin. The circulating glucose level also depends on the peripheral uptake of glucose and the functioning of the liver and its role in gluconeogenesis. Consistently elevated glucose levels signal both an increase in glucagon production and an insufficient amount of effective insulin.

Glycosylated hemoglobin

A normal glycosylated hemoglobin level is 4% to 7%, with acceptable values within 1% of the upper limit of normal;[2] that is, 4% to 7% of the person's hemoglobin contains a glucose group. This laboratory test provides information about the average amount of glucose that has been present in the patient's bloodstream over the previous 3 to 4 months. During the 120-day life span of erythrocytes, the hemoglobin within each cell binds to the available blood glucose through a process known as *glycosylation*. Through this irreversible process, increased levels of circulating glucose cause an increase in glycosylation. This test is not routinely performed as a pancreatic screening tool but rather is used for patients previously diagnosed with diabetes mellitus. It provides information about the degree of hyperglycemia, including the actual increased values over a specific period of time. This test eliminates many variables that normally could affect the accurate interpretation of a glucose test result. Infrequent fasting state, exercise, stress, and medications do not interfere with this test result, nor will the test outcome be influenced by patient compliance or changes in a patient's usual habits initiated only to have a fasting blood glucose value read closer to normal than usual.

Serum ketones

In a serum blood test, the normal ketone levels are 2 to 4 mg/dL of blood and acetone is 0.3 to 2 mg/dL of blood. Ketones are byproducts of fat metabolism. In most cases, when the body uses carbohydrate as its main source of energy, fat metabolism is completed by the liver and only a trace of ketones is found in the blood. Ketone bodies in the blood (ketonemia) is evidenced by a fruity, sweet-smelling odor on the exhaled breath. This odor is the result of the body's attempt to keep the pH within the normal range.

Urine ketones

Normally ketones are not present in the urine; thus the results of urine tests would be negative. As mentioned previously, in the absence of glucose, fats are burned for energy. Lipolysis (fat breakdown) occurs so rapidly that fat metabolism is incomplete, and ketone bodies (acetone, beta-hydroxybutyric acid, and acetoacetic acid) collect in the blood (ketonemia) and are excreted in the urine (ketonuria).

Serum osmolality

Osmolality is a measurement of the number of particles in a solution or the concentration of the solution (this differs from the size or weight of particles in a solution). A search of laboratory data identifies an all-inclusive range for serum osmolality to be 270 to 319 mOsm/kg of water.[3-9] The literature shows that while the different laboratories report various extremes for their ranges, the range itself remains narrow. Serum osmolality is not a routine screening tool for pancreatic dysfunction. It is used commonly to identify the effects of an imbalance in carbohydrate metabolism and to assess fluid volume status.

PITUITARY GLAND

Physical Assessment

Antidiuretic hormone (ADH) controls the amount of fluid lost and retained within the body. Acute dysfunction of the posterior pituitary or the hypothalamus can result in insufficient or excessive ADH production. Thus the clinical manifestions of posterior pituitary dysfunction often manifest as fluid volume deficit (insufficient ADH production) or fluid volume excess (excessive ADH production). The nurse determines the effectiveness of ADH production by conducting a hydration assessment. **Assessment of the patient focuses on three priorities: (1) observation of buccal membrane moisture and skin turgor and moisture, (2) evaluation of vital signs, and (3) measurement of the patient's weight and intake and output.**

Observation of buccal membrane moisture and skin turgor and moisture

Satisfactory fluid balance is easily identified by the presence of moist, shiny buccal membranes. Skin turgor that is resilient and returns to its original position in less than 3 seconds after being pinched or lifted indicates adequate skin elasticity. Skin over the forehead, clavicle, and sternum is the most reliable for testing tissue turgor

because it is less affected by aging and thus more easily assessed for changes related to fluid balance. Edema is absent. A well-hydrated patient has skin in the groin and axilla that is slightly moist to touch.

Evaluation of vital signs

Blood pressure and pulse are monitored frequently. Decreased blood pressure with an increased pulse is characteristic of hypovolemia, whereas elevated blood pressure and rapid, bounding pulse may indicate hypervolemia. Orthostatic hypotension, which occurs when extracellular fluid volume decreases, is identified by a drop in systolic blood pressure of 20 mm Hg and a drop in diastolic blood pressure of 10 mm Hg when the patient changes position from lying to standing.

Measurement of weight and intake and output

Daily weight changes coincide with fluid retention and fluid loss. Sudden changes in weight could result from a change in fluid balance; 1 L of fluid lost or retained is equal to approximately 2.2 pounds (2 pounds, 3 ounces or 1 kg) of weight gained or lost. To use weight as a true determinant of the body's weight changes, all extraneous variables, such as changes in clothing, are eliminated and the same scale is used at the same time each day. Measuring and recording intake and output is a simple task that, when performed accurately and conscientiously on all routes of fluid intake and loss, provides information about the body's fluid balance. Precise intake and output records are used as criteria for fluid replacement therapy. Physical characteristics of urine, such as concentration, color, and specific gravity, are significant factors in assessing the patient's fluid balance. A balanced intake and output, stable weight, and urine specific gravity that falls within the normal range (1.005 to 1.030) all serve as indicators that the patient's hydration status is adequate.

Laboratory Assessment

No single diagnostic test identifies posterior pituitary gland dysfunction. Diagnosis usually is made through an array of laboratory tests combined with the clinical profile of the patient. The tests include both a measurement of the serum antidiuretic hormone that is produced by the hypothalamus and tests that gauge the subsequent release of ADH by the posterior pituitary. Serum and urine osmolality tests measure the effectiveness of ADH in maintaining the correct solute concentration for the particular sample of fluid.

Serum antidiuretic hormone

The result of a blood test for normal levels of serum ADH is 1 to 13.3 pg/ml (picogram, 5 trillionth of a gram). The serum ADH test measures the amount of ADH present in a frozen sample of blood. The direct measurement of ADH is possible by means of a laboratory radioimmunoassay. This test provides accurate results and is used in preference to the water load and water deprivation tests. To prepare a patient for antidiuretic hormone radioimmunoassay testing, all drugs that may alter the release of ADH are withheld for a minimum of 8 hours. Medications that affect ADH levels include morphine sulfate, lithium carbonate, chlorothiazide, carbamazepine, oxytocin, and certain neoplastic and anesthetic agents. Nicotine, alcohol, both positive- and negative-pressure ventilation, and emotional stress can also influence the ADH levels and must be considered in the interpretation of values. The test, read by comparing serum ADH levels with the blood and urine osmolality, is helpful in differentiating the syndrome of inappropriate antidiuretic hormone (SIADH) from central diabetes insipidus (DI). The presence of increased ADH in the bloodstream compared with a low serum osmolality and elevated urine osmolality confirms the diagnosis of SIADH. Reduced levels of serum ADH in a patient with high serum osmolality, hypernatremia, and reduced urine concentration signal central DI.

Urine and serum osmolality

As previously presented, the literature values for serum osmolality range from 270 to 300 mOsm/kg H_2O, with an normal variance from 285 to 300 mOsm/kg H_2O. Osmolality measurements determine the concentration of dissolved particles in a solution. In a healthy person, a change in the concentration of solutes triggers a chain of events to maintain proper dilution. The average value for urine osmolality is within 300 to 800 mOsm/kg H_2O, with the outermost range of 50 to 1200 mOsm/kg H_2O. Increased serum osmolality stimulates the release of ADH, which in turn reduces the amount of water lost at the nephron tubules. Body fluid, thereby, is retained to dilute the particle concentration in the bloodstream. Decreased serum osmolality inhibits the release of ADH, the kidney tubules increase their permeability, and fluid is eliminated from the body in an attempt to regain normal concentration of particles in the bloodstream. The most accurate results of the body's ability to maintain a fluid balance are obtained when urine and blood samples are collected simultaneously.

Water deprivation test

Normal values for the water deprivation test are urine osmolality, 800 mOsm/kg H_2O and serum osmolality, 285 to 300 mOsm/kg H_2O. This test is based on the premise that ADH is released to conserve urinary water when a patient is at risk of becoming dehydrated. The results of this test are useful in diagnosing central diabetes insipidus and SIADH. The procedure for this test purposely withholds all fluids for 24 hours while serum and urine laboratory tests determine the body's response to the pending dehydration. The water deprivation test is rarely done in the intensive care unit because of the time involved and the risks of dehydration to an already severely compromised patient.

Synthetic ADH test

Another test done in place of water deprivation is the administration of a subcutaneous injection of aqueous vasopressin (Pitressin) (synthetic ADH). This test provides information to differentiate the type of diabetes insipidus. The test is performed by measuring urine volume and osmolality on serial urine collections over a 2-hour period. The patient with normal posterior pituitary functioning responds to the exogenous ADH by reabsorbing water at the tubule and raising the urine osmolality slightly. In cases of severe central diabetes insipidus, the urine osmolality rises significantly. (Values are established by the associated laboratory.) A significant rise indicates that the cell receptor sites on the renal tubules are responsive to Pitressin. Test results in which urine osmolality remains unchanged are suggestive of nephrogenic diabetes insipidus, indicating that the target tissue or cell receptor sites are no longer receptive to ADH.

Water load test

The water load test is based on the premise that changes in the concentration of particles in the bloodstream will affect the release of ADH as the body strives to maintain a homeostatic balance. The water load test is helpful in evaluating the function of ADH in both diabetes insipidus and syndrome of inappropriate antidiuretic hormone. In this test, the patient is overhydrated and then a series of blood and urine samples are taken to monitor the sequence of physiologic events leading to a fluid balance. Because of the serious risks of overhydrating the critically ill patient and the potentially lethal effect on patients with cardiac or renal dysfunction, this test is rarely performed in the critical care environment.

Diagnostic Procedures

In addition to laboratory tests, radiographic examination, computed tomography (CT), and magnetic resonance imaging (MRI) are helpful in diagnosing hypothalamic-pituitary disease. Cranial bone fractures that injure the hypophyseal stalk and space-occupying masses, such as tumors or blood clots that interfere with pituitary circulation, are examples of abnormalities identified and studied in diagnostic tests.

Radiologic examination

A basic x-ray examination of the inferior skull views the sella turcica and surrounding bone formation. Bone fractures or tissue swelling at the base of the brain, which are apparent on a radiograph, suggest interference with the vascular supply and nerve impulses to the hypothalamic-pituitary system. Dysfunction may occur if the hypothalamus, the infundibular stalk, or the pituitary is impaired.

Computed tomography

Computed tomography (CT) of the base of the skull (sella turcica) identifies pituitary tumors, blood clots, cysts, nodules, or other tissue masses. A skull CT scan provides more definitive results than does an x-ray test and, whenever possible, is obtained in preference to a skull x-ray film. The 40-minute procedure causes no discomfort except that it requires the patient to be perfectly still. A radioopaque sodium iodine solution may be given intravenously to highlight the hypothalamus, infundibular stalk, and pituitary gland. This dye may cause allergic reactions in iodine-sensitive persons, and the patient must be carefully questioned before the start of the test. Size and shape of the sella turcica and position of the hypothalamus, infundibular stalk, and pituitary gland are identified.

Magnetic resonance imaging

Magnetic resonance imaging (MRI) enables the radiologist to visualize internal organs as well as examine the cellular characteristics of specific tissue. The soft fluid tissue in and immediately surrounding the brain makes the brain especially responsive to MRI scanning. Although the MRI is not a definitive diagnostic test for posterior pituitary hormonal imbalance, its use identifies anatomic disruption of the gland and the surrounding area suggestive of primary causes of diabetes insipidus and SIADH.

THYROID

Physical Examination

The normal-size thyroid gland is not visible or apparent in the anterior neck. Palpation of the neck to reveal a goiter or enlargement of the thyroid gland is not usually done as part of a routine critical care assessment. Assessment of the thyroid gland is accomplished by assessing for the effects of thyroid hormone. Acute dysfunction of the thyroid can result in insufficient or excessive thyroid hormone production. Thus the clinical manifestions of thyroid dysfunction often manifest as hyperthyroidism or hypothyroidism. **Assessment priorities for the patient with thyroid dysfunction focus on observation for signs and symptoms of hyperthyroidism and hypothyroidism.**

Observation of the signs and symptoms of hyperthyroidism

Critical assessment for hyperthyroidism include observation of patient response reflecting increased metabolism, heightened sensitivity to adrenergic receptors, and loss of thermoregulation. Cardiac functioning, including stroke volume and cardiac output, is monitored. Appetite, nausea, vomiting, and diarrhea are assessed as the body attempts to increase food intake and replenish fuel for energy expenditure. Hyperglycemia may result from the change in mobilization of nutrients and imbalance of insulin release. In addition, motility of the gastrointestinal tract is affected by increased thyroid hormones. Observation of the client's tolerance of heat is also important. The patient complains of profuse sweating and being too hot and often follows this report by turning off room heat, opening all windows, and taking off all but minimal clothing and bed linens, even on the coldest days.

Observation of the signs and symptoms of hypothyroidism

Clinical monitoring of the patient with hypothyroidism includes an assessment similar to that for the patient with hyperthyroidism but with different expected outcomes. Critical assessment for hypothyroidism include observation of patient responses to a slowed body metabolism because of decreased oxygen consumption by the tissues. Mental impairment influences judgment, comprehension, and awareness. Bradycardia and reduced cardiac contractility result in diminished cardiac output. The patient is carefully evaluated for heart failure. Hypoventilation and decreased respiratory capacity occur. A distended abdomen, decreased intestinal peristalsis, and constipation are common. The patient with hypothermia has sensations of being cold and will wear layers of clothing and blankets even on the warmest/hottest days.

Laboratory Assessment

Tests most commonly performed on a thyroid panel are listed in Table 22-1. The tests measure the hormonal negative feedback response within the hypothalamic-pituitary axis. Laboratory diagnosis of hyperthyroidism or hypothyroidism is usually based on the ultrasensitive thyroid-stimulating hormone (TSH) (also known as serum thyrotropin assay) and free T_4.[5]

However, the outcome of TSH and free T_4 may be inconclusive in the critically ill patient because hormonal adaptation to the stress of the illness and common problems of protein malnutrition in critical care situations influence thyroid hormone production and distribution throughout the body.[10] Additional disadvantages inherent in the thyroid laboratory tests are the adjustments that need to be made for individual variables in serum protein levels—for example, the elderly patient,[10] the pregnant woman, and persons with hepatitis and acute intermittent porphyria.[11] Concomitant use of certain drugs also must be considered. Heparin, corticosteroids, and dopamine interfere with thyroid test results. Additional interfering drugs are listed in Box 22-2.[7,10,12]

Diagnostic Procedures

Thyroid scanning

Thyroid scanning involves the use of oral radioactive iodine. Iodine-123 is the preferred isotope because of its low-energy, 13-hour output. This short half-life minimizes the patient's exposure to radioactive material. The thyroid-scanning procedure is useful in detecting the presence of ectopic thyroid tissue and thyroid carcinomas. Thyroid scans also identify the presence and amount of viable thyroid glandular tissue after irradiation treatment.

TABLE 22-1

TESTS MOST COMMONLY PERFORMED ON A THYROID PANEL

| TEST | NORMAL ADULT VALUE | CONDITIONS WITH ABNORMAL VALUES | | SPECIAL CONSIDERATION |
		DECREASED	INCREASED	
Serum thyroxine (T_4)	T_4, 4.5-11.5 μg/dL T_4RIA, 5-12 μg/dL	Hypothyroidism Protein malnutrition Anterior pituitary hypofunction	Hyperthyroidism Viral hepatitis Acute/chronic illness	Simple peripheral blood withdrawal Identifies amount of hormone in circulation Bound by serum protein, therefore affected by TBG Affected by pregnancy
Free thyroid index (FT_4I)	Free T_4, 0.8-2.3 ng/dL	Hypothyroidism	Hyperthyroidism	Same as above, except this measures amount of free T_4, the unbound portion of which enters the cells T_3 uptake multiplied by T_4 equals FTI
Serum triiodothyronine (T_3) (T_3RIA)	110-230 ng/dL	Hypothyroidism Malnutrition Trauma Critical illness	Thyrotoxicosis Toxic adenoma Thyroiditis	Simple peripheral blood withdrawal Measured directly by RIA Direct measurement of both bound and free T_3 Values increase in pregnancy
T_3 uptake ratio (T_3 UR) T_3 resin uptake	25%-35% uptake 0.8-1.30 ratio of laboratory result to standard control	Hypothyroidism Active hepatitis Thyroiditis	Hyperthyroidism Nephrosis Malignancy Protein malnutrition	Does not measure T_3 as name implies Indirectly measure TBG available to bind T_3 and T_4; increase in thyrotoxicosis related to increase in thyroid hormone binding Affected by pregnancy Affected by diseases that alter these proteins
Serum thyroid-stimulating hormone (TSH) test	2-5.4 mU/L <3 ng/ml	Secondary hypothyroidism Anterior pituitary disorder, very low levels, 0.005 mU/L, indicate hyperthyroidism	Primary hypothyroidism Cirrhosis	Identifies thyroid vs. pituitary-hypothalamus disorder
Serum thyrotropin-releasing hormone (TRH), stimulation test, or thyrotropin-releasing factor (TRF) test	Serum TSH rises approximately twice its normal level 30 min after IV TRH			Test confirms presence of thyrotoxicosis by measuring response of the pituitary gland's production of TSH 3-4 wk before test, thyroid medication should be discontinued 500 μg of TRH is given IV to mimic the hypothalamus Venous blood samples are taken at intervals as stated by processing laboratory; peak response occurs in 20 min and returns to normal within 2 hr

FTI, Free thyroid index; *RIA*, radioimmunoassay; *TBG*, thyroxine-binding globulin.

BOX 22-2

DRUGS THAT INFLUENCE DIAGNOSTIC THYROID LEVELS

TRIIODOTHYRONINE (T_3)

Increase	Decrease
Methadone	Anabolic steroid
Estrogens	Androgens
Progestins	Salicylates
Amiodarone	Phenytoin
	Lithium
	Reserpine
	Propranolol
	Sulfonamides
	Propylthiouracil
	Methylthiouracil

THYROXINE (T_4)

Increase	Decrease
Oral contraceptives	Phenytoin
Heparin	Steroids
Aspirin	Diphenylhydantoin
Furosemide	Chlorpromazine
Clofibrate	Lithium
Phenylbutazone	Sulfonylurea
Some nonsteroidal	Sulfonamides
antiinflammatory drugs	Reserpine
(NSAIDs)	Chlordiazepoxide
Propranolol	
Corticosteroids	
Amiodarone	

THYROID-STIMULATING HORMONE (TSH)

Increase TSH	Decrease TSH and TSH Response to TRH
Metoclopramide	Glucocorticoids
Iodides	Dopamine
Lithium	Heparin
Potassium iodide	Aspirin
Morphine sulfate	Carbamazepine

THYROXINE-BINDING GLOBULIN (TBG)

Increase	Decrease
Opiates	Androgen therapy
Oral contraceptives	L-Asparaginase
Estrogens	
Clofibrate	
5-Fluorouracil (5-FU)	
Perphenazine	

References

1. Barkauskas VH et al: *Health and physical assessment,* ed 2, St Louis, 1998, Mosby.
2. Peterson KA, Smith CK: The DCCT (Diabetes Control and Complications Trial), *Am Fam Physician* 52:1092, 1995.
3. Ewald MA, McKenzie CR, editors: *Manual of medical therapeutics,* ed 28, Boston, 1995, Little, Brown.
4. Fischbach F: *A manual of laboratory and diagnostic tests,* ed 5, Philadelphia, 1996, JB Lippincott.
5. Ravel R: *Clinical laboratory medicine: clinical application of laboratory data,* ed 6, St Louis, 1995, Mosby.
6. Corbett J: *Laboratory tests and diagnostic procedures with nursing diagnoses,* ed 4, Norwalk, Conn, 1996, Appleton & Lange.
7. Tierney LM, McPhee SJ, Papadakis MA, editors: *Current medical diagnosis and treatment,* ed 37, Stamford, Conn, 1998, Appleton & Lange.
8. Pincus MR, Henry JB: Clinical chemistry. In Henry JB, editor: *Clinical diagnosis and management by laboratory methods,* ed 19, Philadelphia, 1996, WB Saunders.
9. Fauci A, et al, editors: *Harrison's principles of internal medicine,* ed 14, New York, 1998, McGraw-Hill.
10. Shoemaker W, et al, editors: *Textbook of critical care,* ed 4, Philadelphia, 1998, WB Saunders.
11. Pagana KD, Pagana TJ: *Diagnostic and laboratory test reference,* ed 3, St Louis, 1997, Mosby.
12. Tietz N, et al, editors: *Clinical guide to laboratory tests,* ed 3, Philadelphia, 1995, WB Saunders.

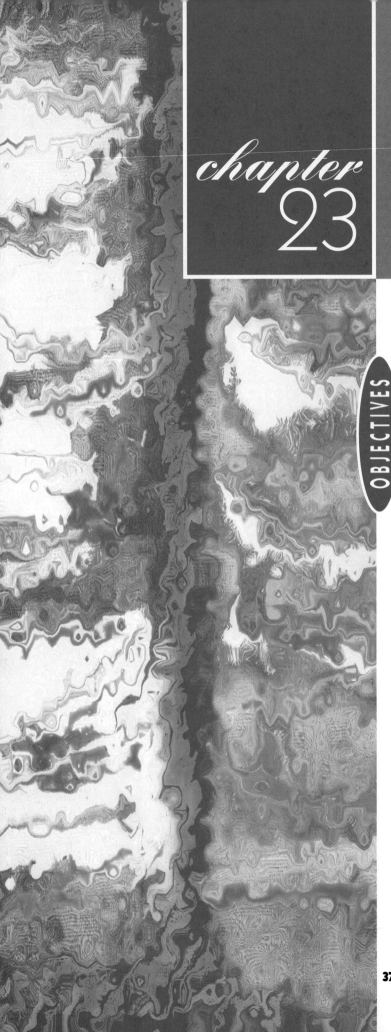

Endocrine Disorders and Therapeutic Management

chapter
23

JoAnn M. Clark

OBJECTIVES

- **Summarize the endocrine responses to the stress of critical illness.**
- **Describe the etiology and pathophysiology of selected endocrine disorders.**
- **Identify the clinical manifestations of selected endocrine disorders.**
- **Explain the treatment of selected endocrine disorders.**
- **Discuss the nursing priorities for managing a patient with selected endocrine disorders.**

Understanding the pathology of a disease, the areas of assessment on which to focus, and the usual medical management allows the critical care nurse to more accurately anticipate and plan nursing interventions. This chapter focuses on endocrine disorders commonly seen in the critical care environment.

STRESS AND CRITICAL ILLNESS

Physiologic changes occur when the individual is confronted with the threat of illness, trauma, or psychologic stress. These changes are initiated when, in an attempt to protect itself from the harm of the stressor, the body mobilizes energy to the cardiopulmonary, endocrine, and nervous systems; the liver; and the muscles. Other systems, such as the reproductive, integumentary, and genitourinary system, are slowed in an attempt to conserve energy. The body's response to stress has a profound effect on both the endocrine and nervous systems. The combined systems' characteristic response pattern to stressors is termed the *neuroendocrine stress response*. The physiologic responses frequently observed by the practitioner to the stress of critical illness are listed in Table 23-1.[1-4]

DIABETIC KETOACIDOSIS

Description and Etiology

Diabetic ketoacidosis (DKA) is a significant community health problem with a major financial impact. Approximately 45,000 to 130,000 hospitalizations for DKA occur annually, based on a population of 10 million persons with diabetes. Of DKA episodes, 20% occur in persons with newly diagnosed diabetes, whereas the other 80% occur after the diagnosis has been made. Individuals 40 years of age and older are most commonly affected by this complication.[5,6] Of all deaths attributed to diabetes, 9% to 14% result from DKA.[7] It is estimated, however, that these deaths occur not from the ketoacidotic state alone but rather from late complications (pneumonia, myocardial infarction, infection) resulting from DKA.[8] Available statistics show that the mortality for patients hospitalized for DKA is 9%, with mortality for females higher than that for males. Furthermore, the death rate from DKA is three times higher in the nonwhite population than in the white population.[7]

Diabetic ketoacidosis is covered under the same DRGs as diabetes mellitus: DRG 295 if the patient's age is between 0 and 35 years, with an average length of stay of 4.1 days, and DRG 294 if the patient is older than 35 years, with an average length of stay of 5.3 days.[9]

Ketoacidosis is a result of hyperglycemia, ketosis, and acidemia without treatment. Counterregulatory hormones, such as glucagon, growth hormone, cortisol, and catecholamines, respond in an attempt to reverse the imbalance, yet only add to the continuing cycle. Box 23-1 lists the etiology of DKA in terms of decreased insulin availability and the presence of increased glucose in the bloodstream.

Changes in self-management of diabetes can influence this ratio, such as a decrease in insulin intake, an increase in dietary intake, or a decrease in routine exercise without adequate adjustment in insulin or diet. Lifestyle changes, such as growth spurts in the adolescent, require an increase in insulin intake as do surgery, infection, and trauma. Emotional stress can increase glucose levels by releasing epinephrine or norepinephrine or both, which then triggers increased glucagon secretion. The person may be continuing a routine insulin dose that becomes, under stress, inadequate for the rate of glucose entry into the bloodstream from gluconeogenesis (formation of glucose from noncarbohydrate sources) and glycogenolysis (breakdown of stored glucose) triggered by the stress hormones. DKA is also seen in patients who use the subcutaneous insulin pump. This device can provide tighter glucose control than subcutaneous injections. However, improper functioning, resulting in insulin leakage or pump failure, initially causes subtle changes in glucose levels.[8,10] The patient, believing that his or her glucose is adequately controlled by the pump, attributes the physi-

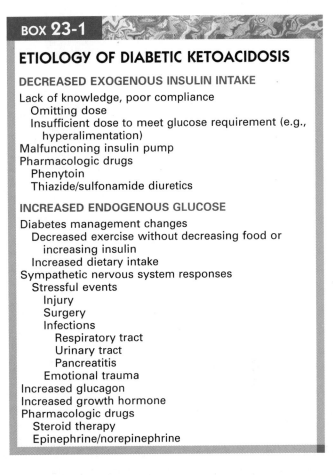

BOX 23-1

ETIOLOGY OF DIABETIC KETOACIDOSIS

DECREASED EXOGENOUS INSULIN INTAKE

Lack of knowledge, poor compliance
  Omitting dose
  Insufficient dose to meet glucose requirement (e.g., hyperalimentation)
Malfunctioning insulin pump
Pharmacologic drugs
  Phenytoin
  Thiazide/sulfonamide diuretics

INCREASED ENDOGENOUS GLUCOSE

Diabetes management changes
  Decreased exercise without decreasing food or increasing insulin
  Increased dietary intake
Sympathetic nervous system responses
  Stressful events
    Injury
    Surgery
    Infections
      Respiratory tract
      Urinary tract
      Pancreatitis
    Emotional trauma
Increased glucagon
Increased growth hormone
Pharmacologic drugs
  Steroid therapy
  Epinephrine/norepinephrine

cal symptoms to extraneous health problems. Tending to trust the functioning of the pump, the patient delays testing serum glucose and urine ketone levels while DKA is progressively developing.

Pathophysiology

Insulin is the metabolic key to the transfer of glucose from the bloodstream into the cell where it can be used immediately for energy or stored to be used at a later time. Without insulin, glucose remains in the bloodstream, and cells are deprived of their energy source. A complex pathophysiologic chain of events follows (Fig. 23-1). The release of glucagon is stimulated when insulin is ineffective in providing the cells with glucose for energy. Glucagon increases the amount of glucose in the bloodstream by breaking down stored glucose (glycogenolysis) and converting noncarbohydrate molecules into glucose (gluconeogenesis) and hyperglycemia occurs. Blood glucose levels for the patient in DKA typically range from 300 to 800 mg/dL of blood. Glucose levels alone do not diagnose DKA; ketoacidosis, which is discussed later, is a major determining factor.

With hyperglycemia, plasma osmolality is increased, and blood becomes hyperosmolar. Cellular dehydration occurs as the hyperosmolar extracellular fluid draws the

TABLE 23-1

ENDOCRINE RESPONSE DURING STRESS

GLAND/ORGAN	HORMONE	RESPONSE
Adrenal cortex	Cortisol	↑Insulin resistance→ ↑glycogenolysis→ ↑glucose circulation ↑Hepatic gluconeogenesis→ ↑glucose available ↑Lipolysis ↑Protein catabolism ↑Sodium,→ ↑water retention to maintain blood plasma osmolality by movement of extravascular fluid to intravascular space Connective tissue fibroblasts→ collagen for poor wound healing
	Glucocorticoid	↓Histamine release→ suppresses immune system ↓Lymphocytes, monocytes, eosinophils, basophils ↑Polymorphonuclear leukocytes→ ↑risk infection ↑Glucose ↓Gastric acid secretion
	Mineralocorticoids	↑Aldosterone→ ↓sodium excretion→ ↓water excretion↓ ↑intravascular volume↓ ↑vasoconstriction↓ ↑blood pressure ↑Potassium excretion→ hypokalemia→ ↑Hydrogen ion excretion→metabolic alkalosis
Adrenal medulla	Epinephrine Norepinephrine	↑Endorphins→ ↓pain
	Epinephrine	↑Metabolic rate to accommodate stress response ↑Liver glycogenolysis→ ↑glucose ↑Insulin (cells are insulin resistant) ↑Cardiac contractility ↑Cardiac output ↑Dilation coronary arteries ↑Blood pressure ↑Heart rate ↑Bronchodilation→ ↑respirations ↑Perfusion to heart, brain, lungs, liver, muscle ↓Perfusion to periphery of body ↓Peristalsis
	Norepinephrine	↑Peripheral vasoconstriction ↑Blood pressure ↑Sodium retention ↑Potassium excretion
Pituitary	All hormones	↑Endogenous opioids→ ↓pain
Anterior pituitary	Adrenocorticotropic hormone	↑Aldosterone→ ↓sodium excretion→ ↓water excretion ↑intravascular volume→ ↑blood pressure ↑Cortisol to ↑blood volume
	Growth hormones	↑Protein anabolism of amino acids to protein ↑Lipolysis→ ↑gluconeogenesis
Posterior pituitary	Antidiuretic hormone	↑Vasoconstriction ↑Water retention→restoration circulating blood volume ↓Urinary output ↑Hypoosmolality
Pancreas	Insulin	Insulin resistance→hyperglycemia
	Glucagon	Directly opposes action of insulin→↑glycolysis ↑Glucose for fuel ↑Glycogenolysis ↑Gluconeogenesis ↑Lipolysis
Thyroid	Thyroxine	↓Routine metabolic demands during stress
Gonads	Sex hormones	Energy and oxygen supply diverted to brain, heart, muscles, liver

↑, Increased; →, causes; ↓, decreased.

more dilute intracellular and interstitial fluid into the vascular space in an attempt to return the plasma osmolality to normal. Dehydration stimulates catecholamine production for further glycogenolysis, lipolysis (breakdown of fats), gluconeogenesis, and ketogenesis (formation of ketones).

Excessive urination (polyuria) and glycosuria occur as a result of the osmotic diuresis. The excess glucose, filtered at the glomeruli, cannot be reabsorbed at the renal tubule and "spills" into the urine. The unreabsorbed solute exerts its own osmotic pull in the renal tubules, and less water is returned to circulation via the collecting

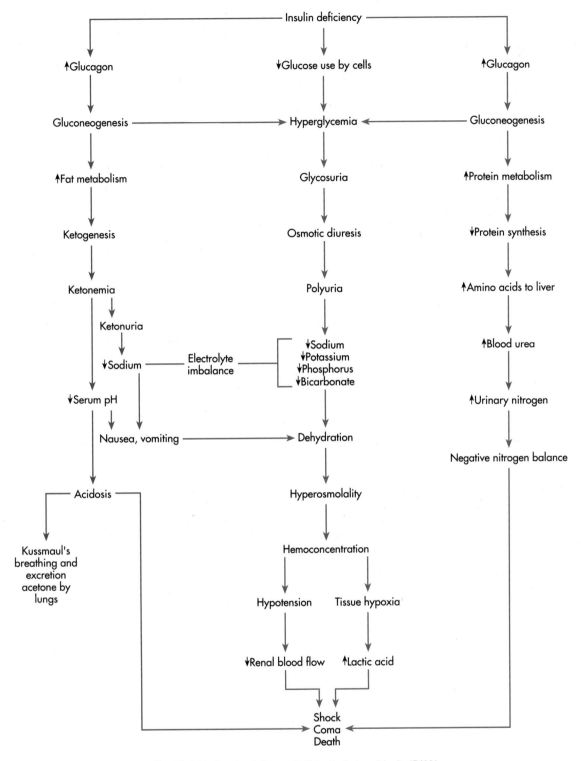

Fig. **23-1** Pathophysiology of diabetic ketoacidosis (DKA).

ducts. As a result, large volumes of water, along with sodium, potassium, and phosphorus, are excreted in the urine, causing fluid volume deficit and electrolyte imbalance. Excessive thirst (polydipsia) occurs as the decrease in circulating blood volume stimulates the osmoreceptors in the hypothalamus and promotes the release of angio-

tensin II. The strong thirst sensation is intended to compensate for the loss of fluids and replenish the circulating blood volume. The fluid volume deficit also stimulates vasoconstriction as a means to preserve blood pressure. Both the vasoconstriction and the extremely elevated levels of glucose impair the delivery of oxygen to the peripheral cells, which impedes the removal of metabolic wastes.

As DKA progresses, gluconeogenesis continues to convert noncarbohydrate molecules into glucose. Keto-acidosis occurs as ketoacid end products accumulate in the blood and rapid, incomplete fatty acid metabolism releases highly acidic substances (acetoacetic acid and beta-hydroxybutyric acid) into the bloodstream (ketone-mia) and the urine (ketonuria). The patient with moderate-to-severe DKA typically has a pH between 7.2 and 7.36.[11] The acid ketones dissociate and yield hydrogen ions (H^+) that accumulate and cause a drop in serum pH. Normally the hydrogen ions react with bicarbonate (HCO_3^-) to produce carbonic acid (H_2CO_3). Carbonic acid dissociates to form water (H_2O) and carbon dioxide (CO_2), which are eliminated through the kidneys and the lungs, respectively. In gluconeogenesis, however, ketones accumulate in the bloodstream faster than they can be metabolized. The bicarbonate and sodium loss through osmotic diuresis prevents the formation of sodium bicarbonate needed to buffer the increasing carbonic acid. The respiratory rate is altered in an attempt to compensate for the carbonic acid build-up. Breathing becomes deep and rapid (Kussmaul's respirations) to release carbonic acid in the form of carbon dioxide. Acetone is exhaled, giving the breath its characteristic "fruity" odor.

Gluconeogenesis stimulates mobilization of protein, and protein catabolism increases. Protein is broken down and converted to glucose in the liver. Continuous, uninterrupted gluconeogenesis leaves no reserve protein available for synthesis and repair of vital body tissues. Nitrogen accumulates as protein is metabolized to urea. Urea, added to the bloodstream, increases the osmotic diuresis and accentuates the dehydration. Loss of muscle mass and reduced resistance to infection occur with impaired protein utilization. The combined states of acidosis and osmotic diuresis lead to a significant loss of phosphorus (yet laboratory serum phosphorus level may not change), further compromising peripheral tissue perfusion. Hypophosphatemia impairs the oxygen function of the hemoglobin by increasing hemoglobin's affinity for oxygen and thereby reducing delivery of oxygen to the cells.[12]

Assessment and Diagnosis

DKA may develop over several hours in a person who has had diabetes for a period of time. In an undiagnosed diabetic patient, it may take days to develop and signal an abrupt onset of the disease.

Clinical manifestations

DKA has a predictable clinical presentation. It is usually preceded by patient complaints of malaise, headache, polyuria, polydipsia, and polyphagia (excessive hunger). Nausea, vomiting, extreme fatigue, dehydration, and weight loss follow. Central nervous system de-pression, with changes in the level of consciousness, can quickly lead to coma. The patient with DKA may be lethargic, stuporous, or unconscious, depending on the degree of fluid-balance disturbance. The physical examination reveals evidence of dehydration, including flushed, dry skin, dry buccal membranes, and skin turgor greater than 3 seconds. Frequently, "sunken eyeballs," resulting from the lack of fluid in the interstitium of the eyeball, are observed. Tachycardia and hypotension may signal profound fluid losses. Kussmaul's air hunger continues to reveal a "fruity" odor of acetone. Normal or subnormal temperatures exist despite volume depletion. An increased temperature at this point may indicate the presence of infection.[10]

Laboratory findings

Urine ketones and bedside fingerstick blood sugar determinations provide rapid confirmation of ketoacidosis in the diabetic patient. Laboratory evidence supporting the ketoacidosis includes low arterial blood pH and low plasma bicarbonate levels.[13] Dehydration manifests by an increased serum osmolality, elevated hematocrit level, marked leukocytosis (regardless of presence of infection), increased blood urea nitrogen (BUN), and a high urine specific gravity. Electrolyte imbalances result from osmotic diuresis, fluid depletion, and the acidosis driving potassium out of the cells. Vomiting and polyuria cause a decrease in serum sodium and potassium levels. Hyponatremia also occurs from the shift of extracellular sodium to intracellular as the potassium is depleted. Serum potassium levels vary, depending on the phase of ketoacidosis. Potassium levels may be elevated as potassium moves from the intercellular compartment to the extracellular compartment in an exchange for hydrogen ions. Hyperkalemia is reduced quickly as potassium is lost from the body by the vomiting, diarrhea, and osmotic diuresis. Potassium is also decreased with the replacement of insulin. Phosphorus levels also may be low, normal, or elevated despite actual serum depletion. Assessment of electrolyte levels must continue throughout the treatment phase inasmuch as both potassium and phosphorus rapidly reenter the cell when fluid and insulin therapy are provided.

Diagnosis of DKA is based on the combination of presenting symptoms, patient history, medical history (Type 1 diabetes mellitus), precipitating factors if known, and results of serum glucose and urine ketone testing. Considering the complexity and potential seriousness of DKA, the diagnosis is straightforward. With a known diabetic patient, a diagnosis of DKA is determined by heavy ketonuria and glycosuria in the presence of hyperglycemia and ketonemia. If the patient is not known to have diabetes, other causes of metabolic acidosis must be differentiated before a course of therapy is begun. Starvation, alcoholism, certain toxic chemicals, lactic acid, and uremia may result in a ketoacidotic state.[8] The treatment plan varies, depending on the cause.

Medical Management

Treatment of the patient in DKA requires an aggressive approach. The major focus of the treatment is aimed at reversing the ketoacidosis and preventing further decompensation. Treatment goals include reversing the dehydration, treating circulatory collapse, restoring the insulin-glucagon ratio to promote the cellular use of glucose, reducing the counterregulatory hormone glucagon, breaking the ketotic cycle, and replenishing electrolytes. In addition to vigorous medical treatment, the practitioner investigates the precipitating causes of ketoacidosis. Unless the precipitating factors are known and resolved, DKA probably will recur. After 10 to 12 hours of effective treatment, the patient's hydration and neurologic and metabolic status should improve dramatically.

Hydration

The patient with DKA is significantly dehydrated, may have lost 5% to 10% of body weight in fluids, and may have a fluid deficit of 3 to 5 L.[14] There is no consensus among medical practitioners on the use of isotonic or hypotonic solution as a replacement for lost fluid. Initially, normal physiologic saline solution may be given to reverse the vascular deficit, hypotension, and extracellular fluid losses. During the first hour of severe dehydration, 1 L is infused. The rate varies, however, depending on urinary output, secondary illnesses, and precipitating factors. To dilute the serum osmolality, infusions of half-strength sodium chloride may follow the initial saline replacement. Because the water deficit exceeds the sodium loss, half-strength sodium chloride can be given at a rate of 300 to 500 ml/hour until the serum osmolality returns to normal and the blood glucose levels decrease.

Insulin administration

Insulin is given simultaneously with intravenous fluids. Refer to Table 23-2 for types of insulin medication and nursing considerations in their administration.[6,12,14,15] A reversal of the ketoacidotic metabolic abnormalities gradually occurs as the patient becomes hydrated and receives insulin. The serum glucose level falls as large quantities of glucose are perfused through the kidneys and removed in the urine. The exogenous insulin complements the fluid therapy and promotes the entry of glucose into the cell (insulin also permits potassium and phosphorus to reenter the cell). Insulin inhibits the release of glucagon, and glucose no longer is poured into the circulation as a result of gluconeogenesis and glycogenolysis. The ketoacidotic cycle gradually is broken because ketoacids no longer are produced as a by-product of incomplete fat metabolism. The serum osmolality is reduced with vigorous fluid replacement, coupled with the reduction of glucose, urea, and ketones circulating in the bloodstream. Osmotic diuresis is reversed as the continuous fluids replace fluid losses, and serum glucose levels return to normal.

Insulin resistance

The patient who does not respond to insulin may have a problem with insulin resistance at the cell receptor site. These patients require a more aggressive approach. A one-time bolus of 0.3 U/kg may be given to saturate the insulin cell receptor sites and compete with the insulin resistance. Replacement of low-dose insulin, 0.1 U/kg/hour (approximately 5 U/hour), is given intravenously (or intramuscularly depending on circulatory perfusion) until acidosis is reversed. Low-dose insulin results in a few serious cases of hypoglycemia.[16]

Electrolyte administration

Hypokalemia may occur as insulin promotes the return of potassium into the cell and acidosis is reduced. Replacement of potassium begins as soon as the potassium shift has stabilized. Insulin treatment also precipitates hypophosphatemia as serum phosphate returns to the cell. Although the need to administer phosphate currently is debated, its use does seem to improve tissue oxygenation and promote the renal excretion of hydrogen ions.[8]

Bicarbonate administration

Replacement of lost bicarbonate is closely monitored. It is given to replace depleted bicarbonate stores in association with a severely acidotic pH. It generally is agreed that bicarbonate is started for clinically severe acidotic states (pH <7.0)[17] and stopped when the pH level reaches 7.20.[18] An indwelling arterial line provides access for hourly sampling of blood gases to evaluate pH and bicarbonate.

Intravenous glucose

Once the serum glucose level is 250 to 300 mg/dL of blood, a 5% dextrose solution is infused.[14] Intravenously administered glucose is necessary to replenish glucose stores because muscle and liver glycogen reserves may have been depleted during gluconeogenesis. Perhaps more importantly, it is necessary to prevent hypoglycemia, which may result from a relative drop in circulating glucose from the infusion of exogenous insulin. In addition, glucose is given to prevent cerebral edema, which may result when free water is drawn across the blood-brain barrier into brain tissue (although several theories exist, the exact mechanism involved in this alteration in the blood-brain barrier is not known).[16] Intravenous glucose level is maintained until the patient no longer requires intravenous fluids and is taking liquids by mouth.

Nursing Management

Nursing management of the patient with diabetic ketoacidosis incorporates a variety of nursing diagnoses (Box 23-2). **Nursing priorities are directed toward administering prescribed fluids, insulin, and electrolytes, monitoring the patient's response to therapy, providing com-**

TABLE 23-2

PARENTERAL* INSULINS AND NURSING IMPLICATIONS FOR USE IN DIABETES MELLITUS

TYPE OF INSULIN	DOSAGE†	ACTION	ONSET, PEAK, AND DURATION	SPECIAL CONSIDERATIONS
Regular insulin (crystalline zinc)	Intravenously (IV) or subcutaneously (SQ)	Insulin replacement therapy; regulates storage and metabolism of protein, carbohydrate, and fats; potent hypoglycemic agent	Onset: within 1 hr Peak: 2-4 hr Duration: 5-8 hr	Only type of insulin suitable for IV use. Also available as regular insulin, human insulin. Do not use if cloudy, colored, or unusually viscous. Insulins prepared from bovine, pork, and human sources. Source determined by patient sensitivity. Human source has least intolerance. Several drugs interact or have potentially related problems with insulin. The reader is referred to a drug information text for further information. Side effect—hypoglycemia

Insulin Lispro	SQ	Insulin replacement	Onset: 10-15 min
			Peak: 45-60 min
			Duration: 1.5-3.5 hrs
				First available synthetic insulin almost *immediately* absorbed.
				  Shorter duration of action than human regular insulin; therefore should be used with longer-acting insulins.
				  Reliable treatment of postprandial hyperglycemia with decreased risk of hypoglycemia.

Insulin zinc suspension (Lente Insulin, Semilente Insulin)	SQ; not for IV use	Insulin replacement hormone	Onset: 1-3 hr Peak: 8-12 hr Duration: 18-28 hr	Also available as insulin zinc, human suspension
Isophane insulin suspension (NPH Insulin)	SQ; not for IV use	Insulin replacement hormone	Onset: 3-4 hr Peak: 6-12 hr Duration: 18-28 hr	Also available as isophane insulin, human
Insulin zinc suspension (Ultralente Insulin)	SQ; not for IV use	Extended action; insulin replacement hormone	Onset: 4-6 hr Peak: 18-24 hr Duration: 36 hr	Also available as extended insulin zinc, human

Isophane insulin, human suspension, and insulin, human injection	SQ; not for IV use	Rapid and intermediate acting	Varies	Combination of insulins:
				  50% isophane insulin human with 50% insulin human Humulin 50/50 (biosynthetic)
				  70% isophane insulin, human with 30% insulin, human injection (Humulin 70/30 biosynthetic), and Novolin

*Parenteral refers to a route other than by mouth (PO).
†Doses are individualized according to patient's age and size.

fort and emotional support, and maintaining surveillance for complications.

Administering prescribed fluids, insulin, and electrolytes

Rapid intravenous fluid replacement requires the use of a volumetric pump. Insulin is given intravenously to the severely dehydrated patient to ensure absorption when inadequate tissue perfusion is present. Throughout the insulin therapy, both patient response and laboratory data are assessed for changes relating to glucose levels. In most patients, serum glucose levels decline approximately 100 mg/dL/hour.[12] When the blood glucose level falls to 250 to 300 mg/dL of blood, a 5% dextrose solution is infused to prevent hypoglycemia. At this time, insulin dosage may be decreased. Administration of regular insulin drip is not discontinued until ketoacidosis subsides, as identified by the arterial blood gases.[12] As glucose lev-

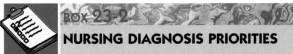

BOX 23-2

NURSING DIAGNOSIS PRIORITIES

Diabetic Ketoacidosis

- Decreased Cardiac Output related to alterations in preload, pp. 467-468
- Fluid Volume Deficit related to absolute loss, p. 486
- Risk for infection, pp. 494-495
- Ineffective Individual Coping related to situational crisis and personal vulnerability, pp. 453-455
- Knowledge Deficit: Discharge Regimen related to lack of previous exposure to information, p. 443

BOX 23-3

CLINICAL MANIFESTATIONS OF HYPOGLYCEMIA AND HYPERGLYCEMIA

HYPOGLYCEMIA	HYPERGLYCEMIA
Restlessness	Excessive thirst
Apprehension	Excessive urination
Irritability	Hunger
Trembling	Weakness
Weakness	Listlessness
Diaphoresis	Mental fatigue
Pallor	Flushed, dry skin
Paresthesia	Itching
Headache	Headache
Hunger	Nausea
Difficulty thinking	Vomiting
Loss of coordination	Abdominal cramps
Difficulty walking	Dehydration
Difficulty talking	Weak, rapid pulse
Visual disturbances	Postural hypotension
Blurred vision	Hypotension
Double vision	Acetone breath odor
Tachycardia	Kussmaul's respirations
Shallow respirations	Rapid breathing
Hypertension	Changes in level of
Changes in level of	consciousness
consciousness	Stupor
Seizures	Coma
Coma	

els, dehydration, and hypotension diminish, insulin is given subcutaneously.

Monitoring the patient's response to therapy

Accurate intake and output measurements must be maintained to record the body's use of fluid. Hourly urine output measures renal functioning and also provides information that helps prevent overhydration or underhydration. Vital signs, especially pulse rate, hemodynamic findings, and blood pressure, are constantly monitored to assess cardiac response to the fluid replacement. Evidence that fluid replacement is effective includes normal central venous pressure (CVP), decreased heart rate, and normal pulmonary artery pressure (PAP). Further evidence of hydration includes a change from the previously weak, thready pulse to a pulse that is strong and full and a change from a previously low blood pressure to a gradual elevation of systolic blood pressure. Respirations are assessed frequently for changes in rate, depth, and fruity "acetone" odor. Reduced respirations also signal a return to adequate fluid balance.

Urine specific gravity determination is performed every 2 hours. Once ketonuria is established, and treatment is initiated, arterial blood gases are performed to evaluate the DKA. Serum osmolality is monitored, and BUN and creatinine levels are assessed for possible renal impairment related to decreased renal perfusion.

Maintaining surveillance for complications

The patient in DKA may experience a variety of complications, including fluid volume overload, hypoglycemia or hyperglycemia, hyperkalemia or hypokalemia, hyponatremia, and cerebral edema. In addition, the patient is at risk for infection.

Fluid volume overload. Fluid overload from rapid volume infusion is a serious complication that can occur in the patient with a compromised cardiovascular or renal system, or both. Neck vein engorgement, dyspnea without exertion, and elevated CVP and PAP, as well as moist lung sounds, signal circulatory overload. Reduc-

tion in the rate and volume of infusion, elevation of the head, and administration of oxygen may be required to manage the increased intravascular volume. Measuring hourly urine is mandatory to assess renal output and adequacy of fluid replacement.

Hypoglycemia or hyperglycemia. Signs of hypoglycemia, such as unexpected behavioral changes, diaphoresis, and tremors, may occur from a relative drop in glucose level. Should hypoglycemia occur, insulin is stopped and the physician is notified immediately. The physical and emotional stressors that the patient experiences during the stay in the critical care unit may induce rebound hyperglycemia. The patient should be closely monitored for signs of hyperglycemia, such as Kussmaul's respirations, dry skin, and fruity, acetone breath odor. Should hypoglycemia occur, the physician is notified immediately (Box 23-3).

Hypokalemia or hyperkalemia. Hypokalemia can occur within the first 4 hours of the rehydration-insulin treatment. Continuous cardiac monitoring is required because potassium affects the heart's electrical condition. Hypokalemia is depicted on the cardiac monitor by ventricular dysrythmias, a prolonged QT interval, a flattened or depressed T wave, and depressed ST segments. Hyperkalemia occurs with acidosis or when potassium deficit is treated too aggressively in patients with renal insufficiency. Hyperkalemia is noted on a cardiac monitor by a large, peaked T wave, flattened P wave, and a broad, slurred QRS complex. Ventricular fibrillation can follow (Box 23-4).

Hyponatremia. Serum sodium levels fall as the sodium replaces the potassium that moves out of the cells. Sodium is eliminated from the body as a result of the osmotic diuresis. In addition, the hyponatremia is compounded by the vomiting and diarrhea that occur during ketoacidosis. Clinical manifestations of hyponatremia include abdominal cramping, apprehension, postural hypotension, and unexpected behavioral changes. Sodium chloride is infused as the initial intravenous solution. Maintenance of the saline infusion depends on clinical manifestations of sodium imbalance plus serum laboratory values.

Cerebral edema. Changes in the patient's neurologic status may be insidious. Alterations in level of consciousness, pupil reaction, and motor function may be the result of fluctuating glucose levels and cerebral fluid shifts. Confusion and sudden complaints of headache are ominous signs that may signal cerebral edema. These observations require immediate action to prevent neurologic damage. Neurologic assessments performed every 4 hours or as needed, coupled with serum osmolality values, serve as an index of the patient's response to the rehydration therapy.

BOX 23-4

CLINICAL MANIFESTATIONS OF HYPOKALEMIA AND HYPERKALEMIA

HYPOKALEMIA	HYPERKALEMIA
Generalized muscle weakness	Impaired muscle activity
Fatigue	Weakness
Diminished to absent reflexes	Muscle pain/cramps
Decreased GI motility	Increased GI motility
Anorexia	Nausea
Abdominal distention	Diarrhea
Paralytic ileus	Intestinal colic
Vomiting	Oliguria
Hypotension	Dizziness
Decreased stroke volume	Bradycardia
Dysrhythmias	Ventricular fibrillation
Weak pulse	Irritability
Respiratory muscle weakness	ECG changes
Shallow respirations	Flattened P wave
Shortness of breath	Large, peaked T wave
Apathy	Broad, slurred QRS complex
Drowsiness	
Depression	
Irritability	
Tetany	
Coma	
ECG changes	
Prolonged QT interval	
Flattened, depressed T wave	
Depressed ST segments	

Risk for infection. Skin care takes on new dimensions for the patient with DKA. Dehydration, hypovolemia, and hypophosphatemia interfere with oxygen delivery at the cell site and contribute to inadequate perfusion and tissue breakdown. Patients must be repositioned every hour to relieve capillary pressure and promote adequate perfusion to body tissues. The typical patient with Type 1 diabetes is either of normal weight or underweight. Bony prominences must be assessed for tissue breakdown and body weight repositioned every hour. Irritation of skin from adhesive tape, shearing force, and detergents is to be avoided. Maintenance of skin integrity prevents unwanted portals of entry for microorganisms.

Oral care, including lip balm, helps keep lips supple and prevents cracking. Prepared sponge sticks or moist gauze pads can be used to moisten oral membranes of the unconscious patient. Swabbing the mouth moistens the tissue and displaces the bacteria that collect when saliva, which has a bacteriostatic action, is curtailed by dehydration. The conscious patient removes bacteria and provides oral comfort with frequent tooth brushing and oral rinsing.

Strict sterile technique is used to maintain all intravenous systems. All venipuncture sites are checked every 4 hours for signs of inflammation, phlebitis, or infiltration. Strict surgical asepsis is used for all invasive procedures. Careful sterile technique is used if urinary catheterization is necessary to obtain urine samples for testing. Catheter care is given every 8 hours.

Patient education

For patients with previously diagnosed diabetes the knowledge level and compliance history are important in formulating a teaching plan. Learning objectives include a definition of hyperglycemia and its causes, harmful effects, and symptoms. Additional objectives include a definition of ketoacidosis and its causes, symptoms, and harmful consequences. The patient and family are expected to learn the principles of diabetes management during illness. They also are expected to know the warning signs that must be brought to the attention of a health care practitioner. Education of the patient and family or other persons involved in the patient's supportive care is the goal of the teaching process.

The patient whose diabetes is newly diagnosed requires teaching about the disease process and self-care management. This instruction is provided once the acute illness is controlled. Comprehensive instruction for patients and families involves various health care personnel, including the nurse, nutritionist, and physician. It is helpful if family members or a specific friend/caregiver attend diabetic sessions as a backup for the client when needed. During this instruction, emphasis is placed on daily maintenance of a chronic disease as well as factors that led to DKA and required admission to a critical care unit. Long-term patient education needs will focus on management of diabetes mellitus.

HYPERGLYCEMIC HYPEROSMOLAR NONKETOTIC SYNDROME

Description and Etiology

Hyperglycemic hyperosmolar nonketotic syndrome (HHNS) is a frequently lethal complication of diabetes mellitus.[13] The hallmarks of HHNS are extremely high levels of plasma glucose, with resulting elevations in hyperosmolality and osmotic diuresis. Ketosis is mild or absent. Inability to replace fluids lost through diuresis or severe diarrhea leads to profound dehydration and changes in level of consciousness. HHNS has a 10% to 50% mortality,[7] which is heightened by other existing disease processes. The severity of symptoms, plus minimal or absent ketosis, distinguishes HHNS from DKA (Table 23-3).

Hyperglycemic hyperosmolar nonketotic syndrome is covered under the same DRGs as diabetes mellitus: DRG 295 if the age is between 0 and 35 years, with an average length of stay of 4.1 days, and DRG 294 if the person is older than 35 years, with an average length of stay of 5.3 days.[9]

HHNS occurs when the pancreas produces a relatively insufficient amount of insulin for the high levels of glucose that flood the bloodstream (Box 23-5). The disorder occurs mainly, although not exclusively, in elderly obese persons with underlying conditions that require medical treatment. The patient may have Type 2 non-insulin–dependent diabetes that is treated with diet and oral hypoglycemic agents. HHNS also can occur in persons with previously undiagnosed and, therefore, untreated diabetes. In either situations, it is possible that some of the manufactured insulin is effective in admitting glucose into the cells for energy. This is a major difference between DKA and HHNS. In HHNS, protein and fats are not used to the same degree as in DKA, and the ketotic cycle is either never started or is very mild.

The extreme hyperglycemia of HHNS can be precipitated by the stress of extensive burns, infection, or other major illness, such as myocardial infarction. The syndrome also may be precipitated by iatrogenic treatments that may increase the serum glucose levels and cause an imbalance in the insulin/glucagon ratio. Such treatments include hyperalimentation, high-calorie enteral feedings, hemodialysis, and peritoneal dialysis. Prescription medications that interfere with pancreatic insulin production may precipitate HHNS, including phenytoin, thiazide diuretics, and diazoxide. Other medications, such as sympathomimetic agents, stimulate gluconeogenesis by in-

TABLE 23-3

GENERAL COMPARISON OF DKA AND HHNS

	DIABETIC KETOACIDOSIS	HYPERGLYCEMIC HYPEROSMOLAR NONKETOTIC SYNDROME
CAUSE	Insufficient exogenous insulin for glucose needs	Insufficient exogenous/endogenous insulin for glucose needs
ONSET	Sudden (hours)	Slow, insidious (days, weeks)
PREDISPOSING FACTORS	Noncompliance to Type I DM, illness, surgery, decreased activity	Elderly with recent acute illness; therapeutic procedures
MORTALITY	9% to 14%	10% to 50%
POPULATION AFFECTED	Type I DM	Type II DM, age >65 yr
CLINICAL MANIFESTATIONS	Similarities: dry mouth, polydipsia, polyuria, polyphagia, dehydration, dry skin, hypotension, weakness, mental confusion, tachycardia, changes in level of consciousness	
	Differences: ketoacidosis: air hunger, acetone breath odor, respirations rapid and deep, nausea, vomiting	No ketosis, no breath odor, respirations rapid and shallow, usually mild nausea and vomiting
LABORATORY TESTS		
Serum glucose	300-800 mg/dL	600-2000 mg/dL
Serum ketones	Strongly positive	Normal or mildly elevated
Serum pH	<7.3	Normal
Serum osmolality	<350 mOsm/L	>350 mOsm/L
Serum sodium	Normal or low	Normal or elevated
Serum potassium	Low, normal, or elevated (total body K^+ is depleted)	Low, normal, or elevated
Serum bicarbonate	<15 mEq/L	Normal
Serum phosphorus	Low, normal, or elevated (may decrease after insulin therapy)	Low, normal, or elevated (may decrease after insulin therapy)
Urine acetone	Strong	Absent or mild

DM, Diabetes mellitus.

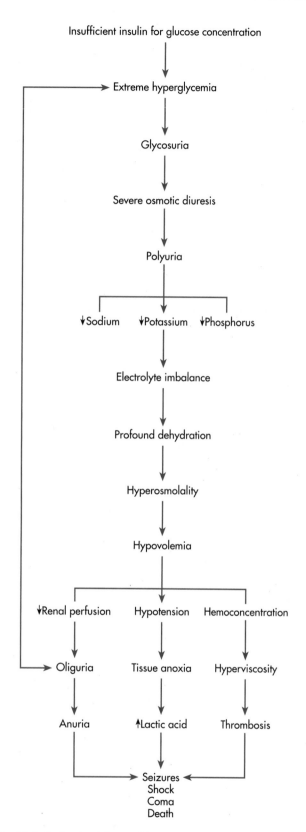

Fig. **23-2** Pathophysiology of hyperglycemic hyperosmolar nonketotic syndrome (HHNS).

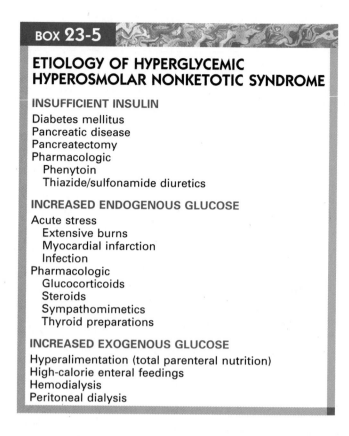

BOX 23-5

ETIOLOGY OF HYPERGLYCEMIC HYPEROSMOLAR NONKETOTIC SYNDROME

INSUFFICIENT INSULIN

Diabetes mellitus
Pancreatic disease
Pancreatectomy
Pharmacologic
    Phenytoin
    Thiazide/sulfonamide diuretics

INCREASED ENDOGENOUS GLUCOSE

Acute stress
    Extensive burns
    Myocardial infarction
    Infection
Pharmacologic
    Glucocorticoids
    Steroids
    Sympathomimetics
    Thyroid preparations

INCREASED EXOGENOUS GLUCOSE

Hyperalimentation (total parenteral nutrition)
High-calorie enteral feedings
Hemodialysis
Peritoneal dialysis

creasing glucose levels through the metabolism of protein and fats.

Pathophysiology

HHNS represents a deficit of insulin and an excess of glucagon (Fig. 23-2). Reduced insulin levels prevent the movement of glucose into the cells, thus allowing glucose to accumulate in the plasma. Glucagon release is triggered by the decreased insulin, and hepatic glucose from glycogenolysis is poured into the circulation. Glucagon also stimulates the metabolism of fat and protein through gluconeogenesis in an attempt to provide cells with an energy source. Excessive glucose, along with the end products of incomplete fat and protein metabolism, collect as debris in the bloodstream. As the number of particles increase in the blood, hyperosmolality increases. In an effort to decrease the serum osmolality, fluid is drawn from the intracellular compartment into the vascular bed. Profound intracellular volume depletion occurs if the patient's thirst sensation is absent or decreased, if the patient is unable to respond to thirst, or if the fluids are inaccessible.

Hemoconcentration persists despite removal of large amounts of glucose in the urine. The glomerular filtration and elimination of glucose by the kidney tubules are ineffective in reducing the serum glucose level sufficiently to maintain normal glucose levels. The hyperosmolality and reduced blood volume stimulate the release of ADH to increase the tubular reabsorption of water. ADH, however, is powerless in overcoming the osmotic pull exerted by the glucose load. Excessive fluid volume is lost at the kidney tubule with simultaneous loss of potassium, sodium, and phosphate in the urine.

Hypovolemia reduces renal circulation, and oliguria develops. Although this process conserves water and preserves the blood volume, it prevents further glucose loss, and hyperosmolality increases. Ketoacidosis is absent or very mild in HHNS despite the level of free fatty acids resulting from gluconeogenesis. It is surmised that the patient may have sufficient insulin present to prevent ketosis.[19]

Failure of the body to regain homeostatic balance further accelerates the life-threatening cycle brought about by hyperglycemia, hyperosmolality, osmotic diuresis, and profound dehydration. To restore homeostasis, the sympathetic nervous system reacts to the body's stress response. Epinephrine, a potent stimulus for gluconeogenesis, is released, and additional glucose is added to the bloodstream. Unless the glycemic diuresis cycle is broken with aggressive fluid replacement, the intracellular dehydration affects fluid and oxygen transport to the brain cells. Central nervous system dysfunctioning may result and lead to coma. Hemoconcentration increases the blood viscosity, which may result in clot formation, thromboemboli, and cerebral, cardiac, and pleural infarcts.[8]

Assessment and Diagnosis

HHNS has a slow, subtle onset. Initially, the symptoms may be nonspecific and may be ignored or attributed to the patient's concurrent disease processes. History reveals polyuria, polydipsia (depending on patient's thirst sensation), and advancing weakness. Medical attention may not be obtained for these nonspecific, nonacute symptoms until the patient is unable to take sufficient fluids to offset the fluid losses. Progressive dehydration follows and leads to mental confusion, convulsions, and coma.

Clinical manifestations

The physical examination may reveal obtundation, with a profound fluid deficit. Signs of severe dehydration include longitudinal wrinkles in the tongue, decreased salivation, and decreased central venous pressure, with increases in pulse and respirations (Kussmaul's air hunger is not present).

Laboratory studies

Serum glucose levels are strikingly elevated, often to double the levels seen in ketoacidosis (reaching 2000 mg/dL). Serum osmolality may reach 350 mOsm/kg,[19] averaging 320 mOsm/kg. Elevated hematocrit and depleted potassium and phosphorus levels result from the osmotic diuresis. Studies have identified an increased hematocrit as a risk factor for both increased insulin resistance and non-insulin–dependent diabetes.[20] Serum electrolyte levels vary, depending on the activity and position of the

electrolyte when the laboratory test is performed. Kidney impairment as a result of the severe reduction in renal circulation is suggested by elevated BUN and creatinine levels. Metabolic acidosis usually is absent. When acidosis is present, it tends to be mild and attributed to other factors. The mild acidosis may be a result of starvation ketosis, a relative increase in lactic acid circulating in the reduced blood volume, or azotemia caused by impaired renal function.[8]

Medical Management

Treatment of the patient in HHNS requires a direct approach. The major focus of the treatment is aimed at interrupting the glycemic diuresis and preventing vascular collapse. The same basic treatment goals used to treat DKA are used for the patient with HHNS: rehydration, restoration of insulin/glucagon ratio, and electrolyte replacement. Aggressive treatment of the underlying causes of HHNS (severe infection, therapeutic procedures, medications) is included in the medical treatment to prevent HHNS recurrence.

Rehydration

Rapid rehydration is the primary intervention. The fluid deficit may be as much as 150 ml/kg of body weight. The average 150-pound adult may lose more than 7 to 10 L of fluid a day.[6,21]

Debate continues regarding whether isotonic or hypotonic solutions are more appropriate for treating the severe fluid deficit. Although an isotonic solution would expand the extracellular fluid and treat hypotension, it could compound the serum osmolality and exceed the body's requirement for sodium. A hypotonic solution would reduce the serum osmolality and provide free water for excretion; however, it could result in hypotonic expansion of the cells. The consensus is to use physiologic normal saline solution (0.9%) for the first 2 L during the first hour of treatment,[21] especially for the patient undergoing circulatory collapse.[8] Once blood pressures are within normal range for the patient, a hypotonic solution may follow. Half-strength hypotonic saline solution (0.45%) subsequently can be used to reduce the serum osmolality. The patient may need replacement of 6 to 10 L of fluid in the first 10 hours.[14] Another parameter for changing from 0.9% to 0.45% is the serum sodium level. Patients with sodium levels equal to or less than 140 mEq/L receive 0.9% normal saline solution;[21] those with levels greater than 140 mEq/L receive 0.45% normal saline solution.[21] Sodium input should not exceed that required to replace the losses. Careful monitoring for sodium and water balance is required to prevent hemolysis as hemoconcentration is reduced.

To prevent relative hypoglycemia, the hydrating solution is changed to 5% dextrose in water, in 0.9% saline solution, or in 0.45% saline solution when the serum glucose levels fall to 250 to 300 mg/dL.

Insulin administration

Intravenously administered insulin usually is given to facilitate the cellular use of glucose and to decrease the serum osmolality more rapidly.[8] Muscle, liver, and adipose cells tend to be receptive to exogenous insulin levels in the patient with HHNS, and the insulin needs are minimal; 10 to 15 U of regular insulin is given intravenously as a bolus. Maintenance doses of insulin to control hyperglycemia vary according to the practitioner. A common practice is to give insulin intravenously at the rate of 0.1 U/kg/hour (this dose mimics the normal physiologic secretion of 30 U/day, which includes upsurges at mealtime)[22] until the glucose falls between 250 and 300 mg. Once glucose levels are at 250 mg/dL, insulin treatment usually is discontinued.

Electrolyte replacement

Increasing the circulating levels of insulin with therapeutic doses of intravenous insulin will promote the rapid return of potassium and phosphorus into the cell. Potassium imbalances disturb the electrocardiographic tracings (see Box 23-4). Continuous cardiac monitoring provides information necessary to maintain or modify electrolyte dosages. Physical changes, such as alterations in gastrointestinal motility and neuromuscular control, also signal the effectiveness of electrolyte replacement. Serial laboratory tests keep the clinician apprised of the fluctuating serum electrolyte levels and provide the basis for electrolyte replacement. Intracellular potassium usually is depleted as dehydration progresses. Increased potassium in the extracellular fluid quickly reenters the cells, however, when insulin is administered. Phosphate levels also are carefully monitored and replaced according to insulin activity.

Nursing Management

Nursing management of the patient with hyperglycemic hyperosmolar nonketotic syndrome incorporates a variety of nursing diagnoses (Box 23-6). **Nursing priorities are directed toward administering prescribed fluids, insulin, and electrolytes, monitoring the patient's response to therapy, providing comfort and emotional support, and maintaining surveillance for complications.**

Administering prescribed fluids, insulin, and electrolytes

Rigorous fluid replacement and low-dose insulin administration are best controlled with electronic volumetric pump devices. Electrolyte replacement orders are based on the patient's response to the treatment plan.

Monitoring the patient's response to therapy

Accurate intake and output measurements must be maintained to record the body's use of fluid. Hourly urine output measures renal functioning and also provides information that helps prevent overhydration or

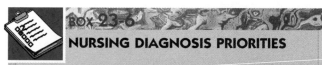

BOX 23-6

NURSING DIAGNOSIS PRIORITIES

Hyperglycemic Hyperosmolar Nonketotic Syndrome

- Decreased Cardiac Output related to alterations in preload, pp. 467-468
- Fluid Volume Deficit related to absolute loss, p. 486
- Risk for Infection, pp. 494-495
- Anxiety related to threat to biologic, psychologic, and/or social integrity, pp. 448-450
- Knowledge Deficit: Discharge Regimen related to previous lack of exposure to information, p. 443

underhydration. Hemodynamic monitoring, including CVP, pulmonary arterial wedge pressure, and PAP, evaluates the degree of dehydration, the effectiveness of the hydration therapy, and the patient's fluid tolerance. Symptoms of circulatory overload include elevated CVP and PAP levels, tachycardia, bounding pulse, dyspnea, tachypnea, lung crackles, and engorged neck veins. Decreasing cardiac output is signaled by hypotension and urine output less than 0.5 ml/kg/hr. Because a preexisting cardiopulmonary or renal problem may exist in the elderly patient, the hemodynamic criteria must be based on the values normal for that patient's age and current medical condition. The nurse is alerted for the clinical manifestations of fluid overload while rehydrating the older patient.

Tests for blood glucose are performed every 30 to 60 minutes at the bedside to determine the effectiveness of treatment. Serum laboratory glucose measurements are usually done every 2 hours along with serum electrolyte determinations. Arterial blood gases are measured at the bedside to rule out the presence of ketoacidosis.

Maintaining surveillance for complications

The patient in HHNS may experience a variety of complications, including dehydration, fluid volume overload, hypoglycemia or hyperglycemia, hyperkalemia or hyperkalemia, and seizures. In addition, the patient is at risk for infection.

Seizures. Alteration in the level of consciousness is directly related to osmotic diuresis and resulting intracellular dehydration. Neurologic assessments, including level of consciousness, pupillary response, motor function, and reflexes, are performed frequently to monitor the patient's response to treatment. Seizure activity may occur as a result of the hyperosmolar state, which interferes with oxygen delivery to the brain cells. Seizure precautions include nursing actions to protect the patient from injury (padded side rails, bed in low position) and to provide an open airway (oral airway, head turned to side without forcibly restraining the patient, suction equipment available). Anticonvulsants, with the exception of phenytoin (which interferes with endogenous insulin [see Table 23-2]), may be ordered. Documentation of seizures includes onset, duration, and description of seizure activity.

Patient education

As the patient's condition improves and the patient and family have received assistance regarding coping strategies, the patient and family become ready to learn. Prevention of recurrence is the major goal. Patients admitted to the critical care area with HHNS and undiagnosed diabetes or those with HHNS with previously diagnosed diabetes will require a teaching plan to include a description of diabetes and how it relates to HHNS. Dietary restrictions, exercise requirements, and medication protocols are all necessary for the patient and/or family member to learn. Additionally, the patient needs to know how a change in daily activities or an illness, such as the flu with nausea or vomiting, will alter the daily diabetes management. Home testing of blood for glucose and signs and symptoms of hyperglycemia and hypoglycemia are part of the learning defense against the complication of diabetes. Patients who use the insulin pump are to have the instructions reviewed.

DIABETES INSIPIDUS

Description and Etiology

Diabetes insipidus (DI) occurs when there is an insufficiency or a hypofunctioning of antidiuretic hormone (ADH). ADH normally stimulates the kidney tubules to reabsorb filtered water when the body needs to increase fluid stores. ADH stimulates the tubules to increase permeability to water when particles in the bloodstream increase in number (rising osmolality) or when blood pressure falls. Persons with inadequately functioning ADH develop unrestricted serum hyperosmolality. An intense thirst and the passage of excessively large quantities of very dilute urine add to the characteristics of the disease.

Diabetes insipidus falls under two different DRGs depending on whether the patient develops complications or comorbid conditions (CC). DRG 300 (Endocrine Disorders With CC) and DRG 301 (Endocrine Disorders Without CC) have average lengths of the stay of 6.6 days and 4.4 days, respectively.[9]

The etiologies of DI are categorized into three types according to cause: central DI, nephrogenic DI, and psychogenic DI (Box 23-7). Central DI occurs when there is an interruption in the synthesis and release of ADH. Central DI is further divided into primary and secondary categories. Primary DI occurs when structural abnormalities within the hypothalamus, infundibular stalk, and posterior pituitary prevent the release of ADH according to the body's inherent signals. Primary DI may result from an inherited familial disorder or from a posterior pituitary system that fails to develop at birth. Primary DI also may be idiopathic or sporadic and occur without apparent cause.[17] Second-

---

BOX 23-7

ETIOLOGY OF DIABETES INSIPIDUS

CENTRAL DIABETES INSIPIDUS
Primary
ADH deficiency from hypothalamic-hypophyseal malformation
  Congenital defect
  Idiopathic

Secondary
ADH deficiency from destruction to the hypothalamic-hypophyseal system
  Trauma
  Infection
  Surgery
  Primary neoplasms
  Metastatic malignancies
  Autoimmune response

NEPHROGENIC DIABETES INSIPIDUS
Inability of kidney tubles to respond to circulating ADH
  Decrease or absence of ADH receptors
  Cellular damage to nephron, especially loop of Henle
  Kidney damage (e.g., hydronephrosis, pyelonephritis, polycystic kidney)
  Untoward response to drug therapy (e.g., lithium carbonate, demeclocycline)

PSYCHOGENIC DIABETES INSIPIDUS
Rare form of water intoxication
  Compulsive water drinking

---

ary DI occurs as a result of trauma to or a pathologic condition of the posterior pituitary functioning unit. Surgery or irradiation to the pituitary gland, traumatic head injury, tumors (malignant and benign), and infections, such as encephalitis, tuberculosis, and meningitis, can potentially interfere with the structure and physiology of the unit and compromise the release of ADH. This is a condition frequently seen in critical care units in patients with head injury or certain types of neurosurgery.

Nephrogenic DI results from the inability of the kidney nephrons to respond to circulating ADH. This may result from diseased kidneys and insensitive or inadequate numbers of receptors on the nephron. Drugs can promote nephrogenic DI by decreasing the responsiveness of the kidney tubules to ADH. Long-term lithium carbonate use is a common cause of nephrogenic NDI.[23] Psychogenic DI is a rare form of the disease that occurs with compulsively drinking more than 5 L of water a day.[23] The infundibular stalk is functioning adequately in psychogenic DI, as are the receptor sites on the kidney nephrons. Long-standing psychogenic DI may closely mimic nephrogenic DI because the kidney tubules develop decreased responsiveness to ADH as a result of prolonged conditioning to hypotonic urine.

Pathophysiology

ADH is released in an effort to maintain blood tonicity and circulating blood volume. Injury to the hypothalamus, infundibular stalk, or posterior pituitary can lead to a disruption in the normal neuroendocrine communication system and resultant secretion of ADH. When ADH is absent, inefficient, or secreted in insufficient amounts, the kidney tubules prevent the reabsorption of urinary substrate and an excessive amount of water is lost to the body, a pathologic condition known as diabetes insipidus (Fig. 23-3). As free water is excreted in urine, the serum osmolality rises and excessive sodium concentration (hypernatremia) in the vascular space stimulates the thirst receptors. Polyuria develops as the kidneys fail to reabsorb tubular fluid and to concentrate the urine. Extremely dilute urine is excreted, and the body is depleted of the fluid necessary for hydration. Urine osmolality and specific gravity decrease. Rising serum osmolality triggers

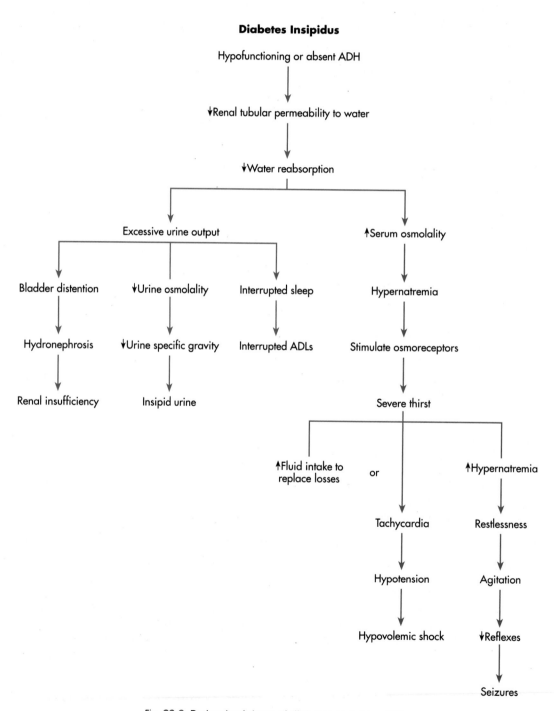

Fig. **23-3** Pathophysiology of diabetes insipidus (DI).

the synthesis and release of ADH. However, the ADH that is released is ineffective or insufficient. Without ADH, the kidney tubules are incapable of conserving enough water to reduce serum sodium.

As the extracellular dehydration ensues, hypotension and hypovolemic shock can occur. Extreme polydipsia develops as the individual attempts to replace lost fluids. The excessive intake of water reduces the serum osmolality to a more normal level and prevents dehydration. The dramatic cycle of polydipsia and polyuria interferes with the person's ability to work, eat, or sleep. Unless the lost fluids are replaced, severe hypernatremia, decreased cerebral perfusion, and severe dehydration lead to seizures, loss of consciousness, and death.

Assessment and Diagnosis

Clinical manifestations

Clinical manifestations of DI may develop gradually or may occur suddenly after head injury or other precipitating diseases. Initially, urine production may exceed 300 ml/hr (polyuria), accompanied by an abnormally low urine osmolality.[24] The diluted urine in DI is "insipid" or tasteless, as opposed to the sweet, honey "mellitus" taste of urine associated with DM.

Laboratory studies

Diagnostic tests used to establish the presence of DI evaluate the body's innate ability to balance fluid and electrolytes (Table 23-4). The tests performed most frequently include a comparison of serum osmolality, urine osmolality, and serum sodium values. The serum osmolality has a narrow range, between 285 and 300 mOsm/kg. Urine osmolality can fluctuate between 300 and 800 mOsm/kg, with extremes ranging from 50 to 1200 mOsm/kg.[24] Severe DI could raise serum osmolality to 330 mOsm/kg, while urine osmolality falls well below

normal.[25,26] Serum sodium levels mirror the high solute concentration within the bloodstream. Unconscious patients or patients unable to respond to the thirst mechanism that accompanies polyuria are at risk of rapid dehydration and hypovolemia if DI is not diagnosed and treated. For these patients a gradual rise in serum sodium level signals the fluid imbalance. Suspect DI in the unconscious patient with hypoosmotic polyuria when the serum sodium level reaches 143 mEq/L before more serious problems with hemoconcentration develop.[26]

Water deprivation test. Laboratory tests are useful in differentiating DI according to cause. In a water deprivation or dehydration test, the patient is deprived of fluids for a 24-hour period. During this time, urine and plasma osmolality measurements are taken. In patients with ADH deficiency the urine is minimally concentrated after dehydration, whereas plasma osmolality rises above 300 mOsm/kg and serum sodium is greater than 145 mEq/L. This test is seldom done in critical care settings because of the potentially serious consequence to the patient who is already volume depleted with an elevated plasma osmolality. Exogenous ADH can be used in urine concentration testing without depriving the patient of fluids. The ADH is given parenterally, after which urine and blood osmolality tests are recorded. While the exogenous ADH test is preferred over the water deprivation test, there are still inherent fluid and sodium risks with this test, and patients with cardiac dysfunction are to be observed cautiously.[27]

Alternate tests may include quantitative analysis of serum ADH. Absent or decreased levels of serum ADH in the presence of hyperosmolar serum and hypoosmolar urine indicate primary and secondary ADH deficiency. Normal serum ADH levels (1.0 to 13.3 pg/ml) accompanying clinical manifestations of DI may indicate nephrogenic DI, in which the kidney tubule is insensitive to ADH. Normal ADH levels with elevated

TABLE 23-4

LABORATORY VALUES AND INTAKE AND OUTPUT FOR PATIENTS WITH DIABETES INSIPIDUS AND SYNDROME OF INAPPROPRIATE ANTIDIURETIC HORMONE

	NORMAL	DIABETES INSIPIDUS	SYNDROME OF INAPPROPRIATE ANTIDIURETIC HORMONE
LAB VALUES			
Serum ADH	1-5 pg/ml	↓in central DI, may be normal with nephrogenic or psychogenic DI	Elevated
Serum osmolality	285-300 mOsm/kg	>300 mOsm/kg	<250 mOsm/kg
Serum sodium	135-145 mEq/L	>145 mEq/L	<120 mEq/L
Urine osmolality	300-1400 mOsm/kg	<300 mOsm/kg	Increased
Urine specific gravity	1.005-1.030	<1.005	>1.030
INTAKE AND OUTPUT			
Urine output	1-1.5 L/24 hr	30-40 L/24 hr	Below normal
Fluid intake	1-1.5 L/24 hr	≥50 L 24 hr	Unchanged

blood osmolality and increased urine output also may suggest pharmacologically induced DI or excessive or compulsive water drinking. The vasopressin (ADH) concentration level may be measured to differentiate the type of DI present.

Medical Management

Treatment of the patient in DI requires an aggressive approach. Treatment goals include restoration of circulating volume and replacement of ADH. In addition, medical management involves treatment of the primary condition that is creating the interference in ADH circulation.

Volume restoration

Fluid replacement is provided in the initial phase of the treatment to prevent circulatory collapse. Patients who are able to drink are given voluminous amounts of fluid orally to balance output. For those unable to take sufficient fluids orally, hypotonic intravenous solutions are rapidly infused and carefully monitored to restore the hemodynamic balance. The amount of fluid lost to the body can be estimated, based on normal fluid stores and usual body weight, using the following formula:

$$\text{Liters body water deficit} = \frac{.6\ (\text{kg wt}) \times (\text{serum sodium} - 140)}{140}$$

The formula assumes that 60% of an individual's weight is fluid, although this is not always exact.[28] The resulting liters of body water deficit can then be used for planning replacement fluids.

ADH replacement

Medications have been used successfully to treat DI[11,15,13,18] (Table 23-5). Patients with primary and secondary DI who are unable to synthesize ADH require exogenous ADH (vasopressin) replacement therapy. One form of the hormone available for short-term substitution is aqueous, synthetic Pitressin. It is administered intramuscularly or subcutaneously or applied topically to the nasal mucosa. Onset of antidiuresis is rapid and lasts up to 8 hours. This drug constricts smooth muscle and can elevate systemic blood pressure. Water intoxication also can occur if the dose is higher than the therapeutic level. Another drug for patients with a mild form of DI is a synthetic analogue of vasopressin, desmopressin acetate (DDAVP). It is administered parenterally or topically, via the nasal mucosa (not inhaled). The drug has fewer side effects than do other vasopressin preparations. It has minimal effects on the smooth muscle tissue and rarely causes hypertension. It is, however, expensive, costing the patient up to $2500/year.[14]

Nursing Management

Nursing management of the patient with diabetes insipidus incorporates a variety of nursing diagnoses (Box 23-8). **Nursing priorities are directed toward administering prescribed fluids and medications, monitoring the patient's response to therapy, providing comfort and emotional support, and maintaining surveillance for complications.**

Administering prescribed fluids and medications

Rapid intravenous fluid replacement requires the use of a volumetric pump. ADH replacement is accomplished with extreme caution in the patient with a history of cardiac disease because vasopressin may cause hypertension and overhydration. At the first signs of cardiovascular impairment, the drug is discontinued and fluid intake is restricted until urine specific gravity is less than 1.015 and polyuria resumes.

Monitoring the patient's response to therapy

Critical assessment and management of the fluid status are the most important concerns for the patient with DI. Intake and output measurement, condition of buccal membranes, skin turgor, daily weights, presence of thirst, and temperature provide a basic assessment list that is vital for the patient unable to regulate fluid needs and fluid lost.

Providing comfort and emotional support

The patient who is unable to satisfy sensations of thirst or to complete any task or self-care activity without the need to urinate is confused and frightened. For patients who are able to verbalize their fears, having someone who is interested and nonjudgmental may help reduce the emotional turmoil. The nurse must recognize the patient's reluctance to engage in any activity because of the polyuria. Having a bedpan or commode constantly available will reduce anxiety for the alert patient who does not have an indwelling urinary catheter.

Maintaining surveillance for complications

Constipation and diarrhea are common problems in the patient with DI. Constipation results from fluid loss and, depending on the patient's status, is treated with dietary fiber, stool softeners, or both. Diarrhea may accompany the abdominal cramping and intestinal hyperactivity associated with vasopressin drug therapy. Untoward effects are brought to the attention of the physician for dose modification.

Patient education

Educating the patient and the family about the disease process and how it affects thirst, urination, and fluid balance will encourage patients to participate in their care and reduce the feelings of hopelessness. Patients who are discharged with the disease are taught, along with their families, the signs and symptoms of dehydration and overhydration. They are taught the procedures for correct daily weight and urine specific gravity measurements. Printed information pertaining to drug actions, side effects, dosages, and timetable is given to the patient, as well as an outline of factors that need to be reported to the physician.

TABLE 23-5

ADH REPLACEMENT THERAPY AND MEDICATIONS FOR DI

	DOSAGE	ACTIONS	SPECIAL CONSIDERATIONS
Desmopressin acetate (DDAVP, nasal spray, Rhinal tube, Rhinyle drops, Stimate)	Nasally, 10-40 μg hs or in divided doses 10 mg/0.1 ml; 100 mg/ml Parenteral, 2-4 mg bid	Treatment of central diabetes insipidus (DI) Antidiuretic—increases water reabsorption in nephron Prevents and controls polydipsia, polyuria Preferred treatment for chronic, long-term DI	Few side effects Observe for nasal congestion, URI, allergic rhinitis Monitor intake and output, urine osmolality, serum sodium level
Vasopressin (Pitressin, Pressyn)	Parenteral, IM, IV, SQ, intrarterial Topical nasal mucosa	Treatment of central DI Antidiuretic Promotes reabsorption of water at kidney tubule Decreases urine output Increases urine osmolality Diagnostic aid Increases gastrointestinal peristalsis	Monitor fluid volume status frequently, especially of elderly Assess cardiac status May precipitate angina, hypertension, myocardial infarction if increased dose given to patient with cardiac history Parenteral extravasation may cause skin necrosis
Lypressin (Diapid)	Intranasal 1-2 sprays (7-14 μg) each nostril qid	Treatment of central DI Synthetic antidiuretic hormone Increases reabsorption of sodium and water in nephron	Proper instillation important for absorption and action of drug Patient to sit upright while holding bottle upright for administration Repeated sprays (>2-3) are ineffective and wasteful; if dose is increased to 2-3 sprays, the time interval between dosing is to be shortened Cough, tightness in chest, shortness of breath
Thiazide diuretics	Varies according to diuretic chosen and size and age of patient	Treatment of nephrogenic DI Leads to mild fluid depletion; increased water and sodium is reabsorbed in the proximal nephron and less fluid travels on to the distal nephron, thereby excreting less water	Varies according to diuretic chosen
Anticompulsive disorder medications, anxietolytics, psychopharmacologic medications	Varies	Treatment of psychogenic DI	Varies according to medication chosen

SYNDROME OF INAPPROPRIATE ANTIDIURETIC HORMONE

Description and Etiology

The opposite of DI is the syndrome of inappropriate antidiuretic hormone (SIADH). The patient with SIADH has ADH secreted into the bloodstream exceeding the amount needed to maintain blood volume and serum osmolality. Excessive water is reabsorbed at the kidney tubule, leading to dilutional hyponatremia. The patient becomes water intoxicated.

SIADH falls under two different DRGs, depending on whether the patient develops complications or comorbid conditions (CC). DRG 300 (Endocrine Disorders With CC) and DRG 301 (Endocrine Disorders Without CC) have average lengths of the stay of 6.6 days and 4.4 days, respectively.[9]

Of the numerous causes of SIADH, many are seen in patients who are critically ill (Box 23-9). Central nervous system injury or disease interfering with the normal functioning of the hypothalamic-pituitary system may cause SIADH. The most common cause, however, is malignant

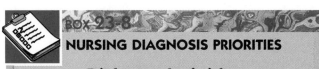

NURSING DIAGNOSIS PRIORITIES

Diabetes Insipidus

- Fluid Volume Deficit related to decreased secretion of ADH, p. 490
- Decreased Cardiac Output related to alterations in preload, pp. 467-468
- Powerlessness related to lack of control over current situation and/or disease process, pp. 455-456
- Knowledge Deficit: Discharge Regimen related to lack of previous exposure to information, p. 443

bronchogenic oat cell carcinoma. This type of malignant cell is capable of synthesizing and releasing ADH. Other carcinomas capable of this autonomous production of ADH involve the pancreas, prostate, duodenum, and thymus. ADH levels also have been elevated in Hodgkin's disease and leukemia. In addition, ectopic endocrine production of ADH is identified in certain nonmalignant pulmonary conditions, such as tuberculosis and pneumonia. Levels of ADH are also increased by positive pressure ventilators that decrease venous return to the thorax, thus stimulating pulmonary baroreceptors to release ADH.[17] Other causes of SIADH are neurologic disorders, such as tetanus, meningitis, and Guillain-Barré syndrome. Anesthesia, stress, pain, and such drugs as cyclophosphamide and chlorpropamide also have been implicated.

Pathophysiology

ADH (vasopressin) is a powerful, complex polypeptide compound. When released into the circulation by the posterior pituitary gland, ADH regulates water and electrolyte balance. In SIADH, profound fluid and electrolyte disturbances result from the unsolicited, continuous release of the hormone into the bloodstream (Fig. 23-4). Rather than providing a water balance within the body, excessive ADH stimulates the kidney tubules to retain fluid, regardless of need. This results in severe overhydration.

Excessive ADH also alters the extracellular fluid's sodium balance. The overhydration causes a dilutional hyponatremia and reduces the sodium concentration to critically low levels.[29] In the healthy adult, hyponatremia inhibits the release of ADH; however, in SIADH the increased levels of circulating ADH are unrelated to the serum sodium. Hyponatremia continues as aldosterone, which is normally released by the adrenal glands to retain sodium, is suppressed. Serum hypoosmolality leads to a shift of fluid from the extracellular fluid space into the intracellular fluid compartment in an attempt to equalize osmotic pressure. Because minimal sodium is present in this fluid, edema usually does not result. Without ADH and aldosterone, water is retained, urine output is diminished, and further sodium is excreted in the urine.

The urine has an increased osmolality from the decreased water excretion. Urinary concentration is also elevated by excess sodium in the urine.[17] It is believed that despite the serum hyponatremia, the increased release of ADH promotes sodium loss through the kidneys into the urine.

Assessment and Diagnosis

Clinical manifestations

The clinical manifestations of SIADH relate to the excess fluid in the extracellular compartment and the proportionate dilution of the circulating sodium. Although edema usually is not present, slight weight gain may occur from the expanded extracellular fluid volume. Hyponatremia initially may be asymptomatic. Early clinical manifestations of dilutional hyponatremia include lethargy, anorexia, nausea, and vomiting. The water and sodium imbalance progresses, with the sodium levels dropping below 120 mEq/L.[16] Progressively deteriorating neurologic signs of hyponatremia then predominate, and the patient is admitted to the critical care unit. Symptoms of severe hyponatremia include the inability to concentrate, mental confusion, apprehension, seizures, loss of consciousness, coma, and death.

Laboratory values

Laboratory values provide the clinical hallmarks of SIADH: serum hypoosmolality with hyponatremia and a urine osmolality greater than would be expected of the hypotonic blood (see Table 23-4). The patient with SIADH characteristically displays a serum hypoosmolality less than 275 mOsm/kg, with urine osmolality that is less than maximally dilute or less than 100 mOsm/kg water.[17] Urine osmolality that is equal to or that exceeds serum osmolality, with urinary sodium greater than 20 mEq/L, demonstrates the SIADH paradox of a very dilute serum with a concentrated urine output.

Water load test. To confirm the diagnosis, a water-load test may be performed. After a period of fasting, a dehydrated patient is overhydrated with water. The urine output and serum osmolality are carefully monitored to discover a decline in serum osmolality resulting from peak moments of overhydration. Patients with SIADH show a decrease in serum osmolality regardless of the fasting state and an inability to secrete dilute urine despite the hydration resulting from the water load.[17] This test is identified as very useful in identifying changes in free water excretion. The test, however, requires that the patient withstand the physical insult of overhydration and for that reason is almost never done in a critical care unit.

Medical Management

In the critical care unit, SIADH often occurs as a secondary disease. Ideally, recognition and treatment of the pri-

BOX 23-9

ETIOLOGY OF SIADH

Malignant disease associated with autonomous
  production of ADH
    Bronchogenic oat cell carcinoma
    Pancreatic adenocarcinoma
    Duodenal, bladder, ureter, prostatic carcinomas
    Lymphosarcoma, Ewing's sarcoma
    Acute leukemia, Hodgkin's disease
    Cerebral neoplasm, thymoma
Central nervous system diseases that interfere with the
  hypothalamic-hypophyseal system and increase the
  production and/or release of ADH
    Head injury
    Brain abscess
    Hydrocephalus
    Pituitary adenoma
    Subdural hematoma
    Subarachnoid hemorrhage
    Cerebral atrophy
    Guillain-Barré syndrome
    Tuberculosis meningitis
    Purulent meningitis
    Herpes simplex encephalitis
    Acute intermittent prophyria
Neurogenic stimuli capable of increasing ADH
    Decreased glomerular filtration rate
    Physical and/or emotional stressors
      Pain
      Fear
      Trauma
      Surgery
      Myocardial infarction
      Acute infection
      Hypotension
      Hemorrhage
      Hypovolemia

Pulmonary diseases believed to stimulate the
  baroreceptors and increase ADH
    Pulmonary tuberculosis
    Viral and bacterial pneumonia
    Empyema
    Lung abscess
    Chronic obstructive lung disease
    Status asthmaticus
    Cystic fibrosis
Endocrine disturbances that hormonally influence ADH
    Myxedema
    Hypothyroidism
    Hypopituitarism
    Adrenal insufficiency—Addison's disease
Medications that mimic, increase the release of, or
  potentiate ADH
    Hypoglycemics
      Insulin
      Tolbutamide
      Chlorpropamide
    Potassium-depicting thiazide diuretics
    Tricyclic antidepressants
      Imipramine
      Amitriptyline
    Phenothiazine
      Fluphenazine
      Thioridazine
    Thioxanthenes
      Thiothixene
      Chlorprothixene
    Chemotherapeutic agents
      Vincristine
      Cyclophosphamide
    Narcotics
    Carbamazepine
    Clofibrate
    Acetaminophen
    Nicotine
    Oxytocin
    Vasopressin
    Anesthetics

mary disease will reduce the production of ADH. If the patient is receiving any of the chemical agents suspected of causing the disease, discontinuing the drug may return ADH levels to normal. Treatment goals include restriction of fluid and replacement of sodium. Certain drugs reduce the effectiveness of ADH on the kidney tubule. Narcotic agonists, such as oxilorphan and butorphanol, are used to reduce the secretion of ADH in many patients with SIADH. The drugs, however, do not seem to be effective in patients with SIADH caused by lung malignancies. Patients with lung malignancies are treated with demeclocycline hydrochloride, an antibacterial tetracycline, and lithium carbonate, an alkali metal salt used primarily to alter psychogenic behavior. These drugs inhibit the tubule response to ADH and decrease the water reabsorption at the tubules.[14]

Fluid restriction

The medical therapy that is most successful (along with treatment of the primary disease) is simple reduction of fluid intake. This is done most successfully for the patient with a moderate increase in the body fluid volume, with hyponatremia. Although fluid restrictions are to be calculated on the basis of individual needs and losses, a general criterion is to restrict fluids to 500 ml less than average daily output.[17]

Sodium replacement

Patients with severe hyponatremia (less than 115 mEq/L) or those with seizures are cautiously infused with 3% to 5% hypertonic saline solution[28] for rapid but temporary correction of the hemodilution caused by the retention of fluid at the tubules and severe sodium loss. It

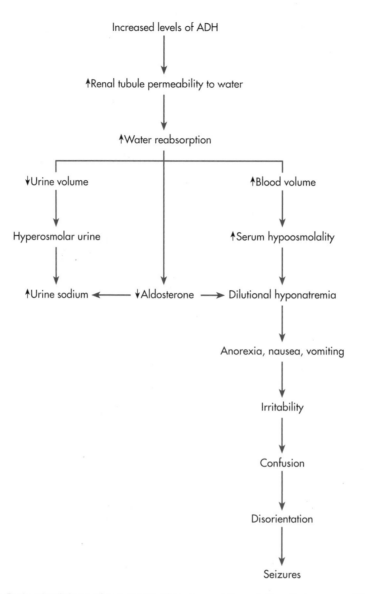

Increased levels of ADH

↓

↑Renal tubule permeability to water

↓

↑Water reabsorption

↓Urine volume   ↑Blood volume

↓   ↓

Hyperosmolar urine   ↑Serum hypoosmolality

↓   ↓

↑Urine sodium ← ↓Aldosterone → Dilutional hyponatremia

↓

Anorexia, nausea, vomiting

↓

Irritability

↓

Confusion

↓

Disorientation

↓

Seizures

Fig. **23-4** Pathophysiology of syndrome of inappropriate antidiuretic hormone (SIADH).

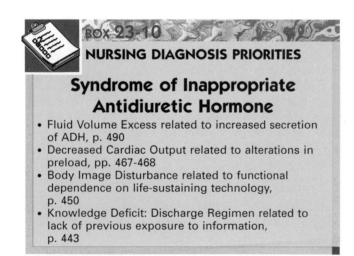

Box 23-10

NURSING DIAGNOSIS PRIORITIES

Syndrome of Inappropriate Antidiuretic Hormone

- Fluid Volume Excess related to increased secretion of ADH, p. 490
- Decreased Cardiac Output related to alterations in preload, pp. 467-468
- Body Image Disturbance related to functional dependence on life-sustaining technology, p. 450
- Knowledge Deficit: Discharge Regimen related to lack of previous exposure to information, p. 443

is considered safe to raise serum sodium levels up to 12 mEq/day for the first 24 to 48 hours while avoiding fatal consequences from neurologic complications. Furosemide may be added to further increase the diuresis of free water and to prevent the risk of pulmonary edema related to the hypertonic saline solution. Hypertonic saline solution is administered very slowly and with extreme caution (1 to 2 ml/kg/hour) until the patient's serum sodium level is increased no greater than 1 to 2 mEq/L/hour.[30] Treatment with a hypertonic saline solution is temporary inasmuch as the sodium is continuously removed from the body through the urine.

Nursing Management

Nursing management of the patient with SIADH incorporates a variety of nursing diagnoses (Box 23-10).

Nursing priorities are directed toward administering and restricting prescribed fluids, monitoring the patient's response to therapy, providing comfort and emotional support, and maintaining surveillance for complications.

Administering and restricting prescribed fluids

Accurate intake and output measurement is required to calculate fluid replacement for the patient with excessive ADH. All fluids are restricted as ordered. Intake that equals urine output may be given until serum sodium level returns to normal. Weights may be taken every 12 hours to gauge fluid retention or loss. Weight gain could signify continual fluid retention, whereas weight loss could indicate loss of body fluid.

Hypertonic saline solution is infused very cautiously. A volumetric pump is used to deliver 1 ml/kg/hour or it is set to deliver a flow rate determined by the serum sodium levels. Hypertonic expansion of the vascular space is a complication of the rapid infusion of hypertonic saline solution that must be avoided. Hypertonic expansion occurs when the hypertonic solution is infused so rapidly that it creates an immediate hyperosmolality of the blood stream. Fluid is drawn from the more diluted intracellular spaces to the bloodstream in an effort to equalize the concentration of particles. The hypertonic solution is discontinued if any signs or symptoms of fluid overload occur.

Monitoring the patient's response to therapy

Thorough, astute nursing assessments are required for care of the patient with SIADH while an attempt is made to correct the fluid and sodium imbalance; the systemic effects of hyponatremia occur rapidly and can be lethal. Evaluation of the patient's neurologic status, especially level of consciousness, occurs every 1 to 2 hours. Frequent assessment of the patient's hydration status is accomplished with serial measurements of urine output, blood and urine sodium levels, urine specific gravity, and urine and blood osmolality. Elimination patterns are assessed because constipation may occur when fluids are restricted.

Providing comfort and emotional support

Frequent mouth care through moistening the buccal membrane may give comfort during the period of fluid restriction.

Maintaining surveillance for complications

The patient with SIADH may experience a variety of complications, including seizures, fluid volume overload, and constipation.

Seizures. Seizure precautions for the patient with SIADH are provided regardless of the degree of hyponatremia. Serum sodium levels may fluctuate rapidly, and neurologic impairment may occur with no apparent warning. The patient's altered neurologic response may also be influenced by the acuity of the primary disease (i.e., central nervous system disease) and not solely by the result of low sodium levels. Seizure precautions include nursing actions to protect the patient from injury (padded side rails, bed in low position when patient is unattended) and to provide an open airway (oral airway, head turned to side without forcibly restraining the patient, suction apparatus). Oxygen is administered as needed.

Fluid volume overload. Blood pressure, CVP, and pulmonary arterial wedge pressure are all expected to be within the normal range of the patient. Clinical manifestations of acute heart failure and pulmonary edema, such as elevated blood pressure, pulmonary artery wedge pressure, and CVP are causes to discontinue the hypertonic saline infusion. Apprehension, abrupt position changes to an upright position to breathe, dyspnea, moist cough, and increased respiratory and pulse rates also indicate the inability of the cardiopulmonary system to accommodate the increased fluid load.

Constipation. An alteration in bowel elimination resulting in constipation may occur from decreased fluid intake and inactivity. Cathartics or low-volume hypertonic enemas may be given to stimulate peristalsis. Tap water or hypotonic enemas should not be given because the water in the enema solution may be absorbed through the bowel and potentiate water intoxication.

Patient education

Rapidly occurring changes in the patient's neurologic status may frighten visiting family members. Sensitivity to the family's unspoken fears can be shown by words that express empathy and by providing time for the patient and family to communicate their feelings. The nurse may discuss the course of the disease, its effect on water balance, the reasons for fluid restrictions, and the family's role in treating SIADH. Teaching the patient and the family alertness to severe thirst and measurement of intake and output along with parameters to notify the physician will encourage independence and involve the family in the patient's care.

References

1. Lennie TA: The metabolic response to injury: current perspectives and nursing implications, *Dimens Crit Care Nurs* 16:79, 1997.
2. Loriavx TC: Endocrine assessment: red flags for those on the front lines, *Nurs Clin North Am* 4:695, 1996.
3. Ober PK, editor: *Endocrinology of critical disease*, Totowa, NJ, 1997, Humana Press.
4. Burr R: Neuroendocrinology. In Noble J, et al, editors: *Textbook of primary care medicine*, ed 2, St Louis, 1996, Mosby.
5. Harris MI: Summary. In Harris MI, et al, editors: *Diabetes in America, National Diabetes Data Group*, ed 2, NIH Publication, No. 95-1468, Washington, DC, 1995, National Institutes of Health, National Institutes of Diabetes and Digestive and Kidney Diseases.
6. Kitabchi AE, Fisher JN: Ketoacidosis and the hyperosmolar hyperglycemic nonketotic state. In Kahn C, Weir G, editors: *Joslin's diabetes mellitus*, ed 13, Philadelphia, 1994, Lea & Febiger.

7. American Diabetes Association: Clinical practice recommendations 1997, *Diabetes Care* 20:S1, 1997.
8. Facui A, et al, editors: *Harrison's principles of internal medicine*, ed 14, New York, 1998, McGraw-Hill.
9. *St. Anthony's DRG guidebook 1998,* Reston, Va, 1997, St Anthony Publishing.
10. Bennett PH: Definition, diagnosis and classification of diabetes and impaired glucose intolerance. In Kahn C, Weir G, editors: *Joslin's diabetes mellitus,* ed 13, Philadelphia, 1994, Lea & Febiger.
11. Karam JH: Pancreatic hormones and diabetes mellitus. In Greenspan FS, Strewler GJ, editors: *Basic and clinical endocrinology,* ed 5, Norwalk, Conn, 1997, Appleton & Lange.
12. Bhasin S, Tom L: Endocrine problems in the critically ill patient. In Bongard FS, Sue DY, editors: *Current critical care: diagnosis and treatment,* Norwalk, Conn, 1994, Appleton & Lange.
13. Ipp E: Diabetes mellitus and the critically ill patient. In Bongard FS, Sue DY, editors: *Current critical care: diagnosis and treatment,* Norwalk, Conn, 1994, Appleton & Lange.
14. Noble SL, et al: Insulin Lispro: a fast-acting insulin analog, *Am Fam Physician* 57:279, 1998.
15. McEvoy GK, editor: *American hospital formulary service drug information 1998,* Bethesda, MD, 1998, American Society of Health-System Pharmacists.
16. Rudy DR, Tzagournis M: Endocrinology. In Rakel RE, editor: *Textbook of family practice,* ed 5, Philadelphia, 1995, WB Saunders.
17. Becker KL, editor: *Principles and practice of endocrinology and metabolism,* ed 2, Philadelphia, 1995, JB Lippincott.
18. Tierney LM, McPhee SJ, Papadakis MA, editors: *Current medical diagnosis and treatment,* Stamford, Conn, 1998, Appleton & Lange.
19. Edelman SV, Henry RR: *Diagnosis and management of type II diabetes,* Caddo, OK, 1997, Professional Communications.
20. Wannamethee SG, Perry IJ, Shaper AG: Hematocrit and risk of non insulin dependent diabetes mellitus, *Diabetes* 45:576, 1996.
21. Unger RH, Foster DW: Diabetes mellitus. In Williams RH, Wilson JD, editors: *Williams textbook of endocrinology,* ed 9, Philadelphia, 1998, WB Saunders.
22. Burge MR, Schade DS: Insulins, *Endocrinol Metab Clin North Am* 26:575, 1997.
23. Bullock B, Rosendahl P: *Pathophysiology: adaptations and alterations in function,* ed 4, Philadelphia, 1996, JB Lippincott.
24. Aron DC, et al: Hypothalamus and pituitary. In Greenspan FS, Strewler, GJ, editors: *Basic and clinical endocrinology,* ed 5, Norwalk, Conn, 1997, Appleton & Lange.
25. Lubin M, et al, editors: *Medical management of the surgical patient,* ed 3, Philadelphia, 1995, JB Lippincott.
26. Szerlip H, et al: Sodium and water. In Noe DA, Rock RC, editors: *Laboratory medicine: the selection and interpretation of clinical laboratory studies,* Baltimore, 1994, Williams & Wilkins.
27. Fischbach F: *A manual of laboratory and diagnostic tests,* ed 5, Philadelphia, 1996, JB Lippincott.
28. Chan PD, Winkle CR, Winkle PJ: *Current clinical strategies,* Fountain Valley, CA, 1995, Current Clinical Strategies Publishing.
29. Guyton AC, Hall JE: *Textbook of medical physiology,* ed 9, Philadelphia, 1996, WB Saunders.
30. Batcheller J: Syndrome of inappropriate antidiuretic hormone secretion, *Crit Care Nurs Clin North Am* 6:687, 1994.

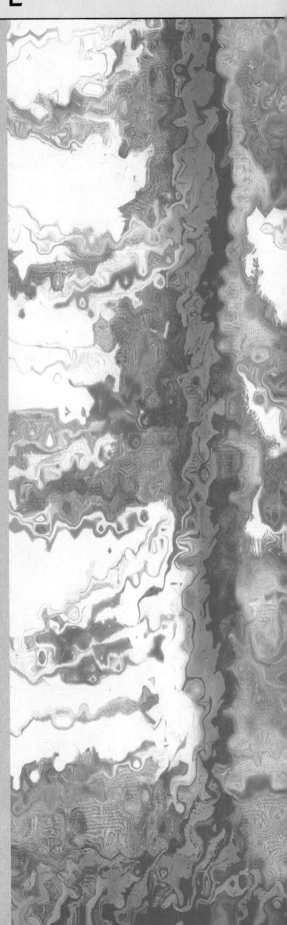

UNIT NINE

MULTISYSTEM ALTERATIONS

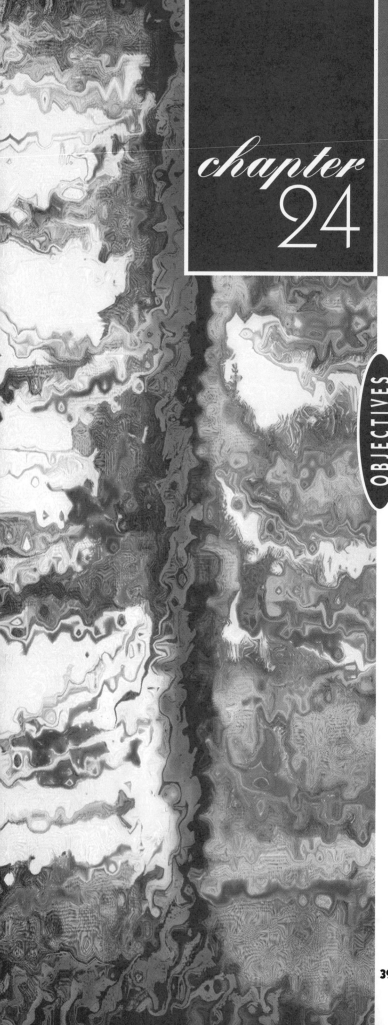

chapter 24

Trauma

Karen Johnson

OBJECTIVES

- **Compare and contrast injuries associated with blunt and penetrating trauma.**

- **Discuss mechanism with injury, pathophysiology, assessment findings, medical management, and nursing management of traumatic injuries to the following sites: head, spinal cord, heart, lungs, and abdomen.**

- **Use assessment findings to identify complications and sequelae of traumatic injuries.**

- **Describe the four phases of trauma care.**

Over the past few decades major advances have been made in the management of patients with traumatic injuries, and significant improvements have been made in their care in both prehospital and emergency department settings. These improvements have affected critical care in that patients with complex, multisystem trauma are admitted to critical care units. These patients require complex nursing care. This chapter reviews nursing management of patients with traumatic injuries, particularly in the critical care setting.

MECHANISMS OF INJURY

Trauma occurs when an external force of energy impacts the body and causes structural or physiologic alterations, or "injuries." External forces can be radiation, electrical, thermal, chemical, or mechanical forms of energy. This chapter focuses on trauma from mechanical energy. Mechanical energy can produce either blunt or penetrating traumatic injuries. Knowledge of the mechanism of injury helps health care providers anticipate and predict potential internal injuries.

Blunt Trauma

Blunt trauma most often is seen with MVAs, contact sports, crush injuries, or falls. Injuries occur because of the forces sustained during a rapid change in velocity (deceleration). To estimate the amount of force a person would sustain in an MVA, multiply the person's weight by miles per hour of speed the vehicle was traveling.[1] A 130-pound woman in a vehicle traveling at 60 miles per hour that hits a brick wall, for example, would sustain 7800 pounds of force within milliseconds. As the body stops suddenly, tissues and organs continue to move forward. This sudden change in velocity causes injuries that result in lacerations or crush injuries of internal body structures.

Penetrating Trauma

Penetrating injuries occur with stabbings, firearms, or impalement on foreign objects that penetrate the skin, with resultant damage to internal structures. Damage is created along the path of penetration. Penetrating injuries can be misleading inasmuch as the outside of the wound does not determine the extent of the internal injury. Bullets can create internal cavities 5 to 30 times larger than the diameter of the bullet.[2]

Several factors determine the extent of damage sustained as a result of penetrating trauma. Different weapons cause different types of injuries. The severity of a gunshot wound depends on the type of gun, type of ammunition used, and the distance and angle from which the gun was fired. Pellets from a shotgun blast expand on impact and cause multiple injuries to internal structures. Handgun bullets, on the other hand, usually damage what is directly in the bullet's path. Once inside the body, the bullet can ricochet off bone and create further damage along its pathway. With penetrating stab wounds, factors that determine the extent of injury include type and length of object used as well as the angle of insertion.

PHASES OF TRAUMA CARE

Prehospital Resuscitation

The goal of prehospital care is immediate stabilization and transportation. Stabilization is accomplished through assessments and interventions related to airway, breathing, and circulation (ABCs). Once stabilized at the scene, the patient is transported to an appropriate medical facility by ground or air transport.

Emergency Department Resuscitation

Primary survey

On arrival of the trauma patient in the emergency department, the primary survey is initiated. During this assessment, life-threatening injuries are discovered and treated. The five steps in the primary survey comprise the ABCs, plus D and E (D, disability [mini-neurologic examination], and E, exposure [undress, with temperature control]) (Table 24-1). The cervical spine must be immobilized in all trauma patients until a cervical spinal cord injury has been definitively ruled out. If the airway is obstructed, foreign bodies are removed. In the presence of ineffective airway clearance, the airway is secured through intubation or cricothyrotomy. Cardiac monitoring is initiated to assess for rhythm disturbances. Life-threatening dysrhythmias are treated according to ACLS protocols. External exsanguination is identified and controlled. A rapid assessment of circulatory status includes assessment of level of consciousness, skin color, and pulse.

Resuscitation phase

After the primary survey, the resuscitation phase begins. Hypovolemic shock is the most common type of shock that occurs in trauma patients.[2] Hemorrhage must be identified and treated rapidly. Vigorous intravenous (IV) fluid replacement is initiated. Large-bore peripheral IV catheters (14 to 16 gauge) or a central venous catheter are inserted. Restoration of volume is accomplished through administration of crystalloid (lactated Ringer's solution), colloid (plasma or albumin), and/or blood products. During the initiation of IV lines, blood samples are drawn. High-flow fluid warmers may be used to deliver warmed IV solutions at rates greater than 1000 ml/minute. If the patient remains unresponsive to bolus intravenous therapy, type-specific blood or O-negative blood may be administered.[2] Transfusion of autologous salvaged blood (autotransfusion) also may be used to replace intravascular volume and to provide oxygen-carrying capacity.

Gastric and urinary catheters are placed, unless contraindicated. Adequate resuscitation is assessed by monitoring for improvement in vital signs (including body temperature), arterial blood gas levels, and urinary output.

Secondary survey

The secondary survey begins when the primary survey is completed, resuscitation initiated, and the patient's ABCs are reassessed.[2] During the secondary survey each body region is thoroughly examined. The history is one of the most important aspects of the secondary survey. Often, head injury, shock, or the use of drugs or alcohol may preclude a good history, so the history must be pieced together from other sources. The prehospital providers (paramedics, emergency medical technicians [EMTs]) usually can provide most of the vital information pertaining to the accident. Specific information that must be elicited pertaining to the mechanism of injury is summarized in Box 24-1.

During the secondary survey, the nurse ensures the completion of special procedures, such as an electrocardiogram (ECG), radiographic studies (chest, cervical spine, thorax, and pelvis), and peritoneal lavage.

TABLE 24-1

PRIMARY SURVEY OF THE TRAUMA PATIENT

SURVEY COMPONENT	NURSING DIAGNOSIS	NURSING ASSESSMENT/CARE
Airway	Airway clearance: Ineffective related to obstruction or actual injury	Look, listen, and feel Immobilize C-spine Position victim/patient: 　Supine 　Sitting 　Log roll Clear airway: 　Jaw thrust 　Chin lift 　Finger sweep 　Suctioning Airway devices: 　Oropharyngeal 　Nasopharyngeal 　Endotracheal tube 　Cricothyrotomy
Breathing	Breathing pattern: Ineffective related to actual injury Gas exchange: Impaired related to Actual injury or disrupted tissue perfusion	Assess for: 　Spontaneous breathing 　Respiratory rate, depth, and symmetry 　Chest wall integrity Administer high-flow oxygen Absent breathing: 　Intubate 　Positive-pressure ventilation Breathing but ineffective: 　Assess and treat life-threatening conditions (e.g., tension pneumothorax, flail chest)
Circulation	Cardiac output, alteration in: Decreased related to actual injury Tissue perfusion, alteration in: Related to actual injury or shock Fluid volume deficit: Related to actual loss of circulating volume	Assess pulse: 　Quality 　Rate No pulse: 　Initiate BCLS 　Initiate ACLS Pulse but ineffective: 　Assess and treat life-threatening conditions (e.g., uncontrolled bleeding, shock) Two large-bore (14- or 16-gauge) IV catheters Fluid replacement ECG monitoring
Disability	Injury potential for: Trauma, spinal cord, and brain related to actual injury	Brief neurologic examination 　Eye opening 　Verbal response 　Motor response 　Pupils Glasgow Coma Scale
Exposure	N/A	To visualize the entire body for inspection, all clothing must be removed

From Beaver BM: *Nurs Clin North Am* 25(1), 1990.

Throughout this survey, the nurse continuously monitors the patient's vital signs and response to medical therapies. Emotional support to the patient and family also is imperative.

Definitive Care/Operative Phase

Once the secondary survey has been completed, specific injuries usually have been diagnosed. Definitive care related to specific injuries is described throughout this chapter. Trauma, often referred to as a *surgical disease* because of the nature and extent of the injuries, usually requires operative management of injuries. After surgery, depending on the patient's status, a transfer to the critical care unit may be indicated.

Critical Care Phase

Critically ill trauma patients are admitted into the critical care unit as direct transfers from the emergency depart-

From Johnson KL: Critical care of the trauma patient. In Neff JA, Kidd PS, editors: *Trauma nursing: the art and science*, St Louis, 1993, Mosby.

BOX 24-1

HISTORY OF MECHANISM OF INJURY

PENETRATING TRAUMA
- Weapon used (handgun, shotgun, rifle, knife)
- Caliber of weapon
- Number of shots fired
- Gender of assailant
- Position of victim and assailant when injury occurred

BLUNT TRAUMA
- Length of fall
- MVA extrication time
- Ejection
- Location in automobile (passenger, driver, front seat, back seat)
- Restraint status (lapbelt, shoulder harness, or combination; unrestrained)
- Speed of automobile(s)/direction of impact
- Occupants (number and morbidity status)

BOX 24-2

FACTORS THAT CONTRIBUTE TO TISSUE HYPOXIA IN THE TRAUMA PATIENT

- Shifts to the left of the oxyhemoglobin dissociation curve (can be secondary to infusion of large volumes of banked blood, hypocarbia or alkalosis, or hypothermia)
- Reduced hemoglobin (secondary to hemorrhage)
- Reduced cardiac output (in the presence of cardiovascular insults)
- Impaired cellular oxygen consumption (associated with metabolic alterations of sepsis)
- Increased metabolic demands (associated with the stress response to injury)

---

ment (ED) or operating room (OR). If surgery is required, the trauma patient is directly admitted to the critical care unit from the OR.[3,4] **Priority nursing care during the critical care phase includes ongoing physical assessments and monitoring the patient's response to medical therapies.**

One of the most important nursing roles is assessment of the balance between oxygen delivery and oxygen demand. Oxygen delivery must be optimized to prevent further system damage. Assessment of circulatory status includes the use of noninvasive and invasive techniques.

Tissue hypoxemia, which is a threat to the trauma patient, results from a variety of factors (Box 24-2). Prevention and treatment of hypoxemia depend on accurate assessment of the adequacy of pulmonary gas exchange, oxygen transport, and cellular oxygen utilization.

HEAD INJURIES

At least 2 million persons incur head injuries each year in the United States, and more than 400,000 patients with head injuries are admitted to hospitals, approximately half of whom were involved in motor vehicle crashes.[5] Approximately 50% of all trauma deaths are associated with head injury, and more than 60% of all vehicular trauma deaths are a result of head injury.[2]

Mechanism of Injury

Head injuries occur when mechanical forces are transmitted to brain tissue. Mechanisms of injury include penetrating or blunt trauma to the head. Penetrating trauma can result from the penetration of a foreign object (e.g., bullet) that causes direct damage to cerebral tissue. Blunt trauma can be the result of deceleration, acceleration, or rotational forces. Deceleration injuries occur when the brain crashes against the skull after it has hit something (e.g., the dashboard of a car). Acceleration injuries occur when the skull has been hit by something (e.g., a baseball bat). In many instances, a head injury can be caused by both acceleration and deceleration. In the combined form, acceleration injuries occur when the skull is hit by a force that causes the brain to move forward to the point of impact, and then, as the brain reverses direction and hits the other side of the skull, deceleration injuries occur.

Pathophysiology

Review of the pathophysiology of head injury can be divided into two categories: primary injury (that which occurs on impact) and secondary injury (that which occurs as a result of the original trauma).

Primary injury

The primary injury occurs at the time of impact as a result of the dynamic forces of acceleration-deceleration or rotation. Primary injuries include contusion, laceration, shearing injuries, or hemorrhage. Primary injury may be mild, with little or no neurologic damage, or severe, with major tissue damage.

Secondary injury

Secondary injury can be caused by further physiologic events that occur after the primary injury. Secondary injury can be caused by hypoxia, hypercapnia, hypotension, cerebral edema, or sustained hypertension. Beyond causing injury to tissue, each of these factors also contributes to significant increases in intracranial pressure (ICP).

Classification

Injuries to the brain are described by the functional changes or losses that occur. Some of the major functional abnormalities seen in head injury are described here.

Skull fractures

Skull fractures are common, but they do not by themselves cause neurologic deficits. Skull fractures can be classified as open (dura is torn) or closed (dura is not torn), or they can be classified as those of the vault or those of the base. Common vault fractures occur in the parietal and temporal regions. Basilar skull fractures usually are not visible on conventional skull films. Assessment findings may include cerebral spinal fluid otorrhea or rhinorrhea, Battle's sign (ecchymosis overlying the mastoid process), or "raccoon eyes" (subconjunctival and periorbital ecchymosis).

The significance of a skull fracture is that it identifies the patient with a higher probability of having or developing an intracranial hematoma. For this reason, all patients with skull fractures are hospitalized for observation.[2] Open skull fractures require surgical intervention to remove bony fragments and to close the dura. The major complications of basilar skull fractures are cranial nerve injury and leakage of cerebrospinal fluid (CSF). CSF leakage may result in a fistula, which increases the possibility of bacterial contamination and resultant meningitis. Because fistula formation may be delayed, patients with a basilar skull fracture are admitted to the hospital for observation and possible surgical intervention.

Concussion

A concussion is a brain injury accompanied by a brief loss of neurologic function, especially loss of consciousness.[2] If loss of consciousness occurs, it may last for seconds to an hour. The neurologic dysfunctions include confusion, disorientation, and sometimes a period of posttraumatic amnesia. Other clinical manifestations that occur after concussion are headache, dizziness, nausea, irritability, inability to concentrate, impaired memory, and fatigue. The diagnosis of concussion is based on the loss of consciousness inasmuch as the brain remains structurally intact despite functional impairment. Patients with a history of 5 or more minutes of loss of consciousness usually are admitted to the hospital for a 24-hour observation period.[2]

Contusion

Contusion, or bruising of the brain, usually is related to acceleration-deceleration injuries, which result in hemorrhage into the superficial parenchyma, often the frontal and temporal lobes. Frontal or temporal contusions can be seen in a coup-contrecoup mechanism of injury (Fig. 24-1). Coup injury affects the cerebral tissue directly under the point of impact. Contrecoup injury occurs in a line directly opposite the point of impact.

The clinical manifestations of contusion are related to the location of the contusion, the degree of contusion, and the presence of associated lesions. Contusions can be small, in which localized areas of dysfunction result in a focal neurologic deficit. Larger contusions can evolve over 2 to 3 days after injury as a result of edema and further hemorrhaging. A large contusion can produce a mass effect that can cause a significant increase in ICP.

Contusions of the tips of the temporal lobe are a common occurrence and are of particular concern. Because the inner aspects of the temporal lobe surround the opening in the tentorium where the midbrain enters the cerebrum, edema in this area can cause rapid deterioration of

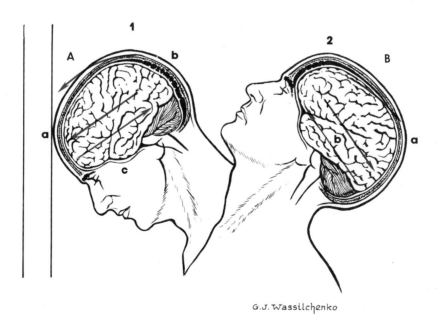

G.J. Wassilchenko

Fig. **24-1** Coup and contrecoup head injury after blunt trauma. **A,** Coup injury: impact against object. *a,* Site of impact and direct trauma to brain. *b,* Shearing of subdural veins. *c,* Trauma to base of brain. **B,** Contrecoup injury: impact within skull. *a,* Site of impact from brain hitting opposite side of skull. *b,* Shearing forces throughout brain. These injuries occur in one continuous motion—the head strikes the wall (coup), then rebounds (contrecoup).

the patient's condition and can lead to herniation. Because of the location, this deterioration can occur with little or no warning at a deceptively low ICP.

Diagnosis of contusion is made by computed tomography (CT) scan. If the CT scan indicates contusion, especially in the temporal area, the nurse must pay particular attention to neurologic assessments and look for subtle changes in pupillary signs or vital signs, irrespective of a stable ICP.

Medical management of cerebral contusions may consist of medical or surgical therapies. Because a contusion can progress over 3 to 5 days after injury, secondary injury may occur. If contusions are small, focal, or multiple, they are treated medically with serial neurologic assessments and possibly ICP monitoring. Larger contusions that produce considerable mass effect require surgical intervention to prevent the increased edema and intracranial pressure as the contusion matures.[2] Outcome of cerebral contusion varies, depending on the location and the degree of contusion.

Hematomas

Hematomas resulting from head injury form a mass lesion and lead to increased ICP. Three types of hematomas are discussed here (Fig. 24-2).

Epidural hematoma. Epidural hematoma (EDH), which is a collection of blood between the inner table of the skull and the outermost layer of the dura, most frequently is associated with skull fractures and middle meningeal artery laceration. A blow to the head that causes a linear skull fracture on the lateral surface of the head may tear the middle meningeal artery. As the artery bleeds, it pulls the dura away from the skull, creating a pouch that expands into the intracranial space.

The incidence of EDH is relatively low. EDH can occur as a result of low-impact injuries (such as falls) or high-impact injuries (such as motor vehicle crashes). EDH occurs from trauma to the skull and meninges rather than from the acceleration-deceleration forces seen in other types of head trauma.

The classic clinical manifestations of EDH include brief loss of consciousness followed by a period of lucidity that may last up to 12 hours. This lucid period is followed by a progressive deterioration in level of consciousness and the development of hemiparesis on the opposite side. A dilated and fixed pupil on the same side as the impact area is a hallmark sign of EDH.[2] The patient may complain of a severe, localized headache and may be sleepy. Diagnosis of EDH is based on clinical symptoms and evidence of a collection of epidural blood identified on CT scan. Treatment of EDH involves surgical intervention to remove the blood and to cauterize the bleeding vessels. Outcome is directly related to the patient's status preoperatively. For patients not in coma, mortality is very low; for those in light coma, mortality is 9%; and for patients in deep coma, mortality is 20%.[6]

Subdural hematoma. Subdural hematoma (SDH), which is the accumulation of blood between the dura and underlying arachnoid membrane, most often is related to a rupture in the bridging veins between the brain and the dura.[2] Acceleration/deceleration and rotational forces are the major causes of SDH, which often is associated with cerebral contusions and intracerebral hemorrhage.

The three types of SDH are based on the time frame from injury to clinical symptoms: acute, subacute, and chronic. Table 24-2 summarizes the time interval and pre-

---

TABLE 24-2

CLASSIFICATION OF SUBDURAL HEMATOMAS

TYPE	TIME INTERVAL	SYMPTOMS
Acute	Within 48 hr	Headache, drowsiness, agitation, confusion, deterioration in LOC, fixed and ipsilateral pupil dilation, contralateral hemiparesis **or** Profound coma
Subacute	2 days to 2 wk	Similar to acute SDH except that symptoms appear more slowly
Chronic	2 wk to months	Progressive lethargy, absent-mindedness, headache, vomiting, seizures, ipsilateral pupil dilation, or contralateral hemiparesis

LOC, Loss of consciousness.

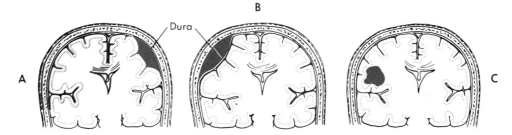

Fig. **24-2** Types of cerebral hematomas. **A,** Subdural hematoma. **B,** Epidural hematoma. **C,** Intracerebral hematoma.

sentation for each type of SDH.[7] Surgical intervention may include craniectomy, craniotomy, or burr hole evacuation. SDH results in a mortality of 22%, which rises to 50% with injuries to other body systems.[8]

Intracerebral hematoma. Intracerebral hematoma (ICH) results when there is bleeding within cerebral tissue. Traumatic causes of ICH include depressed skull fractures, penetrating injuries (bullet, knife), or sudden acceleration/deceleration motion. The ICH acts as a rapidly expanding lesion, and the mortality is high;[9] however, late ICH into the necrotic center of a contused area also is possible. Sudden clinical deterioration of a patient 6 to 10 days after trauma may be the result of ICH.

Medical management of ICH may include surgical or nonsurgical management. Generally it is believed that hemorrhages that do not cause significant ICP problems should be treated nonsurgically. Over time, the hemorrhage may be reabsorbed. If significant problems with ICP occur as a result of the ICH producing a mass effect, surgical removal is necessary. Outcome from ICH depends greatly on the location of the hemorrhage. Size, mass effect, and displacement of other intracranial structures also affect the outcome. ICH results in a mortality between 25% and 72%.[8]

Missile injuries

Missile injuries are caused by objects that penetrate the skull to produce a significant focal damage but little acceleration/deceleration or rotational injury. The injury may be depressed, penetrating, or perforating (Fig. 24-3). Depressed injuries are caused by fractures of the skull, with penetration of bone into cerebral tissue. Penetrating injury is caused by a missile that enters the cranial cavity but does not exit. A low-velocity penetrating injury (knife) may involve only focal damage and no loss of consciousness. A high-velocity missile (bullet) can produce shock waves that are transmitted throughout the brain, in addition to injury caused by the bullet. Perforating injuries are missile injuries that enter and then exit the brain. Perforating injuries have much less ricochet effect but are still responsible for significant injury.

Diffuse axonal injury

Diffuse axonal injury (DAI) covers a wide range of brain dysfunction caused by acceleration/deceleration and rotational forces. This diagnosis usually is reserved for severe dysfunction. Cerebral concussion is the least severe form of diffuse axonal injury. DAI describes prolonged coma from the time of injury that is not the result of mass lesions or ischemia.

The pathophysiology of DAI is related to the stretching and tearing of axons as a result of movement of the brain inside the cranium at the time of impact. The stretching and tearing of axons result in microscopic lesions throughout the brain, but especially deep within cerebral tissue and the base of the cerebrum. Disruption of axonal transmission of impulses results in loss of consciousness. Unless surrounding tissue areas are significantly injured, causing small hemorrhages, DAI is not visible on CT scan. The patient remains in a deep coma, often with decerebrate or decorticate posturing and autonomic dysfunction, including hyperthermia, hypertension, and diaphoresis.

Treatment of DAI includes support of vital functions and maintenance of ICP within normal limits. The outcome after severe DAI is poor because of the extensive dysfunction of cerebral pathways. DAI occurs in 44% of all coma-producing head injuries, with an overall mortality of 33%, but in its most severe form, mortality can be 50%.[2]

Assessment

Neurologic assessment is the most important tool for evaluating the patient with a severe head injury because

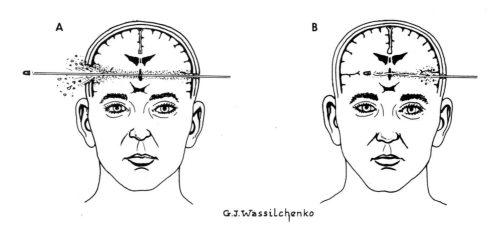

G.J.Wassilchenko

Fig. **24-3** Bullet wounds of the head. Bullet wound or other penetrating missile wounds cause an open (compound) skull fracture and damage to brain tissue. Shock wave effects are transmitted throughout the brain. **A,** Perforating injury. **B,** Penetrating injury.

it can indicate severity of injury, provide prognostic information, and can dictate the speed with which further evaluation and treatment must proceed.[10] The cornerstone of the neurologic assessment is the Glasgow Coma Scale (GCS). To assist with the initial assessment, head injuries are divided into three descriptive categories on the basis of the patient's GCS score and length of the unconscious state.

Degree of injury

Mild injury. Mild head injury is described as a GCS score of 13 to 15, with a loss of consciousness that lasts up to 15 minutes. Patients with mild injury often are seen in the emergency department and discharged home with a family member who is instructed to evaluate the patient routinely and to bring the patient back to the hospital if any further neurologic symptoms should appear.

Moderate injury. Moderate head injury is described as a GCS score of 9 to 12, with a loss of consciousness for up to 6 hours. Patients with this type of head injury usually are hospitalized. They are at high risk for deterioration from increasing cerebral edema and ICP, and, therefore, serial clinical assessments are an important function of the nurse. Hemodynamic and ICP monitoring and ventilatory support often are not required in this group unless other systemic injuries make them necessary. A CT scan usually is performed on admission. Repeat CT scans are indicated if the patient's neurologic status deteriorates.

Severe injury. Patients with a GCS score of 8 or less after resuscitation or those who deteriorate to that level within 48 hours of admission have a severe head injury.[11] Patients with severe head injury often receive ventilatory support along with ICP and hemodynamic monitoring. A CT scan is performed to rule out any mass lesions that can be surgically removed. Patients are placed in a critical care setting for continual assessment, monitoring, and management. Level of consciousness, motor movements, papillary response, respiratory function, and vital signs are all part of a complete neurologic assessment in the patient with severe head injury. Neurologic assessments are ongoing throughout the patient's critical care stay in order to detect any subtle changes in the patient's condition.

Diagnostic procedures

The cornerstone of diagnostic procedures for evaluation of head injuries is the CT scan.[10] The CT scan is a rapid, noninvasive procedure that can provide invaluable information about the presence of mass lesions and cerebral edema. Electrophysiology studies can aid in ongoing assessments of neurologic function. Evoked potentials and electroencephalograph (EEG) are becoming widely used in the diagnosis of head injuries. Magnetic resonance imaging (MRI) appears to be useful in detecting hematomas and cerebral edema.

Medical Management

Surgical management

If a lesion, identified by CT scan, is causing a shift of intracranial contents or increasing ICP, surgical intervention is necessary. A craniotomy is performed to remove the EDH, SDH, or large ICH. Occasionally, if an area of contusion is large, hemorrhagic, and associated with an elevated ICP, a craniotomy for removal of the contused area may be performed to relieve pressure and prevent herniation.

Nonsurgical management

Nonsurgical management includes management of ICP, maintenance of adequate cerebral circulation and oxygenation, and treatment of any complications, such as pneumonia or infection. Medical management can include drainage of CSF through a ventricular catheter, use of diuretics, and/or administration of high-dose barbiturate therapy.

Nursing Management

Priority nursing goals include stabilization of vital signs, prevention of further injury, and reduction of increased ICP. Ongoing nursing assessments are the cornerstone to the care of patients with head injuries. Such assessments are the primary mechanism for determining secondary brain injury from cerebral edema and increased ICP. In addition to astute neurologic assessments, it is critical to monitor ventilatory support, fluid and electrolyte balance, and nutrition.

SPINAL CORD INJURIES

Approximately 10,000 persons annually in the United States sustain permanent spinal cord injury,[12] and among these 60% to 80% are young adult men between 16 and 18 years old.[13] Of those who survive, about half have quadriplegia and half, paraplegia.[14]

Motor vehicle accidents are the most common cause of spinal cord injury, with half of those injuries occurring in persons between the ages 15 and 25 years.[15]

Mechanism of Injury

The type of injury sustained depends on the mechanism of injury. Mechanisms of injury can include hyperflexion, hyperextension, rotation, axial loading (vertical compression), and missile or penetrating injuries.

Hyperflexion

Hyperflexion injury most often is seen in the cervical area, especially at the level of C5 to C6 because this is the most mobile portion of the cervical spine. This type of injury most frequently is caused by sudden deceleration motion, as in head-on collisions. Injury occurs from compression of the cord as a result of fracture fragments or dislocation of the vertebral bodies. Instability of the spinal column occurs because of the rupture or tearing of the posterior muscles and ligaments.

Hyperextension

Hyperextension injuries involve backward and downward motion of the head. With this injury, often seen in rear-end collisions or diving accidents, the spinal cord itself is stretched and distorted. Neurologic deficits associated with this injury often are caused by contusion and ischemia of the cord without significant bony involvement. A mild form of hyperextension is the *whiplash* injury.

Rotation

Rotation injuries often occur in conjunction with a flexion or extension injury. Severe rotation of the neck or body results in tearing of the posterior ligaments and displacement (rotation) of the spinal column.

Axial loading

Axial loading, or vertical compression, injuries occur from vertical force along the spinal cord. This most commonly is seen in a fall from a height in which the person lands on the feet or buttocks. Compression injuries cause burst fractures of the vertebral body that often send bony fragments into the spinal canal or directly into the spinal cord.

Penetrating injuries

Penetrating injury to the spinal cord can be caused by a bullet, knife, or any other object that penetrates the cord. These types of injury cause permanent damage by anatomically transecting the spinal cord.

Pathophysiology

Spinal cord injuries are the result of a mechanical force that disrupts neurologic tissue or its vascular supply, or both. Much like the pathophysiology of head injuries, a primary injury causes a chain of secondary events in response to the injury. Spinal cord damage appears to be the result of these secondary events, which include hemorrhage, vascular damage, structural changes, and subsequent biochemical alterations.

Several events after a spinal cord injury lead to spinal cord ischemia and loss of neurologic function. A cascade of events is initiated by a sudden flux of calcium from extracellular spaces to intracellular spaces.

Functional injury of the spinal cord

Functional injury of the spinal cord refers to the degree of disruption of normal spinal cord function. SCIs are first classified as complete or incomplete and then are further divided into functional injuries.

Complete injury. Complete SCI results in a total loss of sensory and motor function below the level of injury. Regardless of the mechanism of injury, the result is a complete dissection of the spinal cord and its neuro-

chemical pathways, resulting in one of two conditions: quadriplegia or paraplegia.

Quadriplegia. Injuries in the cervical spine region result in quadriplegia. Residual muscle function depends on the specific cervical segments involved. Cervical injuries that occur above C6 result in complete quadriplegia, whereas injuries below C6 produce incomplete quadriplegia with some potential for independence in activities of daily living.[12]

Paraplegia. A complete injury in the thoracolumbar region results in paraplegia. Thoracic L1 and L2 injuries produce paraplegia with variable innervation to intercostal and abdominal muscles.

Incomplete injury. Incomplete SCI results in a mixed loss of voluntary motor activity and sensation below the level of the lesion. Incomplete SCI exists if any function remains below the level of injury. Incomplete injuries can result in one of a variety of syndromes, which are classified according to the degree of motor and sensory loss below the level of injury.

Spinal shock. Spinal shock is a condition that can occur shortly after traumatic injury to the spinal cord. Spinal shock is the complete loss of all normal reflex activity below the level of injury.[2] Manifestations of spinal shock include bradycardia and hypotension. The intensity of spinal shock is influenced by the level of injury, and the duration of this shock state can persist for up to 1 month after injury. Blood pressure support may be required with the use of sympathomimetic drugs.

Autonomic dysreflexia. Autonomic dysreflexia, or autonomic hyperreflexia, is a life-threatening complication that occurs frequently (83% of quadriplegics) in SCI.[16] This condition is caused by a massive sympathetic response to a noxious stimuli (full bladder, line insertions, fecal impaction), which results in bradycardia, hypertension, facial flushing, and headache. A severe vasoconstriction can occur, causing systolic blood pressure to be greater than 200 mm Hg and diastolic blood pressure to reach 130 mm Hg; therefore, prompt recognition is critical to the patient's survival.[16] Treatment is aimed at alleviating the noxious stimuli. If symptoms persist, pharmacologic vasodilating drugs (nitroglycerin, nifedipine, hydralazine) can be administered to reduce blood pressure.

Assessment

Assessment of the patient with a known or suspected SCI must include stabilization of the spinal cord. All trauma patients must be protected from further spinal cord damage until presence of spinal cord injury is ruled out.

Assessment of breathing patterns and gas exchange is made after an airway has been secured. The level of injury dictates the degree of altered breathing patterns and gas exchange. Because complete injuries above the C3 level result in paralysis of the diaphragm,[17] patients with these injuries require ventilatory assistance.

The patient with SCI is assessed for adequate tissue perfusion by means of both invasive and noninvasive hemodynamic monitoring techniques. Cardiac monitoring is required to detect bradycardia and other dysrhythmias that occur in response to reflex vagal activity mediated by the dominant parasympathetic nervous system as well as changes in cardiac rhythm as a result of hypothermia or hypoxia.

The initial neurologic assessment may not be an accurate indication of eventual motor and sensory loss because of spinal shock.[12] It focuses on the rapid and accurate identification of present, absent, or impaired functioning of the motor, sensory, and reflex systems that coordinate and regulate vital functions. A detailed motor and sensory examination includes the assessment of all 32 spinal nerves for evidence of dysfunction. Initial findings must be performed correctly and thoroughly documented in detail so that subsequent serial assessments can rapidly identify deterioration.

Diagnostic procedures

Diagnostic radiographic evaluations can identify the severity of damage to the spinal cord. Initial evaluation includes anteroposterior and lateral views for all areas of the spinal cord. Films of all seven cervical vertebrae and the top of T1 must be obtained to rule out cervicothoracic junction injury.[18] Flexion and extension views can identify subtle ligamentous injuries. CT scan, tomograms, myelography, and MRI also may be used in the diagnostic process.

Medical Management

After assessment and diagnosis of the SCI, medical management begins. The primary treatment goal is to preserve remaining neurologic function. Medical interventions are divided into pharmacologic, surgical, and nonsurgical interventions.

Pharmacologic management

After years of intensive research, high-dose methylprednisolone has been shown to improve neurologic outcome at 6 weeks and 6 months after spinal cord injury if administered within 8 hours of injury.[19] Dosing guidelines are summarized in Box 24-3.[12] Methylprednisolone directly affects the changes that occur within the spinal cord after injury, primarily by preventing posttraumatic spinal cord ischemia, improving energy metabolism, restoring extracellular calcium, and improving nerve impulse conduction.[15]

Surgical management

Surgical intervention provides spinal column stability in the presence of an unstable injury. Unstable injuries include disrupted ligaments and tendons, as well as a vertebral column that cannot maintain normal alignment. Identification and immobilization of unstable injuries are particularly important for the patient with incomplete neurologic deficit. Without adequate stabilization, movement and dislocation of the vertebral column could cause

---

BOX 24-3

ADMINISTRATION OF IV METHYLPREDNISOLONE FOR SPINAL CORD INJURY

Based on drug concentration of 62.5 mg/ml:
1. Administer bolus dose 30 mg/kg IV over 15 minutes.
2. Pause for 45 minutes (administer IV fluid to keep vein open).
3. Begin maintenance dose at 5.4 mg/kg/hr IV for 23 hours.
4. Terminate drug administration 24 hours after bolus dose.

---

a complete neurologic deficit. A variety of surgical procedures may be performed to achieve decompression and stabilization.

Laminectomy. This procedure is the removal of the lamina of the vertebral ring to allow decompression and removal of bony fragments or disk material from the spinal canal.

Spinal fusion. This procedure entails the surgical fusion of two to six vertebral elements to provide stability and to prevent motion. Fusion is accomplished through the use of bone parts or bone chips taken from the iliac crest or by use of wire or acrylic glue.

Rodding. This procedure stabilizes and realigns larger segments of the spinal column by means of a variety of rodding procedures, such as Harrington rods. The rods are attached by screws and glue to the posterior elements of the spinal column. These types of procedures most often are performed to stabilize the thoracolumbar area.

Nonsurgical management

If the injury to the spinal cord is stable, nonsurgical management is the treatment of choice. Nonsurgical management for cervical and thoracolumbar injuries is discussed separately.

Cervical injury. Management of cervical injuries involves the immobilization of the fracture site and realignment of any dislocation. This is accomplished through skeletal traction that involves the use of two-point tongs, which are inserted into the skull through shallow burr holes and are connected to traction weights. Several types of cervical tongs are used. Gardner-Wells and Crutchfield tongs are the most common. These tongs can be applied at the bedside with the use of a local anesthetic.

After the procedure, the patient can be immobilized on a kinetic therapy bed or a regular bed. The kinetic therapy bed is the most popular method used for cervical immobilization because it maintains spinal column alignment while providing constant turning motion to reduce pulmonary and skin breakdown. Use of cervical skeletal traction on a regular bed makes it difficult to provide adequate care to the pulmonary system and skin because of the extensive degree of immobility.

After adequate realignment of the spinal column has occurred through skeletal traction, a halo traction brace often is applied. The halo vest consists of a metal ring secured to the skull with two occipital and two temporal screws. Steel bars anchor the screws to the vest to provide cervical immobilization. The halo traction brace immobilizes the cervical spine, which allows the patient to ambulate and participate in self-care.

Thoracolumbar injury. Nonsurgical management of the patient with a thoracolumbar injury also involves immobilization. Skeletal traction may be used in high thoracic injury. For the most part, misalignment of the spinal canal does not occur in stable injuries of the thoracolumbar spine. Immobilization to allow fractures to heal is accomplished by bedrest (with bed flat) and the use of a plastic or fiberglass jacket, a body cast, or a brace.

Nursing Management

The goal during the critical care phase is to prevent life-threatening complications while maximizing the functioning of all organ systems. **Nursing interventions are aimed at preventing secondary damage to the spinal cord and managing the cardiovascular and respiratory complications of the neurologic deficit.**[20] Because almost all body systems are affected by SCI, nursing management must also include interventions that optimize nutrition, elimination, skin integrity, and mobility. Prevention of complications that can delay the patient's rehabilitation is one of the goals of critical care.[20] In addition, patients with SCI have complex psychosocial needs that require a great deal of emotional support from the critical care nurse.

THORACIC INJURIES

Thoracic injuries involve trauma to the chest wall, lungs, heart, great vessels, and esophagus. Thoracic trauma accounts for 20% to 25% of all traumatic deaths.[21] Most deaths caused by pulmonary trauma occur after the patient reaches the hospital. Thoracic trauma most commonly is the result of a violent crime or MVA.

Mechanism of Injury

Blunt thoracic trauma

Blunt trauma to the chest most frequently is caused by MVAs or falls. The underlying mechanism of injury tends to be a combination of acceleration/deceleration injury and direct transfer mechanics, such as a crush injury. Varying mechanisms of blunt trauma are associated with specific injury patterns. After head-on collisions, drivers have a higher frequency of injury than do back-seat passengers because the driver comes in contact with the steering assembly. Severe thoracic injuries frequently are seen in patients who are unrestrained. Falls from greater than 20 feet are associated with thoracic injury.

Penetrating thoracic injuries

The penetrating object determines the damage sustained from penetrating thoracic trauma. Low-velocity weapons (.22-caliber gun, knife) usually damage only what is in the weapon's direct path. Of particular concern, however, are stab wounds that involve the anterior chest wall between the midclavicular lines, Louis's angle, and the epigastric region inasmuch as these wounds are likely to have entered the mediastinum, heart, and/or the great vessels.[22] High-velocity weapons (rifle, shotgun, or .38 caliber gun) produce more serious injuries. These weapons are associated with massive energy transfer and tissue destruction. Pellets from a shotgun blast cause further damage by expanding and causing multiple injuries.

Specific Thoracic Traumatic Injuries

Chest wall injuries

Rib fractures. Interruption of a single rib is the most minor and the most common chest wall injury associated with blunt thoracic trauma.[23] Fractures of certain ribs or multiple ribs can be more serious. Fractures of certain ribs are associated with more underlying life-threatening injuries. Fractures of the first and second ribs are associated with intrathoracic vascular injuries (brachial plexus, great vessels). Fractures of the seventh through tenth ribs are associated with liver or spleen injuries. The pain of rib fractures can be aggravated by movement associated with respiratory excursion. As a result, the patient often splints, takes shallow breaths, and refuses to cough, which can result in atelectasis and pneumonia.

Flail chest. Flail chest, caused by blunt trauma, disrupts the continuity of chest wall structures. A flail chest occurs when three or more ribs are fractured in two or more places and are no longer attached to the thoracic cage. This results in a free-floating segment of the chest wall. This segment moves independently from the rest of the thorax and results in paradoxical chest wall movement during the respiratory cycle (Fig. 24-4). During inspiration the intact portion of the chest wall expands while the injured part is sucked in. During expiration the chest wall moves in and the flail segment moves out. The physiologic effects of impaired chest wall motion of a flail chest include decreased tidal volume and vital capacity and impaired cough, which lead to hypoventilation and atelectasis.

Ruptured diaphragm. Diaphragmatic rupture is a frequently missed diagnosis in trauma patients because of the subtle and nospecific symptoms this injury produces. The mechanism of injury appears to be a rapid rise in intraabdominal pressure as a result of compression force applied to the lower part of the chest or upper region of the abdomen. This injury can occur when a person is thrown forward over the tip of the steering wheel in a high-speed deceleration accident. The force can cause the diaphragm, which offers little resistance, to rupture or tear. Abdominal viscera then can gradually enter the thoracic cavity, moving from the positive pressure of the abdomen to the negative pressure in the thorax. The

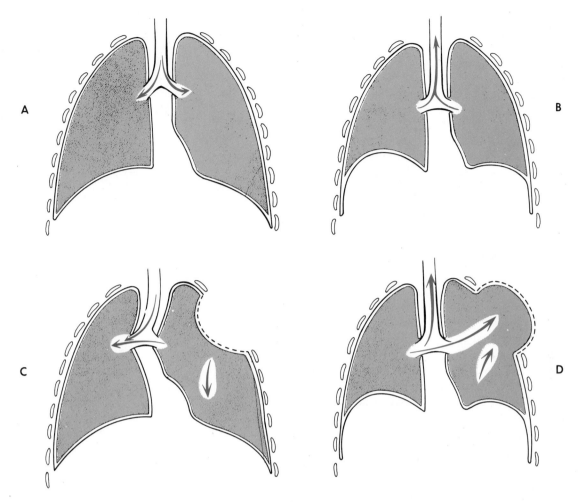

Fig. **24-4** Flail chest. **A,** Normal inspiration. **B,** Normal expiration. **C,** Inspiration: area of lung underlying unstable chest wall sucks in on inspiration. **D,** Same area balloons out on expiration. Note movement of mediastinum toward opposite lung on inspiration. (From Long BC, Phipps WJ, Cassmeyer VL: *Medical-surgical nursing: a nursing process approach,* ed 3, St Louis, 1993, Mosby.)

stomach and colon are the most commonly herniated viscera.[24] Diaphragmatic rupture can be life-threatening. Massive herniation of abdominal contents into the thoracic cavity can compress the lungs and mediastinum, which then hampers venous return and leads to decreased cardiac output. In addition, herniated bowel can become strangulated and perforate.

Pulmonary injuries

Pulmonary contusion. A pulmonary contusion is fundamentally a bruise of the lung. Pulmonary contusion is frequently associated with blunt trauma and other chest injuries such as rib fractures and flail chest. Pulmonary contusions can occur unilaterally or bilaterally. A contusion occurs initially as a hemorrhage followed by alveolar and interstitial edema. The edema can remain rather localized in the contused area or can spread to other lung areas. Inflammation affects alveolar-capillary units. As more units are affected by inflammation, further pathophysiologic events can occur, including decreased compliance, increased pulmonary vascular resistance,

and decreased pulmonary blood flow. These processes result in a ventilation/perfusion imbalance, which results in hypoxemia and poor ventilation that progresses over a 24- to 48-hour period.

Clinical manifestations of pulmonary contusion may take up to 24 to 48 hours to develop. Inspections of the chest wall may reveal ecchymosis at the site of impact. Moist rales may be noted in the contused lung. A cough may be present with blood-tinged sputum. Abnormal lung function can be detected by systemic arterial hypoxemia. The diagnosis is made primarily by chest x-ray consistent with pulmonary infiltrate corresponding to the area of external chest impact that is manifested within 12 to 24 hours of injury.[25] Pulmonary contusions tend to worsen over a 24- to 48-hour period and then slowly resolve unless complications occur (infection, ARDS).[25]

Tension pneumothorax. A tension pneumothorax usually is caused by an injury that perforates the chest wall or pleural space. Air flows into the pleural space with inspiration and becomes trapped. As pressure in the pleural space increases, the lung on the injured side col-

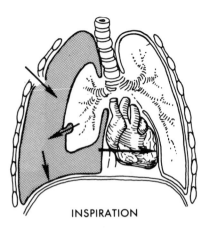
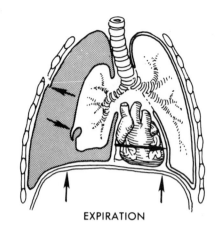

INSPIRATION   EXPIRATION

Fig. **24-5** A tension pneumothorax usually is caused by an injury that perforates the chest wall or pleural space. Air flows into the pleural space with inspiration and becomes trapped. As pressure in the pleural space increases, the lung on the injured side collapses and causes the mediastinum to shift to the opposite side. (From Rosen P, et al: *Emergency medicine: concepts and clinical practice,* ed 3, St Louis, 1992, Mosby.)

lapses and causes the mediastinum to shift to the opposite side (Fig. 24-5). As pressure continues to build, the shift exerts pressure on the heart and thoracic aorta, which results in decreased venous return and decreased cardiac output. Tissue perfusion with oxygenated blood is further hampered because the collapsed lung cannot participate in ventilation.

Clinical manifestations of a pneumothorax include dyspnea or sudden chest pain extending to the shoulders. Tracheal deviation will be noted as the trachea shifts away from the injured side. On the injured side, breath sounds can be decreased or absent. Neck vein distention, cyanosis, and respiratory distress also may be present. Percussion of the chest reveals a hyperresonant sound caused by the trapped air. Diagnosis of tension pneumothorax is made by clinical assessment. There is no time for a chest film inasmuch as this potentially lethal condition must be treated immediately. A large-bore (14-gauge) needle or chest tube is inserted into the affected lung. This procedure allows immediate release of air from the pleural space. A hissing sound is heard as the tension pneumothorax is converted to a simple pneumothorax.

Open pneumothorax. An open pneumothorax, or "sucking chest wound," usually is caused by penetrating trauma. Open communication between the atmosphere and intrathoracic pressure results in immediate lung deflation. Air moves in and out of the hole in the chest, producing a sucking sound heard on inspiration.

Hemothorax. Blunt or penetrating thoracic trauma can cause bleeding into the pleural space to produce a hemothorax (Fig. 24-6). A massive hemothorax can cause a blood loss of more than 1500 ml.[2] The source of bleeding may be the intercostal or internal mammary arteries, lungs, heart, or great vessels. Increasing intrapleural pressure results in a decrease in vital capacity. Increasing vascular blood loss into the pleural space causes decreased venous return and decreased cardiac output.

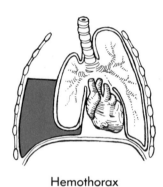

Hemothorax

Fig. **24-6** Blunt or penetrating thoracic trauma can cause bleeding into the pleural space to form a hemothorax.

Assessment findings for patients with a hemothorax include hypovolemic shock and decreased breath sounds in the injured lung. With hemothorax, the neck veins are collapsed and the trachea is at midline. Massive hemothorax can be diagnosed on the basis of clinical manifestations of hypotension associated with the absence of breath sounds and/or dullness to percussion on one side of the chest.[2]

Cardiac injuries

Penetrating cardiac injuries. Penetrating cardiac trauma can occur from mechanical injuries as a result of bullets, knives, or impalements. The chest wall offers little protection to the heart from penetrating trauma. The most common site of injury is the right ventricle because of its anterior position. Mortality from penetrating trauma to the heart is high. Prehospital mortality for penetrating cardiac injuries is 75%, and most deaths occur within 4 or 5 minutes after injury as a result of exsanguination or tamponade.[26]

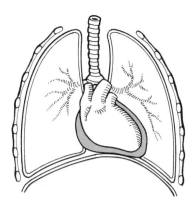

Fig. **24-7** Cardiac tamponade is the progressive accumulation of blood in the pericardial sac.

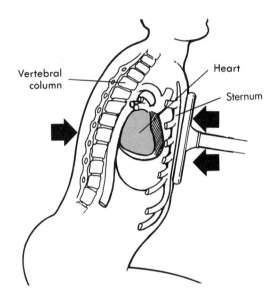

Fig. **24-8** Blunt cardiac trauma. Sudden acceleration (as from contact with the steering wheel) can cause the heart to be thrown against the sternum.

Cardiac tamponade. Cardiac tamponade is the progressive accumulation of blood in the pericardial sac (Fig. 24-7). With cardiac tamponade, a progressive accumulation of blood, 120 to 150 ml, increases the intracardiac pressure and compresses the atria and ventricles. Increased intracardiac pressures lead to decreased venous return and decreased filling pressure, which lead to decreased cardiac output, myocardial hypoxia, cardiac failure, and cardiogenic shock.

Classic assessment findings associated with cardiac tamponade are termed *Beck's triad*—presence of elevated central venous pressure with neck vein distension, muffled heart sounds, and pulsus paradoxus. An ECG may reveal tachycardia with altered QRS complexes.

Blunt cardiac injuries. The most common causes of blunt cardiac trauma include high-speed MVAs, direct blows to the chest, and falls. The heart, because of its mobility and its location between the sternum and thoracic

vertebrae, is susceptible to blunt traumatic injury. Sudden acceleration (as from contact with the steering wheel) can cause the heart to be thrown against the sternum (Fig. 24-8). Sudden deceleration can cause the heart to be thrown against the thoracic vertebrae by a direct blow to the chest (baseball, animal kick, fall). Myocardial contusion is one of the most common injuries sustained as a result of blunt cardiac trauma.

Myocardial contusion. Myocardial cell injury results from the contusion. Histologically, contusions exhibit well-demarcated zones of hemorrhage, which are well-confined to the site of injury, as opposed to a more widespread pattern, as seen with infarction.[27] If the contusion is large enough and has resulted in a large area of myonecrosis, the patient may experience the same complications as those of an acute myocardial infarction. The right ventricle most often is affected because of its proximity to the sternum.

ABDOMINAL INJURIES

Abdominal injury accounts for 10% of trauma fatalities in the United States.[28] Abdominal injuries frequently are associated with multisystem trauma. Injuries to the abdomen are the result of blunt or penetrating trauma. Two major life-threatening conditions that occur after abdominal trauma are hemorrhage and hollow viscus perforation with its associated peritonitis.

Mechanism of Injury

Blunt trauma

Blunt abdominal injuries are common. They result most frequently from MVAs, falls, and assaults. The spleen is the most commonly injured organ in blunt trauma and ranks second to the liver as the source of life-threatening abdominal injury.[29] In MVAs, abdominal injury is more likely to occur when a vehicle is struck from the side. In the passenger position of the front seat, hepatic injury is likely when the point of impact is on the same side as the passenger. A driver is likely to sustain injury to the spleen when the impact is on the driver's side. Seat belts, which substantially reduce morbidity and mortality, also are associated with causing bladder and bowel rupture.[28] Pedestrians hit by motor vehicles are at risk for serious abdominal injuries. Blunt trauma to the thorax can produce injuries to the liver, spleen, and diaphragm. In spinal cord injury, large abdominal arteries and veins can be injured. Deceleration and direct forces can produce retroperitoneal hematomas. Blunt abdominal injuries often are hidden and are more likely to be fatal than are penetrating abdominal injuries.

Penetrating trauma

Penetrating abdominal trauma generally is caused by knives or bullets. The danger of penetrating abdominal trauma is that the outside appearance of the wound does not determine the extent of internal injury. The most commonly injured organs from knife wounds are the liver, spleen, diaphragm, and colon.[30] Gunshot wounds to the abdomen usually are more serious than are stab wounds. A bullet destroys tissue along its path. Once inside the abdomen, a bullet can travel in erratic paths and ricochet off bone. Death from penetrating injuries depends on injury to major vascular structures and resultant intraabdominal hemorrhage.

Assessment

Physical assessment

The location of entry and exit sites associated with penetrating trauma are assessed and documented. Inspection of the patient's abdomen may reveal purplish discoloration of the flanks or umbilicus (Cullen's sign), which is indicative of blood in the abdominal wall. Ecchymosis in the flank area (Turner's sign) may indicate retroperitoneal bleeding or a possible fracture of the pancreas. A hematoma in the flank area is suggestive of renal injury. A distended abdomen may indicate the accumulation of blood, fluid, or gas secondary to a perforated organ or ruptured blood vessel. Serial measurement of abdominal girth can be helpful. The increase of abdominal girth by 1 inch can indicate intraabdominal accumulation of 500 to 1000 ml of blood.[31] Auscultation of the abdomen may reveal friction rubs over the liver or spleen and may indicate rupture. The abdomen is assessed for rebound tenderness and rigidity. Presence of these assessment findings indicates peritoneal inflammation. Referred pain to the left shoulder (Kehr's sign) may indicate a ruptured spleen or irritation of the diaphragm from bile or other material in the peritoneum. Subcutaneous emphysema palpated on the abdomen suggests free air as a result of a ruptured bowel.

Diagnostic procedures

Diagnostic peritoneal lavage (DPL) can exclude or confirm the presence of intraabdominal injury with a high accuracy rate. DPL is indicated for trauma patients with equivocal abdominal findings on physical assessment or for patients who are not alert and oriented enough to provide accurate information or cannot respond appropriately to physical assessments.[32] After the patient's bladder has been emptied, a small incision is made in the abdomen through the skin and into the peritoneum. A small catheter is inserted. If frank blood is encountered, intraabdominal injury is obvious and the patient is taken immediately to the (OR). If gross blood is not initially encountered, a liter of fluid (lactated Ringer's or 0.9% normal saline) is infused through the catheter into the abdomen. The IV bag is then placed in a dependent position and allowed to drain. The drainage fluid is sent to the laboratory for analysis. Positive DPL results signal intraabdominal trauma and usually necessitate surgical intervention.

Abdominal CT scanning can detect retroperitoneal hemorrhage, can localize specific site(s) of abdominal in-

jury, and can determine the relative severity of intraperitoneal or retroperitoneal hemorrhage.[32]

Specific Organ Injuries

Physical assessment findings, DPL, and CT scanning aid in making a diagnosis of specific abdominal organ injury. The medical and nursing management vary according to specific organ injuries. Liver, spleen, bowel, and pancreatic injuries, which are seen more commonly, are discussed here.

Liver injuries

The liver is the primary organ injured in penetrating trauma and the second most commonly injured organ in blunt trauma. Detection of liver injury, as with all intraabdominal injury, is accomplished through the use of physical assessment and DPL or CT scan. Recent evidence supports the view that patients who have sustained blunt liver injuries who are hemodynamically stable and do not require ongoing blood transfusions for their liver injury may be amenable to nonoperative treatment.[33] Patients with penetrating or blunt liver trauma who are hemodynamically unstable usually require surgical intervention to correct the defect. Resection of the devitalized tissue is required for massive injuries.

Spleen injuries

The spleen is the organ most commonly injured by blunt abdominal trauma and is second to the liver as a source of life-threatening hemorrhage. The treatment of an injured spleen is controversial because of the spleen's importance in preventing infection. Hemodynamically stable patients may be monitored in the critical care unit by means of serial hematocrit values and vital signs. Progressive deterioration may indicate the need for operative management. Patients who exhibit hemodynamic instability require operative intervention with splenectomy, partial splenectomy, or splenorraphy.

Intestinal injuries

Intestinal injuries can result from blunt or penetrating trauma. Regardless of mechanism of injury, intestinal contents (bile, stool, enzymes, bacteria) leak into the peritoneum and cause peritonitis. Surgical resection and repair are required. The patient's postoperative course is dictated by the amount of spillage of intestinal contents. The patient is observed for signs of sepsis and abscess or fistula formation.

GENITOURINARY INJURIES

Trauma to the genitourinary (GU) tract seldom occurs as an isolated injury. An associated GU injury must be suspected in any patient with penetrating trauma to the torso; pelvic fracture; blunt trauma to the lower chest or flank; contusions, hematoma, or tenderness over the flank, lower abdomen, or perineum; genital swelling or discoloration; blood at the urethral meatus; hematuria after Foley catheter placement; or difficulty with micturation.[34]

Mechanism of Injury

GU injuries, like all other traumatic injuries, can result from blunt or penetrating trauma. Blunt GU trauma can be caused by deceleration injuries, and penetrating injuries can occur with stabbings or gunshot wounds to the abdomen or back.

Specific Genitourinary Injuries

Renal trauma

Most renal trauma is caused by blunt trauma, resulting in contusions or lacerations without urinary extravasation. Renal injuries are graded to determine the amount of trauma sustained, the care needed, and possible outcomes. CT scan is the most accurate modality available for staging renal injuries because it can assess the extent of parenchymal laceration, urine extravasation, surrounding hemorrhage, and the presence of vascular injury.[34] Contusions and minor lacerations can usually be treated with observation whereas major lacerations and vascular injuries require operative intervention.[34] Postoperative complications can include infection, hemorrhage, infarction, extravasation, calcification, acute tubular necrosis, and hypertension.

Ureteral trauma

Injury to the ureters is the least common result of trauma to the GU tract because the ureters are protected anteriorly by the abdominal contents and musculature and posteriorly by the psoas muscle. The patient with ureteral trauma may complain of flank pain, and hematuria may be a presenting symptom. As in renal trauma, the degree of hematuria is not indicative of the severity of injury. A "missed" ureteral injury can result in intraperitoneal extravasation and produce peritoneal signs. Ureteral injuries are surgically repaired.

Bladder trauma

Most bladder injuries are the result of blunt trauma. Bladder injuries are classified as contusions, extraperitoneal ruptures, intraperitoneal ruptures, or combined injuries. The type of injury that occurs depends not only on the location and strength of the blunt force but also on the volume of urine in the bladder at the time of injury.[35] Urinary extravasation is the hallmark sign of a ruptured bladder. Definitive diagnosis of bladder rupture is made by means of cystographic examination.

PELVIC INJURIES

Because the pelvis protects the lower urinary tract and major blood vessels and nerves of the lower extremities, pelvic trauma can result in life-threatening urologic and neurologic dysfunction and hemorrhage.[36]

Mechanism of Injury

Blunt trauma to the pelvis can be caused by MVAs, falls, or a crushing accident. Most pelvic injuries involve fractures, with or without damage to underlying tissues. Pelvic injuries frequently are associated with motorcycle accidents and accidents that involve pedestrians and vehicles. Any patient who has been ejected from a vehicle must be suspected of having a pelvic fracture.

Assessment

Signs of pelvic fracture include perineal ecchymosis (testicular or labial) indicating extravasation of urine or blood, pain on palpation or "rocking" of the iliac crests, lower limb paresis or hypesthesia, hematuria, and shortening of a lower extremity.

An anteroposterior x-ray film of the pelvis permits classification of a fracture as stable or unstable. Stable fractures usually are breaks in the pelvic ring, sacrum, or coccyx, with no displacement. Unstable fractures are breaks that occur in more than one place or in the acetabulum.

Classification of Pelvic Fractures

Minor fractures

Minor pelvic fractures include breaks of individual bones without a break in continuity of the pelvic ring or a single break in the pelvic ring.

Major fractures

Major pelvic fractures involve double breaks in the pelvic ring. These fractures commonly are seen in patients who are in the critical care unit with multiple trauma. The condition of patients with posterior pelvic fractures is very unstable. The nearby iliac arteries frequently are damaged and can cause massive internal bleeding.

Straddle fracture

The four-ramus, or "straddle," fracture consists of bilateral fractures of the superior and inferior pubic rami. With this fracture comes a high incidence of associated injuries, especially lower urinary tract injuries.

Malgaigne's hemipelvis fracture dislocation

This fracture includes a variety of fracture patterns that have three separate injury components. These fractures always are unstable and the result of severe trauma.

Open fractures

Open pelvic fractures involve an open wound with direct communication between the pelvic fractures and the buttocks, perineum, groin, pubis, or lower flank. The open wound allows contamination. Mortality rates from open pelvic fractures may exceed 50%.[2]

COMPLICATIONS OF TRAUMA

Ongoing nursing assessments are imperative for early detection of complications frequently associated with traumatic injuries (Box 24-4).

Infection remains a major source of mortality and morbidity in critical care units. Of those trauma patients who survive longer than 3 days, infection is a frequent cause of death.[37] The trauma patient is at risk for infection because of contaminated wounds, invasive therapeutic and diagnostic catheters, intubation and mechanical ventilation, host susceptibility, and the critical care environment. The source of sepsis in the trauma patient can be invasive therapeutic and diagnostic catheters or wound contamination with exogenous or endogenous bacteria.

Trauma to the pulmonary system is likely to result in complications because of respiratory failure. This is particularly true if the patient was involved in a high-speed MVA, suffered major blunt trauma, experienced a mean arterial pressure of less than 60 mm Hg for a period of time, had 20% or more of blood volume replaced, or experienced a decrease in level of consciousness. Respiratory insufficiency is one of the most common complications after multiple trauma.

Pulmonary embolism (PE) occurs in 4% to 22% of all trauma patients. All trauma patients face the greatest risk for developing a PE in the first 2 weeks after injury. Those who are at high risk for developing a PE include patients with spinal cord injury, pelvic fracture, and lower extremity fracture with delayed orthopedic fixation.

Fat embolism syndrome (FES) can occur as a complication of orthopedic trauma. The syndrome is characterized by pulmonary system dysfunction. FES appears to develop as a result of fat droplets that leak from fractured bone and embolize to the lungs. The droplets are broken down into free fatty acids that are toxic to the pulmonary microvascular membranes. Damage to these membranes results in edema, inactivation of surfactant, and atelecta-sis. Fat droplets further activate a coagulation cascade that results in thrombocytopenia. The lung becomes highly edematous and hemorrhagic. The clinical presentation is almost indistinguishable from ARDS.

Life-threatening gastrointestinal (GI) bleeding as a result of stress ulcers is infrequent but associated with high mortality. The patient with multiple traumatic injuries is particularly at risk for developing this complication. The pathophysiology of stress ulceration is thought to be caused by a variety of factors, including mucosal barrier breakdown, decreased mucosal blood flow, increased intraluminal acid, decreased epithelial regeneration, and lowered intramural pH. Prevention of stress ulcer development is accomplished through the use of histamine$_2$ antagonists, antacids, and sucralfate.

Assessment and ongoing monitoring of renal function are critical to the survival of the trauma patient. The etiology of posttraumatic renal failure is complex and may involve a variety of factors.

Patients with a crush injury are susceptible to the development of myoglobinuria, with subsequent secondary renal failure. Crush injuries can result in arterial trauma. Loss of arterial blood flow, particularly to the extremities, results in the loss of oxygen transport to distal tissues and ischemia. This initiates a cascade of events that leads to necrosis of skeletal muscle cells. As cells die, intracellular contents—particularly potassium and myoglobin—are released. As myoglobin circulates in the cardiovascular system, it causes acute renal tubular blockade and subsequent renal failure. Myoglobinuria frequently develops within 6 hours after injury.

Compartment syndrome is a condition in which increased pressure within a limited space compromises circulation, resulting in ischemia and necrosis of tissues within that space. Among those at high risk for the development of compartment syndrome are patients with lower extremity trauma, including fractures, penetrating trauma, vascular ruptures, massive tissue injuries, or venous obstruction.

Clinical manifestations of compartment syndrome include obvious swelling and tightness of an extremity, paresis, and pain in the affected extremity. Diminished pulses and decreased capillary refill do not reliably identify compartment syndrome because they may be intact until after irreversible changes have occurred. Elevated intracompartmental pressures confirm the diagnosis.

Despite improvements in care, venous thromboembolism remains a significant source of morbidity and mortality in the trauma patient.[38] Trauma patients are at risk for developing venous thrombosis because of endothelial injury, coagulopathy, immobility, and bedrest. Trauma patients are at the greatest risk for developing thromboembolism early in their hospitalization.

Nursing assessment of the multiple injury patient in the critical care unit may reveal missed diseases or missed injuries. Missed "diseases" may include preexisting undiagnosed medical illnesses, such as endocrine disorders (diabetes, hypothyroidism), myocardial infarction,

---

BOX 24-4

COMPLICATIONS OF TRAUMA

Infection
Sepsis
Pulmonary complications
• Respiratory failure
• Fat embolism syndrome (FES)
Gastrointestinal complications
• Hemorrhage
• Acalculous cholecystitis
Renal complications
• Renal failure
• Myoglobinuria
Vascular complications
• Compartment syndrome
• Venous thromboembolism
Missed injury
Multiple organ dysfunction syndrome (MODS)

hypertension, respiratory insufficiency, renal insufficiency, or malnutrition.

Occasionally injuries may not be diagnosed in the precritical care phases. Injuries can be subtle or masked, preventing an accurate diagnosis. In the critical care unit, a missed injury may be suspected if the patient fails to show appropriate response to medical or surgical intervention.

Multiple organ dysfunction syndrome (MODS) is a clinical syndrome of progressive dysfunction of organ systems. Trauma patients are at high risk for systemic inflammatory response syndrome (SIRS) and MODS because of circulatory shock occurring with tissue hypoxemia, tissue injury, and infection.[39] Organ dysfunction can be the result of *primary MODS,* which is caused by direct traumatic injury such as that which occurs with acute lung dysfunction because of pulmonary contusion. Organ dysfunction that occurs latently in the trauma patient's course is the result of *secondary MODS,* or uncontrolled systemic inflammation with resultant organ dysfunction (see Chapter 25).

Although any number of diagnosis-related groups (DRGs) may apply to the trauma patient, depending on the underlying cause and comorbidities, the following lengths of stay may be anticipated: DRG 444 (Traumatic injury), 4.8 days; DRG 487 (Multiple significant trauma), 8.3 days; DRG 83 (Major chest trauma), 5.9 days; and DRG 2 (Craniotomy for trauma), 10.6 days.[40]

Nursing Management of Trauma Patients

Trauma patients present unique challenges to critical care nurses. Often, multiple organs or body systems are affected, which necessitates continuous monitoring and assessment of various potential problems. Priorities for nursing management of trauma patients are listed in Box 24-5.

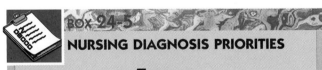

BOX 24-5

NURSING DIAGNOSIS PRIORITIES

Trauma

Decreased Adaptive Capacity: Intracranial related to failure of normal intracranial compensatory mechanisms, p. 480

Decreased Cardiac Output related to vasodilation and bradycardia secondary to sympathetic blockage of neurogenic (spinal) shock after spinal cord injury above T6 level, p. 470

Ineffective Breathing Pattern related to decreased lung expansion secondary to thoracic trauma (ruptured diaphragm, pneumothorax, hemothorax, rib fractures, pulmonary contusion, flail chest, penetrating and blunt cardiac injuries), p. 473

Risk for Infection (risk factors: invasive monitoring devices), p. 494

Ineffective Individual Coping related to situational crisis and personal vulnerability, p. 453

References

1. Robertson L: Motor vehicles, *Pediatr Clin North Am* 32:87, 1985.
2. American College of Surgeons: *Advanced trauma life support,* ed 5, Chicago, 1993, American College of Surgeons.
3. Boggs RL: Multiple system trauma: nursing implications, *J Adv Med Surg Nurs* 2(1):1, 1989.
4. Meyer AA, Trunkey DD: Critical care as an integral part of trauma care, *Crit Care Nurs Clin North Am* 2(4):673, 1986.
5. Gennarelli TA: Triage of head injured patients. In Trunkey DD, Lewis FR, editors: *Current therapy of trauma,* ed 3, Philadelphia, 1991, BC Decker.
6. Keenan K: The role of nursing assessment of traumatic events in sudden injury, illness and death, *Crit Care Nurs Clin North Am* 7:483, 1995.
7. Ammons AM: Cerebral injuries and intracranial hemorrhages as a result of trauma, *Nurs Clin North Am* 25(1):23, 1990.
8. Stand PE: Diagnostic and therapeutic concerns in head injured patients, *J Am Acad Phys Assist* 1(2):112, 1988.
9. Childs SA: Musculoskeletal trauma: implications for critical care nursing practice, *Crit Care Nurs North Am* 6:483, 1994.
10. Valadka AB: *Evaluating and monitoring head injury: jugular bulb and non-invasive CNS monitoring. Proceedings from Trauma and Critical Care 1996,* American College of Surgery Western States Committee on Trauma, 1996.
11. Walleck-Jastremski CA: Traumatic brain injury: assessment and treatment, *Crit Care Nurse Clin North Am* 6:472, 1994.
12. Hughes MC: Critical care nursing for the patient with a spinal cord injury, *Crit Care Nurs Clin North Am* 2(1):33, 1990.
13. Walker M: Acute spinal cord injury, *N Engl J Med* 324:1885, 1991.
14. Hickey JV: *The clinical practice of neurological and neurosurgical nursing,* ed 3, Philadelphia, 1992, JB Lippincott.
15. Nayduch D, Lee A, Butler D: High dose methylprednisolone after acute spinal cord injury, *Crit Care Nurs* 14(4):69, 1994.
16. Nolan S: Current trends in the management of acute spinal cord injury, *Crit Care Nurse Q* 17(1):64, 1994.
17. Kocan MJ: Pulmonary considerations in the critical care phase, *Crit Care Nurs Clin North Am* 2(3):369, 1990.
18. Richmond TS: Spinal cord injury, *Nurs Clin North Am* 25(1):57, 1990.
19. Bracken MB, et al: A randomized controlled trial of methylprednisolone or naloxone in the treatment of acute spinal cord injury, *N Engl J Med* 322:1405, 1990.
20. Walleck CA: Neurologic considerations in the critical care phase, *Crit Care Nurs Clin North Am* 2(3):357, 1990.
21. Johnson SB, Kearney PK, Smith MD: Echocardiography in the evaluation of thoracic trauma, *Surg Clin North Am* 75:193, 1995.
22. Ross SE, Cernaianu AC: Epidemiology of thoracic injuries: mechanisms of injury and pathophysiology, *Top Emerg Med* 12(1):1, 1990.
23. Hammond SG: Chest injuries in the trauma patient, *Nurs Clin North Am* 25(1):35, 1990.
24. Andrew L: Difficult diagnoses in blunt thoraco-abdominal trauma, *J Emerg Nurs* 15(5):399, 1989.
25. Moore FA, Haenel JB, Moore EE: Blunt pulmonary injury. In Maull, et al, editors: *Advances in trauma and critical care,* vol 8, St Louis, 1993, Mosby.
26. Feliciano DV, Mattox KL: The heart. In Trunkey DD, Lewis FR, editors: *Current therapy of trauma,* ed 3, Philadelphia, 1991, BC Decker.
27. Christensen MA, Sutton KR: Myocardial contusion: new concepts in diagnosis and management, *Am J Crit Care* 2:28, 1993.
28. Merrill CR, Sparger G: Current thoughts on blunt abdominal trauma, *Top Emerg Med* 12(2):21, 1990.

29. Carrico CJ: The spleen. In Trunkey DD, Lewis FR, editors: *Current therapy of trauma*, ed 3, Philadelphia, 1991, BC Decker.
30. Wagner MM: The patient with abdominal injuries, *Nurs Clin North Am* 25(1):45, 1990.
31. Shoemaker W, Ayers S, Grenvick A: *Textbook of critical care*, ed 2, Philadelphia, 1988, WB Saunders.
32. Wachtel T: Critical care concepts in the management of abdominal trauma, *Crit Care Nurse Q* 17(2):34, 1994.
33. Pacher HL, et al: The status of nonoperative management of blunt hepatic injuries in 1995: a multicenter experience with 404 patients, *J Trauma* 40(1):31-38, 1996.
34. Cyer HG: *Emergency center evaluation of urologic trauma. Proceedings from Trauma and Critical Care 1996.* American College of Surgery Western States Committee on Trauma, 1996.
35. Frevele G: Urinary tract injuries due to blunt abdominal trauma, *Phys Assist* 13(2):123, 1989.
36. Ruhl JM: Pelvic trauma, *RN* July:50, 1991.
37. Martin MT: Wound management and infection control after trauma: implications for the intensive care setting, *Crit Care Nurs Q* 11(2):43, 1988.
38. Rogers FB: Venous thromboembolism in trauma patients, *Surg Clin North Am* 75:279, 1995.
39. Fitzsimmons L: Consequences of trauma: systemic inflammation and multiple organ dysfunction, *Crit Care Nurse Q* 17(2):74, 1994.
40. *St. Anthony's DRG Guidebook 1998*, Reston VA, 1997, St. Anthony Hospital.

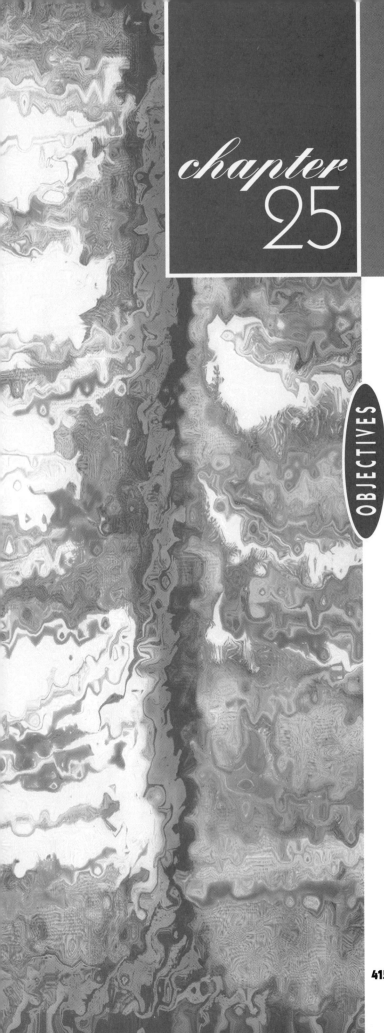

chapter 25

Shock and Multiple Organ Dysfunction Syndrome

Kathleen M. Stacy
and Lorraine Fitzsimmons

OBJECTIVES

- Describe generalized shock response and systemic inflammatory response.

- List the etiologies of hypovolemic, cardiogenic, anaphylactic, neurogenic, and septic shock and multiple organ dysfunction syndrome.

- Explain the pathophysiology of hypovolemic, cardiogenic, anaphylactic, neurogenic, and septic shock and multiple organ dysfunction syndrome.

- Identify the clinical manifestations of hypovolemic, cardiogenic, anaphylactic, neurogenic, and septic shock and multiple organ dysfunction syndrome.

- Outline the important aspects of the medical management of hypovolemic, cardiogenic, anaphylactic, neurogenic, and septic shock and multiple organ dysfunction syndrome.

- Summarize the nursing priorities for managing a patient with hypovolemic, cardiogenic, anaphylactic, neurogenic, and septic shock and multiple organ dysfunction syndrome.

Shock is an acute, widespread process of impaired tissue perfusion that results in cellular, metabolic, and hemodynamic derangements. Impaired tissue perfusion occurs when an imbalance develops between cellular oxygen supply and cellular oxygen demand. This imbalance can occur for a variety of reasons and eventually results in cellular dysfunction, multiple organ dysfunction syndrome (MODS), and death. This chapter presents an overview of the general shock response, or shock syndrome, followed by a discussion of the different shock states and MODS.

SHOCK SYNDROME

Description and Etiology

Shock is a complex pathophysiologic process that often results in multiple organ dysfunction syndrome (MODS) and death. All types of shock eventually result in impaired tissue perfusion and the development of acute circulatory failure or shock syndrome. Shock syndrome is a generalized systemic response to inadequate tissue perfusion.[1] It consists of four different stages: initial, compensatory, progressive, and refractory. Progression through each stage varies with the patient's prior condition, duration of initiating event, response to therapy, and correction of underlying cause.[2]

Shock can be classified as hypovolemic, cardiogenic, or distributive, depending on the pathophysiologic cause. Hypovolemic shock results from a loss of circulating or intravascular volume. Cardiogenic shock results from the impaired ability of the heart to pump. Distributive shock results from maldistribution of circulating blood volume and can be further classified as septic, anaphylactic, and neurogenic. Septic shock is the result of microorganisms entering the body. Anaphylactic shock is the result of a severe antibody-antigen reaction. Neurogenic shock is the result of the loss of sympathetic tone.[3,4]

Pathophysiology

During the initial stage, cardiac output (CO) is decreased and tissue perfusion is impaired. As the blood supply to the cells decreases, the cells switch from aerobic to anaerobic metabolism as a source of energy. Anaerobic metabolism produces small amounts of energy but large amounts of lactic acid. Lactic acidemia quickly develops and causes more cellular damage.[2,5]

During the compensatory stage, an attempt is made by the body's homeostatic mechanisms to improve tissue perfusion. The compensatory mechanisms are mediated by the sympathetic nervous system (SNS) and consist of neural, hormonal, and chemical responses. Neural compensation includes an increase in heart rate (HR) and contractility, arterial and venous vasoconstriction, and shunting of blood to the vital organs. Hormonal compensation includes activation of the renin response and stimulation of the anterior pituitary and adrenal medulla. Activation of the renin response results in the production of angiotensin II, which causes vasoconstriction and the release of aldosterone and antidiuretic hormone (ADH), leading to sodium and water retention. Stimulation of the anterior pituitary results in the secretion of adrenocorticotropic hormone (ACTH), which in turn stimulates the adrenal cortex to produce glucocorticoids, causing a rise

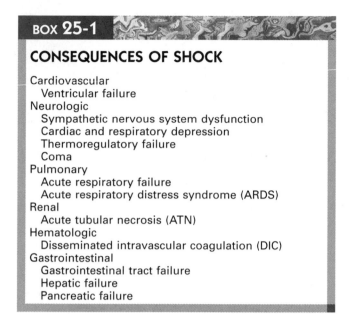

BOX 25-1

CONSEQUENCES OF SHOCK

Cardiovascular
   Ventricular failure
Neurologic
   Sympathetic nervous system dysfunction
   Cardiac and respiratory depression
   Thermoregulatory failure
   Coma
Pulmonary
   Acute respiratory failure
   Acute respiratory distress syndrome (ARDS)
Renal
   Acute tubular necrosis (ATN)
Hematologic
   Disseminated intravascular coagulation (DIC)
Gastrointestinal
   Gastrointestinal tract failure
   Hepatic failure
   Pancreatic failure

in blood glucose levels. Stimulation of the adrenal medulla causes the release of epinephrine and norepinephrine, which further enhance the compensatory mechanisms. Chemical compensation includes hyperventilation to neutralize lactic acidosis.[2,5]

During the progressive stage, the compensatory mechanisms start to fail and the shock cycle is perpetuated. At the cellular level, the small amount of energy created by anaerobic metabolism is not enough to keep the cell functional, and irreversible damage begins to occur. The sodium-potassium pump in the cell membrane fails, causing the cell and its organelles to swell. Cellular energy production comes to a complete halt as the mitochondria swell and rupture. At this point the problem becomes one of oxygen utilization instead of oxygen delivery. Even if the cell were to receive more oxygen, it would be unable to use it because of damage to the mitochondria. The cell's digestive organelles swell, resulting in leakage of destructive enzymes into the cell. Autodigestion occurs with ensuing cell death.[5] Every system in the body is affected by this process[6] (Box 25-1).

During the refractory stage, shock becomes unresponsive to therapy and is considered irreversible. As the individual organ systems die, MODS, defined as failure of two or more body systems, occurs. Death is the final outcome.[2] Regardless of etiologic factors, death occurs from impaired tissue perfusion because of the failure of the circulation to meet the oxygen needs of the cell.[7]

Assessment and Diagnosis

The patient with a systolic blood pressure (SBP) less than 90 mm Hg accompanied by either tachycardia or bradycardia and altered mental status is considered to be in a shock state.[8] Clinical manifestations will differ, however, according to the underlying cause and the stage of the shock and are related to both the cause and the patient's response to shock.[9] (See individual shock sections for a discussion of clinical assessment and diagnosis of the patient in shock.)

Medical Management

Treatment of the patient in shock requires an aggressive approach. The major focus of the treatment of shock is the improvement and preservation of tissue perfusion. Adequate tissue perfusion depends on an adequate supply of oxygen being transported to the tissues and the cell's ability to use it. Oxygen transport is influenced by pulmonary gas exchange, CO, and hemoglobin level. Oxygen utilization is influenced by the internal metabolic environment. Management of the patient in shock focuses on supporting oxygen transport and oxygen utilization.[1,7]

Adequate pulmonary gas exchange is critical to oxygen transport. Establishing and maintaining an adequate airway are the first steps in ensuring adequate oxygenation. Once the airway is patent, emphasis is placed on improving ventilation and oxygenation. Therapies include administration of supplemental oxygen and mechanical ventilatory support.[5,8,10]

An adequate CO and hemoglobin level are crucial to oxygen transport. CO depends on HR, preload, afterload, and contractility. A variety of fluids and drugs are used to manipulate these parameters. The types of fluids used include both crystalloids and colloids. The categories of drugs used include vasoconstrictors, vasodilators, positive inotropes, and antidysrhythmic agents.[5,8]

Indicated for decreased preload related to intravascular volume depletion, fluid administration can be accomplished by use of either a crystalloid or colloid solution or both. Crystalloids are balanced electrolyte solutions that may be hypotonic, isotonic, or hypertonic. Examples of crystalloid solutions are normal saline, lactated Ringer's, and 5% dextrose in water. Colloids are protein- or starch-containing solutions. Examples of colloid solutions are blood and blood components and pharmaceutic plasma expanders, such as hetastarch, dextran, and mannitol. The choice of fluid depends on the situation. Advantages of colloids include faster restoration of intravascular volume and use of smaller amounts. Colloids stay in the intravascular space as opposed to crystalloids, which readily leak into the extravascular space. Disadvantages include expense, allergic reactions, and difficulties in typing and cross-matching blood. Colloids also can leak out of damaged capillaries and cause a variety of additional problems, particularly in the lungs.[5,10-13] Blood should be used to augment oxygen transport if the patient's hemoglobin level is low.[1]

Vasoconstrictor agents are used to increase afterload by increasing systemic vascular resistance (SVR) and improving the patient's blood pressure level. Vasodilator agents are used to decrease preload or afterload, or both, by decreasing venous return and SVR. Positive inotropic agents are used to increase contractility. Antidysrhythmic

agents are used to influence HR. Box 25-2 provides examples of each of these agents.[5,10,14]

An optimal metabolic environment is very important to oxygen utilization. Once the oxygen is delivered to the cells, they have to be able to use it. The major metabolic derangement seen in shock is lactic acidosis. Interventions to correct lactic acidosis include correcting the cause, reestablishing perfusion, inducing hyperventilation, and, in severe cases, administering sodium bicarbonate.[15] The role of sodium bicarbonate in the treatment of acidosis is controversial because of the associated risks of using it. It is usually reserved for severe cases that are refractory to other treatments. The risks include rebound increase in lactic acid production, development of a hyperosmolar state, production of fluid overload resulting from excessive sodium, shifting of the oxyhemoglobin dissociation curve to the left, and rapid cellular electrolyte shifts.[16]

The patient also should be started on a nutritional support therapy. The type of nutritional supplementation initiated varies according to the cause of shock and should be tailored to the individual patient's need, as indicated by the underlying condition and laboratory data. The enteral route generally is preferred over the parenteral.[17]

BOX 25-2

EXAMPLES OF THE DIFFERENT AGENTS USED IN THE TREATMENT OF SHOCK

VASOCONSTRICTOR AGENTS
Epinephrine (Adrenalin)
Norepinephrine (Levophed)
Alpha-range dopamine (Intropin)
Metaraminol (Aramine)
Phenylephrine (Neo-Synephrine)
Ephedrine

VASODILATOR AGENTS
Nitroprusside (Nipride, Nitropress)
Nitroglycerin (Nitrol, Tridil)
Hydralazine (Apresoline)
Labetalol (Normodyne, Trandate)

INOTROPIC AGENTS
Beta-range dopamine (Intropin)
Dobutamine (Dobutrex)
Amrinone (Inocor)
Epinephrine (Adrenalin)
Isoproterenol (Isuprel)
Norepinephrine (Levophed)
Digoxin (Lanoxin)

ANTIDYSRHYTHMIC AGENTS
Lidocaine (Xylocaine)
Bretylium (Bretylol)
Procainamide (Promestyl)
Labetalol (Normodyne, Trandate)
Verapamil (Calan, Isoptin)
Esmolol (Brevibloc)
Diltiazem (Cardizem)

Nursing Management

The nursing management of a patient in shock is a complex and challenging responsibility. It requires an in-depth understanding of the pathophysiology of the disease and the anticipated effects of each intervention as well as a solid understanding of the nursing process.[18] (Individual shock sections contain separate discussions of specific interventions for the patient in shock.)

The psychosocial needs of the patient and family dealing with shock are extremely important. These needs, which differ with each patient and family, are based on situational, familial, and patient-centered variables. **Nursing priorities are directed toward providing information on patient status, explaining procedures and routines, supporting the family, encouraging the expression of feelings, facilitating problem-solving and decision-making, involving the family in the patient's care, and establishing contacts with necessary resources.**[19]

HYPOVOLEMIC SHOCK

Description and Etiology

Hypovolemic shock occurs from inadequate fluid volume in the intravascular space. The lack of adequate circulating volume leads to decreased tissue perfusion and initiation of the general shock response. Hypovolemic shock is the most commonly occurring form of shock.[2,13]

BOX 25-3

ETIOLOGIC FACTORS IN HYPOVOLEMIC SHOCK

ABSOLUTE

Loss of whole blood
  Trauma
  Surgery
  Gastrointestinal bleeding
Loss of plasma
  Thermal injuries
  Large lesions
Loss of other bodily fluids
  Severe vomiting
  Severe diarrhea
  Massive diuresis

RELATIVE

Loss of intravascular integrity
  Ruptured spleen
  Long bone or pelvic fractures
  Hemorrhagic pancreatitis
  Hemothorax or hemoperitoneum
  Arterial dissection
Increased capillary membrane permeability
  Sepsis
  Anaphylaxis
  Thermal injuries
Decreased colloidal osmotic pressure
  Severe sodium depletion
  Hypopituitarism
  Cirrhosis
  Intestinal obstruction

Hypovolemic shock can result from either absolute or relative hypovolemia. Absolute hypovolemia occurs when there is an external loss of fluid from the body, including whole blood, plasma, or any other body fluid. Relative hypovolemia occurs when there is an internal shifting of fluid from the intravascular space to the extravascular space. This can result from a loss in intravascular integrity, increased capillary membrane permeability, or decreased colloidal osmotic pressure[2,13] (Box 25-3).

Pathophysiology

Hypovolemia results in a loss of circulating fluid volume. A decrease in circulating volume leads to a decrease in venous return, which in turn results in a decrease in end-diastolic volume or preload. Preload is a major determinant of stroke volume (SV) and CO. A decrease in preload results in a decrease in SV and CO. The decrease in CO leads to inadequate cellular oxygen supply and impaired tissue perfusion[2,13] (Fig. 25-1).

Assessment and Diagnosis

The clinical manifestations of hypovolemic shock vary, depending on the severity of fluid loss and the patient's ability to compensate for it. The first, or initial, stage occurs with a fluid volume loss up to 15% or an actual volume loss up to 750 ml. Compensatory mechanisms maintain CO, and the patient appears symptom-free.[4,11,13]

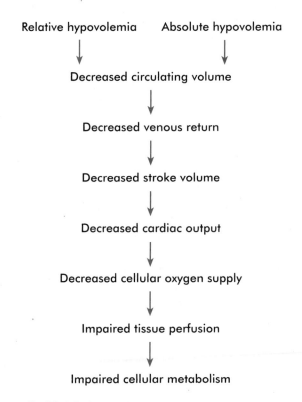

Fig. **25-1** Pathophysiology of hypovolemic shock.

The second, or compensatory, stage occurs with a fluid volume loss of 15% to 30% or an actual volume loss of 750 to 1500 ml.[11] CO falls, resulting in the initiation of a variety of compensatory responses. HR increases in response to increased SNS stimulation. The pulse pressure (PP) narrows as the diastolic blood pressure increases because of vasoconstriction. Respiratory rate (RR) and depth increase in an attempt to improve oxygenation. Arterial blood gas (ABG) specimens drawn during this phase reveal respiratory alkalosis and hypoxemia, as evidenced by a low $PaCO_2$ and a low PaO_2, respectively. Urine output (UO) starts to decline as renal perfusion decreases. Urine sodium decreases while urine osmolarity and specific gravity increase as the kidneys start to conserve sodium and water. The patient's skin becomes pale and cool, with delayed capillary refill because of peripheral vasoconstriction. Jugular veins appear flat as a result of decreased venous return. Decreased cerebral perfusion causes a change in level of consciousness (LOC). The patient may appear disoriented, confused, restless, anxious, or irritable.[9,11,13]

The third, or progressive, stage occurs with a fluid volume loss of 30% to 40% or an actual volume loss of 1500 to 2000 ml.[11] The compensatory mechanisms become overwhelmed, and impaired tissue perfusion develops. HR continues to increase, and dysrhythmias develop as myocardial ischemia ensues. Respiratory distress occurs as the pulmonary system deteriorates. ABG values during this phase reveal respiratory and metabolic acidosis and hypoxemia, as evidenced by a high $PaCO_2$, low bicarbonate (HCO_3^-), and low PaO_2, respectively. Decreased renal perfusion results in the development of oliguria. Blood urea nitrogen (BUN) and serum creatinine levels start to rise as the kidneys begin to fail. The patient's skin becomes ashen, cold, and clammy, with marked delayed capillary refill. The patient appears lethargic as cerebral perfusion decreases and LOC continues to deteriorate.[9,11,13]

The fourth, or refractory, stage occurs with a fluid volume loss of greater than 40% or an actual volume loss of more than 2000 ml.[11] The compensatory mechanisms completely deteriorate, and organ failure occurs. Severe tachycardia and hypotension ensue. Peripheral pulses are absent, and because of marked peripheral vasoconstriction, capillary refill does not occur. The skin appears cyanotic, mottled, and extremely diaphoretic. The patient becomes unresponsive, and a variety of clinical manifestations associated with failure of the different body systems develop.[11,13]

Assessment of the hemodynamic parameters of a patient in hypovolemic shock reveals a decreased CO and cardiac index (CI). Loss of circulation volume leads to a decrease in venous return to the heart, which results in a decrease in the preload of the right and left ventricles. This is evidenced by a decline in the right atrial pressure (RAP) and pulmonary artery wedge pressure (PAWP). Vasoconstriction of the arterial system results in an increase in the afterload of the heart as evidenced by an increase in the systemic vascular resistance (SVR).[9,13]

Medical Management

The major goals of therapy are to correct the cause of the hypovolemia and to restore tissue perfusion. This approach includes identifying and stopping the source of fluid loss and vigorously administering fluid to replace circulating volume.[20] Fluid administration can be accomplished with use of either a crystalloid or a colloid solution, or a combination of both. The type of solution used usually depends on the type of fluid lost.[10-13]

Another therapy available for assisting with resuscitation of the patient in hypovolemic shock is autotransfusion. Autotransfusion is the collection and administration of the patient's own blood. It has been particularly useful in managing the patient with hypovolemic shock caused by chest trauma and hemorrhage.[21]

Nursing Management

Prevention of hypovolemic shock is one of the primary responsibilities of the nurse in the critical care area. Preventive measures include the identification of patients at risk and constant assessment of the patient's fluid balance. Accurate monitoring of intake and output and daily weights are essential components of preventive nursing care. Early identification and treatment result in decreased mortality.[22]

The patient in hypovolemic shock may have any number of nursing diagnoses, depending on the progression of the process (Box 25-4). **Nursing priorities are directed toward minimizing fluid loss, enhancing volume replacement, providing comfort and emotional support, and maintaining surveillance for complications.** Measures to minimize fluid loss include limiting blood sampling, observing lines for accidental disconnection, and applying direct pressure to bleeding sites. Measures to enhance volume replacement include insertion of large-diameter peripheral intravenous catheters, rapid administration of prescribed fluids, and positioning the patient with the legs elevated, trunk flat, and head and shoulders above the chest. In addition, monitoring the patient for clinical manifestations of fluid overload is critical to preventing further problems.

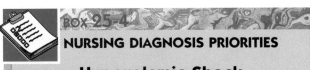

BOX 25-4

NURSING DIAGNOSIS PRIORITIES

Hypovolemic Shock

- Fluid Volume Deficit related to absolute loss, p. 486
- Fluid Volume Deficit related to relative loss, pp. 486-487
- Decreased Cardiac Output related to alterations in preload, pp. 467-468
- Anxiety related to threat to biologic, psychologic, and/or social integrity, pp. 448-450

CARDIOGENIC SHOCK

Description and Etiology

Cardiogenic shock is the result of failure of the heart to pump blood forward effectively. It can occur with dysfunction of either the right or the left ventricle or both. The lack of adequate pumping function leads to decreased tissue perfusion and initiation of the general shock response.[3,23] It occurs in approximately 7% to 10% of the patients with an acute myocardial infarction (MI), and the mortality rate is 65% to 90%.[23]

Cardiogenic shock can result from primary ventricular ischemia, structural problems, and dysrhythmias.[23] The most common cause is acute MI resulting in the loss of 40% or more of the functional myocardium. The damage to the myocardium may occur after one massive MI, or it may be cumulative as a result of several smaller MIs.[3,23,24] Structural problems of the cardiopulmonary system and dysrhythmias also may cause cardiogenic shock if they disrupt the forward motion of the blood through the heart (Box 25-5).[2,23,24]

Pathophysiology

Cardiogenic shock results from the impaired ability of the ventricle to pump blood forward, which leads to a decrease in SV and an increase in the blood left in the ventricle at the end of systole. The decrease in SV results in a decrease in CO, which leads to decreased cellular oxygen supply and impaired tissue perfusion. When the underlying problem involves the left ventricle, the increase in end-systolic volume results in the back-up of blood into the pulmonary system and the subsequent development of pulmonary edema. Pulmonary edema causes impaired gas exchange and decreased oxygenation of the arterial blood, which further impairs tissue perfusion (Fig. 25-2). Death may result from cardiopulmonary collapse.[3,23,24]

Assessment and Diagnosis

A variety of clinical manifestations occur in the patient in cardiogenic shock, depending on etiologic factors in pump failure, the patient's underlying medical status, and the severity of the shock state. Some clinical manifestations are caused by failure of the heart as a pump, whereas many relate to the overall shock response (Box 25-6).

Initially the clinical manifestations relate to the decline in CO. These signs and symptoms include SBP less than 90 mm Hg; decreased sensorium; cool, pale, moist skin; and UO less than 30 ml/hr. The patient also may complain of chest pain. Once the compensatory mechanisms are activated, tachycardia develops to compensate for the fall in CO. A weak, thready pulse develops, and heart sounds may reveal a diminished S_1 and S_2 as a result of the decrease in contractility. Respiratory rate increases to improve oxygenation. ABG values at this time indicate respiratory alkalosis as evidenced by a decrease in $Paco_2$. Urinalysis findings demonstrate a

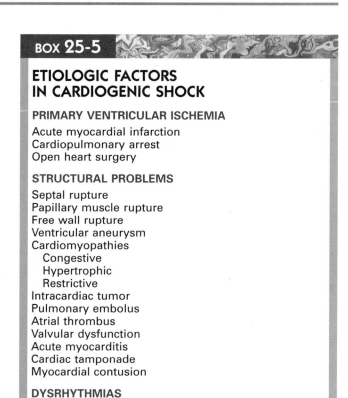

BOX 25-5

ETIOLOGIC FACTORS IN CARDIOGENIC SHOCK

PRIMARY VENTRICULAR ISCHEMIA

Acute myocardial infarction
Cardiopulmonary arrest
Open heart surgery

STRUCTURAL PROBLEMS

Septal rupture
Papillary muscle rupture
Free wall rupture
Ventricular aneurysm
Cardiomyopathies
    Congestive
    Hypertrophic
    Restrictive
Intracardiac tumor
Pulmonary embolus
Atrial thrombus
Valvular dysfunction
Acute myocarditis
Cardiac tamponade
Myocardial contusion

DYSRHYTHMIAS

Bradydysrhythmias
Tachydysrhythmias

decrease in urine sodium and an increase in urine osmolarity and specific gravity as the kidneys start to conserve sodium and water. The patient also may experience a variety of dysrhythmias, depending on the underlying problem.[9,23]

In the patient with left ventricular failure, a variety of additional clinical manifestations may be seen. Auscultation of the lungs may disclose crackles and rhonchi, indicating the development of pulmonary edema. Hypoxemia occurs as evidenced by a fall in Pao_2 as measured by ABG values. Heart sounds may reveal an S_3 and S_4. If right-sided failure occurs, jugular venous distention may become evident.[24]

Once the compensatory mechanisms become overwhelmed and impaired tissue perfusion develops, a variety of other clinical manifestations appear. Myocardial ischemia progresses as evidenced by continued increases in HR, dysrhythmias, and chest pain. The pulmonary system starts to deteriorate, which leads to respiratory distress. ABG values during this phase reveal respiratory and metabolic acidosis and hypoxemia as indicated by a high $Paco_2$, low HCO_3^-, and low Pao_2, respectively. Renal failure occurs as exhibited by the development of anuria and increases in BUN and serum creatinine levels. Cerebral hypoperfusion manifests as decreasing LOC.[23]

Assessment of the hemodynamic parameters of a patient in cardiogenic shock reveals a decreased CO and a CI less than 2.2 L/min/m[2].[24] Inadequate pumping action leads to a decrease in SV, which results in an increase in

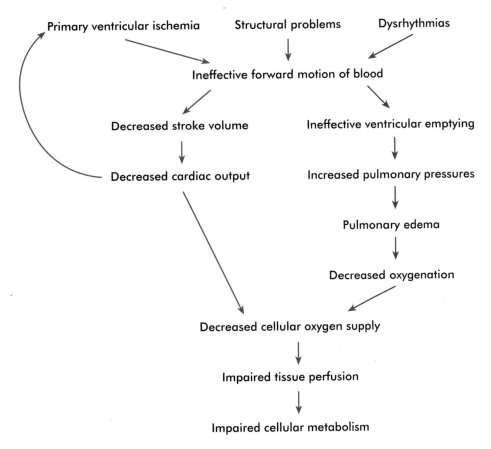

Fig. **25-2** Pathophysiology of cardiogenic shock.

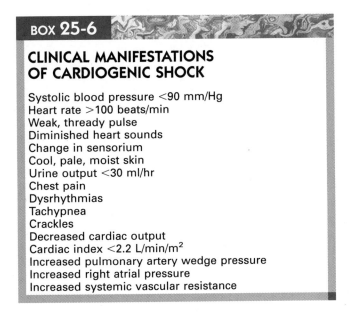

BOX 25-6

CLINICAL MANIFESTATIONS OF CARDIOGENIC SHOCK

Systolic blood pressure <90 mm/Hg
Heart rate >100 beats/min
Weak, thready pulse
Diminished heart sounds
Change in sensorium
Cool, pale, moist skin
Urine output <30 ml/hr
Chest pain
Dysrhythmias
Tachypnea
Crackles
Decreased cardiac output
Cardiac index <2.2 L/min/m²
Increased pulmonary artery wedge pressure
Increased right atrial pressure
Increased systemic vascular resistance

the left ventricular end-diastolic pressure (LVEDP). This is reflected in an increase in the PAWP. Compensatory vasoconstriction results in an increase in the afterload of the heart as evidenced by an increase in the SVR. If right ventricular failure is present, the RAP also will be increased.[9,24]

Medical Management

The major goals of therapy are to treat the underlying cause, enhance the effectiveness of the pump, and improve tissue perfusion. This approach includes identifying the etiologic factors of pump failure and administering pharmacologic agents to enhance CO. Inotropic agents are used to increase contractility, whereas vasodilating agents and diuretics are used for afterload and preload reduction, respectively. Antidysrhythmic agents should be used to suppress or control dysrhythmias that can affect CO.[10,25]

Once the cause of pump failure has been identified, measures should be taken to correct the problem if possible. If the problem is related to an acute MI, measures should be taken to increase myocardial oxygen supply and decrease myocardial oxygen demand. Therapies to increase myocardial oxygen supply include supplemental oxygen, intubation and mechanical ventilation, and coronary artery vasodilator agents, such as nitroglycerine. In addition, thrombolytic agents, coronary angioplasty, intracoronary stents, or coronary artery bypass surgery may also be used. Therapies to decrease myocardial demand include activity restrictions, analgesics, and sedatives.[10,24]

Two other therapies available to improve the effectiveness of the pumping action of the heart are the intraaortic balloon pump (IABP) and the ventricular assist device

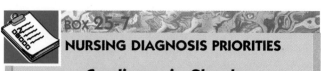

(VAD). The IABP is a temporary measure to decrease myocardial workload by improving myocardial supply and decreasing myocardial demand. It achieves this goal by improving coronary artery perfusion and reducing left ventricular afterload. The VAD is a temporary external pump that takes the place of the patient's ventricle, allowing it to heal.[24]

Nursing Management

Prevention of cardiogenic shock is one of the primary responsibilities of the nurse in the critical care area. Preventive measures include the identification of patients at risk and constant assessment of the patient's cardiopulmonary status.[22] Patients who require IABP therapy need to be observed frequently for complications. Complications include emboli formation, infection, rupture of the aorta, thrombocytopenia, improper balloon placement, bleeding, improper timing of the balloon, balloon rupture, and circulatory compromise of the cannulated extremity.[26]

The patient in cardiogenic shock may have any number of nursing diagnoses depending on the progression of the process (Box 25-7). **Nursing priorities are directed toward limiting myocardial oxygen consumption, enhancing myocardial oxygen supply, providing comfort and emotional support, and maintaining surveillance for complications.** Measures to limit myocardial oxygen consumption include administering analgesics and sedatives, positioning the patient for comfort, limiting activities, offering support to reduce anxiety, providing a calm and quiet environment, and teaching the patient about his or her condition. Measures to enhance oxygen myocardial supply include administering supplemental oxygen, monitoring the patient's respiratory status, and administering prescribed medications.

ANAPHYLACTIC SHOCK

Description and Etiology

Anaphylactic shock, a type of distributive shock, is the result of an immediate hypersensitivity reaction. It is a life-threatening event that requires prompt intervention.

The severe antibody-antigen response leads to decreased tissue perfusion and initiation of the general shock response.[2,27-29]

Anaphylactic shock is caused by an antibody-antigen response. Almost any substance can cause a hypersensitivity reaction. These substances, known as antigens, can be introduced by injection or ingestion or through the skin or respiratory tract. A number of antigens have been identified that can cause a reaction in a hypersensitive person. This list includes foods, food additives, diagnostic agents, biologic agents, drugs, venoms, and environmental agents, such as latex (Boxes 25-8 and 25-9).[3,28,29]

Pathophysiology

The antibody-antigen response (immunologic stimulation) or the direct triggering (nonimmunologic activation) of the mast cells results in the release of biochemical mediators. These mediators include histamine, eosinophilic chemotactic factor of anaphylaxis (ECF-A), neutrophilic chemotactic factor of anaphylaxis (NCF-A), proteinases, heparin, serotonin, leukotrienes (formerly known as slow-reacting substance of anaphylaxis), prostaglandins, and platelet-activating factor. The activation of the biochemical mediators causes vasodilation, increased capillary permeability, bronchoconstriction, excessive mucus secretion, coronary vasoconstriction, inflammation, cutaneous reactions, and constriction of the smooth muscle in the intestinal wall, bladder, and uterus. Coronary vasoconstriction causes severe myocardial depression. Cutaneous reactions cause stimulation of nerve endings followed by itching and pain.[29]

ECF-A promotes chemotaxis of eosinophils, thus facilitating the movement of eosinophils into the area. During allergic reactions, eosinophils phagocytose the antibody-antigen complex and other inflammatory debris and release enzymes that inhibit vasoactive mediators, such as histamine and leukotrienes. In addition, secondary mediators are produced that either enhance or inhibit the already released biochemical mediators. Bradykinin, a secondary mediator, increases capillary permeability, facilitates vasodilation, and contracts smooth muscles.[29]

Peripheral vasodilation results in decreased venous return. Increased capillary membrane permeability results in the loss of intravascular volume and the development of relative hypovolemia. Decreased venous return results in decreased end-diastolic volume and SV. The decline in SV leads to a fall in CO and impaired tissue perfusion. Death may result from airway obstruction or cardiovascular collapse, or both[3,27-29] (Fig. 25-3).

Assessment and Diagnosis

Anaphylactic shock is a severe systemic reaction that can affect any number of organ systems. A variety of clinical manifestations occur in the patient in anaphylactic shock, depending on the extent of multisystem involvement.

BOX 25-8

ETIOLOGIC FACTORS IN ANAPHYLACTIC SHOCK

Foods
  Eggs and milk
  Fish and shellfish
  Nuts and seeds
  Legumes and cereals
  Citrus fruits
  Chocolate
  Strawberries
  Tomatoes
  Other
Food additives
  Food coloring
  Preservatives
Diagnostic agents
  Iodinated contrast dye
  Sulfobromophthalein (Bromsulphalein) (BSP)
  Dehydrocholic acid (Decholin)
  Iopanoic acid (Telepaque)
Biologic agents
  Blood and blood components
  Insulin and other hormones
  Gamma globulin
  Seminal plasma

Enzymes
  Vaccines and antitoxins
Environmental agents
  Pollens, molds, and spores
  Sunlight
  Animal hair
Drugs
  Antibiotics
  Aspirin
  Narcotics
  Dextran
  Vitamins
  Local anesthetic agents
  Muscle relaxants
  Barbiturates
  Other
Venoms
  Bees and wasps
  Snakes
  Jellyfish
  Spiders
  Deer flies
  Fire ants

BOX 25-9

LATEX ALLERGIES

Latex is the milky sap of the rubber tree *Hevea brasilliensis*. It is treated with preservatives, accelerators, stabilizers, and antioxidants to make a more elastic, stable rubber. Reactions to products containing latex can be triggered by either the latex protein or by an additive used in the manufacturing process.

Latex reactions can be classified into three different categories—irritation (nonallergic inflammation occurring when the skin is abraded), delayed hypersensitivity (non-IgE-mediated response to the chemical agents added during the manufacturing process), or immediate sensitivity (IgE-mediated response to latex proteins). Although the overall prevalence of latex allergy in the general population is only 1%, it is much higher (28% to 67%) in selected groups, such as patients with neural tube defects (spina bifida, myelomeningocele, lipomyelomeningocele) or congenital urologic disorders, those who have undergone multiple surgeries or who have a history of allergy to anesthetic drugs, and health care, rubber industry, or glove manufacturing plant workers.

Five routes of exposure to latex proteins have resulted in systemic reactions—cutaneous (contact with moist skin), mucous membranes (mouth, vagina, urethra, or rectum), internal tissue (during surgery and other invasive procedures), intravascular, and inhalation (exposure to anesthesia equipment or endotracheal tubes or through the aerosolization of glove powder). It has been postulated that the latex allergen adheres to the cornstarch or powder and is released into the air with the manipulation of rubber gloves.

The American Academy of Allergy and Immunology has published guidelines for providing care to persons with latex allergy. All persons at risk for latex allergy should have a careful history and should complete a standardized latex allergy questionnaire. A history suggestive of reactivity to latex includes local swelling or itching after blowing up balloons, after dental examinations, contact with rubber gloves, vaginal or rectal examinations, using condoms or diaphragms, and contact with other rubber products. Other historical information that may suggest increased risk of latex allergy includes hand eczema; previous, unexplained anaphylaxis; oral itching after eating bananas, chestnuts, kiwis, and avocados; and multiple surgical procedures in infancy. Patients at high risk should be offered clinical testing for latex allergy.

The patient with a latex allergy should be cared for in a latex-free environment. That is an environment in which there are no latex gloves used and no direct patient contact with other latex devices.[30,31]

The symptoms usually start to appear within minutes of exposure to the antigen, peak within 15 to 30 minutes, and resolve over the next several hours (Box 25-10).[28]

The cutaneous effects usually appear first and include pruritus, generalized erythema, urticaria, and angioedema. Commonly seen on the face and in the oral cavity and lower pharynx, angioedema develops as a result of fluid leaking into the interstitial space. The patient may appear restless, uneasy, apprehensive, anxious, and complain of being warm. Respiratory effects include the de-

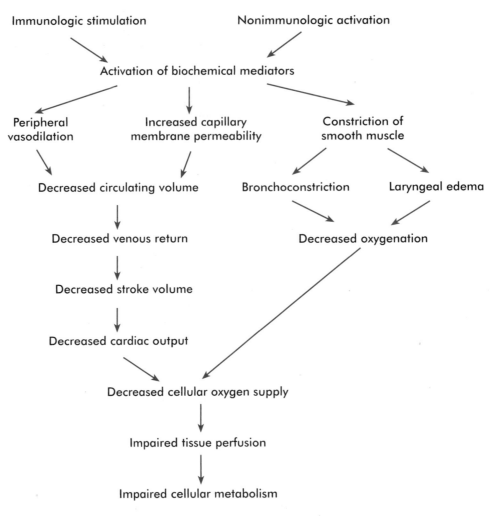

Fig. **25-3** Pathophysiology of anaphylactic shock.

velopment of laryngeal edema, bronchoconstriction, and mucus plugs. Clinical manifestations of laryngeal edema include inspiratory stridor, hoarseness, a sensation of fullness or a lump in the throat, and dysphagia. Bronchoconstriction causes dyspnea, wheezing, and chest tightness.[9,29-31] In addition, gastrointestinal and genitourinary manifestations may develop as a result of smooth muscle contraction. These include vomiting, diarrhea, cramping, abdominal pain, urinary incontinence, and vaginal bleeding.[27-29]

As the anaphylactic reaction progresses, hypotension and reflex tachycardia develop. This occurs in response to massive vasodilation and loss of circulating volume. Jugular veins appear flat as right ventricular end-diastolic volume is decreased. The eventual outcome is circulatory failure and shock.[9,27-29] The patient's level of consciousness may deteriorate to unresponsiveness.[29]

Assessment of the hemodynamic parameters of a patient in anaphylactic shock reveals a decreased CO and CI. Venous vasodilation and massive volume loss lead to a decrease in preload, which results in a decline in the RAP and PAWP. Vasodilation of the arterial system re-

sults in a decrease in the afterload of the heart, as evidenced by a decrease in the SVR.[9]

Medical Management

The goals of therapy are to remove the offending antigen, reverse the effects of the biochemical mediators, and promote adequate tissue perfusion. When the hypersensitivity reaction occurs as a result of administration of medications, dye, blood, or blood products, the infusion should be immediately discontinued. Many times it is not possible to remove the antigen because it is unknown or has already entered the patient's system.[28]

Reversal of the effects of the biochemical mediators involves the preservation and support of the patient's airway, ventilation, and circulation. This is accomplished through oxygen therapy, intubation, mechanical ventilation, and administration of drugs and fluids. Epinephrine is given to promote bronchodilation and vasoconstriction and to inhibit further release of biochemical mediators.[28,32] It usually is administered intravenously or via endotracheal tube. The dose is 0.1 mg/kg of 1:10,000 di-

BOX 25-10

CLINICAL MANIFESTATIONS OF ANAPHYLACTIC SHOCK

CARDIOVASCULAR

Hypotension
Tachycardia

RESPIRATORY

Lump in throat
Dysphagia
Hoarseness
Stridor
Wheezing
Rales and rhonchi

CUTANEOUS

Pruritus
Erythema
Urticaria
Angioedema

NEUROLOGIC

Restlessness
Uneasiness
Apprehension
Anxiety
Decreased level of consciousness

GASTROINTESTINAL

Nausea
Vomiting
Diarrhea

GENITOURINARY

Incontinence
Vaginal bleeding

SUBJECTIVE COMPLAINTS

Sensation of warmth
Dyspnea
Abdominal cramping and pain
Itching

HEMODYNAMIC PARAMETERS

Decreased cardiac output (CO)
Decreased cardiac index (CI)
Decreased right atrial pressure (RAP)
Decreased pulmonary artery wedge pressure (PAWP)
Decreased systemic vascular resistance (SVR)

BOX 25-11

NURSING DIAGNOSIS PRIORITIES

Anaphylactic Shock

- Fluid Volume Deficit related to relative loss, pp. 486-487
- Decreased Cardiac Output related to alterations in preload, pp. 467-468
- Decreased Cardiac Output related to alterations in afterload, pp. 468-469
- Ineffective Breathing Pattern related to decreased lung expansion, pp. 473-474
- Ineffective Family Coping: Compromised related to critically ill family member, pp. 452-453

Nursing Management

Prevention of anaphylactic shock is one of the primary responsibilities of the nurse in the critical care area. Preventive measures include the identification of patients at risk and cautious assessment of the patient's response to the administration of drugs, blood, and blood products. A complete and accurate history of the patient's allergies is an essential component of preventive nursing care. In addition to a list of the allergies, a detailed description of the type of response for each one should be obtained.[22]

The patient in anaphylactic shock may have any number of nursing diagnoses, depending on the progression of the process (Box 25-11). **Nursing priorities are directed toward facilitating ventilation, enhancing volume replacement, providing comfort and emotional support, and maintaining surveillance for complications.** Measures to facilitate ventilation include positioning the patient to assist with breathing and instructing the patient to breathe slowly and deeply. Measures to enhance volume replacement include inserting large-diameter peripheral intravenous catheters, rapidly administering prescribed fluids, and positioning the patient with the legs elevated, trunk flat, and head and shoulders above the chest. Measures to promote comfort include administering medications to relieve itching, applying warm soaks to skin, and, if necessary, covering the patient's hands to discourage scratching. In addition, observing the patient for clinical manifestations of a delayed reaction is critical to preventing further problems.

NEUROGENIC SHOCK

Description and Etiology

Neurogenic shock, a type of distributive shock, is the result of the loss or suppression of sympathetic tone. Its onset is within minutes, and it may last for days, weeks, or months depending on the cause.[33] The lack of sympathetic tone leads to decreased tissue perfusion and initiation of the general shock response. Neurogenic shock is the rarest form of shock.[3,34]

lution IV over at least 3 to 5 minutes or 10 ml of 1:10,000 dilution endotracheally. Diphenhydramine (Benadryl), 1 to 2 mg/kg IV every 6 to 8 hours, is used to block the histamine response. Corticosteroids may also be given with the goal of preventing a delayed reaction and stabilizing capillary membranes.[32] Fluid replacement is accomplished by use of either a crystalloid or colloid solution. In addition, positive inotropic agents and vasoconstrictor agents may be necessary to reverse the effects of myocardial depression and vasodilation.[10,27,28,32]

Neurogenic shock can be caused by anything that disrupts the sympathetic nervous system (SNS). The problem can occur as the result of interrupted impulse transmission or blockage of sympathetic outflow from the vasomotor center in the brain.[3,34] The most common cause is a spinal cord injury above the level of T6, this is also known a spinal shock.[35] Other causes include spinal anesthesia, drugs, emotional stress, pain, and CNS dysfunction.[3]

Pathophysiology

Loss of sympathetic tone results in massive peripheral vasodilation, inhibition of the baroreceptor response, and impaired thermoregulation. Arterial vasodilation leads to a decrease in SVR and a fall in blood pressure. Venous vasodilation leads to decreased venous return because of pooling of blood in the venous circuit. A decreased venous return results in a decrease in end-diastolic volume or preload. A decrease in preload results in a decrease in SV and CO, and relative hypovolemia develops. The fall in blood pressure and CO leads to inadequate or impaired tissue perfusion.[33,35] Inhibition of the baroreceptor response results in loss of compensatory reflex tachycardia. The HR does not increase to compensate for the fall in CO, which further compromises tissue perfusion.[36] Impaired thermoregulation occurs because of loss of vasomotor tone in the cutaneous blood vessels that dilate and constrict to maintain body temperature. The patient becomes poikilothermic, or dependent on the environment for temperature regulation[33,36] (Fig. 25-4).

Assessment and Diagnosis

The patient in neurogenic shock usually presents with hypotension, bradycardia, hypothermia, and warm, dry skin. The decreased blood pressure results from massive peripheral vasodilation. The decreased HR is caused by inhibition of the baroreceptor response and unopposed parasympathetic control of the heart. Hypothermia occurs from uncontrolled heat loss peripherally. The warm, dry skin occurs as a consequence of pooling of blood in the extremities and loss of vasomotor control in surface vessels of the skin that control heat loss.[33,35]

Assessment of the hemodynamic parameters of a patient in neurogenic shock reveals a decreased CO and CI. Venous vasodilation leads to a decrease in preload, which results in a decline in the RAP and PAWP. Vasodilation of the arterial system causes a decrease in the afterload of the heart as evidenced by a decrease in the SVR.[34]

Medical Management

The goals of therapy are to treat or remove the cause, prevent cardiovascular instability, and promote optimal tissue perfusion. Cardiovascular instability can occur from hypovolemia, hypothermia, hypoxia, and dysrhythmias.

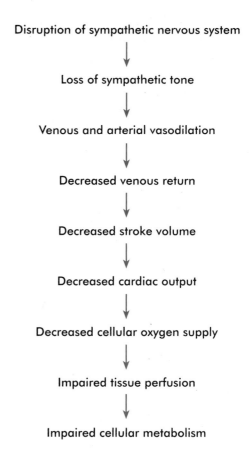

Fig. **25-4** Pathophysiology of neurogenic shock.

Specific treatments are aimed at preventing or correcting these problems as they occur.

Hypovolemia is treated with careful fluid resuscitation. The minimal amount of fluid is administered to ensure adequate tissue perfusion. Volume replacement is initiated for SBP lower than 90 mm Hg, urine output less than 30 ml/hr, or changes in mental status that indicate decreased cerebral tissue perfusion. The patient is carefully observed for evidence of fluid overload.[35] Vasopressors may be used as necessary to maintain blood pressure and organ perfusion.[34]

Hypothermia is treated with warming measures and environmental temperature regulation. The goal is to maintain normothermia and avoid large swings in the patient's body temperature.[36]

The treatment of hypoxia varies with the underlying cause. Chest wall paralysis, retained secretions, pulmonary edema, and suctioning contribute to the development of hypoxia. Management of this problem may include ventilatory support, vigorous pulmonary hygiene, and supplemental oxygen. Continuous pulse oximetry monitoring also may be helpful in recognizing hypoxia early, before complications arise. The major dysrhythmia seen in neurogenic shock is bradycardia, which should be treated with atropine.[33,36]

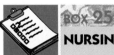

Nursing Management

Prevention of neurogenic shock is one of the primary responsibilities of the nurse in the critical care area. This includes the identification of patients at risk and constant assessment of the neurologic status. Vigilant immobilization of spinal cord injuries and slight elevation of the head of bed of the patient after spinal anesthesia are essential components of preventive nursing care. Early identification allows for early treatment and decreased mortality.[22]

The patient in neurogenic shock may have any number of nursing diagnoses, depending on the progression of the process (Box 25-12). **Nursing priorities are directed toward treating hypovolemia, maintaining normothermia, preventing hypoxia, providing comfort and emotional support, and maintaining surveillance for complications.** Venous pooling in the lower extremities promotes the formation of deep vein thrombosis (DVT) which can result in a pulmonary embolism. All patients at risk for DVT should be started on prophylaxis therapy. DVT prophylatic measures include monitoring of calf and thigh measurements, passive range of motion, application of antiembolic stockings and/or sequential pneumatic stockings, and administration of prescribed anticoagulation therapy.

SEPTIC SHOCK

Description and Etiology

Septic shock, a form of distributive shock, occurs when microorganisms invade the body. The primary mechanism of this type of shock is the maldistribution of blood flow to the tissues, with some areas being overperfused and others being underperfused.[4,37] The incidence of sepsis is estimated at more than 400,000 cases annually in the United States, with the mortality rate for septic shock being estimated between 40% and 60%.[38]

A variety of terms may be used to describe the condition the patient with an infection experiences. In 1991, at the American College of Chest Physicians/Society of Critical Care Medicine Consensus Conference, definitions were developed to describe to these conditions (Box 25-13).[39]

Septic shock is caused by a wide variety of microorganisms including gram-negative and gram-positive aerobes, anaerobes, fungi, and viruses. The source of these microorganisms is varied. Exogenous sources include the hospital environment and members of the health care team.

Endogenous sources include the patient's skin, gastrointestinal (GI) tract, respiratory tract, and genitourinary tract. Gram-negative bacteria are responsible for more than half of the cases of septic shock.[5,38,40,41] Toxic shock

PRECIPITATING FACTORS ASSOCIATED WITH SEPTIC SHOCK

INTRINSIC FACTORS

Extremes of age
Co-existing diseases
  Malignancies
  Burns
  Acquired immune deficiency syndrome (AIDS)
  Diabetes
  Substance abuse
  Dysfunction of one or more of the major body
    systems
Malnutrition

EXTRINSIC FACTORS

Invasive devices
Drug therapy
Fluid therapy
Surgical and traumatic wounds
Surgical and invasive diagnostic procedures
Immunosuppressive therapy

syndrome is an example of gram-positive shock due to *Staphylococcus aureus*.[42]

Sepsis and septic shock are associated with a wide variety of intrinsic and extrinsic precipitating factors (Box 25-14). All these factors interfere directly or indirectly with the body's anatomic and physiologic defense mechanisms. Several of the intrinsic factors are not modifiable or are very difficult to control. Several of the extrinsic factors may be required for diagnosis and management. All critically ill patients are, therefore, at risk for the development of septic shock.[38,41,42]

Pathophysiology

Septic shock is a complex systemic response that is initiated when a microorganism enters the body and stimulates the inflammatory/immune system. Shed protein fragments and the release of toxins and other substances from the microorganism activate the plasma enzyme cascades (complement, kallikrein/kinin, coagulation and fibrinolytic factors) as well as platelets, neutrophils, and macrophages. In addition, the toxins damage the endothelial cells. Once activated, these systems and cells release a variety of mediators that target various organs throughout the body.[41,43,44]

These mediators initiate a chain of complex interactions that are controlled by numerous feedback mechanisms. Eventually the immune system is overwhelmed, the feedback mechanisms fail, and a process that was designed to protect the body actually harms the body.[5,43] Once the mediators are activated, a variety of physiologic and pathophysiologic events occur that affect capillary membrane permeability, clotting, the distribution of blood flow to the tissues and organs, and the metabolic

state of the body. Subsequently, a systemic imbalance between cellular oxygen supply and demand develops that results in cellular hypoxia, damage, and death[5,38,44] (Fig. 25-5).

Assessment and Diagnosis

The patient in septic shock may present with a variety of clinical manifestations (Box 25-15). During the initial stage, massive vasodilation occurs in both the venous and arterial beds. Dilation of the venous system leads to a decrease in venous return to the heart, which results in a decrease in the preload of the right and left ventricles. This is evidenced by a decline in the RAP and PAWP. Dilation of the arterial system results in a decrease in the afterload of the heart as evidenced by a decrease in the SVR. The patient's blood pressure falls in response to the reduction in preload and afterload. The patient's skin becomes pink, warm, and flushed as a result of the massive vasodilation.[9,38,41,44]

The HR rises to compensate for the hypotension and in response to increased metabolic, SNS, and adrenal gland stimulation. This results in a normal to high CO and CI. The PP widens as the diastolic blood pressure decreases because of the vasodilation, and the SBP increases because of the elevated CO. A full, bounding pulse develops. Myocardial contractility is decreased, as evidenced by a decline in the left ventricular stroke work index (LVSWI), an effect of myocardial depression factor.[9,41,47]

In the lungs, ventilation/perfusion mismatching develops as a result of pulmonary vasoconstriction and the formation of pulmonary microemboli. Hypoxemia occurs, and the RR increases to compensate for the lack of oxygen. Crackles develop as increased pulmonary capillary membrane permeability leads to pulmonary interstitial edema.[38]

Level of consciousness starts to change as a result of decreased cerebral perfusion, immune mediator activation, hyperthermia, and lactic acidosis. The patient may appear disoriented, confused, combative, or lethargic. Urine output declines because of decreased perfusion of the kidneys. The patient's temperature is elevated in response to pyrogens released from the invading microorganisms, immune mediator activation, and increased metabolic activity.[9,38,41]

Arterial blood gas values during this phase reveal respiratory alkalosis, hypoxemia, and metabolic acidosis. This is demonstrated by a low PaO_2, low $PaCO_2$, and low HCO_3^- respectively. The respiratory alkalosis is caused by the patient's increased RR. As the patient becomes fatigued, the RR decreases and the $PaCO_2$ increases, resulting in respiratory acidosis. The metabolic acidosis is the result of lack of oxygen to the cells and the development of lactic acidemia. The mixed venous oxygen saturation (SvO_2) is increased because of maldistribution of the circulating blood volume and impaired cellular metabolism.[38]

The WBC count is elevated as part of the immune response to the invading microorganisms. In addition, the

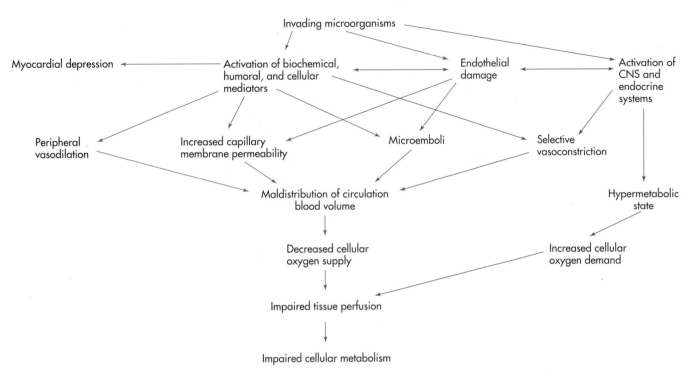

Fig. **25-5** Pathophysiology of septic shock.

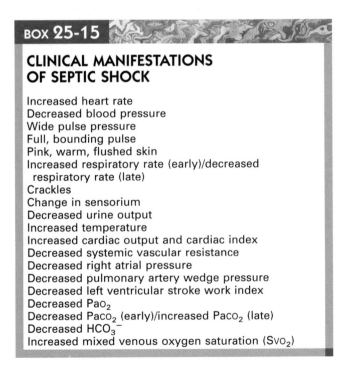

CLINICAL MANIFESTATIONS OF SEPTIC SHOCK

Increased heart rate
Decreased blood pressure
Wide pulse pressure
Full, bounding pulse
Pink, warm, flushed skin
Increased respiratory rate (early)/decreased respiratory rate (late)
Crackles
Change in sensorium
Decreased urine output
Increased temperature
Increased cardiac output and cardiac index
Decreased systemic vascular resistance
Decreased right atrial pressure
Decreased pulmonary artery wedge pressure
Decreased left ventricular stroke work index
Decreased PaO_2
Decreased $PaCO_2$ (early)/increased $PaCO_2$ (late)
Decreased HCO_3^-
Increased mixed venous oxygen saturation (SvO_2)

white blood cell differential reveals an increase in immature neutrophils (shift to the left). This occurs because the body has to mobilize increasing numbers of WBCs to fight the infection.[41] Increased serum glucose also occurs as part of the hypermetabolic response and the development of insulin resistance.[46] As impaired tissue perfusion

develops, a variety of other clinical manifestations appear, indicating the development of MODS.[38]

Medical Management

The goals of treatment are to control the infection, reverse the pathophysiologic responses, and promote metabolic support. This approach includes identifying and treating the infection, supporting the cardiovascular system and enhancing tissue perfusion, and initiating nutritional therapy. In addition, dysfunction of the individual organ systems must be prevented.

One of the first measures that must be taken in the treatment of septic shock is finding and eradicating the cause of the infection. Blood, urine, sputum, and wound cultures should be obtained to find the location of the infection. Antibiotic therapy should be initiated as soon as possible. If the microorganism is unknown, a broad-spectrum antibiotic should be administered. Once the microorganism is identified, an antibiotic more specific to the microorganism should be started. Administration of antibiotics can be particularly hazardous in gram-negative shock because more endotoxin is released from the cell walls when the microorganisms die. This further aggravates the entire septic process. Surgical intervention to debride infected or necrotic tissue or to drain abscesses also may be necessary to facilitate removal of the septic source.[47]

Another important measure in the treatment of septic shock is to support the cardiovascular system and enhance tissue perfusion. Specific interventions are aimed at increasing cellular oxygen supply and decreasing cellular oxygen demand. These treatments include administration of fluids, vasoconstrictor and positive inotropic agents, as well as ventilatory support, temperature control, and reversal of acidosis.[41,47]

Aggressive fluid administration to augment intravascular volume and increase preload is very important during the initial phase. Crystalloids or colloids may be used, depending on the patient's condition. The amount of fluid that is administered may vary, but generally the goal is to restore the patient's the PAWP to the 15 to 18 mm Hg range. The administration of vasoconstrictor agents is indicated to reverse the massive peripheral vasodilation. These agents help increase the SVR and augment the patient's blood pressure. Positive inotropic agents are used to increase contractility and treat myocardial depression. All these medications are titrated to the patient's response.[41,47]

To optimize oxygenation and ventilation, intubation and mechanical ventilation are required. Ventilator settings should be adjusted to provide the patient with a PaO_2 greater than 70 mm Hg and a pH within the normal range. Temperature control also is necessary to decrease the metabolic demands created by hyperthermia. Antipyretic agents and cooling measures often are used.[41,47]

The initiation of nutritional therapy is critical in the management of the patient in septic shock. The goal is to improve the patient's overall nutritional status, enhance the immune system, and promote wound healing. The ideal nutritional supplement for the patient in septic shock should be high in protein because of the metabolic derangements that develop in the hypermetabolic state. The amount of protein calories given depends on the patient's nitrogen balance. In early sepsis, the mix of nonprotein calories may be divided evenly between carbohydrates and fats. In the later stages, significant alterations in fat metabolism occur and the lipid content should be limited to 10% to 15% of the total nonprotein calories. The lipid emulsion should contain long-chain fatty acid triglycerides for their protein-sparing effects.[47]

Nursing Management

Prevention of septic shock is one of the primary responsibilities of the nurse in the critical care area. These measures include the identification of patients at risk and reduction of their exposure to invading microorganisms. Hand washing, aseptic technique, and an understanding of how microorganisms can invade the body are essential components of preventive nursing care. Early identification allows for early treatment and decreased mortality.[22]

The patient in septic shock may have any number of nursing diagnoses, depending on the progression of the process (Box 25-16). **Nursing priorities are directed toward administering prescribed antibiotics, fluids, and vasoactive agents; preventing the development of concomitant infections; facilitating nutritional support; providing comfort and emotional support; and main-**

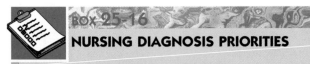

NURSING DIAGNOSIS PRIORITIES

Septic Shock

- Decreased Cardiac Output related to alterations in preload, pp. 467-468
- Decreased Cardiac Output related to alterations in afterload, pp. 468-469
- Decreased Cardiac Output related to alterations in contractility, p. 469
- Impaired Gas Exchange related to ventilation/perfusion mismatching or intrapulmonary shunting, p. 476
- Anxiety related to threat to biologic, psychologic, or social integrity, pp. 448-450

taining surveillance for complications. Continual observation to detect subtle changes indicating the progression of the septic process is also very important.

MULTIPLE ORGAN DYSFUNCTION SYNDROME

Description and Etiology

MODS results from progressive physiologic failure of several interdependent organ systems. It is defined as the "presence of altered organ function in an acutely ill patient such that homeostasis cannot be maintained without intervention."[39] Dysfunction of one organ may amplify dysfunction in another. Organ dysfunction may be absolute or relative and occurs over varying time periods. MODS is the major cause of morbidity in the critically ill patient and may account for up to 80% of all mortalities in the critical care unit. MODS is a leading cause of late mortality after trauma.

Lack of consensus regarding acceptable definitions for organ dysfunction, the number of organs involved, and the duration of organ dysfunction has hampered an accurate account of organ dysfunction in critically ill patients. About 7% to 15% of critically ill patients experience dysfunction in at least two organ systems. Patient outcome is directly related to the number of organs that fail. Failure of three or more organs is associated with a 90% to 95% mortality rate.[48]

Although various patient populations are at risk for organ dysfunction, trauma patients are particularly vulnerable because they frequently experience prolonged episodes of circulatory shock with tissue hypoxemia, tissue injury, and infection.[49] Other high-risk patients include those who have experienced a shock episode associated with a ruptured aneurysm, acute pancreatitis, sepsis, burns, or surgical complications.[49-51] Patients age 65 years and older are at increased risk secondary to their decreased organ reserve.[49]

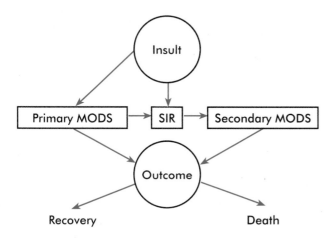

Fig. 25-6 Different causes and results of primary and secondary multiple organ dysfunction syndrome (MODS). *SIR,* systemic inflammatory response. (From American College of Chest Physicians/Society of Critical Care Medicine Consensus Conference Committee: Definitions for sepsis and organ failure and guidelines for the use of innovative therapies in sepsis, *Crit Care Med* 20:868, 1992.)

Pathophysiology

Organ dysfunction may be a direct consequence of the insult (primary MODS) or can manifest latently and involve organs not directly affected in the initial insult (secondary MODS) (Fig. 25-6). Patients can experience both primary and secondary MODS.

Primary MODS

Primary MODS "directly results from a well-defined insult in which organ dysfunction occurs early and is directly attributed to the insult itself."[39] Direct insults initially cause localized inflammatory responses. Examples of primary MODS include the immediate consequences of trauma, such as pulmonary contusion, pulmonary dysfunction after aspiration or inhalation injury, and renal dysfunction as a result of rhabdomyolysis or emergency aortic surgery.[39,52] Primary MODS generally results in one of three patient outcomes: recovery, a stable hypermetabolic state, or death.[48]

Secondary MODS

Secondary MODS is a consequence of widespread systemic inflammation that results in dysfunction of organs not involved in the initial insult.[39,52] The focus of the following discussion pertains to the relationship between systemic inflammatory response syndrome (SIRS) and secondary MODS.

Secondary MODS develops latently after a variety of insults. The early impairment of organs normally involved in immunoregulatory function, such as the liver and gastrointestinal (GI) tract, intensifies the host response to an insult.[49,53-55]

SIRS is a common initiating event in the development of secondary MODS. The systemic inflammatory response, a continuous process, is an abnormal host

response characterized by generalized inflammation in organs remote from the initial insult.[56] SIRS pertains to the widespread inflammation or clinical response to inflammation occurring in patients with a variety of insults. Clinical conditions and manifestations associated with SIRS are listed in Box 25-17. These insults produce similar or identical systemic inflammatory responses, even in the absence of infection. SIRS is present when two or more of four clinical manifestations are present in the high-risk patient (Box 25-13). Manifestations of SIRS must represent an acute alteration from the patient's normal baseline and must not be related to other causes (e.g., neutropenia from chemotherapy or leukopenia). When SIRS is a result of infection, the term *sepsis* is used. Organ dysfunction or failure, such as acute lung injury, acute renal failure, and MODS, are complications of SIRS.[39,52]

When SIRS is not contained, several consequences may occur that lead to organ dysfunction, including intense, uncontrolled activation of inflammatory cells (neutrophils, macrophages, lymphocytes), direct damage of vascular endothelium, disruption of immune cell function, persistent hypermetabolism, and maldistribution of circulatory volume to organ systems.[50,53,54,56] Consequently, inflammation becomes a systemic self-perpetuating process that is inadequately controlled and results in organ dysfunction.[53-55,57,58]

However, not all patients develop MODS from SIRS. The development of MODS appears to be associated with failure to control the source of inflammation or infection; a persistent perfusion-deficit, supply-dependent oxygen consumption (VO_2); or the continued presence of necrotic tissue.[59] Normally, under steady-state conditions, VO_2 is relatively constant and independent of oxygen delivery (DO_2) unless delivery becomes severely impaired. The relationship is known as supply-independent oxygen consumption. VO_2 is about 25% of DO_2. Consequently, a percentage of oxygen is not used (physiologic reserve). SIRS/MODS patients often develop supply-dependent oxygen consumption in which VO_2 becomes dependent on DO_2, rather than demand, at a normal or high DO_2. When VO_2 does not equal demand, a tissue oxygen debt develops, subjecting organs to failure.

The definitive clinical course of secondary MODS has not been completely identified. Clinical observations suggest that organ dysfunction may occur in a progressive pattern; however, organs may fail simultaneously.[49,50,55,60,61] Renal dysfunction, for example, may occur concurrently with hepatic dysfunction. The lungs generally are the first major organs affected. After the initial insult and resuscitation, patients develop a persistent hypermetabolism, a metabolic consequence of sustained systemic inflammation and physiologic stress, followed closely by pulmonary dysfunction, manifested as acute respiratory distress syndrome (ARDS).

Hypermetabolism accompanies SIRS but may not occur immediately after insult. Hypermetabolism generally lasts for 14 to 21 days. During hypermetabolism, changes occur in cellular anabolic and catabolic function, resulting in autocatabolism. Autocatabolism manifests as a severe decrease in lean body mass, severe weight loss, anergy, and increased cardiac output and VO_2. The patient experiences profound alterations in carbohydrate, protein, and fat metabolism.[62] Concurrently, GI, hepatic, and immunologic dysfunction may occur, which intensifies the SIRS. Clinical manifestations of cardiovascular instability and central nervous system dysfunction may be present. Ongoing perfusion deficits and septic foci continue to perpetuate SIRS. About 25% to 40% of patients die during hypermetabolism.[51] The development of renal and hepatic failure is a preterminal event in MODS.[51] Patients with decreased physiologic organ reserve may manifest signs and symptoms of organ dysfunction earlier than previously healthy patients.[63] Survivors may develop generalized polyneuropathy and a chronic form of pulmonary disease from ARDS, complicating recovery.[64] These patients often require prolonged, expensive rehabilitation.

Secondary MODS results from altered regulation of the patient's acute immune and inflammatory responses. Dysregulation, or failure to control the host inflammatory response, leads to the excessive production of inflammatory cells and biochemical mediators that cause widespread damage to vascular endothelium and organ damage.[65] The critically ill patient's compromised immune state also fosters an environment conducive to organ failure.

The inflammatory and immune responses implicated in SIRS and MODS are mediated by certain cells and biochemicals that in turn affect cellular activity. As outlined in Box 25-18, mediators associated with SIRS and MODS

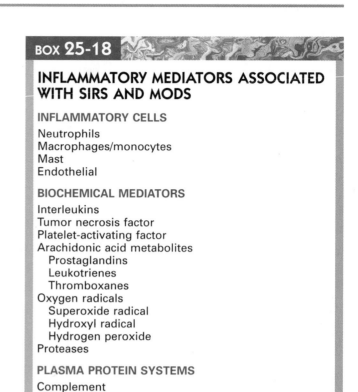

BOX 25-18

INFLAMMATORY MEDIATORS ASSOCIATED WITH SIRS AND MODS

INFLAMMATORY CELLS

Neutrophils
Macrophages/monocytes
Mast
Endothelial

BIOCHEMICAL MEDIATORS

Interleukins
Tumor necrosis factor
Platelet-activating factor
Arachidonic acid metabolites
   Prostaglandins
   Leukotrienes
   Thromboxanes
Oxygen radicals
   Superoxide radical
   Hydroxyl radical
   Hydrogen peroxide
Proteases

PLASMA PROTEIN SYSTEMS

Complement
Kinin/kallikrein
Coagulation

can be classified as either inflammatory cells, plasma protein systems, or inflammatory biochemicals. Activation of one mediator often leads to activation of another. Plasma levels are not always indicative of cellular levels. The biologic activity of inflammatory cells, biochemical mediators, and plasma protein systems and how they work in concert to cause SIRS and MODS are not yet totally defined.

Assessment and Diagnosis

Secondary MODS is a systemic disease with organ-specific manifestations. Organ dysfunction is influenced by numerous factors, including organ host defense function, response time to the injury, metabolic requirements, organ vasculature response to vasoactive drugs, and organ sensitivity to damage and physiologic reserve. The responses of the gastrointestinal (GI), hepatobiliary, cardiovascular, pulmonary, renal, and coagulation systems are discussed in the following text. Clinical manifestations of organ dysfunction are outlined in Box 25-19.

Gastrointestinal dysfunction

The GI tract plays an important role in MODS. GI organs normally have immunoregulatory functions. Consequently, GI dysfunction amplifies SIRS and gut damage, which may lead to bacterial translocation and endogenous endotoxemia.[53-55,57,58]

Three specific mechanisms link the GI tract and latent organ dysfunction. First, hypoperfusion and/or shock-

BOX 25-19

CLINICAL MANIFESTATIONS OF ORGAN DYSFUNCTION

GASTROINTESTINAL

Abdominal distention
Intolerance to enteral feedings
Paralytic ileus
Upper/lower GI bleeding
Diarrhea
Ischemic colitis
Mucosal ulceration
Decreased bowel sounds
Bacterial overgrowth in stool

LIVER

Jaundice
Increased serum bilirubin (hyperbilirubinemia)
Increased liver enzymes (AST, ALT, LDH, alkaline phosphatase)
Increased serum ammonia
Decreased serum albumin
Decreased serum transferrin

GALLBLADDER

Right upper quadrant tenderness/pain
Abdominal distention
Unexplained fever
Decreased bowel sounds

METABOLIC/NUTRITIONAL

Decreased lean body mass
Muscle wasting
Severe weight loss
Negative nitrogen balance
Hyperglycemia
Hypertriglyceridemia
Increased serum lactate
Decreased serum albumin, serum transferrin, preabumin
Decreased retinol-binding protein

IMMUNE

Infection
Decreased lymphocyte count
Anergy

PULMONARY

Tachypnea
ARDS pattern of respiratory failure (dyspnea, patchy infiltrates, refractory hypoxemia, respiratory acidosis, abnormal O_2 indexes)
Pulmonary hypertension

RENAL

Increased serum creatinine, BUN levels
Oliguria, anuria, or polyuria consistent with prerenal azotemia or acute tubular necrosis
Urinary indexes consistent with prerenal azotemia or acute tubular necrosis

CARDIOVASCULAR
Hyperdynamic

Decreased pulmonary capillary wedge pressure
Decreased systemic vascular resistance
Decreased right atrial pressure
Decreased left ventricular stroke work index
Increased oxygen consumption
Increased cardiac output, cardiac index, heart rate

Hypodynamic

Increased systemic vascular resistance
Increased right atrial pressure
Increased left ventricular stroke work index
Decreased oxygen delivery and consumption
Decreased cardiac output and cardiac index

CENTRAL NERVOUS SYSTEM

Lethargy
Altered level of consciousness
Fever
Hepatic encephalopathy

COAGULATION/HEMATOLOGIC

Thrombocytopenia
DIC pattern

AST, Aspartate aminotransferase; *ALT,* alanine aminotransferase; *LDH,* lactate dehydrogenase.

like states damage the normal GI mucosa barrier. The GI tract is extremely vulnerable to oxygen metabolite–induced reperfusion injury. Endothelial injury and GI lesions occur in response to mediator-induced tissue damage. In addition, ischemic events and the absence of feedings can disrupt the normal metabolism of the gastric/intestinal lumen and the normal protective function of the gut barrier.[55,65]

Second, the translocation of normal GI bacteria via a "leaky gut" into the systemic circulation initiates and perpetuates an inflammatory focus in the critically ill patient. The GI tract harbors organisms that present an inflammatory focus when translocated from the gut into the portal circulation and are inadequately cleared by the liver. Hepatic macrophages respond to the presence of enteric organisms by producing tissue-damaging amounts of tumor necrosis factor (TNF). Bacterial translocation has been associated with paralytic ileus and drugs commonly used in the critically ill patient, including antibiotics, antacids, and histamine blockers.[55]

The third mechanism linking the GI tract and organ dysfunction is colonization. The oropharynx of the critically ill patient becomes colonized with potentially pathogenic organisms from the GI tract. Pulmonary aspiration of colonized sputum presents an inflammatory focus. Antacids, histamine antagonists, and antibiotics also increase colonization of the upper GI tract.[55,66]

Hepatobiliary dysfunction

The liver plays a vital role in host homeostasis related to the acute inflammatory response. In addition, the liver responds to SIRS by selectively changing carbohydrate

(CHO), fat, and protein metabolism. Consequently, hepatic dysfunction after a critical insult threatens the patient's survival.

The liver normally controls the inflammatory response by several mechanisms. Kupffer's cells, which are hepatic macrophages, detoxify substances that might normally induce systemic inflammation, as well as vasoactive substances that cause hemodynamic instability. Failure to detoxify gram-negative bacteria translocated from the GI tract causes endotoxemia, perpetuates SIRS, and may lead to MODS. Additionally, the liver produces proteins and antiproteases to control the inflammatory response; however, hepatic dysfunction limits this response.[53,54]

The liver and gallbladder are extremely vulnerable to ischemic injury. Ischemic hepatitis occurs after a prolonged period of physiologic shock and is associated with centrilobular hepatocellular necrosis. The degree of hepatic damage is related directly to the severity and duration of the shock episode. Terms such as shock liver and posttraumatic hepatic insufficiency have been used to describe ischemic hepatitis. Both anoxic and reperfusion injury damage hepatocytes and the vascular endothelium.[67] Patients at high risk for ischemic hepatitis after a hypotensive event include those with a history of cardiac failure and/or cardiac dysrhythmias. Clinical manifestations of hepatic insufficiency are evident 1 to 2 days after the insult. Jaundice and transient elevations in serum transaminase and bilirubin levels occur. Hyperbilirubinemia results from hepatocyte anoxic injury and an increased production of bilirubin from the hemoglobin catabolism. Ischemic hepatitis may either resolve spontaneously or progress to fulminant hepatic failure. Although ischemic hepatitis is not a life-threatening complication, it can contribute to patient morbidity and mortality as a component of MODS.[67] Researchers have recently proposed that serum bilirubin is a valid indicator of hepatic dysfunction in MODS because it significantly differentiates MODS survivors from nonsurvivors.[68]

Acalculous cholecystitis manifests 3 to 4 weeks after an insult. Its pathogenesis is unclear but may be related to ischemic reperfusion injury, narcotics, and cystic duct obstruction as a result of hyperviscous bile. Mediator-induced gallbladder dysfunction associated with acalculous cholecystitis may be related to the release of thromboxane A_2 and leukotrienes (vasoactive substances) into the microcirculation in response to a damaged endothelium, aggregated platelets, and neutrophils. Clinical manifestations of acalculous cholecystitis may mimic acute cholecystitis with gallstones. Patients may demonstrate vague symptoms, including right upper quadrant pain and tenderness. Critical to the detection of acalculous cholecystitis is the recognition of abdominal distention, unexplained fever, loss of bowel sounds, and a sudden deterioration in the patient's condition. About 50% of patients with acalculous cholecystitis have gallbladder gangrene, and 10% have gallbladder perforation. Consequently, a cholecystectomy may be performed.[69]

Hypermetabolism accompanies SIRS and is commonly referred to as the "metabolic response to injury." During hypermetabolism and SIRS, the liver perpetuates select changes in metabolism, including increased gluconeogenesis, glucogenesis, lipogenesis, and increased production of acute phase reactant proteins. Concurrently, the liver decreases synthesis of proteins, particularly albumin and transferrin. This metabolic response is partially mediated by interleukin-1 (IL-1), TNF, select arachidonic acid (AA) metabolites, and the stress hormones.[61]

Pulmonary dysfunction

The lungs, a frequent and early target organ for mediator-induced injury, are usually the first organs affected in secondary MODS. Acute pulmonary dysfunction in secondary MODS manifests as acute respiratory distress syndrome (ARDS). Patients who develop MODS generally develop ARDS; however, not all patients with ARDS develop secondary MODS. ARDS patients who develop SIRS/sepsis concurrently with acute respiratory failure are at the greatest risk for MODS.[50]

ARDS generally occurs 24 to 72 hours after the initial insult. Patients initially exhibit a low-grade fever, tachycardia, dyspnea, and mental confusion. As dyspnea, hypoxemia, and the work of breathing increase, intubation and mechanical ventilation are required. Pulmonary function is acutely disrupted, resulting in refractory hypoxemia secondary to intrapulmonary shunting, decreased pulmonary compliance, altered airway mechanics, and radiographic evidence of noncardiogenic pulmonary edema. ARDS is also associated with severe hypermetabolism equated to running an 8-minute mile, 24 hours a day, 7 days a week.[59]

Mediators associated with ARDS include AA metabolites, toxic oxygen metabolites, proteases, TNF, platelet activating factor (PAF), and interleukins.[56,64] Intense mediator activity damages the pulmonary vascular endothelium and the alveolar epithelium, resulting in surfactant deficiency, mild pulmonary hypertension, and increased lung water (noncardiogenic pulmonary edema) resulting from increased pulmonary capillary permeability. Pulmonary hypertension and hypoxic pulmonary vasoconstriction occur secondary to loss of the vascular bed.

Attempts to quantify the severity of pulmonary dysfunction in ARDS have led to the development of an acute lung injury scoring system. Variables included in the score are chest x-ray findings, the magnitude of hypoxemia using the PaO_2/FIO_2 ratio, pulmonary compliance during mechanical ventilation, and the use of positive endexpiratory pressure (PEEP) with mechanical ventilation. The total score is intended to provide an index of pulmonary dysfunction.[70] Attempts to predict outcome in MODS patients and quantify the magnitude of pulmonary dysfunction using scoring systems are ongoing.

Renal dysfunction

Acute renal failure is a common manifestation of MODS. The kidney is highly vulnerable to reperfusion injury. Consequently, renal ischemic-reperfusion injury may be a major cause of renal dysfunction in MODS. The patient may demonstrate oliguria or anuria secondary to decreased renal perfusion and relative hypovolemia. The condition may become refractory to diuretics, fluid challenges, and dopamine. Additional signs and symptoms include azotemia, decreased creatinine clearance, abnormal renal indices, and fluid and electrolyte imbalances. Prerenal oliguria may progress to acute tubular necrosis, necessitating hemodialysis or other renal therapies. The frequent use of nephrotoxic drugs during critical illness also intensifies the risk of renal failure.[71] Researchers have proposed that the serum creatinine is a valid indicator of renal function because it significantly differentiates MODS survivors from nonsurvivors.[68]

Cardiovascular dysfunction

The initial cardiovascular response in SIRS/sepsis is myocardial depression; decreased right atrial pressure and systemic vascular resistance (SVR); and increased venous capacitance, VO_2, cardiac output (CO), and heart rate (HR). Despite an increased CO, myocardial depression occurs and is accompanied by decreased SVR, increased HR, and ventricular dilation. These compensatory mechanisms help maintain CO during the early phase of SIRS/sepsis. An inability to increase CO in response to a low SVR may indicate myocardial failure or inadequate fluid resuscitation and is associated with increased mortality. VO_2 may be twice normal and may be flow-dependent. Mediators implicated in the hyperdynamic response include bradykinin, select AA metabolites, PAF, endogenous opioids, and beta-adrenergic stimulators.[49,72-74]

As MODS progresses, cardiac failure develops. Cardiac dysfunction is characterized by ventricular dilation, decreased diastolic compliance, and decreased systolic contractile function. Cardiovascular function becomes vasopressor-dependent. Cardiac failure may be caused by immune mediators, TNF, acidosis, or myocardial depressant factor (MDF), a substance secreted by the pancreas. TNF has a myocardial-depressant effect and is associated with myocardial depression during septic shock.[75] Myocardial depression is exacerbated by myocardial hypoperfusion from a low CO state and persistent lactic acidosis. Cardiogenic shock and biventricular failure occur and lead to death.

Coagulation system dysfunction

Failure of the coagulation system manifests as disseminated intravascular coagulation (DIC). It results in simultaneous microvascular clotting and hemorrhage in organ systems because of the depletion of clotting factors and excessive fibrinolysis. As depicted in Fig. 25-7, cell injury and damage to the endothelium initiate the intrinsic or extrinsic coagulation pathways. The endothelium is closely involved in DIC. Several relationships have been proposed. Endotoxins may roughen and expose the endothelial lining of blood vessels and consequently stimu-

late clotting. Low-flow states during hypotensive episodes may damage vessel endothelium and release tissue thromboplastin, with subsequent activation of the extrinsic pathway. A variety of clinical conditions, such as trauma, burns, and radiographic procedures, can also cause damage to the local endothelium and activation of the intrinsic coagulation pathway.[60,76]

DIC is a complex, consumptive coagulopathy that occurs in patients with a variety of disorders, including sepsis, tissue injury, and shock and is an overstimulation of the normal coagulation process. Thrombosis and fibrinolysis are magnified to life-threatening proportions. The initial alteration in DIC is a generalized state of systemic hypercoagulation that produces organ ischemia. All organs, particularly the skin, lungs, and kidneys, are involved.[60,76] The thrombotic clinical manifestations of DIC are presented in Box 25-20.

Hemorrhage is the second pathophysiologic alteration in DIC. The lysis of clots (fibrinolysis) normally is initiated by the coagulation cascade. The intensity of the thrombosis enhances an equally intense lysis; however, clot lyse cannot effectively maintain blood vessel patency. As depicted in Fig. 25-7, the production of fibrin split products exerts further anticoagulant effects, and hemorrhage ensues. Clotting factors, platelets, fibrinogen, and thrombin are consumed in large quantities during the thrombosis. Consequently, coagulation substances are depleted. The hemorrhagic signs and symptoms of DIC are presented in Box 25-20.

The abnormal clotting studies in patients with DIC may indicate thrombocytopenia; prolonged clotting times; depressed levels of clotting factors, particularly Factor VII; and fibrinogen/fibrin and high levels of breakdown products of fibrinogen and fibrin (fibrin degradation products, D-dimer). Medical management of DIC includes immediate treatment of the underlying cause; transfusion of blood products, such as red blood cells, platelets, and fresh frozen plasma, to correct the clotting factor deficiencies; and cryoprecipitate to treat hypofibrinogenemia. The use of heparin therapy in DIC remains controversial. Heparin must be used with caution; however, it is contraindicated in patients with bleeding in critical areas such as the cranium. Antifibrinolytic agents may be used concurrently with heparin therapy but generally are contraindicated because of the risk of thrombotic complications. Strict adherence to bleeding precautions is essential to minimize tissue and vascular trauma.[60,76]

Medical Management

The goals of therapy are prevention and treatment of infection, maintenance of tissue oxygenation, nutritional/metabolic support, and support for individual organs.[49,50,71,77] The use of investigational therapies may be part of the patient's clinical management.

Elimination of the source of inflammation or infection can reduce mortality.[51] Therefore surgical procedures

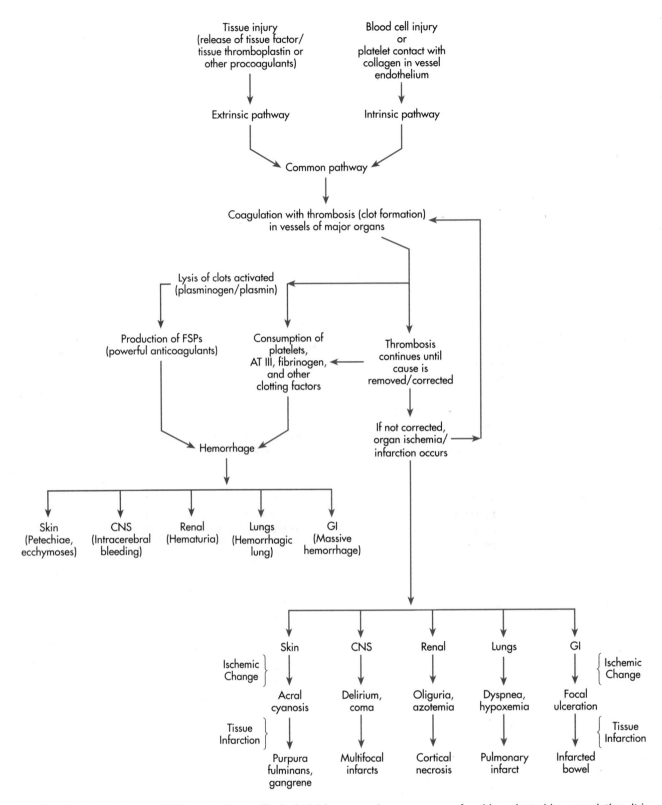

Fig. **25-7** Pathophysiology of DIC. Lysis of clots (fibrinolysis) is a natural consequence of and is activated by coagulation. It is intensified in patients with DIC. DIC is known as a consumptive coagulopathy. During thrombosis, clotting factors are used to form clots. During fibrinolysis, clotting factors are destroyed inside the clot. The end result is a depletion of coagulation substances. *FSP,* Fibrin split products or fibrin degradation products. (Modified from Carr M: Disseminated intravascular coagulation: pathogenesis, diagnosis, and therapy, *J Emer Med* 5:316, 1987.)

BOX 25-20

CLINICAL MANIFESTATIONS OF DIC

THROMBOTIC CLINICAL MANIFESTATIONS

Skin involvement
  Red, indurated areas along vessel wall
  Purpura fulminans (diffuse skin infarction)
  Acral cyanosis
  Necrosis of fingers, toes, nose, and genitalia
Cool, pale extremities with mottling, cyanosis, or
  edema
Renal involvement
  Renal failure
Cerebral infarcts or hemorrhage
Focal neurologic deficits (e.g., hemiplegia or loss of
  vision)
Nonspecific changes (e.g., altered loss of
  consciousness, confusion, headache, or seizures)
Bowel infarction
Melena, hematemesis, abdominal distention, or
  absent or hyperactive bowel sounds
Thrombophlebitis
Pulmonary embolism

HEMORRHAGIC CLINICAL MANIFESTATIONS

Spontaneous hemorrhage into body cavities and skin
  surfaces
Classic symptom of oozing or bleeding from
  invasive-line insertion sites or from body orifices.
Bleeding from body orifices such as the rectum,
  vagina, urethra, nose, and ears, as well as from the
  lung and gastrointestinal tract
Petechiae, purpura, or ecchymosis
Gingival, nasal, or scleral hemorrhage on physical
  examination
Hemorrhaging into all body cavities, including the
  abdomen, retroperitoneal space, cranium, and thorax

such as early fracture stabilization, removal of infected organs or tissue, and burn excision may be helpful in limiting the inflammatory response. Appropriate antibiotics are needed if the focus cannot be removed surgically.

Despite compliance with meticulous infection control practices, critically ill patients may "infect" themselves. As previously noted, bacterial contamination of the highly vulnerable respiratory tract and pneumonia can result from the colonization of GI tract bacteria. New approaches to infection control have been proposed, including selective decontamination of the GI tract with enteral antibiotics to prevent nosocomial infections, topical antibiotics in the oral pharynx to prevent colonization, monoclonal antibodies against endotoxin, and passive antibody protection.[43,70] Gut decontamination and prevention of oral pharyngeal colonization reduce the incidence of infection; however, morbidity from MODS is not significantly affected.[66]

New approaches to infection and inflammation control currently are being investigated, including immunotherapy. Immunotherapy is antibody therapy that lessens the SIRS to microbes (antiinflammatory immunotherapy) and is based on the principle that antibodies directed against endotoxin can prevent the endotoxin from stimulating SIRS.[78]

Hypoperfusion and resultant organ hypoxemia frequently occur in patients at high risk for MODS, subjecting essential organs to failure. Therefore effective fluid resuscitation and early recognition of supply-dependent VO_2 is essential. Patients at risk for MODS require pulmonary artery catheterization, frequent measurements of DO_2 and VO_2, and arterial lactate levels to guide therapy. Arterial lactate levels provide information regarding the severity of impaired perfusion and the presence of lactic acidosis[58] and differ significantly in MODS survivors and nonsurvivors. Failure to maintain adequate oxygenation to vital organs results in organ dysfunction. Despite adequate DO_2, VO_2 may not meet the needs of the body during MODS. Patients with ARDS and sepsis frequently manifest supply-dependent oxygen consumption and are unable to use oxygen appropriately despite normal delivery.[72,73,79,80] Possible causes of this flow-dependent VO_2 include abnormal mitochondrial function, redistribution of blood flow to organs, decreased SVR (secondary to prostaglandins), maldistribution of blood flow, microembolization, and capillary obstruction.[77,79]

Interventions that decrease oxygen demand and increase oxygen delivery are essential. Decreasing oxygen demand may be accomplished by sedation, mechanical ventilation, temperature and pain control, and rest. DO_2 may be increased by maintaining normal hematocrit and PaO_2 levels, using PEEP, increasing preload or myocardial contractility to enhance CO, or reducing afterload to increase CO. Many critical care clinicians advocate the maintenance of a supranormal DO_2 to increase VO_2; however, this therapeutic measure has not significantly improved survival, except in select groups of trauma patients.[59]

Hypermetabolism in SIRS/MODS results in profound weight loss, cachexia, and loss of organ function. The goal of nutritional support is the preservation of organ structure and function. Although nutritional support may not alter the course of organ dysfunction, it prevents generalized nutritional deficiencies and preserves gut integrity. The enteral route is preferable to parenteral support.[48,81] Enteral feedings are given distal to the pylorus to prevent pulmonary aspiration. Enteral feedings may limit bacterial translocation. In addition to early nutritional support the pharmacologic properties of enteral feeding formulas may limit SIRS for select critical care populations. Supplementation of enteral feedings with glutamine and arginine may be beneficial. Enteral feedings with omega-3 fatty acids may lessen SIRS.[81-84]

Recent guidelines have been proposed regarding nutritional support during SIRS for trauma patients. Patients are to receive 25 to 30 kcal/kg/day, with 3 to 5 g/kg/day as glucose. The respiratory quotient is monitored and maintained under 0.9. Long-chain polyunsaturated fatty acids (less than 1.5 g/kg/day) and amino acids (1.5 mg/kg/day) are given. Fat emulsions are limited to 0.5 to 1 g/kg/day to prevent iatrogenic immunosuppression associated with lipids and fat overload syndromes. Plasma transferrin and prealbumin levels are used to monitor hepatic protein synthesis.[61] Efficient protein use must be assessed via nitrogen balance studies.

Organ-specific interventions have not been highly effective in improving survival in MODS. Although organ-specific therapies such as mechanical ventilation and hemodialysis are needed for immediate survival, future medical management must target and control the effects of mediators that cause SIRS and MODS. Animal model studies continue to provide information regarding the efficacy of drugs that prevent organ dysfunction. Several experimental drugs and agents are currently being tested in human clinical trials. However, the initial enthusiasm about inflammatory therapies has been dampened, with many clinical trials reporting negative findings.

Nursing Management

Preventive measures include a multitude of assessment strategies to detect early organ manifestations of this syndrome. Patients who continue to experience sites of inflammation, septic foci, and inadequate tissue perfusion may be at higher risk. Hand washing, aseptic technique, and an understanding of how microorganisms can invade the body are essential components of preventive nursing care.

Nursing management of the patient with acute MODS incorporates a variety of nursing diagnoses (Box 25-21). **Nursing priorities are directed toward preventing the development of infections, facilitating tissue oxygen delivery and limiting tissue oxygen demand, facilitating nutritional support, providing comfort and emotional support, and maintaining surveillance for complications.** Patients are assessed closely for inflammation and infection. Subtle expressions of infection warrant investigation. Nursing measures include strict adherence to standards of practice to prevent infection. Practices related to infection control with invasive hemodynamic monitoring, urinary catheters, endotracheal tubes, intracranial pressure monitoring devices, total parenteral nutrition, and wound care must be stringent to prevent further infection. Measures to limit tissue oxygen consumption include administering analgesics and sedatives, positioning the patient for comfort, limiting activities, offering support to reduce anxiety, providing a calm and quiet environment, and teaching the patient about his or her condition. Measures to enhance tissue oxygen supply include administering supplemental oxygen, monitoring the patient's respiratory status, and administering prescribed fluids and medications.

References

1. Barone JE, Snyder AB: Treatment strategies in shock: use of oxygen transport measurement, *Heart Lung* 20:81, 1991.
2. Rice V: Shock, a clinical syndrome: an update. II. The stages of shock, *Crit Care Nurs* 11(5):74, 1991.
3. Rice V: Shock, a clinical syndrome: an update. I. An overview of shock, *Crit Care Nurs* 11(4):20, 1991.
4. Houston MC: Pathophysiology of shock, *Crit Care Nurs Clin North Am* 2:143, 1990.
5. Astiz ME, Rackow EC, Weil MH: Pathophysiology and treatment of circulatory shock, *Crit Care Clin* 9:183, 1993.
6. McMahon K: Multiple organ failure: the final complication of critical illness, *Crit Care Nurs* 15(6):20, 1995.
7. Shoemaker WC: Pathophysiology, monitoring and therapy of circulatory problems, *Crit Care Nurs Clin North Am* 6:295, 1994.
8. Nawas YN, Balk RA: General approach to shock, *Clin Geriatr Med* 10:185, 1994.
9. Summers G: The clinical and hemodynamic presentation of the shock patient, *Crit Care Nurs Clin North Am* 2:161, 1990.
10. Rice V: Shock, a clinical syndrome: an update. III. Therapeutic management, *Crit Care Nurs* 11(6):34, 1991.
11. Sommers MS: Fluid resuscitation following multiple trauma, *Crit Care Nurs* 10(10):74, 1990.
12. Kuhn MM: Colloids vs crystalloids, *Crit Care Nurs* 11(5):37, 1991.
13. Daleiden A: Pathophysiology and treatment of hemorrhagic shock during the early postoperative period, *Crit Care Nurs Q* 16:45, 1993.
14. Burns KM: Vasoactive drug therapy in shock, *Crit Care Nurs Clin North Am* 2:167, 1990.
15. Lorenz A: Lactic acidosis: a nursing challenge, *Crit Care Nurs* 9(4):64, 1989.
16. Arieff AI: Managing metabolic acidosis: update on the sodium bicarbonate controversy, *J Crit Illness* 8:224, 1993.
17. Kuhn MM: Nutritional support for the shock patient, *Crit Care Nurs Clin North Am* 2:201, 1990.
18. Lancaster LE, Rice V: Nursing care planning: overview and application to the patient in shock, *Crit Care Nurs Clin North Am* 2:279, 1990.
19. Jillings CR: Shock: psychosocial needs of the patient and family, *Crit Care Nurs Clin North Am* 2:325, 1990.
20. Britt LD, et al: Priorities in the management of profound shock, *Surg Clin North Am* 76:645, 1996.
21. Blansfield J: Emergency autotransfusion in hypovolemia, *Crit Care Nurs Clin North Am* 2:195, 1990.
22. Rice V: Shock, a clinical syndrome: an update. IV. Nursing care of the shock patient, *Crit Care Nurs* 11(7):28, 1991.

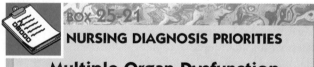

NURSING DIAGNOSIS PRIORITIES

Multiple Organ Dysfunction Syndrome

- Impaired Gas Exchange related to ventilation/perfusion mismatching or intrapulmonary shunting, p. 476
- Altered Renal Tissue Perfusion related to decreased renal blood flow, p. 485
- Altered Myocardial Tissue Perfusion related to decreased myocardial oxygen supply and/or increased myocardial oxygen demand, p. 466
- Altered Nutrition: Less Than Body Requirements related to increased metabolic demands or lack of exogenous nutrients, p. 460
- Risk for Infection, pp. 494-495
- Acute Confusion related to sensory overload, sensory deprivation, and sleep pattern disturbance, pp. 444-448
- Ineffective Family Coping: Compromised related to critically ill family member, pp. 452-453

23. Chatterjee K, et al: Gaining ground on cardiogenic shock, *Patient Care* 28(15):24, 1994.

24. Alpert JS, Becker RC: Mechanisms and management of cardiogenic shock, *Crit Care Clin* 9:205, 1993.

25. Zaloga GP, et al: Pharmacologic cardiovascular support, *Crit Care Clin* 9:335, 1993.

26. Schott KE: Intra-aortic balloon counterpulsation as a therapy for shock, *Crit Care Nurs Clin North Am* 2:187, 1990.

27. Crnkovick DJ, Carlson RW: Anaphylaxis: an organized approach to management and prevention, *J Crit Illness* 8:332, 1993.

28. Atkinson TP, Kaliner MA: Anaphylaxis, *Med Clin North Am* 76:841, 1992.

29. Mackan MD: Managing the patient with anaphylaxis. Part 1. Mechanisms and manifestations, *Emer Med* 27(2):68, 1995.

30. Sussman GL, Beezhold DH: Allergy to latex rubber, *Ann Intern Med* 122:43, 1995.

31. Steelman VM: Latex allergy precautions, *Nurs Clin North Am* 30:457, 1995.

32. Mackan MD: Managing the patient with anaphylaxis. Part 2. Therapeutic strategies, *Emer Med* 27(3):20, 1995.

33. Schwenker D: Cardiovascular considerations in the critical care phase, *Crit Care Nurs Clin North Am* 2:363, 1990.

34. Walleck CA: Neurological considerations in the critical care phase, *Crit Care Nurs Clin North Am* 2:357, 1990.

35. Atkinson PP, Atkinson JLD: Spinal shock, *Mayo Clin Proc* 71:384, 1996.

36. Kidd PS: Emergency management of spinal cord injuries, *Crit Care Nurs Clin North Am* 2:349, 1990.

37. Vincent JL, Van Der Linden P: Septic shock: particular type of acute circulatory failure, *Crit Care Med* 18:S70, 1990.

38. Hazinski MF, et al: Epidemiology, pathophysiology and clinical presentation of gram-negative sepsis, *Am J Crit Care* 2:224, 1993.

39. American College of Chest Physicians/Society of Critical Care Medicine Consensus Conference Committee: Definitions for sepsis and organ failure and guidelines for the use of innovative therapies in sepsis, *Crit Care Med* 20:864, 1992.

40. Hoyt NJ: Preventing septic shock: infection control in the intensive care unit, *Crit Care Nurs Clin North Am* 2:287, 1990.

41. Rackow EC, Astiz ME: Mechanisms and management of septic shock, *Crit Care Clin* 9:219, 1993.

42. Creehan PA: Toxic shock syndrome: an opportunity for nursing intervention, *J Obstet Gynecol Neonatal Nurs* 24:557, 1995.

43. Secor VH: The inflammatory/immune response in critical illness: role of the systemic inflammatory response syndrome, *Crit Care Nurs Clin North Am* 6:251, 1994.

44. Crowley SR: The pathogenesis of septic shock, *Heart Lung* 25:124, 1996.

45. Lawler DA: Hormonal response in sepsis, *Crit Care Nurs Clin North Am* 6:265, 1994.

46. Ackerman MH, Evans NJ, Ecklund MM: Systemic inflammatory response syndrome, sepsis, and nutritional support, *Crit Care Nurs Clin North Am* 6:321, 1994.

47. Wiessner WH, Casey LC, Zbilut JP: Treatment of sepsis and septic shock: a review, *Heart Lung* 24:380, 1995.

48. Cipolle MD, Pasquale MD, Cerra F: Secondary organ dysfunction from clinical perspective to molecular mediators, *Crit Care Clin* 8:261, 1993.

49. Matuschak GM: Multiple systems organ failure: clinical expression, pathogenesis, and therapy. In Hall JB, Schmidt GA, Wood LD, editors: *Principles of critical care*, New York, 1992, McGraw-Hill.

50. Cerra FB: The multiple organ failure syndrome, *Hosp Pract* 25(15):169, 1990.

51. Cerra FB: The syndrome of hypermetabolism and multiple systems organ failure. In Hall JB, Schmidt GA, Wood LD, editors: *Principles of critical care*, New York, 1992, McGraw-Hill.

52. Bone RC, Sprung CL, Sibbald WJ: Definitions for sepsis and organ failure, *Crit Care Med* 20:724, 1992.

53. Pinsky MR: Multiple systems organ failure: malignant intravascular inflammation, *Crit Care Clin* 5:195, 1989.

54. Pinsky MR, Matuschak GM: Multiple systems organ failure: failure of host defense homeostasis, *Crit Care Clin* 5:199, 1989.

55. Deitch EA: Gut failure: its role in the multiple organ failure syndrome. In Deitch EA, editor: *Multiple organ failure: pathophysiology and basic concepts of therapy*, New York, 1990, Thieme Medical.

56. Bone RC: Toward a theory regarding the pathogenesis of the systemic inflammatory response syndrome: what we do and do not know about cytokine regulation, *Crit Care Med* 24:163, 1996.

57. Rote NS: Inflammation. In McCance KL, Huether SE, editors: *Pathophysiology: the biologic basis for disease in adults and children*, ed 3, St Louis, 1998, Mosby.

58. Yurt RW, Lowry SF: Role of the macrophage and endogenous mediators in multiple organ failure. In Deitch EA, editor: *Multiple organ failure: pathophysiology and basic concepts of therapy*, New York, 1990, Thieme Medical.

59. Bishop M, et al: Prospective trial of supranormal values in severely traumatized patients, *Crit Care Med* 20:S93, 1992 (abstract).

60. Bell TN: Disseminated intravascular coagulation and shock, *Crit Care Nurs Clin* 2:255, 1990.

61. Cerra FB: Hypermetabolism-organ failure syndrome: a metabolic response to injury, *Crit Care Clin* 5:289, 1989.

62. Cerra FB: Nutritional pharmacology: its role in the hypermetabolism-organ failure syndrome, *Crit Care Med* 18:S154, 1990.

63. Waxman K: Postoperative multiple organ failure, *Crit Care Clin* 3:429, 1987.

64. Knaus WA, Wagner DP: Multiple systems organ failure: epidemiology and prognosis, *Crit Care Clin* 5:221, 1989.

65. Zimmerman JJ, Ringer TV: Inflammatory host responses in sepsis, *Crit Care Clin* 8:163, 1992.

66. Van Saene HK, Stoutenbeek CC, Stoller JK: Selective decontamination of the digestive tract in the intensive care unit: current status and future prospects, *Crit Care Med* 20:691, 1992.

67. Vickers SM, Bailey RW, Bulkley GB: Ischemic hepatitis. In Marston A, et al, editors: *Splanchnic ischemia and multiple organ failure*, St Louis, 1989, Mosby.

68. Marshall JC, et al: Multiple organs dysfunction score: a reliable descriptor of a complex clinical outcome, *Crit Care Med* 23:1638, 1995.

69. Haglund UH, Arvidsson D: Acute acalculous cholecystitis. In Marston A, et al, editors: *Splanchnic ischemia and multiple organ failure*, St Louis, 1989, Mosby.

70. Murray JF, et al: An expanded definition of the adult respiratory distress syndrome, *Am Rev Respir Dis* 138:720, 1988.

71. Gamelli RL, Silver GM: Acute renal failure. In Deitch EA, editor: *Multiple organ failure: pathophysiology and basic concepts of therapy*, New York, 1990, Thieme Medical.

72. Berstern A, Sibbald WJ: Circulatory disturbances in multiple systems organ failure, *Crit Care Clin* 5:233, 1989.

73. Shoemaker WC, Kram HB, Appel PL: Therapy of shock based on pathophysiology, monitoring, and outcome prediction, *Crit Care Med* 18:S19, 1990.

74. Vincent JL, De Backer D: Initial management of circulatory shock as prevention of MSOF, *Crit Care Clin* 5:369, 1989.

75. Kumar A, et al: Tumor necrosis factor produces depression of myocardial cell contraction in vitro, *Crit Care Med* 20:S52, 1992 (abstract).

76. Guyton AC: *Textbook of medical physiology*, ed 9, Philadelphia, 1996, WB Saunders.

77. Macho JR, Luce JM: Rational approach to the management of multiple systems organ failure, *Crit Care Clin* 5:379, 1989.

78. Sheagren JN: Mechanism-oriented therapy for multiple systems organ failure, *Crit Care Clin* 5:393, 1989.

79. Feustel PJ, et al: Oxygen delivery and consumption in head-injured and multiple trauma patients, *J Trauma* 30:30, 1990.

80. Edwards JD: Use of survivors' cardiopulmonary values as therapeutic goals in septic shock, *Crit Care Med* 17:1098, 1989.

81. Lehman S: Nutritional support in the hypermetabolic patient, *Crit Care Nurs Clin North Am* 5:97, 1993.

82. Daly JM, Lieberman MD, Goldfine L: Enteral nutrition with supplemental arginine, RNA, and omega-3 fatty acids in patients after operation: immunologic, metabolic and clinical outcome, *Surgery* 112:56, 1992.

83. Keithley J, Eisenberg P: The significance of enteral nutrition in the intensive care unit patient, *Crit Care Nurs Clin North Am* 5:23, 1993.

84. Moore FA, Felicano DV, Andrassy RJ: Early enteral feeding compared with parenteral reduces postoperative septic complications, *Ann Surg* 216:172, 1992.

NURSING MANAGEMENT PLANS OF CARE

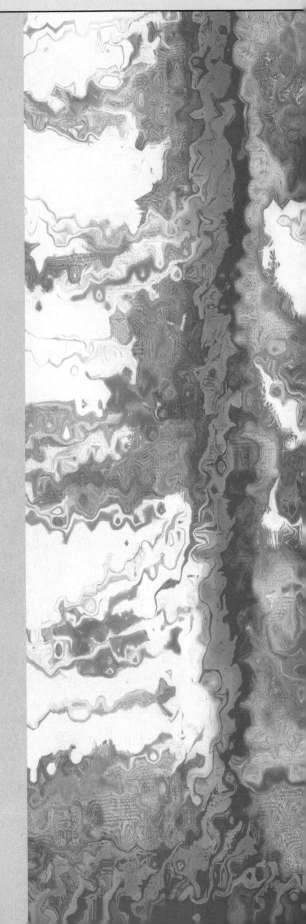

NURSING MANAGEMENT OF PATIENT EDUCATION

NURSING MANAGEMENT PLAN OF CARE	KNOWLEDGE DEFICIT

DEFINITION

Absence or deficiency of cognitive information related to a specific topic.

Knowledge Deficit _____ (Specify) Related to Cognitive/Perceptual Learning Limitations (e.g., sensory overload, sleep deprivation, medications, anxiety, sensory deficits, language barrier)

DEFINING CHARACTERISTICS

- Verbalized statement of inadequate knowledge of skills
- Verbalization of inadequate recall of information
- Verbalization of inadequate understanding of information
- Evidence of inaccurate follow-through of instructions
- Inadequate demonstration of a skill
- Lack of compliance with prescribed behavior

OUTCOME CRITERIA

- Patient participates actively in necessary and prescribed health behaviors.
- Patient verbalizes adequate knowledge or demonstrates adequate skills.

NURSING INTERVENTIONS AND *RATIONALE*

1. Continue to monitor the assessment parameters listed under "Defining Characteristics."
2. Determine specific cause of patient's cognitive or perceptual limitation. (See also nursing management plans of care, Impaired Verbal Communication, p. 483; Anxiety, p. 448; Sleep Pattern Disturbance, p. 458; and Acute Confusion, p. 444.)
3. Provide uninterrupted rest period before teaching session *to decrease fatigue and encourage optimal state for learning and retention.*
4. Manipulate environment as much as possible *to provide quiet and uninterrupted learning sessions:*
   Ensure lights are bright enough to see teaching aids but not too bright.
   Close door if necessary *to provide quiet environment.*
   Schedule care and medications *to allow uninterrupted teaching periods.*
   Move patient to quiet, private room for teaching *if possible.*

5. Adapt teaching sessions and materials to patient's and family's levels of education and ability to understand:
   Provide printed material appropriate to reading level.
   Use terminology understood by the patient.
   Provide printed materials in patient's primary language *if possible.*
   Use interpreters during teaching sessions *when necessary.*
6. Teach only present-tense focus during periods of sensory overload.
7. Determine potential effects of medications on ability to retain or recall information. Avoid teaching critical content while patient is taking sedatives, analgesics, or other medications affecting memory.
8. Reinforce new skills and information in several teaching sessions. Use several senses when possible in teaching session (e.g., see a film, hear a discussion, read printed information, and demonstrate skills related to self-injection of insulin).
9. Reduce patient's anxiety:
   Listen attentively and encourage verbalization of feelings.
   Answer questions as they arise in a clear and succinct manner.
   Elicit patient's concerns and address those issues first.
   Give only correct and relevant information.
   Continually assess response to teaching session and discontinue if anxiety increases or physical condition becomes unstable.
   Provide nonthreatening information before more anxiety-producing information is presented.
   Plan for several teaching sessions so information can be divided into small manageable packages.

NURSING MANAGEMENT PLAN OF CARE — **KNOWLEDGE DEFICIT—cont'd**

Knowledge Deficit _____ (Specify) Related to Lack of Previous Exposure to Information

DEFINING CHARACTERISTICS

- Verbalized statement of inadequate knowledge or skills
- New diagnosis or health problem requiring self-management or care
- Lack of prior formal or informal education about the specific health problem
- Demonstration of inappropriate behaviors related to management of health problem

OUTCOME CRITERIA

- Patient verbalizes adequate knowledge about or performs skills related to disease process, its causes, factors related to onset of symptoms, and self-management of disease or health problem.
- Patient actively participates in health behaviors required for performance of a procedure or in those behaviors enhancing recovery from illness and preventing recurrence or complications.

NURSING INTERVENTIONS AND *RATIONALE*

1. Continue to monitor the assessment parameters listed under "Defining Characteristics."
2. Determine existing level of knowledge or skill.
3. Assess factors affecting the knowledge deficit:
   Learning needs, including patient's priorities and the necessary knowledge and skills for safety
   Learning ability of client, including language skills, level of education, ability to read, preferred learning style
   Physical ability to perform prescribed skills or procedures; consider effect of limitations imposed by treatment such as bedrest, restriction of movement by intravenous or other equipment, or effect of sedatives or analgesics
   Psychologic effect of stage of adaptation to disease
   Activity tolerance and ability to concentrate
   Motivation to learn new skills or gain new knowledge

4. Reduce or limit barriers to learning:
   Provide consistent nurse-patient contact *to encourage development of trusting and therapeutic relationship.*
   Structure environment *to enhance learning;* control unnecessary noise, interruptions.
   Individualize teaching plan *to fit patient's current physical and psychologic status.*
   Delay teaching until patient is ready to learn.
   Conduct teaching sessions during period of day when patient is most alert and receptive.
   Meet patient's immediate learning needs as they arise (e.g., give brief explanation of procedures when they are performed).
5. Promote active participation in the teaching plan by the patient and family:
   Solicit input during development of plan.
   Develop mutually acceptable goals and outcomes.
   Solicit expression of feelings and emotions related to new responsibilities.
   Encourage questions.
6. Conduct teaching sessions, using the most appropriate teaching methods:
   Discussion
   Lecture
   Demonstration/return demonstration
   Use of audiovisual or printed educational materials
7. Repeat key principles and provide them in printed form *for reference at a later time.*
8. Give frequent feedback to patient when practicing new skills.
9. Use several teaching sessions when appropriate. *New information and skills should be reinforced several times after initial learning.*
10. Initiate referrals for follow-up if necessary:
    Health educators
    Home health care
    Rehabilitation programs
    Social services
11. Evaluate effectiveness of teaching plan, based on patient's ability to meet preset goals and objectives, and determine need for further teaching.

NURSING MANAGEMENT OF PSYCHOSOCIAL ALTERATIONS

NURSING MANAGEMENT PLAN OF CARE	ACUTE CONFUSION

DEFINITION

The abrupt onset of a cluster of global, transient changes and disturbances in attention, cognition, psychomotor activity level of consciousness, and/or sleep/wake cycle.

Acute Confusion Related to Sensory Overload, Sensory Deprivation, and Sleep Pattern Disturbance

DEFINING CHARACTERISTICS

(At least two of the following)

Early Symptoms

- Sudden onset of global cognitive function impairment (from hours to days)
- Restlessness, agitation, and combative behavior
- Drowsiness (can lead to loss of consciousness)
- Slurring of speech, inappropriate statements or "word salad," mumbling or inappropriate gestures
- Short attention span (needs questions repeated); inability to learn new material
- Disordered awake-sleep cycle
- Disorientation to person, time, place, and situation
- Difficulty in separating dreams from reality (may experience bizarre dreams/nightmares)
- Anger at staff for continued questions about his or her orientation

Later Symptoms

- Symptoms that tend to fluctuate throughout the day and night
- Early symptoms continue and may be more frequent and of longer duration
- Illusions
- Hallucinations
- Extreme agitation (e.g., attempts to climb out of bed, pull out catheters, rip off dressings)
- Calling out in loud voice, swearing, or attempting to bite or hit people who approach patient

CONTRIBUTING FACTORS

- Fluid and electrolyte imbalances
- Potential for organ dysfunction (hepatic, renal, gastrointestinal, cardiac, respiratory) caused by inadequate oxygenation
- Delay in metabolism and excretion of drugs, thus prolonging half-life and increasing drugs' effect or interaction with other drugs
- Immune-suppressant drug side effects
- Narcotic analgesics
- Hypersensitivity to drugs
- Surgical time (or time on bypass equipment) more than 4 hours of duration
- Stressors in critical care unit
- Physical and mental status of patient before surgery (preexisting medical conditions such as diabetes, epilepsy, neoplasm)
- Withdrawal symptoms, such as those from alcohol, drugs, or amphetamines
- Availability of social/spiritual/family support

NURSING INTERVENTIONS AND RATIONALE

1. Continue to monitor the assessment parameters listed under "Defining Characteristics." In addition, determine and document the patient's dominant spoken language, his or her literacy, and the language(s) in which he or she is literate. Determine and document his or her premorbid degree of orientation, cognitive capabilities, and any sensory-perceptual deficits. *It is sometimes the case that people are not literate in their spoken language or, less commonly, that they are literate only in their second language. These situations can result in unfortunate errors in the appraisal of patients' ability to communicate in writing and in estimating the extent of their orientation. Similarly, assuming that the patients were or were not fully oriented before critical care admission bases the nurse's assessment on possibly erroneous assumptions.*

For sensory overload

1. Initiate each nurse-patient encounter by calling the patient by name and identifying yourself by name. *This fosters reality orientation and assists the patient in filtering irrelevant or impersonal conversation.*
2. Assess the patient's immediate physical environment from his or her viewpoint, and explain equipment, its sounds, and its therapeutic purpose. Demonstrate audible and visual alarms, and explain the possible alarm conditions. *This decreases alienation of the patient from the technologic environment and reduces the inherent sense of fear and urgency accompanying alarm conditions.*

NURSING MANAGEMENT PLAN OF CARE	ACUTE CONFUSION—cont'd

NURSING INTERVENTIONS AND RATIONALE—cont'd

For sensory overload—cont'd

3. For each procedure performed, provide "preparatory sensory information" (i.e., explain procedures in relation to the sensations the patient will experience, including duration of sensations). *Preparatory sensory information enhances learning and lessens anticipatory anxiety.*

4. Limit noise levels. Certainly, audible alarms cannot and must not be silenced, and many critical, albeit noisy, activities must take place in the critical care area. It has been shown, however, that noise levels produced by clinical personnel exceed those levels designated as "acceptable" and are often greater than those generated by technologic devices. Staff conversations must be kept soft enough that they are inaudible to the patient whenever possible. Critical care personnel are to assume that everything said at or around a patient's bedside is intended for that patient's awareness and that it will be interpreted as pertaining to him or her. *As in the discussion that follows, conversations about the patient but not to him or her foster depersonalization and delusions of reference.*

5. Well-enforced noise limits need to exist for nighttime.

6. Readjust alarm limits on physiologic monitoring devices as the patient's condition changes (improves or deteriorates) *to lessen unnecessary alarm states.*

7. Consider use of head phones and audio cassette or compact disc player with patient's favorite and/or subliminal or classical music. *This can effectively filter out assaultive noise of the critical care environment and supplant it with familiar, soothing sounds and rhythms.*

8. Modify lighting. Day-night cycles need to be simulated with environmental lighting. At no time should overhead fluorescent lights be abruptly turned on without either warning the patient, assisting him or her out of the supine position, and/or shielding his or her eyes with gauze or a face cloth. *Continuous bright lighting sustains anxiety and promotes circadian rhythm desynchronization.*

9. To the extent possible, shield patients from viewing urgent and emergent events in the critical care unit. *Resuscitation efforts, albeit difficult to conceal, engender fear in the patient and a sense of instability and vulnerability (e.g., "I'm next").* When such an event occurs, the nurse needs to elicit the patient's cognitive and emotional reaction; thoughts, impressions, and feelings need to be shared and misconceptions clarified. A useful approach for the nurse in this interchange is that of emphasizing the differences between the patient at hand and the one resuscitated (e.g., "He was considerably older," "more unstable," "had serious lung disease").

10. Ensure patients' privacy, their modesty, and, at the very least, their dignity. Physical exposure and nudity, although seeming to pale in importance alongside such priorities as physiologic assessment and stabilization, are primal indignities in all individuals. Patients must be kept minimally exposed. When, in the course of assessment and intervention, it becomes necessary to expose the patient, the nurse is to first verbally apologize for this necessity. *To be naked is to feel vulnerable; to be vulnerable is to feel fearful. In this regard, fear is an emotion concomitant to critical care that is preventable through nursing intervention.*

For sensory deprivation

1. Provide reality orientation in four spheres (person, place, time, and situation) at more frequent intervals than when testing. Convey this information in the context of routine conversation. *Sample statements:* "Mr. Clark, this is Tuesday morning and you're in University Hospital. Your heart surgery was yesterday morning, and you're doing well. My name is Joe, and I'm your nurse today." *The patient is made to feel patronized by repetitions such as, "Do you know where you are?"* Given the effects of general anesthesia, narcotic analgesics, sedatives, and sleep, it is fully expected that some degree of disorientation will exist normally.

2. Ensure the patient's visual access to a calendar. (Of interest, the design of most state-of-the-art critical care units now reflects many of the principles of sensory stimulation. One such coronary care unit was designed with a large wall clock facing the patient. A patient who had spent more than 1 week in this unit later reflected that one of the most "distressing, frustrating" aspects of his stay in the coronary care unit was the monotonous, inescapable attention to the clock and its painfully slow documentation of the passing of time.)

3. Apprise the patient of daily news events and the weather.

4. Touch patients for the express purpose of communicating caring. Hold their hands, stroke their

Continued

NURSING INTERVENTIONS AND RATIONALE—cont'd

For sensory deprivation—cont'd

brows, rub the skin on an aspect of their arms. *Touch is the universal language of caring. In the setting of critical care, in which there is considerable physical body manipulation, it is useful and important to contrast assaultive touch with comforting touch.* Touch can be used as a technique for distraction from painful stimuli when used in conjunction with uncomfortable procedures.

5. Foster liberal visitation by family and significant others. Encourage significant others to touch the patient as consistent with their individual comfort level and cultural norms.

6. Structure and identify opportunities for the patient to exercise decision-making skills, however small. *Although not so designated, patients with sensory alterations experience a type of "cognitive deprivation" as well.*

7. Assist patients to find meaning in their experiences. Explain the therapeutic purpose of all that they are asked to do for themselves and all that is done with them and for them. Avoid statements such as, "Will you turn to that side for me?" or "I need you to swallow this medication." *These statements implicitly convey that the maneuver has some value for the nurses versus the patients.* Similarly, use "thank you" judiciously. *This simple salutation, when used indiscriminately, suggests something was done to benefit the nurses and not the patients.* Patients need to find meaning and to identify their roles in the experience of critical illness and critical care. The sensations that constitute this experience and those that do not are made bearable and intelligible when attached to the larger picture of their conditions, treatment, and progress.

For sleep pattern disturbances

For excellent management strategies of sleep pattern disturbance, see nursing management plan of care, Sleep Pattern Disturbance, pp. 458-459.

For management of the patient experiencing hallucinations

1. Approach the patient with a calm, matter-of-fact demeanor. *The goal of this interaction is for the nurse to demonstrate external control. This helps decrease the anxiety and fear that generally accompany hallucinations and allows the patient to feel safe. Anxiety is transferrable.*

2. Address the patient by name. *This is a useful presentation of reality because self-identity is the last sphere of orientation to vanish.*

3. In responding to the patient's description of the hallucination, DO NOT deny, argue, or attempt to disprove the existence of the perceived event. *Statements such as, "There are no voices coming from that air vent" or, "Look, I'm brushing my hand across the wall, and there are no bugs" confuse the patient further, because the hallucination, although frightening, is his or her perceived reality.*

4. Express to the patient that your experiences are dissimilar, and acknowledge how frightening his or hers must be. *Sample statement:* "I don't hear (see, etc.) what you do, but I know how frightening such an experience must be to you. I'm Joe, your nurse, and I'm going to stay with you until the voices (etc.) go away." Remain with any patient who is experiencing a hallucination. *Feelings of fear and anxiety often accelerate when a patient is left alone. He or she needs someone to represent a nonthreatening reality. In addition, validating the patient's feelings demonstrates acceptance and sensitivity to the experience and promotes trust.*

5. DO NOT explore the content of the hallucination with the patient by asking about its nature or character. *The nurse is the patient's link with reality. Pursuit of a detailed description of a hallucination may signify to the patient that the nurse accepts his or her sensory distortion as factual. This may further confuse the patient and distance him or her more from reality.* The nurse can help bridge the gap between the patient's misperception and reality by addressing the feelings (e.g., fear, anxiety) and/or meanings (e.g., danger, death) engendered by the hallucination. Determination of how the misperception affects the patient emotionally; acknowledgment of those feelings, and a calm, controlled, matter-of-fact approach will provide the trust and comfort he or she needs to tolerate this frightening experience. In other words, deal with the intent more than the content of the hallucination. *The resultant decrease in anxiety will enable the patient to focus more accurately on his or her immediate environment.*

---

*An exception is the patient who the nurse suspects is experiencing auditory hallucinations (i.e., hearing "voice commands"). To ascertain that the voices are not telling the patient to harm himself or herself, it is appropriate for the nurse to ask simply and concretely, "What are the voices saying?"

NURSING MANAGEMENT PLAN OF CARE	**ACUTE CONFUSION—cont'd**

NURSING INTERVENTIONS AND RATIONALE—cont'd

For management of the patient experiencing hallucinations—cont'd

6. Talk concretely with the patient about things that are really happening. *Sample statements:* "How does your chest incision feel this afternoon, Mr. Clark?" "Your sister Kate was here to see you, but you were sleeping. She went down to the cafeteria and will be back." "Your secretions are a little easier for you to cough up today." *Interpretation of reality-based stimuli by the nurse encourages the patient to focus on actual circumstances and discourages a preoccupation with sensory misperceptions.*

7. There may be circumstances in which it is appropriate for the nurse simply to distract the patient by changing the topic. This tactic is useful in situations of escalating anxiety and confusion or when all else fails. Topics need to consist of basic themes that are universally understood and culturally congruent, such as music, food, or weather. They may also be topics of special interest to the patient, such as hobbies, crafts, or sports. Topics that evoke strong emotions, such as politics, religion, or sexuality, are to be avoided with most patients. *This is especially true of the patient with reality distortions; sometimes hallucinations and delusions are expressions of repressed conflicts associated with religious, sexual, or aggressive issues. Pursuit of such subjects could increase confusion and anxiety.*

8. The use of touch: *Touch presents a nonthreatening external reality and can therefore be useful in the management of patients with sensory alterations. However, in the patient experiencing hallucinations (as well as delusions and illusions), touch can be readily misinterpreted as, for instance, aggression or pain, or it can actually provide the basis for a tactile illusion.* Therefore the use of touch as an intervention strategy is to be avoided in any patient who demonstrates escalating anxiety or paranoid, suspicious, or mistrustful thoughts.

9. Types of hallucinations include the following: auditory—voices or running commentaries, with self-destructive messages; visual—persons or images that appear threatening; olfactory—smells that may be interpreted as poisonous gases; gustatory—tastes that seem peculiar or harmful; and tactile—touch that feels unusual or unnatural.

10. Specific management strategies for patients experiencing hallucinations:
    - Auditory hallucinations
      a. Patient behaviors: Head cocked as if listening to an unseen presence; lips moving.
      b. Therapeutic nurse responses: "Mr. Clark, you appear to be listening to something." If patient acknowledges voices: "I don't hear any voices, but I know this is troubling you. The voices will go away. Nothing is going to harm you. I'm Joe, your nurse, and I'll be here with you."
      c. Nontherapeutic nurse responses: "Tell me about your conversations with these voices." "To whom do the voices belong—anyone you know?"
    - Visual hallucinations
      a. Patient behaviors: Staring into space as if focused on an unseen object; startled movements and anxious facial expression.
      b. Therapeutic nurse responses: "Mr. Clark, something seems to be troubling you. Tell me what it is." If patient states he visualizes people, images, or the devil in his environment and implies a sense of danger, respond, "There are only nurses and doctors here, Mr. Clark. I know this must be upsetting, but these images will go away. We're here with you in the hospital. Nothing will happen to you."
      c. Nontherapeutic nurse responses: "Describe the people you see. What are they wearing?" "What does the devil mean in your life? What about God?"

For management of the patient experiencing delusions

1. Explain all unseen noises, voices, and activity simply and clearly. *They readily feed a delusional system. Sample statements:* "That is Dr. Smith. He's come to see you and other patients here in the hospital." "The voices and activity you hear are from the bedside of the patient behind this curtain. He's being helped by one of the nurses."

2. Avoid the "negative challenge" (e.g., "Nobody here stole your belongings" or "Doctors and nurses do not harm people") of the patient's delusion. Similarly, avoid defending the referents of the patient's belief: "Nurses are good" and "Doctors mean well." *Remember, a delusion is a belief, albeit false, that cannot be changed with logic. To attempt this change is to challenge the*

Continued

NURSING MANAGEMENT PLAN OF CARE — ACUTE CONFUSION—cont'd

NURSING INTERVENTIONS AND *RATIONALE*—cont'd

For management of the patient experiencing delusions—cont'd

patient's belief system and thereby escalate his or her anxiety, further blurring the boundaries between reality and the patient's internally based "logic."

3. For the patient with persecutory delusions who refuses food, fluids, or medications because of a belief they have been poisoned or tainted, permit the refusal unless it is a life-threatening event. Try again in 20 minutes; allow the patient to choose an alternative selection of food or to read the label on the unit's medication. Coercion, show of force, or engaging in complicated, logical justifications will only heighten the patient's suspiciousness and possibly reinforce the delusional belief. *When the patient feels more in control, he or she need not rely on the "paradoxical" quality of the delusion to feel equipped with a false sense of power. His or her power instead is derived from making reality-based decisions.*

4. Staff members should be particularly careful not to engage in unnecessary laughter or whispering within view of the delusional patient. *The delusional patient is hypervigilant, scanning the environment for evidence to corroborate or confirm his or her belief that staff members are colluding against him or her; clearly, laughter and whispers easily suggest this belief, this delusion of reference. This rationale pertains to the patient experiencing hallucinations and/or illusions as well.*

5. Observe the principles detailed in the third intervention under management of the patient experiencing hallucinations, p. 446.

For management of the patient experiencing illusions

1. As with the management of delusions, the nurse simply and briefly interprets reality-based stimuli for the patient in a calm, matter-of-fact manner. *Seen and unseen noises, voices, activity, and people can provide the stimulus for a sensory misinterpretation, an illusion.*

2. The immediate environment of the patient must provide as low a level of stimulation as possible. Nursing interventions detailed previously under "Sensory Overload" are especially relevant here.

3. The theme of the nurse's verbal approach to the patient experiencing illusions is similar to that outlined for hallucinations and delusions: address the feelings and meanings associated with the experience, not the content of the sensory misinterpretation.
   - Patient behaviors: Eyes darting, startled movements; frightened facial expression. "I know who you are. You're the devil come to take me to hell."
   - Therapeutic nurse responses: "I'm Joe, your nurse. I know this experience is troubling for you. You're in the hospital, and no one here will harm you."
   - Nontherapeutic nurse responses: "There are no such things as devils or angels." "Do you think the devil would be dressed in white?" *The first nontherapeutic nurse response carries a parental tone (i.e., "you know better than that"), thus infantilizing the patient and adding to his or her feelings of powerlessness over the environment. The second nontherapeutic response reflects obvious logic, which is not in the patient's sensory domain; therefore it cannot be processed and only adds to his or her confused state.*

4. Observe the principles detailed under the fifth item in management of the patient experiencing hallucinations, p. 446.

NURSING MANAGEMENT PLAN OF CARE — ANXIETY

DEFINITION

A vague, uneasy feeling of discomfort or dread accompanied by an autonomic response; the source is often nonspecific or unknown to the individual; a feeling of apprehension caused by anticipation of danger.

Anxiety Related to Threat to Biologic, Psychologic, and/or Social Integrity

DEFINING CHARACTERISTICS

Subjective
- Verbalizes increased muscle tension
- Expresses frequent sensation of tingling in hands/feet
- Relates continuous feeling of apprehension
- Expresses preoccupation with a sense of impending doom
- States has difficulty falling asleep
- Repeatedly expresses concerns about changes in health status and outcome of illness

NURSING MANAGEMENT PLAN OF CARE   ANXIETY—cont'd

NURSING INTERVENTIONS AND RATIONALE—cont'd

Objective

- Psychomotor agitation (fidgeting, jitteriness, restlessness)
- Tightened, wrinkled brow
- Strained (worried) facial expression
- Hypervigilance (scans environment)
- Startles easily
- Distractibility
- Sweaty palms
- Fragmented sleep patterns
- Tachycardia
- Tachypnea

OUTCOME CRITERIA

- Patient effectively uses learned relaxation strategies.
- Patient demonstrates significant decrease in psychomotor agitation.
- Patient verbalizes reduction in tingling sensations in hands and feet.
- Patient is able to focus on the tasks at hand.
- Patient expresses positive, futuristic plans to family and staff.
- Patient's heart rate and rhythm remain within limits commensurate with physiologic status.

NURSING INTERVENTIONS AND RATIONALE

1. Continue to monitor the assessment parameters listed under "Defining Characteristics."
2. Instruct the patient in the following simple, effective relaxation strategies:
   - If not contraindicated cardiovascularly, tense and relax all muscles progressively from toes to head.
   - Perform slow, deep-breathing exercises.
   - Focus on a single object or person in the environment.
   - Listen to soothing music or relaxation tapes with eyes closed.

   Progressive toe-to-head relaxation releases the muscular tension that may be a stress-related effect resulting from the threat or change in the patient's health status and outcome of illness. Deep-breathing exercises provide slow, rhythmic, controlled breathing patterns that relax the patient and distract him or her from the effects of his or her illness and hospitalization. Focusing on a single object or person helps the patient dismiss the myriad of disorienting stimuli from his or her visual-perceptual field, which can have a dizzying, distorted effect. A clear sensorium allows him or her to feel more

in control of his or her environment. Music or words expressed in soft, low tones tend to produce soothing, relaxing effects that counteract or inhibit escalating anxiety and provide respites from the patient's situational crisis. Closed eyes eliminate distracting, visual stimuli and promote a more restful environment.

3. Actively listen to and accept the patient's concerns regarding the threats from his or her illness, outcome, and hospitalization. *Active listening and unconditional acceptance validate the patient as a worthwhile individual and assure him or her that his or her concerns, no matter how great, will be addressed. Knowledge that he or she has an avenue for ventilation will assuage anxiety.*

4. Help the patient distinguish between realistic concerns and exaggerated fears through clear, simple explanations. *Sample statements:* "Your lab results show that you're doing OK right now." "The shortness of breath you're experiencing is not unusual." "The pain you described is expected, and this medication will relieve it." *A patient who is informed about his or her progress and is reassured about expected symptoms and management of care will be better equipped to maintain a more realistic perspective of his or her illness and its outcome. Thus anxiety emanating from imagined or exaggerated fears will likely be assuaged or averted.*

5. Provide simple clarification of environmental events and stimuli that are not related to the patient's illness and care. *Sample statements:* "That loud noise is coming from a machine that is helping another patient." "The visitor behind the curtain is crying because she's had an upsetting day." "That gurney is here to bring another patient to x-ray." *Clarification of events and stimuli that are unrelated to the patient helps to disengage him or her from the extant anxiety-provoking situations surrounding him or her, thus avoiding further anxiety and apprehension.*

6. Assist the patient in focusing on building on prior coping strategies to deal with the effects of his or her illness and care. *Sample statements:* "What methods have helped you get through difficult times in the past?" "How can we help you use those methods now?" (See nursing management plan of care, Ineffective Individual Coping, pp. 453-455, for interventions that assist patients to use coping strategies effectively.) *Use of previously successful coping strategies in conjunction with newly learned techniques arms the patient with an arsenal of weapons against*

Continued

NURSING MANAGEMENT PLAN OF CARE	ANXIETY—cont'd

NURSING INTERVENTIONS AND RATIONALE—cont'd

anxiety, providing him or her with greater control over his or her situational crisis and decreased feelings of doom and despair.

7. Give the patient permission to deny or suppress the effects of his or her illness and hospitalization with which he or she cannot cope or control. *Sample statements:* "It's perfectly OK to ignore things you can't handle right now."

"How can we help ease your mind during this time?" "What are some things or tasks that may help distract you?" *Adaptive denial can be helpful in reducing feelings of anxiety in patients with life-threatening illness.* Bigus* reports that in studies of two groups of patients with myocardial infarction, the group that used adaptive denial demonstrated significantly fewer symptoms of state anxiety than those patients who failed to use it.

*From Bigus KM: *West J Nurs Res* 3:150, 1981.

NURSING MANAGEMENT PLAN OF CARE	BODY IMAGE DISTURBANCE

DEFINITION

Confusion in mental picture of one's physical self.

Body Image Disturbance Related to Functional Dependence on Life-Sustaining Technology (ventilator, dialysis, IABP, halo traction)

DEFINING CHARACTERISTICS

- Actual change in function requiring permanent or temporary replacement
- Refusal to verify actual loss
- Verbalization of the following: feelings of helplessness, hopelessness, powerlessness, fear of failure to wean from technology

OUTCOME CRITERIA

- Patient verifies actual change in function.
- Patient does not refuse or fight technologic intervention.
- Patient verbalizes acceptance of expected change in lifestyle.

NURSING INTERVENTIONS AND RATIONALE

1. Continue to monitor the assessment parameters listed under "Defining Characteristics." In addition, assess patient's response to the technologic intervention.
2. Assess responses of family and significant others. *Body image is derived from the "reflected appraisals" of family and significant others.*
3. Provide information needed by patient and family.
4. Promote trust, security, comfort, and privacy.
5. Recognize anxiety. Allow and encourage its expression. *Anxiety is the most predominant emotion accompanying body image alterations.*
6. Assist patient to recognize his or her own functioning and performance in the face of technology. For example, assist the patient to distinguish spontaneous breaths from mechanically delivered breaths. *This activity will assist in weaning the patient from the ventilator when feasible. To establish realistic, accurate body boundaries, a patient needs help to separate himself or herself from the technology that is supporting his or her functioning. Any participation or function on the part of the patient during periods of dependency is helpful in preventing and/or resolving an alteration in body image.*
7. Plan for discontinuation of the treatment (e.g., weaning from ventilator). Explain procedure that will be followed, and be present during its initiation.
8. Plan for transfer from the critical care environment.
9. Document care, ensuring an up-to-date management plan is available for all involved caregivers.

NURSING MANAGEMENT PLAN OF CARE	BODY IMAGE DISTURBANCE—cont'd

Body Image Disturbance Related to Actual Change in Body Structure, Function, or Appearance

DEFINING CHARACTERISTICS

- Actual change in appearance, structure, or function
- Avoidance of looking at body part
- Avoidance of touching body part
- Hiding or overexposing body part (intentional or unintentional)
- Trauma to nonfunctioning part
- Change in ability to estimate spatial relationship of body to environment
- Verbalization of the following:
    Fear of rejection or reaction by others
    Negative feelings about body
    Preoccupation with change or loss
    Refusal to participate in or to accept responsibility for self-care of altered body part
- Personalization of part or loss with a name
- Depersonalization of part or loss by use of impersonal pronouns
- Refusal to verify actual change

OUTCOME CRITERIA

- Patient verbalizes the specific meaning of the change to him or her.
- Patient requests appropriate information about self-care.
- Patient completes personal hygiene and grooming daily with or without help.
- Patient interacts freely with family or other visitors.
- Patient participates in the discussions and conferences related to planning his or her medical and nursing management in the critical care unit and transfer from the unit.
- Patient talks with trained visitors (support group representatives) at least twice about his or her loss.

NURSING INTERVENTIONS AND RATIONALE

1. Continue to monitor the assessment parameters listed under "Defining Characteristics." In addition, assess patient's mental, physical, and emotional state; recognize assets, strengths, response to illness, position in Lee's phases, coping mechanisms, past experience with stress, and support systems.
2. Appraise the response of family and significant others. *Body image is derived from the "reflected appraisals" of family and significant others.*
3. Determine the patient's goals and readiness for learning.
4. Provide the necessary information to help the patient and family adapt to the change. Clarify misconceptions about future limitations.
5. Permit and encourage the patient to express the significance of the loss or change; note nonverbal behavioral responses.
6. Allow and encourage the patient's expression of anxiety. *Anxiety is the most predominant emotional response to a body image disturbance.*
7. Recognize and accept the use of denial as an adaptive defense mechanism when used early and temporarily.
8. Recognize maladaptive denial as that which interferes with the patient's progress and/or alienates support systems. Use confrontation.
9. Provide an opportunity for the patient to discuss sexual concerns.
10. Touch the affected body part *to provide patient with sensory information about altered body structure and/or function.*
11. Encourage and provide movement of altered body part *to establish kinesthetic feedback. This enables the person to know his or her body as it now exists.*
12. Prepare the patient to look at the body part. Call the body part by its anatomical name (e.g., stump, stoma, limb) as opposed to "it" or "she." *The use of impersonal pronouns increases a sense of fantasy and depersonalization of the body part.*
13. Allow the patient to experience excellence in some aspect of physical functioning—walking, turning, deep breathing, healing, self-care—and point out progress and accomplishment. *This helps to balance the patient's sense of dysfunction with function.*
14. Avoid false reassurance. Acknowledge the difficulty of incorporating the altered body part or function into one's body image. *This evidences the nurse's sensitivity and promotes trust.*
15. Talk with the patient about his or her life, generativity, and accomplishments. *Patients with disturbances in body image frequently see themselves in a distortedly "narrow" sense. Encouraging a wider focus of themselves and their life reduces this distortion.*
16. Help the patient explore realistic alternatives.
17. Recognize that incorporating a body change into one's body image takes time. Avoid setting unrealistic expectations and *thereby inadvertently reinforcing a low self-esteem.*
18. Suggest the use of additional resources such as trained visitors who have mastered situations similar to those of the patient. Refer patient to a psychiatric liaison nurse or psychiatrist if needed.

| NURSING MANAGEMENT PLAN OF CARE | INEFFECTIVE FAMILY COPING: COMPROMISED |

DEFINITION

A usually supportive primary person (family member or close friend) is providing insufficient, ineffective, or compromised support, comfort, assistance, or encouragement that may be needed by the client to manage or master adaptive tasks related to his or her health challenge.

Ineffective Family Coping: Compromised Related to Critically Ill Family Member

DEFINING CHARACTERISTICS

- Disruption of usual family functions and roles.
- Inability to accept or deal with crisis situation; use of defense mechanisms (e.g., denial, anger); unrealistic expectations of patient's outcome and care provided; judgmental toward health care providers.
- Nonrecognition that family is in state of crisis.
- Inappropriate emotional outbursts; arguments among family and with others; inability to respond to each other's feelings or support each other.
- Misinterpretation of information; short attention span with repeated questions about information already provided; members do not share information with each other.
- Inability to make decisions regarding changes in family structure or about course of care for ill member; noncooperation among family members.
- Expressions of grief, hopelessness, powerlessness, and isolation; do not seek or respond to support services.
- Hesitancy to spend time with ill person in the critical care unit, or inappropriate behavior when visiting (may upset patient.)
- Neglect of own personal health; fatigue, apathy; refuse offers for respite time.

OUTCOME CRITERIA

- The family will express an understanding of course/prognosis of illness, therapies, and alternative measures.
- The family will diminish or resolve conflicts and cooperate in decision making.
- The family will develop trust and mutual support for each member and form a cohesive unit.
- The family will support ill person in making decisions (if capable) or respect prior wishes regarding provision of health care.
- Family efforts will be directed toward a purpose and readjust to changes in life patterns and role functions. Members will accept responsibility for changes.
- The family will identify and use effective coping strategies.
- The family will identify and use available resources as needed to facilitate resolution of the crisis.

- The family will have a sense of control and confidence in meeting personal and collective needs.

NURSING INTERVENTIONS AND *RATIONALE*

1. Identify family's perception of the crisis situation. Determine family structure; roles; developmental phase; and ethnic, cultural, and belief factors that may affect communication with family and the plan of care. Identify strengths of family. *All initial nursing interventions should be directed toward resolving the crisis situation. Understanding and use of family theory principles will facilitate this process and individualize care.*
2. Provide honest and accurate information in language persons can understand. Give updated information as appropriate. Listen! *This facilitates open communication between family and health care providers, projects a caring attitude and concern for them and patient, and assists family in making decision and being involved with the plan and goals of care.*
3. Encourage liberal visitation with patient. Prepare family for what they will observe in a technical environment before the visit. Inform them about patient's appearance, behaviors (etc.) that may be distressing to them. Explain the etiology of patient responses to stimuli, (e.g., pain, trauma, surgery, medication) and explain that these behaviors are being monitored and are usually temporary. Encourage them to touch the patient and let the patient know of their presence. *This prevents a strong emotional reaction to an unfamiliar and frightening situation; involves family as support to each other and to patient; demonstrates the nurse's concern for them as persons; and facilitates satisfaction with care being provided for their loved one.*
4. Identify and support effective coping behaviors. *This aids in family's sense of control and resolution of helplessness/powerlessness.*
5. Observe for signs of fatigue and the need for emotional/spiritual support and respite from hospital waiting routine. Encourage family to verbalize feelings. Provide information on available resources. Alert interdisciplinary team members (social, psychologic/spiritual) to family

NURSING INTERVENTIONS AND RATIONALE—cont'd

needs. Provide pager device (if available), or obtain phone numbers when family leaves hospital premises. *This provides support, comfort; facilitates hope; resolves sense of isolation; gives sense of security; and diminishes guilt feelings for attending to personal needs.*

6. Instruct family in simple caregiving techniques and encourage participation in patient's care. *This facilitates a sense of "normalcy" to experience, self-confidence, and assurance that good care is being provided.*

7. Serve as advocate for patient and family. Teach family how to negotiate with the health care delivery system and include them in health care team conferences when appropriate. *This facilitates informed decision making; promotes control, satisfaction; and permits mutual goal setting.*

8. Consider nonbiologic or nonlegal family relationships. Encourage contact with patient and participation in care. *This facilitates holistic care and support of emotional ties and demonstrates respect for the family unit and relationships.*

9. Provide emotional support, compassion when patient's condition worsens or deteriorates. *The use of touch and expression of concern for the patient and family conveys comfort and trust in the health care provider and respect and assurance that the family's loved one will receive appropriate care and attention.*

NURSING MANAGEMENT PLAN OF CARE   **INEFFECTIVE INDIVIDUAL COPING**

DEFINITION

Inability to form valid appraisal of stressors, inadequate choices of practiced responses, and/or inability to use available resources.

Ineffective Individual Coping Related to Situational Crisis and Personal Vulnerability

DEFINING CHARACTERISTICS

- Verbalization of inability to cope. *Sample statements:* "I can't take this anymore." "I don't know how to deal with this."
- Ineffective problem solving (problem lumping). *Sample statements:* "I have to eliminate salt from my diet. They tell me I can no longer mow the lawn. This hospitalization is costing a mint. What about my kids' future? Who's going to change the oil in the car? This is an incredible amount of time away from work."
- Ineffective use of coping mechanisms.
   Projection: blames others for illness or pain.
   Displacement: directs anger and/or aggression toward family. *Sample statement:* "Get out of here. Leave me alone." Curses, shouts, or demands attention; strikes out or throws objects.
   Denial of severity of illness and need for treatment.
- Noncompliance. *Examples:* activity restriction; refusal to allow treatment or to take medications.
- Suicidal thoughts (verbalizes desire to end life).
- Self-directed aggression. *Examples:* disconnects or attempts to disconnect life-sustaining equipment; deliberately tries to harm self.

- Failure to progress from dependent to more independent state (refusal or resistance to care for self).

OUTCOME CRITERIA

- Patient verbalizes beginning ability to cope with illness, pain, and hospitalization. *Sample statements:* "I'm trying to do the best I can." "I want to help myself get better."
- Patient demonstrates effective problem solving (lists and prioritizes problems from most to least urgent).
- Patient uses effective behavioral strategies to manage the stress of illness and care.
- Patient demonstrates interest or involvement in illness or environment. *Examples:* patient does the following:
   Requests medications when anticipating pain.
   Questions course of treatment, progress, and prognosis.
   Asks for clarification of environmental stimuli and events.
   Seeks out supportive individuals in his or her environment.
   Uses coping mechanisms and strategies more effectively to manage situational crisis.
   Demonstrates significant reduction in impulsive, angry, or aggressive outbursts (projection, shouting, cursing) directed toward family.

Continued

NURSING MANAGEMENT PLAN OF CARE — INEFFECTIVE INDIVIDUAL COPING—cont'd

OUTCOME CRITERIA—cont'd

Verbalizes futuristic plans, with cessation of self-directed aggressive acts and suicidal thoughts. Willingly complies with treatment regimen. Begins to participate in self-care.

NURSING INTERVENTIONS AND RATIONALE

1. Continue to monitor the assessment parameters listed under "Defining Characteristics."
2. Actively listen and respond to patient's verbal and behavioral expressions. *Active listening signifies unconditional respect and acceptance for the patient as a worthwhile individual. It builds trust and rapport, guides the nurse toward problem areas, encourages the patient to express concerns, and promotes compliance.*
3. Offer effective coping strategies to help the patient better tolerate the stressors related to his or her illness and care. Give permission to vent feelings in a safe setting. *Sample statements:* "I don't blame you for feeling angry or frustrated." "Others who are ill like you have expressed similar feelings." "I will listen to anything you want to share with me." "We don't have to talk; I'd like to sit here with you." "It's perfectly OK to cry." *Individuals who are provided with opportunities to express their feelings will be better able to release pent-up emotions and derive a greater sense of relief and comfort. Thus they are less likely to resort to overly impulsive, aggressive acts, which may harm self or others.*
4. Inform the family of the patient's need to displace anger occasionally but that you will be working with the patient to help him or her release his or her feelings in a more constructive, effective way. *Family members who are well-informed are better equipped to cope with their loved one's emotional anguish and outbursts. They are less likely to waste energy on feelings of guilt, fear, anger, or despair and can use their strength to help the patient in more constructive ways. The knowledge that their loved one is being cared for emotionally, as well as physically, will offer family members a greater sense of comfort and understanding. They will feel nurtured and respected by the nurse's attempt to include them in the process.*
5. With the patient, list and number problems from most to least urgent. Assist him or her in finding immediate solutions for most urgent problems; postpone those that can wait; delegate some to family members; and help him or her acknowledge problems that are beyond his or her control. *Listing and numbering problems in an organized fashion help break them down into more manageable "pieces" so that the patient is better able to identify solutions for those that are solvable and to suppress those that are less relevant or not amenable to interventions.*
6. Identify individuals in the patient's environment who best help him or her to cope, as well as those who do not. Validate your observations with the patient. *Sample statements:* "I notice you seemed more relaxed during your daughter's visit." "After the clergy left, you were able to sleep a bit longer than usual; would you like to see him more often?" "Your grandson was a bit upset today; I'll be glad to talk to him if you like." *Supportive persons can invoke a calming effect on the patient's physiologic and psychologic states. Conversely, well-meaning but nonsupportive individuals can have a deleterious effect on the patient's ability to cope and must be carefully screened and counseled by the nurse.*
7. Teach the patient effective cognitive strategies to help him or her better manage the stress of critical illness and care. Help him or her construct pleasant thoughts, situations, or images that can simultaneously inhibit unpleasant realities. *Examples:* a day at the beach, a walk in the park, drinking a glass of wine, or being with a loved one. *Pleasant thoughts or images constructed during critical illness and care tend to inhibit or reduce the intensity of the unpleasant, stressful effects of the experience.*
8. Assist the patient in using coping mechanisms more effectively so he or she can better manage his or her situational crisis:
   Suppression of problems beyond his or her control.
   Compensation for illness and its effects; focusing on his or her strengths, interests, family, and spiritual beliefs.
   Adaptive displacement of anger, fear, or frustration through healthy, verbal expressions to staff.
   Effective use of coping mechanisms helps to assuage the patient's painful feelings in a safe setting. Thus the patient is strengthened and need not resort to the use of more ineffective defenses to eliminate anxiety.
9. Initiate a suicidal assessment if the patient verbalizes the desire to die, states that life is not worth living, or exhibits self-directed aggression. *Sample statement:* "We know this is a bad time for you. You're saying repeatedly that you want

NURSING MANAGEMENT PLAN OF CARE   INEFFECTIVE INDIVIDUAL COPING—cont'd

NURSING INTERVENTIONS AND RATIONALE—cont'd

to die. Are you planning to harm yourself?" If the response is yes, remain with the patient, alert staff members, and provide for psychiatric consultation as soon as possible. Continue to express concern to the patient and protect him or her from harm. *Suicidal thoughts as a result of ineffective coping or exhaustion of coping devices are not an uncommon occurrence in critically ill patients. If the mood state is distressing enough, a patient may seek relief by attempting a self-destructive act. Although the patient may not imminently have the energy to succeed in his or her attempt, voicing specific*

plans signifies a depressed mood state and a depletion of coping strategies. Thus immediate intervention is needed, since the attempt may be successful when the patient's energy is restored.

10. Encourage the patient to participate in self-care activities and treatment regimen in accordance with his or her level of progress. Offer praise for his or her efforts toward self-care. *Patients who take an active role in their own treatment and progress are less apt to feel like helpless or powerless victims. This greater sense of control over their illness and environment will guide them more swiftly toward becoming as independent as possible.*

NURSING MANAGEMENT PLAN OF CARE   POWERLESSNESS

DEFINITION

Perception that one's own action will not significantly affect an outcome; a perceived lack of control over a current situation or immediate happening.

Powerlessness Related to Lack of Control Over Current Situation and/or Disease Progression

DEFINING CHARACTERISTICS

Severe
- Verbal expressions of having no control or influence over situation
- Verbal expressions of having no control or influence over outcome
- Verbal expressions of having no control over self-care
- Depression over physical deterioration that occurs despite patient's compliance with regimens
- Apathy

Moderate
- Nonparticipation in care or decision making when opportunities are provided
- Expressions of dissatisfaction and frustration about inability to perform previous tasks and/or activities
- Lack of progress monitoring
- Expressions of doubt about role performance
- Reluctance to express true feelings, fearing alienation from caregivers
- Passivity
- Inability to seek information about care
- Dependence on others that may result in irritability, resentment, anger, and guilt
- No defense of self-care practices when challenged

Low
- Passivity

OUTCOME CRITERIA

- Patient verbalizes increased control over situation by wanting to do things his or her way.
- Patient actively participates in planning care.
- Patient requests needed information.
- Patient chooses to participate in self-care activities.
- Patient monitors progress.

NURSING INTERVENTIONS AND RATIONALE

1. Continue to monitor the assessment parameters listed under "Defining Characteristics." In addition, assess the patient's feelings and perception of the reasons for lack of power and sense of helplessness.
2. Determine as far as possible the patient's usual response to limited control situations. Determine through ongoing assessment the patient's usual locus of control (i.e., believes that influence over his or her life is exerted by luck, fate, powerful persons [external locus of control] or that influence is exerted through personal choices, selfeffort, self-determination [internal locus of control]).
3. Support patient's physical control of the environment by involving him or her in care activities; knock before entering room if appropriate; ask permission before moving personal belong

Continued

NURSING MANAGEMENT PLAN OF CARE — POWERLESSNESS—cont'd

NURSING INTERVENTIONS AND *RATIONALE*—cont'd

ings. Inform the patient that, although an activity may not be to his or her liking, it is necessary. *This gives the patient permission to express dissatisfaction with the environment and regimen.*

4. Personalize the patient's care using his or her preferred name. *This supports the patient's psychologic control.*
5. Provide the therapeutic rationale for all the patient is asked to do for himself or herself and for all that is being done for and with him or her. Reinforce the physician's explanations; clarify misconceptions about the illness situation and treatment plans. *This supports the patient's cognitive control.*
6. Include patient in care planning by encouraging participation and allowing choices wherever possible (e.g., timing of personal care activities and deciding when pain medicines are needed). Point out situations in which no choices exist.
7. Provide opportunities for the patient to exert influence over himself or herself and his or her body, thereby affecting an outcome. For example, share with the patient the nurse's assessment of his or her breath sounds and explain that they can be improved by self-initiated deep breathing exercises. *Feedback that the patient has been successful in helping clear his or her lungs reinforces the influence he or she does retain.*

8. Encourage family to permit patient to do as much independently as possible *to foster perceptions of personal power.*
9. Assist the patient to establish realistic short-term and long-term goals. *Setting unrealistic or unattainable goals inadvertently reinforces the patient's perception of powerlessness.*
10. Document care to provide for continuity *so that the patient can maintain appropriate control over the environment.*
11. Assist the patient to regain strength and activity tolerance as appropriate, *thus increasing a sense of control and self-reliance.*
12. Increase the sensitivity of the health team members and significant others to the patient's sense of powerlessness. Use power over the patient carefully. Use the words "must," "should," and "have to" with caution, *because they communicate coercive power and imply that the objects of "musts" and "shoulds" are of benefit to the nurse versus the patient.*
13. Plan with the patient for transfer from the critical care unit to the intermediate unit and eventually to home.

NURSING MANAGEMENT PLAN OF CARE — SELF-ESTEEM DISTURBANCE

DEFINITION

Negative self-evaluation/feelings about self or self-capabilities, which may be directly or indirectly expressed.

Self-Esteem Disturbance Related to Feelings of Guilt About Physical Deterioration

DEFINING CHARACTERISTICS

- Inability to accept positive reinforcement
- Lack of follow-through
- Nonparticipation in therapy
- Not taking responsibility for self-care (i.e., self-neglect)
- Self-destructive behavior
- Lack of eye contact

OUTCOME CRITERIA

- Patient verbalizes feelings of self-worth.
- Patient maintains positive relationships with significant others.
- Patient manifests active interest in appearance by completing personal grooming daily.

NURSING INTERVENTIONS AND *RATIONALE*

1. Continue to monitor the assessment parameters listed under "Defining Characteristics." In addition, assess the meaning of health-related situation. How does the patient feel about himself or herself, the diagnosis, and the treatment? How does the present fit into the larger context of his or her life?
2. Assess the patient's emotional level, interpersonal relationships, and feelings about himself or herself. Recognize the patient's uniqueness (how the hair is worn, preference for name used).
3. Help the patient discover and verbalize feelings and understand the crisis by listening and providing information.

NURSING MANAGEMENT PLAN OF CARE	SELF-ESTEEM DISTURBANCE—cont'd

NURSING INTERVENTIONS AND *RATIONALE*—cont'd

4. Assist the patient to identify strengths and positive qualities that increase the sense of self-worth. Focus on past experiences of accomplishment and competency. Help the patient with positive self-reinforcement. Reinforce the obvious love and affection of family and significant others.

5. Assess coping techniques that have been helpful in the past. Help the patient decide how to handle negative or incongruent feedback about the situation.

6. Encourage visits from family and significant others. Facilitate interactions and ensure privacy. Help family members entering the critical care unit by explaining what they will see. Increase visitors' comfort with equipment; offer chairs and other courtesies.

7. Encourage the patient to pursue interest in individual or social activities, even though difficult in the critical care unit.

8. Reflect caring, concern, empathy, respect, and unconditional acceptance in nurse-patient relationships.

9. Remember that for the patient the nurse is a significant other who provides important appraisals of the patient and who can facilitate the change process.

10. Help the family support the patient's self-esteem.

11. Provide for continuity of nurse assignment to ensure consistent contacts that can *facilitate support of the patient's self-esteem.*

NURSING MANAGEMENT OF SLEEP ALTERATIONS

NURSING MANAGEMENT PLAN OF CARE	SLEEP PATTERN DISTURBANCE

DEFINITION

Time limited disruption of sleep (natural, periodic suspension of consciousness) amount and quality.

Sleep Pattern Disturbance Related to Fragmented Sleep

DEFINING CHARACTERISTICS

- Decreased sleep during one block of sleep time
- Daytime sleepiness
- Sleep deprivation
  Less than one half of normal total sleep time
  Decreased slow-wave, or REM sleep
- Anxiety
- Fatigue
- Restlessness
- Disorientation and hallucinations
- Combativeness
- Frequent wakenings
- Decreased arousal threshold

OUTCOME CRITERIA

- Patient's total sleep time approximates patient's normal.
- Patient can complete sleep cycles of 90 minutes without interruption.
- Patient has no delusions, hallucinations, illusions.
- Patient has reality-based thought content.
- Patient is oriented to four spheres.

NURSING INTERVENTIONS AND *RATIONALE*

1. Continue to monitor the assessment parameters listed under "Defining Characteristics."
2. Assess normal sleep pattern on admission and any history of sleep disturbance or chronic illness that may affect sleep or sedative/hypnotic use. Promote normal sleep activity while patient is in critical care unit. Assess sleep effectiveness by asking patient how his or her sleep in the hospital compares with sleep at home. (See Chapter 4, Psychosocial Alterations, for management of acute confusion.)
3. Minimize awakenings *to allow for at least 90-minute sleep cycles.* Continually assess the need to awaken the patient, particularly at night. Distinguish between essential and nonessential nursing tasks. Organize nursing management to allow for maximum amount of uninterrupted sleep while ensuring close monitoring of the patient's condition. Whenever possible, monitor physiologic parameters without waking the patient. Coordinate awakenings with other departments, such as respiratory therapy, laboratory, and x-ray, *to minimize sleep interruptions.*
4. Minimize noise, particularly that of the staff and noisy equipment. Reduce the level of environmental stimuli.
5. Plan nap times to assist in equilibrating the normal total sleep time. Discourage or prevent catnaps (sleep lasting longer than 90 minutes at a time) *because these physically refresh the individual and thereby decrease the stimulus for longer sleep cycles in which REM sleep is obtained.* Early morning naps, however, may be beneficial in promoting REM sleep *because a greater proportion of early morning sleep is allocated to REM activity.*
6. Promote comfort, relaxation, and a sense of well-being. Treat pain. Eliminate stressful situations before bedtime. Use of relaxation techniques, imagery, backrubs, or warm blankets may be helpful. Other interventions may include increased privacy or a private room and providing the patient with his or her own garments or coverings. Individual patients may prefer quiet or may prefer the background noise of the television *to best promote sleep.*
7. Be aware of the effects of commonly used medications on sleep. *Many sedative and hypnotic medications decrease REM sleep.* Sedative and analgesic medications should not be withheld, but rather, drugs that minimally disrupt sleep are to be used to complement comfort measures, with dosages reduced gradually as the medication is no longer necessary. Do not abruptly withdraw REM suppressing medications, *because this can result in "REM rebound."*
8. Foods containing tryptophan (e.g., milk or turkey) may be appropriate *because these promote sleep.*
9. Be aware that the best treatment for sleep deprivation is prevention.

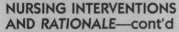

| NURSING MANAGEMENT PLAN OF CARE | SLEEP PATTERN DISTURBANCE—cont'd |

NURSING INTERVENTIONS AND *RATIONALE*—cont'd

10. Facilitate staff awareness that sleep is essential and health promoting. Assess the critical care unit for sleep-reducing stimuli and work to minimize them.

11. Document amount of uninterrupted sleep per shift, especially sleep episodes lasting longer than 2 hours. This can be effectively documented as part of the 24-hour flow sheet and reported routinely, shift to shift. *Sleep pattern disturbance is diagnosed, treated, and resolved more efficiently when formally documented in this manner.*

Sleep Pattern Disturbance Related to Circadian Desynchronization

DEFINING CHARACTERISTICS

- Sleep is out of synchronization with biologic rhythms, resulting in sleeping during the day and awakening at night
- Anxiety and restlessness
- Decreased arousal threshold

OUTCOME CRITERIA

- Majority of patient's sleep time will fall during low cycle of the circadian rhythm (normally at night).

NURSING INTERVENTIONS AND *RATIONALE*

1. Continue to monitor the assessment parameters listed under "Defining Characteristics."
2. Assist patient to maintain normal day-night cycles by decreasing lighting, noise, and sensory stimulation at night and critically evaluating the need to awaken the patient at night. Maintain a regular schedule for external time cues, such as mealtimes and favorite television shows.
3. Increase activity during the daytime to stimulate wakefulness. Increased physical activity until 2 hours before bedtime is useful in *promoting naturally induced sleep.* Limiting caffeine intake after early afternoon will promote sleep in the evening.
4. Do not schedule routine procedures at night.
5. Be aware that cardiac dysrhythmias can be precipitated by the decreased arousal threshold secondary to desynchronization.
6. If desynchronization occurs, plan for resynchronization by maintaining constancy in day-night pattern for at least 3 days (may require 5 to 12 days to reacclimatize). Plan for activities during the day *to stimulate wakefulness* and use comfort measures (comfortable body position, warm blankets, backrub, etc.) *to promote sleep* at night. Resynchronization is characteristically associated with chronic fatigue, malaise, and a decreased ability to perform life tasks.

NURSING MANAGEMENT OF NUTRITIONAL ALTERATIONS

NURSING MANAGEMENT PLAN OF CARE	ALTERED NUTRITION: LESS THAN BODY REQUIREMENTS

DEFINITION

The state in which an individual is experiencing an intake of nutrients insufficient to meet metabolic needs.

Altered Nutrition: Less than Body Requirements Related to Lack of Exogenous Nutrients and Increased Metabolic Demand

DEFINING CHARACTERISTICS

- Unplanned weight loss of 20% of body weight within the past 6 months
- Serum albumin <3.5 g/dL
- Total lymphocytes <1500 mm^3
- Anergy
- Negative nitrogen balance
- Fatigue; lack of energy and endurance
- Nonhealing wounds
- Daily caloric intake less than estimated nutritional requirements
- Presence of factors known to increase nutritional requirements (e.g., sepsis, trauma, multiple organ dysfunction syndrome [MODS])
- Maintenance of NPO status for >7-10 days
- Long-term use of 5% dextrose intravenously
- Documentation of suboptimal calorie counts
- Drug or nutrient interaction that might decrease oral intake (e.g., chronic use of bronchodilators, laxatives, anticonvulsives, diuretics, antacids, narcotics)
- Physical problems with chewing, swallowing, choking, and salivation and presence of altered taste, anorexia, nausea, vomiting, diarrhea, or constipation

OUTCOME CRITERIA

- Patient exhibits stabilization of weight loss or weight gain of ½ pound daily.
- Serum albumin is >3.5 g/dL.
- Total lymphocytes are >1500 mm^3.
- Patient has positive response to cutaneous skin antigen testing.
- Patient is in positive nitrogen balance.
- Wound healing is evident.
- Daily caloric intake equals estimated nutritional requirements.
- Increased ambulation and endurance are evident.

NURSING INTERVENTIONS AND RATIONALE

1. Monitor patient during physical care for signs of nutritional deficiencies.
2. Measure admission height and weight.
3. Weigh patient daily.
4. Ensure that specimens for biochemical tests of nutritional status are collected properly and on time.
5. Administer parenteral and enteral solutions as prescribed.
6. Control infusion rate of parenteral and enteral solutions through infusion control devices and check rate every hour.
7. Flush enteral feeding tubes every 4 hours *to maintain patency.*
8. Document oral intake through calorie counts.
9. Perform serial assessments of patient's strength, endurance, conditions of wounds.

NURSING MANAGEMENT RELATED TO PAIN

NURSING MANAGEMENT PLAN OF CARE	ACUTE PAIN

DEFINITION

An unpleasant sensory and emotional experience arising from actual or potential tissue damage or described in terms of such damage; sudden or slow onset of any intensity from mild to severe with an anticipated or predictable end and a duration of less than 6 months.

Acute Pain Related to Transmission and Perception of Cutaneous, Visceral, Muscular, or Ischemic Impulses

DEFINING CHARACTERISTICS

Subjective
- Patient verbalizes presence of pain
- Patient rates pain on scale of 1 to 10 using a visual analog scale

Objective
- Increase in BP, pulse, and respirations
- Pupillary dilation
- Diaphoresis, pallor
- Skeletal muscle reactions (grimacing, clenching fists, writhing, pacing, guarding or splinting affected part)
- Apprehensive, fearful appearance
- May not exhibit any physiologic change

OUTCOME CRITERIA

NOTE: Outcome is highly variable, depending on individual patient and pain circumstance factors.
- Patient verbalizes that pain is reduced to a tolerable level or is removed.
- Patient's pain rating on scale of 1 to 10 is lower.
- BP, heart rate, and respiratory rate return to baseline 5 minutes after administration of IV narcotic or 20 minutes after administration of intramuscular (IM) narcotic.

NURSING INTERVENTIONS AND *RATIONALE*

1. Modify variables that heighten the patient's experience of pain.
   - Explain to the patient that frequent, detailed, and seemingly repetitive assessments will be conducted *to allow the nurse to better understand the patient's pain experience, not because the existence of pain is in question.*
   - Explain the factors responsible for pain production in the individual. Estimate the expected duration of the pain if possible.
   - Explain diagnostic and therapeutic procedures to the patient in relation to sensations the patient should expect to feel.
   - Reduce the patient's fear of addiction by ex-

plaining the difference between drug tolerance and drug addiction. Drug tolerance is a physiologic phenomenon in which a drug dose begins to lose effectiveness after repeated doses; drug dependence is a psychologic phenomenon in which narcotics are used regularly for emotional, not medical, reasons.
   - Instruct patient to ask for pain medication when pain is beginning and not to wait until it is intolerable.
   - Explain that the physician will be consulted if pain relief is inadequate with the present medication.
   - Instruct patient in the importance of adequate rest, especially when it reduces pain *to maintain strength and coping abilities and to reduce stress.*
2. Collaborate with physician regarding pharmacologic interventions:
   - For postsurgical or posttraumatic cutaneous, muscular, or visceral pain, perform the following:
     a. Medicate with narcotic maximally to break the pain cycles as long as level of consciousness and vital signs are stable: check patient's previous response to similar dosage and narcotic.
     NOTE: First dose received postoperatively is usually reduced by one half *to evaluate patient's individual response to medication.*
     b. Continuous pain requires continuous analgesia.
       (1) Establish optimal analgesic dose that brings optimal pain relief.
       (2) Offer pain medication at prescribed regular intervals rather than making patient ask for it *to maintain more steady blood levels.*
       (3) Consider waking patient to avoid loss of opiate blood levels during sleep.

Continued

NURSING MANAGEMENT PLAN OF CARE **ACUTE PAIN—cont'd**

NURSING INTERVENTIONS AND RATIONALE—cont'd

c. If administering medication on prn basis, give it when patient's pain is just beginning, rather than at its peak. Advise patient to intercept pain, not endure it, or it may take several hours and higher doses of narcotics to relieve pain, leading to a cycle of undermedication and pain alternating with overmedication and drug toxicity.

d. Perform rehabilitation exercises (turn, deep breathe, leg exercises, ambulate) shortly before peak of drug effect *because this will be the optimal time for the patient to increase activity with the least risk of increasing pain.*

e. When making the transition from one drug to another or from IM or IV to PO medications, the use of an equianalgesic chart is helpful. Equianalgesic means *approximately* the same pain relief. Many consider the IM and IV dose of medications equianalgesic; however, others recommend using one half the IM dose for the IV dose. To effectively use analgesics, each patient requires an individualized choice of drug, dose, time interval, and route. Close monitoring of the patient's response is needed to determine if the right analgesic choice was made.

f. To assess effectiveness of pain medication, do the following:
    (1) Reevaluate pain 5 minutes after IV and 20 minutes after IM medication administration, observe patient's behavior, and ask patient to rate pain on scale of 1 to 10.
    (2) Collaborate with physician to add or delete other medications that potentiate the action of analgesics, such as antiemetics, hypnotics, sedatives, or muscle relaxants.
    (3) Observe for indicators of undertreatment: report of pain not relieved; observed restlessness, sleeplessness, irritability, and anorexia; decreased activity level.
    (4) Observe for indicators of overtreatment: hypotension or bradycardia; respiratory rate <10/min; excessive sedation.

g. If IV patient-controlled analgesia (PCA) is used, perform the following:
(NOTE: Patient-controlled analgesia allows patients to administer small doses of their prescribed medication when they feel the need. Constant levels of the drug in the bloodstream mean lower doses can be used to obtain analgesia. Pain control is improved because the patient is in control and experiences less fear of unrelieved pain. Reduced net narcotic use is noted, as is less sedation. Critical care patients appropriate for patient-controlled analgesia are those who are alert, such as burn patients, trauma patients without head injury, and some postoperative patients.)
    (1) Instruct the patient on what the drug is, the dose, and how often it can be self-administered by pushing the button to activate the PCA machine. For example, "When you have pain, instead of asking the nurse to bring medication, push the button that activates the machine and a small dose of the pain medicine will be injected into your IV line. You can keep your pain under control by administering additional medicine as soon as your pain begins to return or increases. Also, push the button before undertaking a painful activity, such as ambulation. Try to balance your pain relief against sleepiness, and don't activate the machine if you start to feel sleepy. If your pain medicine seems to stop working despite pushing the button several times, call the nurse to check your IV. If you are not receiving adequate pain relief, the nurse will call your doctor."
    (2) Monitor vital signs, especially BP and respiratory rate, every hour for the first 4 hours, and assess postural heart rate and BP before initial ambulation.
    (3) Monitor respirations every 2 hours while patient is on patient-controlled analgesia.
    (4) If patient's respirations decrease to <10/min or if patient is overly sedated, anticipate IV administration of naloxone.

NURSING INTERVENTIONS AND *RATIONALE*—cont'd

h. If epidural narcotic analgesia is used, do the following:

(NOTE: The delivery of narcotics, such as morphine or fentanyl, by epidural route to specific receptors in the spinal cord selectively blocks pain impulses to the brain for up to 24 hours. Effective analgesia can be obtained without many of the negative side effects or serum narcotic concentrations.)

(1) Keep patient's head elevated 30 to 45 degrees after injection *to prevent respiratory depressant effects.*

(2) Observe closely for respiratory depression up to 24 hours after injection. Monitor respiratory rate every 15 minutes for 1 hour; every 30 minutes for 7 hours; and every 1 hour for the remaining 16 hours.

(3) Assess for adequate cough reflex.

(4) Avoid use of other CNS depressants, such as sedatives.

(5) Observe for reports of pruritus, nausea, or vomiting.

(6) Anticipate administration of naloxone for respiratory depression (and smaller doses of naloxone for pruritus).

(7) Assess for and treat urinary retention.

(8) Assess epidural catheter site for local infection. Keep catheter taped securely *to prevent catheter migration.*

• For peripheral vascular ischemic pain (hypothetical vascular occlusion of leg), do the following:

a. Correctly identify and differentiate ischemic pain from other types of pain.

NOTE: Ischemic pain is usually a burning, aching pain made worse by exercise and lessened or relieved by rest. Eventually the pain occurs at rest. Coldness and pallor of extremity may be noted, especially if the limb is elevated above the heart level. Rubor and mottling of the skin may be evident from prolonged tissue anoxia and inability of damaged vessels to constrict. Eventually cyanosis and gangrenous tissue will be evident. Chronic ischemia leads to trophic changes in the limb, such as flaking skin, brittle nails, hair, leg ulcers, and cellulitis.

b. Administer pain medications and evaluate their effectiveness as previously described. Remember that the pain of ischemia is chronic and continuous and can make the patient irritable and depressed.

c. Treat the cause of the ischemic pain, and institute measures to increase circulation to the affected part.

3. Initiate nonpharmacologic interventions:

• Treat contributing factors; provide explanations (see intervention number 1 at beginning of this care plan).

• Apply comfort measures.

a. Use relaxation techniques, such as back rubs, massage, warm baths, music and aroma-therapy. Use blankets and pillows *to support the painful part and reduce muscle tension.* Encourage slow, rhythmic breathing.

b. Encourage progressive muscle relaxation techniques.

(1) Instruct patient to inhale and tense (tighten) specific muscle groups, then relax the muscles as exhalation occurs.

(2) Suggest an order for performing the tension-relaxation cycle (e.g., start with facial muscles and move down body, ending with toes).

c. Encourage guided imagery.

(1) Ask patient to recall an experienced image that is very pleasurable and relaxing and involves at least two senses.

(2) Have patient begin with rhythmic breathing and progressive relaxation, then travel mentally to the scene.

(3) Have the patient slowly experience the scene—how it looks, sounds, smells, feels.

(4) Ask patient to practice this imagery in private.

(5) Instruct the patient to end the imagery by counting to three and saying, "Now I'm relaxed." If person does not end the imagery and falls asleep, the purpose of the technique is defeated.

d. If TENS unit is prescribed by physician, do the following:

(NOTE: TENS is a battery-operated unit that serves as a nerve stimulator. It produces mild,

Continued

NURSING MANAGEMENT PLAN OF CARE   ACUTE PAIN—cont'd

NURSING INTERVENTIONS AND *RATIONALE*—cont'd

tingling sensations as it blocks incisional pain messages to the brain. It is sometimes used as part of the pain relief program for the post-surgical patient.)

(1) Take the TENS unit, patient pamphlet, and teaching electrodes to the patient before surgery to explain the process.

(2) Apply electrodes to skin, and instruct patient in proper use of unit. Let patient experience how the TENS unit should feel when activated. Refer to manufacturer's directions for proper application and operation of TENS unit.

(3) Electrodes are usually placed by the physician on the skin alongside the operative incision at the close of the surgical procedure in the operating room. The unit is usually used for 3 to 5 days as an adjunct to medications.

(4) When the patient is awake and alert, readjust the amplitude or output of the TENS unit to the patient's comfort as necessary. Keep the TENS unit on continuously unless ordered otherwise. Occasionally, percutaneous epi-

dural nerve stimulation is used when more than one nerve root is involved in producing pain. Again, patients are able to control their pain by adjusting the rate and frequency of a millivoltage electrical current stimulator affixed externally.

e. Assist with biofeedback, which represents a wide range of behavioral techniques that provide the patient with information about changes in body functions of which the person is usually unaware. For example, information used to reduce muscle contraction is obtained by an electromyogram recorded from body surface electrodes. Changes in blood flow are produced by monitoring skin temperature changes. The person using biofeedback tries to change the display of information in the desired direction by actions such as reducing muscle tension, by reducing or altering blood flow to a particular area. The critical care nurse should be familiar with the theoretic concepts of biofeedback and should support the patient in maximizing pain control through whatever techniques are successful for that patient.

NURSING MANAGEMENT OF CARDIOVASCULAR ALTERATIONS

NURSING MANAGEMENT PLAN OF CARE	ACTIVITY INTOLERANCE

DEFINITION

The state in which an individual has insufficient physiologic or psychologic energy to endure or complete required or desired daily activities.

Activity Intolerance Related to Cardiopulmonary Dysfunction

DEFINING CHARACTERISTICS

- Chest pain on activity
- Electrocardiographic changes on activity
- Heart rate elevations 30 beats/minute (bpm) above baseline on activity; heart rate elevations 15 bpm above baseline on activity for patients on beta-blockers or calcium channel blockers
- Heart rate elevations above baseline 5 minutes after activity
- Breathlessness on activity
- SpO_2 <92% on activity
- Postural hypotension when moving from supine to upright position
- Subjective fatigue on activity

OUTCOME CRITERIA

- Heart rate elevations are <20 bpm above baseline on activity and are <10 bpm above baseline on activity for patients on beta-blockers or calcium channel blockers.

- Heart rate returns to baseline 5 minutes after activity.
- Chest pain is absent on activity.
- The patient has subjective tolerance to activity.

NURSING INTERVENTIONS AND RATIONALE

1. Encourage active or passive range-of-motion exercises while the patient is in bed *to keep joints flexible and muscles stretched.* Teach patient to refrain from holding breath while performing exercises. *Avoid the Valsalva maneuver.*
2. Encourage performance of muscle-toning exercises at least 3 times daily, *because a toned muscle uses less oxygen when performing work than an untoned muscle.*
3. Progress ambulation.
4. Teach patient to take pulse *to determine activity tolerance:* take pulse for full minute before exercise, then for 10 seconds and multiply by 6 at exercise peak.

Activity Intolerance Related to Prolonged Immobility or Deconditioning

DEFINING CHARACTERISTICS

- Systolic blood pressure (SBP) drop >20 mm Hg; heart rate increase >20 bpm on postural change
- Vertigo on postural change
- Syncope on postural change

OUTCOME CRITERIA

- SBP drop is <10 mm Hg; heart rate increase is <10 bpm on postural change.
- Vertigo or syncope is absent on postural change.

NURSING INTERVENTIONS AND RATIONALE

1. Instruct and assist in the following bed exercises: straight leg raises, dorsiflexion/plantar

flexion, and quadriceps setting and gluteal setting exercises *to increase muscular and vascular tone.*
2. Determine that the patient is hydrated to 24-hour fluid requirements per body surface area (BSA) *to increase preload and thus stroke volume and cardiac output.* Hydrate accordingly if not contraindicated by cardiac or renal disorders.
3. Assist with postural changes accomplished in increments:
   Head of bed to 45 degrees and hold until symptom free

Continued

NURSING MANAGEMENT PLAN OF CARE — ACTIVITY INTOLERANCE—cont'd

NURSING INTERVENTIONS AND RATIONALE—cont'd

Head of bed to 90 degrees and hold until symptom free
Dangle until symptom free
Stand until symptom free and ambulate

4. As soon as it is medically safe, assist patient to sit at bedside for meals.
5. When treating pain with narcotic analgesics, plan ambulation to occur well before peak action of drug.

NURSING MANAGEMENT PLAN OF CARE — ALTERED TISSUE PERFUSION

DEFINITION

A decrease in oxygen resulting in the failure to nourish the tissues at the capillary level.

Altered Myocardial Tissue Perfusion Related to Decreased Myocardial Oxygen Supply and/or Increased Myocardial Oxygen Demand

DEFINING CHARACTERISTICS

- Angina for more than 30 minutes
- ST segment elevation on 12-lead electrocardiogram (ECG)
- Elevation of cardiac enzymes
- Apprehension

OUTCOME CRITERIA

- Absence of angina.
- Normalization of ST segment on 12-lead ECG without the appearance of new Q waves.
- Cardiac enzymes within normal range.

NURSING INTERVENTIONS AND RATIONALE

1. Collaborate with the physician regarding the administration of the following medications:
   - Oxygen to maintain SpO$_2$ >92% *to increase myocardial oxygen supply.*
   - Sublinqual nitroglycerin, intravenous nitroglycerin, and intravenous morphine *to alleviate angina, decrease myocardial oxygen demand, and increase myocardial oxygen supply.*
   - Aspirin *to decrease blood viscosity.*
   - Heparin *to prevent recurrent thrombosis.*
   - Thrombolytic therapy *to promote coronary artery clot lysis and increase myocardial oxygen supply.*
   - Beta-blockers and angiotensin-converting enzyme inhibitors *to decrease myocardial oxygen demand.*

2. Collaborate with physician regarding need for intraaortic balloon pump therapy *to increase myocardial oxygen supply and decrease myocardial oxygen demand.*
3. Collaborate with physician regarding the need for emergency cardiac catheterization and percutaneous transluminal coronary angioplasty or coronary artery bypass surgery *to increase myocardial oxygen supply.*
4. Maintain patient on bedrest, with bedside commode privileges, for the first 6 to 12 hours to decrease myocardial oxygen demand. Advance ambulation as tolerated over the next 48 hours.
5. Instruct patient to avoid the Valsalva maneuver *because this can cause rapid changes in heart rate and blood pressure and precipitate dysrhythmias.*
6. Monitor patient's blood pressure and heart rate and rhythm as many conditions may precipitate hypotension and dysrhythmias *that may impair myocardial oxygen supply.* Collaborate with physician regarding administration of vasoactive and/or antidysrhythmic medications.
7. Maintain surveillance for signs of decreased cardiac output *to facilitate the early identification and treatment of complications.*

| NURSING MANAGEMENT PLAN OF CARE | ALTERED TISSUE PERFUSION—cont'd |

Altered Peripheral Tissue Perfusion Related to Decreased Peripheral Blood Flow

RISK FACTORS

- Femoral artery cannulation for interventional cardiology or vascular procedures, intraaortic balloon pump (IABP), or hemodynamic monitoring catheters
- Radial artery cannulation or puncture
- Acute arterial thrombus
- Orthopedic trauma to an extremity

DEFINING CHARACTERISTICS

- Weak and/or unequal peripheral pulses
- Delayed capillary refill
- Ischemic pain from extremity
- Cool skin on extremity
- Pale extremity
- Paresthesias from extremity

OUTCOME CRITERIA

- Peripheral pulses are full and equal bilaterally.
- Capillary refill is equal bilaterally.
- There is no ischemic pain.
- There is equal skin temperature in both extremities.
- The skin is pink and warm in both extremities.
- Paresthesias are absent.

NURSING INTERVENTIONS AND *RATIONALE*

1. Observe cannulation/injury site to prevent hematoma formation or bleeding.
2. Do not bend limb at cannulation/injury site.
3. Notify physician of any changes in peripheral pulses, pallor, paresthesias, or pain in the extremity.
4. Prepare for return to surgery, peripheral arterial embolectomy, or peripheral lytic therapy.
5. In consultation with physician, medicate for pain from limb ischemia.

| NURSING MANAGEMENT PLAN OF CARE | DECREASED CARDIAC OUTPUT |

DEFINITION

A state in which the blood pumped by the heart is inadequate to meet the metabolic demands of the body

Decreased Cardiac Output Related to Alterations in Preload

DEFINING CHARACTERISTICS

- Cardiac output <4.0 L/min
- Cardiac index <2.5 L/min/m^2
- Heart rate >100 bpm
- Urine output <30 ml/hr or 0.5 ml/kg/hr
- Decreased mentation, restlessness, agitation, confusion
- Diminished peripheral pulses
- Blue, gray, or dark purple tint to tongue and sublingual area
- Systolic blood pressure <90 mm Hg
- Subjective complaints of fatigue

Reduced Preload
- Right atrial pressure <2 mm Hg
- Pulmonary artery wedge pressure <5 mm Hg

Excessive Preload
- Right atrial pressure >6 mm Hg
- Pulmonary artery wedge pressure >12 mm Hg

OUTCOME CRITERIA

- Cardiac output 4.0-8.0 L/min
- Cardiac index 2.5-4.0 L/min/m^2
- Right atrial pressure 2-8 mm Hg
- Pulmonary artery wedge pressure 5-12 mg Hg

NURSING INTERVENTIONS AND *RATIONALE*

1. Collaborate with physician regarding the administration of oxygen to maintain an SpO$_2$ >92% *to prevent tissue hypoxia.*
2. Maintain surveillance for signs of decreased tissue perfusion and acidosis *to facilitate the early identification and treatment of complications.*
3. Monitor fluid balance and daily weights *to facilitate regulation of the patient's fluid balance.*

For Reduced Preload Secondary to Volume Loss
4. Collaborate with physician regarding the administration of crystalloids, colloids, blood, and blood products *to increase circulating volume.*
5. Limit blood sampling, observe intravenous lines for accidental disconnection, apply direct pressure to bleeding sites, and maintain normal body temperature *to minimize fluid loss.*
6. Position patient with legs elevated, trunk flat, and head and shoulders above the chest *to enhance venous return.*

Continued

**NURSING MANAGEMENT
PLAN OF CARE**   **DECREASED CARDIAC OUTPUT—cont'd**

NURSING INTERVENTIONS AND RATIONALE—cont'd

7. Encourage oral fluids (as appropriate), administer free water with tube feedings, and replace fluids that are lost through wound or tube drainage *to promote adequate fluid intake.*
8. Maintain surveillance for signs of fluid volume excess and adverse effects of blood and blood product administration *to facilitate the early identification and treatment of complications.*

For Reduced Preload Secondary to Venous Dilation

9. Collaborate with physician regarding the administration of vasoconstrictors *to increase venous return.*
10. Maintain surveillance for adverse effects of vasoconstrictor therapy *to facilitate the early identification and treatment of complications.*
11. If patient is hyperthermic, administer tepid bath, hypothermia blanket, and/or ice bags to axilla and groin *to decrease temperature and promote vas,.oconstriction.*

For Excessive Preload Secondary to Volume Overload

12. Collaborate with physician regarding the administration of the following:
    - Diuretics *to remove excessive fluid.*

- Vasodilators *to decrease venous return.*
- Inotropes *to increase myocardial contractility.*

13. Restrict fluid intake and double concentrate intravenous drips *to minimize fluid intake.*
14. Position patient in semi-Fowler's or high-Fowler's position *to reduce venous return.*
15. Maintain surveillance for signs of fluid volume deficit and adverse effects of diuretic, vasodilator, and inotropic therapies *to facilitate the early identification and treatment of complications.*

For Excessive Preload Secondary to Venous Constriction

16. Collaborate with physician regarding the administration of vasodilators *to promote venous dilation.*
17. Maintain surveillance for adverse effects of vasodilator therapy *to facilitate the early identification and treatment of complications.*
18. If patient is hypothermic, wrap patient in warm blankets or apply hyperthermia blanket *to increase temperature and promote vasodilation.*

Decreased Cardiac Output Related to Alterations in Afterload

DEFINING CHARACTERISTICS

- Cardiac output <4.0 L/min
- Cardiac index <2.5 L/min/m^2
- Heart rate >100 bpm
- Urine output <30 ml/hr
- Decreased mentation, restlessness, agitation, confusion
- Diminished peripheral pulses
- Blue, gray, or dark purple tint to tongue and sublingual area
- Systolic blood pressure <90 mm Hg
- Subjective complaints of fatigue

Reduced Afterload

- Pulmonary vascular resistance <100 dynes/sec/cm^{-5}
- Systemic vascular resistance <800 dynes/sec/cm^{-5}

Excessive Afterload

- Pulmonary vascular resistance >250 dynes/sec/cm^{-5}

- Systemic vascular resistance >1200 dynes/sec/cm^{-5}

OUTCOME CRITERIA

- Cardiac output 4.0-8.0 L/min
- Cardiac index 2.5-4.0 L/min/m^2
- Pulmonary vascular resistance 80-250 dynes/sec/cm^{-5}
- Systemic vascular resistance 800-1200 dynes/sec/cm^{-5}

NURSING INTERVENTIONS AND RATIONALE

1. Collaborate with physician regarding the administration of oxygen to maintain an SpO$_2$ >92% *to prevent tissue hypoxia.*
2. Maintain surveillance for signs of decreased tissue perfusion and acidosis *to facilitate the early identification and treatment of complications.*

For Reduced Afterload

3. Collaborate with physician regarding the administration of vasoconstrictors *to promote arterial*

NURSING MANAGEMENT PLAN OF CARE   DECREASED CARDIAC OUTPUT—cont'd

NURSING INTERVENTIONS AND RATIONALE—cont'd

vasoconstriction and prevent relative hypovolemia. If decreased preload is present, implement nursing management plan of care, Decreased Cardiac Output Related to Alterations in Preload, pp. 467-468.

4. Maintain surveillance for adverse effects of vasoconstrictor therapy *to facilitate the early identification and treatment of complications.*

5. If patient is hyperthermic, administer tepid bath, hypothermia blanket, and/or ice bags to axilla and groin *to decrease temperature and promote vasoconstriction.*

For Excessive Afterload

6. Collaborate with physician regarding the administration of vasodilators *to promote arterial vasodilation.*

7. Collaborate with physician regarding initiation of intraaortic balloon pump therapy *to facilitate afterload reduction.*

8. Promote rest and relaxation and decrease environmental stimulation *to minimize sympathetic stimulation.*

9. Maintain surveillance for adverse effects of vasodilator therapy *to facilitate the early identification and treatment of complications.*

10. If patient is hypothermic, wrap patient in warm blankets or apply hyperthermia blanket *to increase temperature and promote vasodilation.*

11. If patient is in pain, treat pain *to reduce sympathetic stimulation.* Implement nursing management plan of care, Acute Pain Related to Transmission and Perception of Cutaneous, Visceral, Muscular, or Ischemic Impulses, pp. 461-464.

Decreased Cardiac Output Related to Alterations in Contractility

DEFINING CHARACTERISTICS

- Cardiac output <4.0 L/min
- Cardiac index <2.5 L/min/m^2
- Heart rate >100 bpm
- Urine output <30 ml/hr
- Decreased mentation, restlessness, agitation, confusion
- Diminished peripheral pulses
- Blue, gray, or dark purple tint to tongue and sublingual area
- Systolic blood pressure <90 mm Hg
- Subjective complaints of fatigue
- Right ventricular stroke work index <7 g/m^2/beat
- Left ventricular stroke work index <35 g/m^2/beat

OUTCOME CRITERIA

- Cardiac output 4.0-8.0 L/min
- Cardiac index 2.5-4.0 L/min/m^2
- Right ventricular stroke work index 7-12 g/m^2/beat
- Left ventricular stroke work index 35-85 g/m^2/beat

NURSING INTERVENTIONS AND RATIONALE

1. Collaborate with physician regarding the administration of oxygen to maintain an SpO$_2$ >92% *to prevent tissue hypoxia.*

2. Maintain surveillance for signs of decreased tissue perfusion and acidosis *to facilitate the early identification and treatment of complications.*

3. Ensure preload is optimized. If preload is reduced or excessive, implement nursing management plan of care, Decreased Cardiac Output Related to Alterations in Preload, pp. 467-468.

4. Ensure afterload is optimized. If afterload is reduced or excessive, implement nursing management plan of care, Decreased Cardiac Output Related to Alterations in Afterload, pp. 468-469.

5. Ensure electrolytes are optimized. Collaborate with physician regarding the administration of electrolyte replacement therapy *to enhance cellular ionic environment.*

6. Collaborate with physician regarding the administration of inotropes *to enhance myocardial contractility.*

7. Maintain surveillance for adverse effects of inotropic therapy *to facilitate the early identification and treatment of complications.*

8. If myocardial ischemia present, implement nursing management plan of care, Altered Tissue Perfusion, p. 466.

Continued

NURSING MANAGEMENT PLAN OF CARE	DECREASED CARDIAC OUTPUT—cont'd

Decreased Cardiac Output Related to Alterations in Heart Rate or Rhythm

DEFINING CHARACTERISTICS

- Cardiac output <4.0 L/min
- Cardiac index <2.5 L/min/m^2
- Heart rate >100 bpm
- Urine output <30 ml/hr or 0.5 ml/kg/hr
- Decreased mentation, restlessness, agitation, confusion
- Diminished peripheral pulses
- Blue, gray, or dark purple tint to tongue and sublingual area
- Systolic blood pressure <90 mm Hg
- Subjective complaints of fatigue
- Heart rate <60 bpm
- Dysrhythmias

OUTCOME CRITERIA

- Cardiac output 4.0-8.0 L/min
- Cardiac index 2.5-4.0 L/min/m^2
- Absence of dysrhythmias or return to baseline
- Heart rate >60 bpm

NURSING INTERVENTIONS AND RATIONALE

1. Collaborate with physician regarding the administration of oxygen to maintain an SpO$_2$ >92% *to prevent tissue hypoxia.*
2. Ensure electrolytes are optimized. Collaborate with physician regarding the administration of electrolyte therapy *to enhance cellular ionic environment and avoid precipitation of dysrhythmias.*
3. Collaborate with physician and pharmacist regarding patient's current medications and their effect on heart rate and rhythm *to identify any prodysrhythmic or bradycardiac side effects.*
4. Maintain surveillance for signs of decreased tissue perfusion and acidosis *to facilitate the early identification and treatment of complications.*
5. Monitor ST segment continuously *to determine changes in myocardial tissue perfusion.* If myocardial ischemia is present, implement nursing management plan of care, Altered Tissue Perfusion, p. 466.

For Lethal Dysrhythmias or Asystole

6. Initiate Advanced Cardiac Life Support interventions (see Appendix A) and notify physician immediately.

For Nonlethal Dysrhythmias

7. Collaborate with physician regarding administration of antidysrhythmic therapy, synchronized cardioversion, and/or overdrive pacing *to control dysrhythmias.*
8. Maintain surveillance for adverse effects of antidysrhythmic therapy *to facilitate the early identification and treatment of complications.*

For Heart Rate <60 bpm

9. Collaborate with physician regarding the initiation of temporary pacing *to increase heart rate.*

NURSING MANAGEMENT OF PULMONARY ALTERATIONS

NURSING MANAGEMENT PLAN OF CARE	DYSFUNCTIONAL VENTILATORY WEANING RESPONSE

DEFINITION

A state in which an individual cannot adjust to lowered levels of mechanical ventilator support, which interrupts and prolongs the weaning process.

Dysfunctional Ventilatory Weaning Response (DVWR) Related to Physical, Psychologic, or Situational Factors

DEFINING CHARACTERISTICS

Mild DVWR
Responds to lowered levels of mechanical ventilator support with:
- Restlessness
- Slight increased respiratory rate from baseline
- Expressed feelings of increased need for oxygen; breathing discomfort; fatigue; warmth
- Queries about possible machine malfunction
- Increased concentration on breathing

Moderate DVWR
Responds to lowered levels of mechanical ventilator support with:
- Slight baseline increase in blood pressure <20 mm Hg
- Slight baseline increase in heart rate <20 beats/min
- Baseline increase in respiratory rate <5 breaths/min
- Hypervigilence to activities
- Inability to respond to coaching
- Inability to cooperate
- Apprehension
- Diaphoresis
- Eye widening "wide-eyed look"
- Decreased air entry on auscultation
- Color changes; pale, slight cyanosis
- Slight respiratory accessory muscle use

Severe DVWR
Responds to lowered levels of mechanical ventilator support with:
- Agitation
- Deterioration in arterial blood gases from current baseline
- Baseline increase in blood pressure >20 mm Hg
- Baseline increase in heart rate >20 beats/min
- Respiratory rate increases significantly from baseline
- Profuse diaphoresis
- Full respiratory accessory muscle use
- Shallow, gasping breaths

- Paradoxical abdominal breathing
- Discoordinated breathing with the ventilator
- Decreased level of consciousness
- Adventitious breath sounds, audible airway secretions
- Cyanosis

OUTCOME CRITERIA
- Airway is clear.
- Underlying disorder is resolving.
- Patient is rested, and pain is controlled.
- Nutritional status is adequate.
- Patient has feelings of perceived control, situational security, and trust in the nurses.
- Patient is able to adapt to selected level of ventilator support without undue fatigue.

NURSING INTERVENTIONS AND *RATIONALE*
1. Communicate interest and concern for the patient's well-being and demonstrate confidence in ability to manage weaning process *to instill trust in the patient.*
2. Use normalizing strategies (e.g., grooming, dressing, mobilizing, social conversation) *to reinforce patient's self-esteem and feelings of identity.*
3. Identify parameters of the patient's usual functioning before the weaning process begins *to facilitate early identification of problems.*
4. Identify patient's strengths and resources that can be mobilized *to enhance the patient's coping and maximize the weaning effort.*
5. Note concerns that adversely affect the patient's comfort and confidence, and manage them discretely *to facilitate the patient's ease.*
6. Praise successful activities, encourage a positive outlook, and review the patient's positive progress to date *to increase patient's perceived self-efficacy.*
7. Inform patient of his or her situation and weaning progress *to permit the patient as much control as possible.*

Continued

NURSING MANAGEMENT PLAN OF CARE

DYSFUNCTIONAL VENTILATORY WEANING RESPONSE—cont'd

NURSING INTERVENTIONS AND *RATIONALE*—cont'd

8. Teach patient about the weaning process and how he or she can participate in the process.
9. Negotiate daily weaning goals with patient *to gain cooperation.*
10. Position patient with the head of the bed elevated *to optimize respiratory efforts.*
11. Coach patient in breath control by regular demonstrations of slow, deep, rhythmic patterns of breathing *to assist with dyspnea.*
12. Remain visible in the room and reassure patient that help is immediately available if needed *to reduce the patient's anxiety and fearfulness.*
13. Encourage patient to view weaning trials as a form of training, regardless of whether the weaning goal is achieved *to avoid discouragement.*
14. Encourage patient to maintain emotional calmness by reassuring, being present, comforting, talking down if emotionally aroused, and reinforcing the idea that he or she can and will succeed.
15. Monitor the patient's status frequently *to avoid undue fatigue and anxiety.*
16. Provide regular periods of rest by reducing activities, maintaining or increasing ventilator support, and providing oxygen as needed before fatigue advances.
17. Provide distraction (e.g., visitors, radio, television, conversation) when the patient's concentration starts to create tension and increases anxiety.
18. Ensure adequate nutritional support, sufficient rest and sleep time, and sedation or pain control to *promote the patient's optimal physical and emotional comfort.*
19. Start weaning early in the day *when the patient is most rested.*
20. Restrict unnecessary activities and visitors who do not cooperate with weaning strategies *to minimize energy demands on the patient during the weaning process.*
21. Coordinate necessary activities *to promote adequate time for rest or relaxation.*
22. Monitor the patient's underlying disease process *to ensure it is stabilized and under control.*
23. Advocate for additional resources (e.g., sedation, analgesia, rest) needed by the patient *to maximize comfort status.*
24. Develop and adhere to an individualized plan of care *to promote the patient's feelings of control.*

NURSING MANAGEMENT PLAN OF CARE

INEFFECTIVE AIRWAY CLEARANCE

DEFINITION

Inability to clear secretions or obstructions from the respiratory tract to maintain a clear airway.

Ineffective Airway Clearance Related to Excessive Secretions or Abnormal Viscosity of Mucus

DEFINING CHARACTERISTICS

- Abnormal breath sounds (displaced normal sounds, adventitious sounds, diminished or absent sounds)
- Ineffective cough with or without sputum
- Tachypnea, dyspnea
- Verbal reports of inability to clear airway

OUTCOME CRITERIA

- Cough produces thin mucus.
- Lungs are clear to auscultation.
- Respiratory rate, depth, and rhythm return to baseline.

NURSING INTERVENTIONS AND *RATIONALE*

1. Assess sputum for color, consistency, and amount.
2. Assess for clinical manifestations of pneumonia.
3. Provide for maximal thoracic expansion by repositioning, deep breathing, splinting, and pain management *to avoid hypoventilation and atelectasis.* If hypoventilation is present, implement nursing management plan of care, Ineffective Breathing Pattern Related to Decreased Lung Expansion, pp. 473-474.
4. Maintain adequate hydration by administering oral and intravenous fluids (as ordered) *to thin secretions and facilitate airway clearance.*
5. Provide humidification to airways via oxygen delivery device or artificial airway *to thin secretions and facilitate airway clearance.*
6. Administer bland aerosol every 4 hours *to facilitate expectoration of sputum.*

NURSING MANAGEMENT PLAN OF CARE   INEFFECTIVE AIRWAY CLEARANCE—cont'd

NURSING INTERVENTIONS AND *RATIONALE*—cont'd

7. Collaborate with the physician regarding the administration of the following:
   - Bronchodilators *to treat or prevent broncho-spasms and facilitate expectoration of mucus*
   - Mucolytics and expectorants *to enhance mobilization and removal of secretions*
   - Antibiotics *to treat infection*
8. Assist with directed coughing exercises *to facilitate expectoration of secretions.* If patient is unable to perform cascade cough, consider using huff cough (patients with hyperactive airways), end-expiratory cough (patient with secretions in distal airway), or augmented cough (patient with weakened abdominal muscle).
   - Cascade cough—Instruct patient to do the following:
     a. Take a deep breath and hold it for 1 to 3 seconds
     b. Cough out forcefully several times until all air is exhaled
     c. Inhale slowly through the nose
     d. Repeat once
     e. Rest and then repeat as necessary
   - Huff cough—Instruct patient to do the following:
     a. Take a deep breath and hold it for 1 to 3 seconds
     b. Say the word "huff" while coughing out several times until air is exhaled
     c. Inhale slowly through the nose
     d. Repeat as necessary
   - End-expiratory cough—Instruct patient to do the following:
     a. Take a deep breath and hold it for 1 to 3 seconds

   b. Exhale slowly
   c. At the end of exhalation, cough once
   d. Inhale slowly through the nose
   e. Repeat as necessary or follow with cascade cough
   - Augmented cough—Instruct patient to do the following:
     a. Take a deep breath and hold it for 1 to 3 seconds
     b. Perform one or more of the following maneuvers to increase intraabdominal pressure:
        1) Tighten knees and buttocks
        2) Bend forward at the waist
        3) Place a hand flat on the upper abdomen just under the xiphoid process and press in and up abruptly during coughing
        4) Keep hands on the chest wall and press inward with each cough
     c. Inhale slowly through the nose
     d. Rest and repeat as necessary
9. Suction nasotracheally or endotracheally as necessary *to assist with secretion removal.*
10. Reposition patient at least every 2 hours or use continuous lateral rotation therapy *to mobilize and prevent stasis of secretions.*
11. Consider chest physiotherapy (postural drainage and/or chest percussion) three to four times per day in a patient with large amounts of sputum *to assist with the expulsion of retained secretions.*
12. Allow rest periods between coughing sessions, chest physiotherapy, suctioning, or any other demanding activities *to promote energy conservation.*

NURSING MANAGEMENT PLAN OF CARE   INEFFECTIVE BREATHING PATTERN

DEFINITION

Inspiration and/or expiration that does not provide adequate ventilation.

Ineffective Breathing Pattern Related to Decreased Lung Expansion

DEFINING CHARACTERISTICS

- Abnormal respiratory patterns (hypoventilation, hyperventilation, tachypnea, bradypnea, obstructive breathing)
- Abnormal ABG values (increased $PaCO_2$, decreased pH)

- Unequal chest movement
- Shortness of breath, dyspnea

OUTCOME CRITERIA

- Respiratory rate, rhythm, and depth return to baseline.
- Minimal or absent use of accessory muscles.

Continued

NURSING MANAGEMENT PLAN OF CARE — INEFFECTIVE BREATHING PATTERN—cont'd

OUTCOME CRITERIA

- Chest expands symmetrically.
- ABG values return to baseline.

NURSING INTERVENTIONS AND RATIONALE

1. Treat pain, if present, *to prevent hypoventilation and atelectasis.* Implement nursing management plan of care, Acute Pain Related to Transmission and Perception of Cutaneous, Visceral, Muscular, or Ischemic Impulses, pp. 461-464.
2. Position patient in high-Fowler's or semi-Fowler's position *to promote diaphragmatic descent and maximal inhalation.*
3. Assist with deep breathing exercises and incentive spirometry with sustained maximal inspiration 5 to 10 times/hr *to help reinflate collapsed portions of the lung.*
   - Deep breathing—Instruct patient to do the following:
     a. Sit up straight or lean forward slightly while sitting on edge of bed or chair (if possible)
     b. Take a slow, deep breath in
     c. Pause slightly or hold breath for at least 3 seconds
     d. Exhale slowly
     e. Rest and repeat
   - Incentive spirometry—Instruct patient to do the following:
     a. Exhale normally
     b. Place lips around the mouthpiece and close mouth tightly around it
     c. Inhale slowly and as deeply as possible, noting the maximum volume of air inspired
     d. Hold maximum inhalation for 3 seconds
     e. Take the mouthpiece out of mouth and slowly exhale
     f. Rest and repeat
4. Assist physician with intubation and initiation of mechanical ventilation as indicated.

Ineffective Breathing Pattern Related to Musculoskeletal Fatigue or Neuromuscular Impairment

DEFINING CHARACTERISTICS

- Unequal chest movement
- Shortness of breath, dyspnea
- Use of accessory muscles
- Tachypnea
- Thoracoabdominal asynchrony
- Abnormal ABG values (increased $PaCO_2$, decreased pH)
- Nasal flaring
- Assumption of 3-point position

OUTCOME CRITERIA

- Respiratory rate, rhythm, and depth return to baseline.
- Minimal or absent use of accessory muscles.
- Chest expands symmetrically.
- ABG values return to baseline.

NURSING INTERVENTIONS AND RATIONALE

1. Prevent unnecessary exertion *to limit drain on patients' ventilatory reserve.*
2. Instruct patient in energy-saving techniques *to conserve patient's ventilatory reserve.*
3. Assist with pursed-lip and diaphragmatic breathing techniques *to facilitate diaphragmatic descent and improved ventilation.*
   - Diaphragmatic breathing—Instruct patient to do the following:
     a. Sit in the upright position
     b. Place one hand on the abdomen just above the waist and the other on the upper chest
     c. Breathe in through the nose and feel the lower hand push out; the upper hand should not move
     d. Breathe out through pursed lips and feel the lower hand move in
4. Position patient in high-Fowler's or semi-Fowler's position *to promote diaphragmatic descent and maximal inhalation.*
5. Assist physician with intubation and initiation of mechanical ventilation as indicated.

NURSING MANAGEMENT PLAN OF CARE   INABILITY TO SUSTAIN SPONTANEOUS VENTILATION

DEFINITION

A state in which the response pattern of decreased energy reserves results in an individual's inability to maintain breathing adequate to support life.

Inability to Sustain Spontaneous Ventilation Related to Respiratory Muscle Fatigue or Metabolic Factors

DEFINING CHARACTERISTICS

- Dyspnea and apprehension
- Increased metabolic rate
- Increased restlessness
- Increased use of accessory muscles
- Decreased tidal volume
- Increased heart rate
- Abnormal arterial blood gas (ABG) values (decreased PaO_2, increased $PaCO_2$, decreased pH, decreased SaO_2)
- Decreased cooperation

OUTCOME CRITERIA

- Metabolic rate and heart rate are within patient's baseline.
- Eupnea.
- ABG values are within patient's baseline.

NURSING INTERVENTIONS AND *RATIONALE*

1. Collaborate with the physician regarding the application of pressure support to the ventilator *to assist patient in overcoming the work of breathing imposed by the ventilator and endotracheal tube.*
2. Carefully snip excess length from the proximal end of the endotracheal tube *to decrease dead space and thereby decrease the work of breathing.*
3. Collaborate with the physician and dietitian to ensure that at least 50% of the diet's nonprotein caloric source is in the form of fat versus carbohydrates *to prevent excess carbon dioxide production.*
4. Collaborate with the physician and respiratory therapist regarding the best method of weaning for individual patients *because each situation is different, and a variety of weaning options are available.*

5. Collaborate with the physician and physical therapist regarding a progressive ambulation and conditioning plan *to promote overall muscle conditioning and respiratory muscle functioning.*
6. Determine the most effective means of communication for patient *to promote independence and reduce anxiety.*
7. Develop a daily schedule and post it in patient's room *to coordinate care and facilitate patient's involvement in the plan.*
8. Treat pain, if present, *to prevent respiratory splinting and hypoventilation.* Implement nursing management plan of care, Acute Pain Related to Transmission and Perception of Cutaneous, Visceral, Muscular, or Ischemic Impulses, pp. 461-464.
9. Ensure that patient receives at least 2- to 4-hour intervals of uninterrupted sleep in a quiet, dark room. Collaborate with the physician and respiratory therapist regarding the use of full ventilatory support at night *to provide respiratory muscle rest.*
10. Place patient in semi-Fowler's position or in a chair at the bedside *for best use of ventilatory muscles and to facilitate diaphragmatic descent.*
11. Explain the weaning procedure to the patient before the initial trial *so that patient will understand what to expect and how to participate.*
12. Monitor patient during the weaning trial for evidence of respiratory muscle fatigue *to avoid overtiring patient.*
13. Provide diversional activity during the weaning trial *to reduce patient's anxiety.*
14. Collaborate with physician and respiratory therapist regarding the removal of the ventilator and artificial airway when patient has been successfully weaned.

NURSING MANAGEMENT PLAN OF CARE | IMPAIRED GAS EXCHANGE

DEFINITION

Excess or deficit in oxygenation and/or carbon dioxide elimination at the alveolar-capillary membrane.

Impaired Gas Exchange Related to Ventilation/Perfusion Mismatching or Intrapulmonary Shunting

DEFINING CHARACTERISTICS

- Abnormal ABG values (decreased PaO_2, decreased SaO_2)
- Somnolence
- Neurobehavioral changes (restlessness, irritability, confusion)
- Central cyanosis

OUTCOME CRITERIA

- ABG values are within patient's baseline.
- Absence of central cyanosis.

NURSING INTERVENTIONS AND *RATIONALE*

1. Initiate continuous pulse oximetry or monitor SpO_2 every hour.
2. Collaborate with physician on the administration of oxygen to maintain an SpO_2 >90%
   a. Administer supplemental oxygen via appropriate oxygen delivery device *to increase driving pressure of oxygen in the alveoli.*
   b. If supplemental oxygen alone is not effective, administer constant positive airway pressure or mechanical ventilation with positive end-expiratory pressure *to open collapsed alveoli and increase the surface area for gas exchange.*
3. Position patient to optimize ventilation/ perfusion matching
   a. For patient with unilateral lung disease, position with the good lung down *because*

gravity will improve perfusion to this area, and this will best match ventilation with perfusion.
   b. For patient with bilateral lung disease, position with the right lung down *because this lung is larger than the left and affords a greater area for ventilation and perfusion,* or change position every 2 hours, favoring positions that improve oxygenation.
   c. Avoid any position that seriously compromises oxygenation status.
4. Perform procedures only as needed and provide adequate rest and recovery time in between *to prevent desaturation.*
5. Collaborate with the physician regarding the administration of the following:
   - Sedatives *to decrease ventilator asynchrony and facilitate patient's sense of control*
   - Neuromuscular blocking agents *to prevent ventilator asynchrony and decrease oxygen demand*
   - Analgesics *to treat pain if present.* Implement nursing management plan of care, Acute Pain Related to Transmission and Perception of Cutaneous, Visceral, Muscular, or Ischemic Impulses, pp. 461-464.
6. If secretions are present, implement nursing management plan of care, Ineffective Airway Clearance Related to Excessive Secretions or Abnormal Viscosity of Mucus, pp. 472-473.

Impaired Gas Exchange Related to Alveolar Hypoventilation

DEFINING CHARACTERISTICS

- Abnormal ABG values (decreased PaO_2, increased $PaCO_2$, decreased pH, decreased SaO_2)
- Somnolence
- Neurobehavioral changes (restlessness, irritability, confusion)
- Tachycardia or dysrhythmias
- Central cyanosis

OUTCOME CRITERIA

- ABG values within patient's baseline.
- Absence of central cyanosis.

NURSING INTERVENTIONS AND *RATIONALE*

1. Initiate continuous pulse oximetry or monitor SpO_2 every hour.
2. Collaborate with physician on the administration of oxygen to maintain an SpO_2 >90%
   a. Administer supplemental oxygen via appropriate oxygen delivery device *to increase driving pressure of oxygen in the alveoli.*
   b. If supplemental oxygen alone is not effective, administer constant positive airway pressure or mechanical ventilation with positive end-expiratory pressure *to open*

NURSING MANAGEMENT PLAN OF CARE   IMPAIRED GAS EXCHANGE—cont'd

NURSING INTERVENTIONS AND *RATIONALE*—cont'd

collapsed alveoli and increase the surface area for gas exchange.

3. Prevent hypoventilation
    a. Position patient in high-Fowler's position or semi-Fowler's position *to promote diaphragmatic descent and maximal inhalation.*
    b. Assist with deep breathing exercises and/or incentive spirometry with sustained maximal inspiration 5 to 10 times/hr *to help reinflate collapsed portions of the lung.* See

nursing management plan of care, Ineffective Breathing Pattern Related to Decreased Lung Expansion, pp. 473-474, for further instructions.
    c. Treat pain, if present, *to prevent hypoventilation and atelectasis.* Implement nursing management plan of care, Acute Pain Related to Transmission and Perception of Cutaneous, Visceral, Muscular, or Ischemic Impulses, pp. 461-464.
4. Assist physician with intubation and initiation of mechanical ventilation as indicated.

NURSING MANAGEMENT PLAN OF CARE   RISK FOR ASPIRATION

DEFINITION

A state in which an individual is at risk for entry of gastrointestinal secretions, oropharyngeal secretions, or solids or fluids into tracheobronchial passages.

RISK FACTORS

*   Impaired laryngeal sensation or reflex
    Reduced level of consciousness
    Immediately after extubation
*   Impaired pharyngeal peristalsis or tongue function
    Neuromuscular dysfunction
    Central nervous system dysfunction
    Head or neck surgery
*   Impaired laryngeal closure or elevation
    Laryngeal nerve dysfunction
    Artificial airways
    Gastrointestinal tubes
*   Increased gastric volume
    Delayed gastric emptying
    Enteral feedings
    Medication administration
*   Increased intragastric pressure
    Upper abdominal surgery
    Obesity
    Pregnancy
    Ascites
*   Decreased lower esophageal sphincter pressure
    Increased gastric acidity
    Gastrointestinal tubes
*   Decreased antegrade esophageal propulsion
    Trendelenburg or supine position
    Esophageal dysmotility
    Esophageal structural defects or lesions

OUTCOME CRITERIA

*   Normal breath sounds or no change in patient's baseline breath sounds.

*   ABG values remain within patient's baseline.
*   No evidence of gastric contents in lung secretions.

NURSING INTERVENTIONS AND *RATIONALE*

1. Assess gastrointestinal function *to rule out hypoactive peristalsis and abdominal distention.*
2. Position patient with head of bed elevated 30 degrees *to prevent gastric reflux through gravity.* If head elevation is contraindicated, position patient in right lateral decubitus position *to facilitate passage of gastric contents across the pylorus.*
3. Maintain patency and functioning of nasogastric suction apparatus *to prevent accumulation of gastric contents.*
4. Provide frequent and scrupulous mouth care *to prevent colonization of the oropharynx with bacteria and inoculation of the lower airways.*
5. Ensure that endotracheal/tracheostomy cuff is properly inflated *to limit aspiration of oropharyngeal secretions.*
6. Treat nausea promptly; collaborate with physician on an order for antiemetic *to prevent vomiting and resultant aspiration.*

Additional Interventions for Patients Receiving Continuous or Intermittent Enteral Tube Feedings

7. Position patient with head of bed elevated 45 degrees *to prevent gastric reflux.* If a head-down position becomes necessary at any time, interrupt the feeding 30 minutes before the position change.

Continued

| NURSING MANAGEMENT PLAN OF CARE | RISK FOR ASPIRATION—cont'd |

NURSING INTERVENTIONS AND RATIONALE—cont'd

8. Check placement of feeding tube either by auscultation or radiographically at regular intervals (e.g., before administering intermittent feedings and after position changes, suctioning, coughing episodes, or vomiting) *to ensure proper placement of the tube.*
9. Instill blue food coloring to feeding solutions *to assist with identification of gastric contents in pulmonary secretions.*

10. Monitor patient for signs of delayed gastric emptying *to decrease potential for vomiting and aspiration.*
    a. For large-bore tubes, check residuals of tube feedings before intermittent feedings and every 4 hours during continuous feedings. Consider withholding feedings for residuals greater than 150% of the hourly rate (continuous feeding) or greater than 50% of the previous feeding (intermittent feeding).
    b. For small-bore tubes, observe abdomen for distention, palpate abdomen for hardness or tautness, and auscultate abdomen for bowel sounds.

NURSING MANAGEMENT OF NEUROLOGIC ALTERATIONS

| NURSING MANAGEMENT PLAN OF CARE | ALTERED CEREBRAL TISSUE PERFUSION |

DEFINITION

A decrease in oxygen resulting in the failure to nourish the tissues at the capillary level.

Altered Cerebral Tissue Perfusion Related to Vasospasm or Hemorrhage

DEFINING CHARACTERISTICS

Hemorrhage
- Aneurysm grading system according to Hunt and Hess
  Grade I: minimal bleed
    Asymptomatic or minimal headache
    Slight nuchal rigidity
  Grade II: mild bleed
    Moderate-to-severe headache
    Nuchal rigidity
    Minimal neurologic deficit (for example, possible cranial nerve palsies—oculomotor [cranial nerve III] most common; unilateral pupillary dilation, ptosis, and dysconjugate gaze)
  Grade III: moderate bleed
    Drowsiness
    Confusion
    Nuchal rigidity
    Possible mild focal neurologic deficits
  Grade IV: moderate-to-severe bleed
    Extremely decreased level of consciousness, stupor
    Possible moderate-to-severe hemiparesis
    Possible early posturing (decorticate or decerebrate)
  Grade V: severe bleed
    Profound coma
    Posturing
    Moribund appearance
- Pathologic reflexes resulting from meningeal irritation
  Kernig's sign: resistance to full extension of the leg at the knee when the hip is flexed
  Brudzinski's sign: flexion of the hip and knee during passive neck flexion
  Photophobia
  Nausea and vomiting

Vasospasm
- Worsening headache
- Confusion and decreasing level of consciousness
- Focal motor deficits such as unilateral weakness of extremities
- Speech deficits such as slurring, receptive, or expressive aphasia
- Increasing BP

OUTCOME CRITERIA

- Patient is oriented to time, place, person, and situation.
- Pupils are equal and normoreactive.
- BP is within patient's norm.
- Motor function is bilaterally equal.
- Headache, nausea, and vomiting are absent.
- Patient verbalizes importance of and displays compliance with reduced activity.

NURSING INTERVENTIONS AND RATIONALE

1. Assess for indicators of increased intracranial pressure (ICP) and brain herniation (see nursing management plan of care, Decreased Adaptive Capacity: Intracranial Related to Failure of Normal Intracranial Compensatory Mechanism, pp. 480-481). *ICP will increase during vasospasm only when caused by the edema resulting from brain infarction.*
2. If hypertensive-hypervolemic therapy is prescribed, administer crystalloid and colloid IV fluids and monitor pulmonary artery wedge pressure (PAWP), pulmonary artery diastolic (PAD) pressure, systemic vascular resistance (SVR), and BP to achieve and maintain prescribed parameters. Systolic blood pressure is usually maintained at 150-160 mm Hg.
3. Monitor lung sounds and chest x-ray reports because of *the risk of pulmonary edema associated with fluid overload.*
4. Anticipate administration of calcium channel blockers such as nifedipine *to decrease peripheral vascular resistance and cause vasodilation.*
5. Rebleeding is a potential complication of aneurysm rupture; to prevent rebleeding, the following interventions constitute subarachnoid precautions:
   - Ensure bedrest in a quiet environment *to lessen external stimuli.*

Continued

NURSING MANAGEMENT PLAN OF CARE | **ALTERED CEREBRAL TISSUE PERFUSION—cont'd**

NURSING INTERVENTIONS AND *RATIONALE*—cont'd

- Maintain a darkened room *to lessen symptoms of photophobia.*
- Restrict visitors and instruct them to keep conversation as nonstressful as possible.
- Administer prescribed sedatives as needed *to reduce anxiety and promote rest.*
- Administer analgesics as prescribed *to relieve or lessen headache.*

- Provide a soft, high-fiber diet and stool softeners *to prevent constipation, which can lead to straining and increased risk of rebleeding.*
- Assist with activities of daily living (feeding, bathing, dressing, toileting).
- Avoid any activity that could lead to increased ICP; ensure that patient does not flex hips beyond 90 degrees and avoids neck hyperflexion, hyperextension, or lateral hyperrotation *that could impede jugular venous return.*

NURSING MANAGEMENT PLAN OF CARE | **DECREASED ADAPTIVE CAPACITY: INTRACRANIAL**

DEFINITION

A clinical state in which intracranial fluid dynamic mechanisms that normally compensate for increases in intracranial volumes are compromised, resulting in repeated, disproportionate increases in intracranial pressure in response to a variety of noxious and nonnoxious stimuli.

Decreased Adaptive Capacity: Intracranial Related to Failure of Normal Intracranial Compensatory Mechanisms

DEFINING CHARACTERISTICS

- ICP >15 mm Hg, sustained for 15-30 minutes
- Headache
- Vomiting, with or without nausea
- Seizures
- Decrease in Glasgow Coma Scale score of 2 or more points from baseline
- Alteration in level of consciousness, ranging from restlessness to coma
- Change in orientation: disoriented to time and/or place and/or person
- Difficulty or inability to follow simple commands
- Increasing systolic blood pressure of more than 20 mm Hg with widening pulse pressure
- Bradycardia
- Irregular respiratory pattern (e.g., Cheyne-Stokes, central neurogenic hyperventilation, ataxic, apneustic)
- Change in response to painful stimuli (e.g., purposeful to inappropriate or absent response)
- Signs of impending brain herniation:
  Hemiparesis or hemiplegia
  Hemisensory changes
  Unequal pupil size (1 mm or more difference)
  Failure of pupil to react to light
  Dysconjugate gaze and inability to move one eye beyond midline if third, fourth, or sixth cranial nerves involved
  Loss of oculocephalic or oculovestibular reflexes
  Possible decorticate or decerebrate posturing

OUTCOME CRITERIA

- ICP is ≤15 mm Hg.
- Cerebral perfusion pressure (CPP) is >60 mm Hg.
- Absence of clinical signs of increased ICP as previously described.

NURSING INTERVENTIONS AND *RATIONALE*

1. Maintain adequate CPP.
   a. With physician's collaboration, maintain BP within patient's norm by administering volume expanders, vasopressors, or antihypertensives.
   b. Reduce ICP.
      - Elevate head of bed 30 to 45 degrees *to facilitate venous return.*
      - Maintain head and neck in neutral plane (avoid flexion, extension, or lateral rotation) *to enhance venous drainage from the head.*
      - Avoid extreme hip flexion.
      - With physician's collaboration, administer steroids, osmotic agents, and diuretics.
      - Drain cerebrospinal fluid (CSF) according to protocol if ventriculostomy is in place.
      - Assist patient to turn and move self in bed (instruct patient to exhale while turning or pushing up in bed) *to avoid isometric contractions and Valsalva maneuver.*

| NURSING MANAGEMENT PLAN OF CARE | DECREASED ADAPTIVE CAPACITY: INTRACRANIAL—cont'd |

NURSING INTERVENTIONS AND *RATIONALE*—cont'd

2. Maintain patent airway and adequate ventilation and supply oxygen *to prevent hypoxemia and hypercarbia.*

3. Monitor arterial blood gas (ABG) values and maintain PaO_2 >80 mm Hg, $PaCO_2$ at 25-35 mm Hg, and pH at 7.35-7.45 *to prevent cerebral vasodilation.*

4. Avoid suctioning beyond 10 seconds at a time; hyperoxygenate and hyperventilate before and after suctioning.

5. Plan patient care activities and nursing interventions around patient's ICP response. Avoid unnecessary additional disturbances and allow patient up to 1 hour of rest between activities as frequently as possible. *Studies have shown the direct correlation between nursing care activities and increases in ICP.*

6. Maintain normothermia with external cooling or heating measures as necessary. Wrap hands, feet, and male genitalia in soft towels before cooling measures *to prevent shivering and frostbite.*

7. With physician's collaboration, control seizures with prophylactic and as necessary (PRN) anti-convulsants. *Seizures can greatly increase the cerebral metabolic rate.*

8. With physician's collaboration, administer sedatives, barbiturates, or paralyzing agents *to reduce cerebral metabolic rate.*

9. Counsel family members to maintain calm atmosphere and avoid disturbing topics of conversation (e.g., patient condition, pain, prognosis, family crisis, financial difficulties).

10. If signs of impending brain herniation are present, do the following:
    - Notify physician at once.
    - Be sure head of bed is elevated 45 degrees and patient's head is in neutral plane.
    - Slow mainline intravenous (IV) infusion to keep open rate.
    - If ventriculostomy catheter is in place, drain CSF as ordered.
    - Prepare to administer osmotic agents and/or diuretics.
    - Prepare patient for emergency computed tomographic (CT) head scan and/or emergency surgery.

| NURSING MANAGEMENT PLAN OF CARE | UNILATERAL NEGLECT |

DEFINITION

The state in which an individual is perceptually unaware of and inattentive to one side of the body.

Unilateral Neglect Related to Perceptual Disruption

DEFINING CHARACTERISTICS

- Neglect of involved body parts and/or extrapersonal space
- Denial of the existence of the affected limb or side of body
- Denial of hemiplegia or other motor and sensory deficits
- Left homonymous hemianopia
- Difficulty with spatial-perceptual tasks
- Left hemiplegia

OUTCOME CRITERIA

- Patient is safe and free from injury.
- Patient is able to identify safety hazards in the environment.
- Patient recognizes disability and describes physical deficits present (e.g., paralysis, weakness, numbness).

- Patient demonstrates ability to scan the visual field to compensate for loss of function or sensation in affected limb(s).

NURSING INTERVENTIONS AND *RATIONALE*

1. Adapt environment to patient's deficits *to maintain patient safety.*
   - Position the patient's bed with the unaffected side facing the door.
   - Approach and speak to the patient from the unaffected side. If the patient must be approached from the affected side, announce your presence as soon as entering the room *to avoid startling the patient.*
   - Position the call light, bedside stand, and personal items on the patient's unaffected side.
   - If the patient will be assisted out of bed, simplify the environment *to eliminate hazards*

Continued

NURSING INTERVENTIONS AND RATIONALE—cont'd

by removing unnecessary furniture and equipment.

- Provide frequent reorientation of the patient to the environment.
- Observe the patient closely and anticipate his or her needs. In spite of repeated explanations, the patient may have difficulty retaining information about the deficits.
- When patient is in bed, elevate his or her affected arm on a pillow *to prevent dependent edema and support the hand in a position of function.*

2. Assist the patient to recognize the perceptual defect.
- Encourage the patient to wear any prescription corrective glasses or hearing aids *to facilitate communication.*
- Instruct the patient to turn the head past midline to view the environment on the affected side.
- Encourage the patient to look at the affected side and to stroke the limbs with the unaffected hand. Encourage handling of the affected limbs *to reinforce awareness of the affected side.*
- Instruct the patient to always look for the affected extremity or extremities when performing simple tasks *to know where it is at all times.*
- After pointing to them, have the patient name the affected parts.
- Encourage the patient to use self-exercises (e.g., lifting the affected arm with the good hand).
- If the patient is unable to discriminate between the concepts of "right" and "left," use descriptive adjectives such as "the weak arm," "the affected leg," or "the good arm" to refer to the body. Use gestures not just words to indicate right and left.

3. Collaborate with the patient, physician, and rehabilitation team *to design and implement a beginning rehabilitation program for use during critical care unit stay.*
- Use adaptive equipment (braces, splints, slings) as appropriate.
- Teach the patient the individual components of any activity separately, then proceed to integrate the component parts into a completed activity.

- Instruct the patient to attend to the affected side, if able, and to assist with the bath or other tasks.
- Use tactile stimulation *to reintroduce the arm or leg to the patient.* Rub the affected parts with different textured materials *to stimulate sensations (warm, cold, rough, soft).*
- Encourage activities that require the patient to turn the head toward the affected side and retrain the patient to scan the affected side and environment visually.
- If patient is allowed out of bed, cue him or her with reminders to scan visually when ambulating. Assist and remain in constant attendance because *the patient may have difficulty maintaining correct posture, balance, and locomotion.* There may be vertical-horizontal perceptual problems, with the patient leaning to the affected side to align with the perceived vertical. Provide sitting, standing, and balancing exercises before getting the patient out of bed.
- Assist patient with oral feedings.
  a. Avoid giving patient any very hot food items that could cause injury.
  b. Place the patient in an upright sitting position if possible.
  c. Encourage the patient to feed himself or herself; if necessary, guide the patient's hand to the mouth.
  d. If the patient is able to feed himself or herself, place one dish at a time in front of the patient. When the patient is finished with the first, add another dish. Tell the patient what he or she is eating.
  e. Initially place food in the patient's visual field; then gradually move the food out of the field of vision and teach the patient to scan the entire visual field.
  f. When the patient has learned to visually scan the environment, offer a tray of food with various dishes.
  g. Instruct the patient to take small bites of food and to place the food in the unaffected side of the mouth.
  h. Teach the patient to sweep out pockets of food with the tongue after every bite *to eliminate retained food in the affected side of the mouth.*
  i. After meals or oral medications, check the patient's oral cavity for pockets of retained material.

NURSING MANAGEMENT PLAN OF CARE	UNILATERAL NEGLECT—cont'd

NURSING INTERVENTIONS AND RATIONALE—cont'd

4. Initiate patient and family health teaching.
   - Assess to ensure that both the patient and the family understand the nature of the neurologic deficits and the purpose of the rehabilitation plan.

- Teach the proper application and use of any adaptive equipment.
- Teach the importance of maintaining a safe environment and point out potential environmental hazards.
- Instruct family members how to facilitate relearning techniques (e.g., cueing, scanning visual fields).

NURSING MANAGEMENT PLAN OF CARE	IMPAIRED VERBAL COMMUNICATION

DEFINITION

The state in which an individual experiences a decreased, delayed, or absent ability to receive, process, transmit, and use a system of symbols (anything that has meaning, i.e., transmits meaning).

Impaired Verbal Communication Related to Cerebral Speech Center Injury

DEFINING CHARACTERISTICS

- Inappropriate or absent speech or responses to questions
- Inability to speak spontaneously
- Inability to understand spoken words
- Inability to follow commands appropriately through gestures
- Difficulty or inability to understand written language
- Difficulty or inability to express ideas in writing
- Difficulty or inability to name objects

OUTCOME CRITERION

- Patient is able to make basic needs known.

NURSING INTERVENTIONS AND RATIONALE

1. Consult with physician and speech pathologist *to determine the extent of the patient's communication deficit (e.g., if fluent, nonfluent, or global aphasia is involved).*
2. Have the speech therapist post a list of appropriate ways to communicate with the patient in the patient's room *so that all nursing personnel can be consistent in their efforts.*
3. Assess the patient's ability to comprehend, speak, read, and write.
   - Ask questions that can be answered with a "yes" or a "no." If a patient answers "yes" to a question, ask the opposite (e.g., "Are you hot?" "Yes." "Are you cold?" "Yes."). *This may help determine if in fact the patient understands what is being said.*
   - Ask simple, short questions, and use gestures, pantomime, and facial expressions to give the patient additional clues.

- Stand in the patient's line of vision, giving a good view of your face and hands.
- Have the patient try to write with a pad and pencil. Offer pictures and alphabet letters at which to point.
- Make flash cards with pictures or words depicting frequently used phrases (e.g., glass of water, bedpan).
4. Maintain an uncluttered environment, and decrease external distractions *that could hinder communication.*
5. Maintain a relaxed and calm manner, and explain all diagnostic, therapeutic, and comfort measures before initiating them.
6. Do not shout or speak in a loud voice. *Hearing loss is not a factor in aphasia, and shouting will not help.*
7. Have only one person talk at a time. *It is more difficult for the patient to follow a multisided conversation.*
8. Use direct eye contact, and speak directly to the patient in unhurried, short phrases.
9. Give one-step commands and directions, and provide cues through pictures or gestures.
10. Try to ask questions that can be answered with a "yes" or a "no," and avoid topics that are controversial, emotional, abstract, or lengthy.
11. Listen to the patient in an unhurried manner, and wait for his or her attempt to communicate.
    - Expect a time lag from when you ask the patient something until the patient responds.
    - Accept the patient's statement of essential words without expecting complete sentences.
    - Avoid finishing the sentence for the patient if possible.

Continued

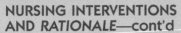

IMPAIRED VERBAL COMMUNICATION—cont'd

NURSING INTERVENTIONS AND *RATIONALE*—cont'd

- Wait approximately 30 seconds before providing the word the patient may be attempting to find (except when the patient is very frustrated and needs something quickly, such as a bedpan).
- Rephrase the patient's message aloud *to validate it.*
- Do not pretend to understand the patient's message if you do not.

12. Encourage the patient to speak slowly in short phrases and to say each word clearly.
13. Ask the patient to write the message, if able, or draw pictures if only verbal communication is affected.
14. Observe the patient's nonverbal clues for validation (e.g., answers "yes" but shakes head "no").
15. When handing an object to the patient, state what it is, *since hearing language spoken is necessary to stimulate language development.*
16. Explain what has happened to the patient, and offer reassurance about the plan of care.
17. Verbally address the problem of frustration over inability to communicate, and explain that patience is needed for both the nurse and the patient.
18. Maintain a calm, positive manner, and offer reassurance (e.g., "I know this is very hard for you, but it will get better if we work on it together").
19. Talk to the patient as an adult. Be respectful, and avoid talking down to the patient.
20. Do not discuss the patient's condition or hold conversations in the patient's presence without including him or her in the discussion. *This may be the reason some aphasic patients develop paranoid thoughts.*
21. Do not exhibit disapproval of emotional utterances or spontaneous use of profanity; instead, offer calm, quiet reassurance.
22. If the patient makes an error in speech, do not reprimand or scold but try to compliment the patient by saying, "That was a good try."
23. Delay conversation if the patient is tired. *The symptoms of aphasia worsen if the patient is fatigued, anxious, or upset.*
24. Be prepared for emotional outbursts and tears in patients who have more difficulty in expressing themselves than with understanding. The patient may become depressed, refuse treatment and food, ignore relatives, and push objects away. Comfort the patient with statements such as, "I know it's frustrating and you feel sad, but you are not alone. Other people who have had strokes have felt the way you do. We will be here to help you get through this."

NURSING MANAGEMENT OF RENAL ALTERATIONS

NURSING MANAGEMENT PLAN OF CARE | **ALTERED RENAL TISSUE PERFUSION**

DEFINITION

The state in which an individual experiences altered renal blood flow.

Altered Renal Tissue Perfusion Related to Decreased Renal Blood Flow

DEFINING CHARACTERISTICS

Initial Stages
- Decreased mean arterial pressure (MAP) <60 mm Hg
- Low cardiac output (CO) <4.0 L/min
- Low cardiac index (CI) <2.2 L/min/m^2
- Decreased urinary output

Later Stages
- Anuria or oliguria
- Decreased urinary creatinine clearance
- Increased serum creatinine
- Increased blood urea nitrogen (BUN)
- Electrolyte abnormalities: $\uparrow K^+$, $\downarrow Na^+$
- Increased MAP, pulmonary artery wedge pressure (PAWP), pulmonary artery diastolic (PAD) pressure, central venous pressure (CVP) secondary to fluid overload
- Sinus tachycardia
- Metabolic acidosis
- Crackles on lung auscultation
- Engorged neck veins
- Fluid weight gain
- Pitting edema
- Mental status changes
- Anemia

OUTCOME CRITERIA
- CO is >4.0 L/min.
- CI is >2.2 L/min/m^2.
- MAP, PAWP, PAD, CVP are within normal limits for patient.
- Electrolytes are within normal range.
- Serum creatinine and BUN are within normal range.
- Normal acid-base imbalance.
- Normal level of consciousness.
- Lungs are clear on auscultation.
- Urinary output to normal limits or patient stable on dialysis.
- Hemoglobin and hematocrit values are stable.

NURSING INTERVENTIONS AND *RATIONALE*

Initial Stages
1. Increase MAP 70 mm Hg **to restore renal perfusion pressure.**
2. Increase CO >4.0 L/min **to increase renal blood flow.**
3. Increase CI >2.5 L/min **to increase renal blood flow.**

Later Stages
1. Monitor hourly urinary output.
2. Administer prescribed diuretics.
3. Measure daily weight.
4. Restrict fluids as appropriate for urine output or dialysis/CRRT filtrate removal.
5. Assist with hemodialysis (if required by patient) **to remove excess fluid.**
6. Assist with hemodialysis (if required by patient) **to maintain electrolyte balance.**
7. Maintain oxygenation by keeping lungs clear of fluid.
8. Maintain skin integrity by frequent repositioning or air mattress bed.
9. Minimize risk of infection by sterile dialysis catheter care.
10. Orient patient to time and place.
11. Minimize blood withdrawals.
12. Monitor blood levels of drugs cleared by kidneys or dialysis.
13. Educate patient and family about renal failure, medications, and dialysis.

NURSING MANAGEMENT PLAN OF CARE — FLUID VOLUME DEFICIT

DEFINITION

The state in which an individual experiences decreased intravascular, interstitial, and/or intracellular fluid.

Fluid Volume Deficit Related to Absolute Loss

DEFINING CHARACTERISTICS

- Cardiac output (CO) <4 L/min
- Cardiac index (CI) <2.2 L/min
- Pulmonary artery wedge pressure (PAWP), pulmonary artery diastolic pressure (PAD) less than normal or less than baseline, central venous pressure (CVP) less than normal or less than baseline (PAWP <6 mm Hg)
- Tachycardia
- Narrowed pulse pressure
- Systolic blood pressure (BP) <100 mm Hg
- Urinary output <30 ml/hour
- Pale, cool, moist skin
- Apprehensiveness

OUTCOME CRITERIA

- Patient's CO is >4 L/min and CI is >2.2 L/min.
- Patient's PAWP, PAD, and CVP are normal or back to baseline level.
- Patient's pulse is normal or back to baseline.
- Patient's systolic blood pressure is >90.
- Patient's urinary output is >30 ml/hour.

NURSING INTERVENTIONS AND RATIONALE

1. Continue to monitor the assessment parameters listed under "Defining Characteristics." In addition, a serum lactate level >2 mOsm/L is believed to represent cellular perfusion failure at its earliest stage.
2. Secure airway and administer high-flow oxygen.
3. Place patient in supine position with legs elevated *to increase preload.* Consider using low-Fowler's position with legs elevated for patient with head injury.
4. For fluid repletion use the 3:1 rule, replacing three parts of fluid for every unit of blood lost.
5. Administer crystalloid solutions using the fluid challenge technique: infuse precise aliquots of fluid (usually 5 to 20 ml/min) over 10-minute periods; monitor cardiac loading pressures serially *to determine successful challenging.* If the PAWP or PAD elevates more than 7 mm Hg above beginning level, the infusion should be stopped. If the PAWP or PAD rises only to 3 mm Hg above baseline or falls, another fluid challenge should be administered.
6. Replete fluids first before considering use of vasopressors, *since vasopressors increase myocardial oxygen consumption out of proportion to the reestablishment of coronary perfusion in the early phases of treatment.*
7. When blood is available or its need is indicated, replace it with fresh packed red cells and fresh frozen plasma *to keep clotting factors intact.*
8. Move or reposition patient minimally *to decrease or limit tissue oxygen demands.*
9. Evaluate patient's anxiety level and intervene through patient education or sedation *to decrease tissue oxygen demands.*
10. Be alert for the possibility of acute respiratory distress syndrome (ARDS) development in the ensuing 72 hours.

Fluid Volume Deficit Related to Relative Loss

DEFINING CHARACTERISTICS

- Pulmonary artery wedge pressure (PAWP), pulmonary artery diastolic pressure (PAD), central venous pressure (CVP) less than normal or less than baseline
- Tachycardia
- Narrowed pulse pressure
- Systolic blood pressure (BP) <100 mm Hg
- Urinary output <30 ml/hour
- Increased hematocrit level

OUTCOME CRITERIA

- The patient's PAWP, PAD, and CVP are normal or back to baseline.
- Systolic BP is >90 mm Hg.
- Urinary output is >30 ml/hour.
- The patient's hematocrit level is normal.

NURSING INTERVENTIONS AND RATIONALE

1. Continue to monitor the assessment parameters listed under "Defining Characteristics." In addi-

NURSING MANAGEMENT PLAN OF CARE	FLUID VOLUME DEFICIT—cont'd

NURSING INTERVENTIONS AND *RATIONALE*—cont'd

tion, inspect soft tissues *to determine the presence of edema.*

2. With physician's collaboration, administer intravenous (IV) fluid replacements (usually normal

saline solution or lactated Ringer's solution) at a rate sufficient *to maintain urinary output >30 ml/hour.* Colloid solutions are avoided in the initial phases (but can be used later) because of the possibility of increased edema formation *as a result of the increased capillary permeability.*

NURSING MANAGEMENT PLAN OF CARE	FLUID VOLUME EXCESS

DEFINITION

The state in which an individual experiences increased fluid retention and edema.

Fluid Volume Excess Related to Renal Dysfunction

DEFINING CHARACTERISTICS

- Weight gain that occurs during a 24- to 48-hour period
- Dependent pitting edema
- Ascites in severe cases
- Fluid crackles on lung auscultation
- Exertional dyspnea
- Oliguria or anuria
- Hypertension
- Engorged neck veins
- Decrease in urinary osmolality as renal failure progresses
- Central venous pressure (CVP) >15 cm of H_2O
- Pulmonary artery wedge pressure (PAWP) 20-25 mm Hg

OUTCOME CRITERIA

- Weight returns to baseline.
- Edema or ascites is absent or reduced to baseline.
- Lungs are clear to auscultation.
- Exertional dyspnea is absent.
- Blood pressure returns to baseline.

- Heart rate returns to baseline.
- Neck veins are flat.
- Mucous membranes are moist.

NURSING INTERVENTIONS AND *RATIONALE*

1. Continue to monitor the assessment parameters listed under "Defining Characteristics."
2. Promote skin integrity of edematous areas by frequent repositioning and elevation of areas where possible. Avoid massaging pressure points or reddened areas of skin *because this results in further tissue trauma.*
3. Plan patient care to provide rest periods *to not heighten exertional dyspnea.*
4. Weigh patient daily at same time in same clothing, preferably with the same scale.
5. Instruct the patient about the correlation between fluid intake and weight gain, using commonly understood fluid measurements such as ingesting 4 cups (1000 ml) of fluid results in an approximate 2-pound weight gain in the anuric patient.

NURSING MANAGEMENT OF GASTROINTESTINAL ALTERATIONS

NURSING MANAGEMENT PLAN OF CARE	IMPAIRED SWALLOWING

DEFINITION

Abnormal functioning of the swallowing mechanism associated with deficits in oral, pharyngeal, or esophageal structure or function.

Impaired Swallowing Related to Neuromuscular Impairment, Fatigue, and Limited Awareness

DEFINING CHARACTERISTICS

- Evidence of difficulty swallowing
  Drooling
  Difficulty handling oral secretions
  Absence of gag, cough, and/or swallow reflex
  Moist, wet, gurgling voice quality
  Decreased tongue and mouth movements
  Presence of dysarthria
  Difficulty handling solid foods:
    Uncoordinated chewing or swallowing
    Stasis of food in the oral cavity
    Wet-sounding voice or change in voice quality
    Sneezing, coughing, or choking with eating
    Delay in swallowing of more than 5 seconds
    Change in respiratory pattern
  Difficulty handling liquids:
    Momentary loss of voice or change in voice quality
    Nasal regurgitation of liquids
    Coughing with drinking
- Evidence of aspiration
  Hypoxemia
  Productive cough
  Frothy sputum
  Wheezing, crackles, or rhonchi
  Temperature elevation

OUTCOME CRITERIA

- Absence of evidence of swallowing difficulties.
- Absence of evidence of aspiration.

NURSING INTERVENTIONS AND *RATIONALE*

1. Collaborate with physician and speech therapist regarding a swallowing evaluation and rehabilitation program *to decrease the incidence of aspiration.*
2. Collaborate with physician and dietitian regarding a nutritional assessment and nutritional plan *to ensure that the patient is receiving enough nutrition.*
3. Place the patient in an upright position with the head midline and the chin slightly down *to keep food in the anterior portion of the mouth and to prevent it from falling over the base of the tongue into the open airway.*
4. Provide patient with single-textured soft foods (e.g., cream cereals) that maintain their shape *because these foods require minimal oral manipulation.*
5. Avoid particulate foods (e.g., hamburger) and foods containing more than one texture (e.g., stew) *because these foods require more chewing and oral manipulation.*
6. Avoid dry foods (e.g., popcorn, rice, crackers) and sticky foods (e.g., peanut butter, bananas) *because these foods are difficult to manipulate orally.*
7. Provide patient with thick liquids (e.g., fruit nectar, yogurt) *because thick liquids are more easily controlled in the mouth.*
8. Thicken thin liquids (e.g., water, juice) with a thickening preparation or avoid them *because thin liquids are easily aspirated.*
9. Place foods in the uninvolved side of the mouth *because oral sensitivity and function are greatest in this area.*
10. Avoid the use of straws *because they can deposit the liquid too far back in the mouth for the patient to handle.*
11. Serve foods and liquids at room temperature *because the patient may be overly sensitive to heat or cold.*
12. Offer solids and liquids at different times *to avoid swallowing solids before being properly chewed.*
13. Provide oral hygiene after meals *to clear food particles from the mouth that could be aspirated.*
14. Collaborate with physician and pharmacist regarding oral medication administration *to adjust medication regimen to prevent aspiration and choking and to ensure all prescribed medications are swallowed.*

NURSING MANAGEMENT PLAN OF CARE   **IMPAIRED SWALLOWING—cont'd**

NURSING INTERVENTIONS AND *RATIONALE*—cont'd

15. Crush tablets (if appropriate) and mix with food that is easily formed into a bolus, use thickened liquid medications (if available), and/or embed small capsules into food *to facilitate oral medication administration.*

16. Inspect mouth for residue following all medication administration *to ensure medication has been swallowed.*

17. Educate patient and family on the swallowing problem, rehabilitation program, and emergency measures for choking.

NURSING MANAGEMENT OF ENDOCRINE ALTERATIONS

NURSING MANAGEMENT PLAN OF CARE	FLUID VOLUME DEFICIT

DEFINITION

State in which an individual experiences decreased intravascular, interstitial, and/or intracellular fluid. This refers to dehydration, water loss without changes in sodium.

Fluid Volume Deficit Related to Decreased Secretion of ADH

DEFINING CHARACTERISTICS

- Polyuria (15 L/day)
- Serum sodium 145 mEq/L (particularly in patient who is not drinking to replace losses)
- Intense thirst
- Polydipsia (alert patient)
- Urinary specific gravity <1.005
- Urinary osmolality <300 mOsm/kg
- Plasma osmolality >300 mOsm/kg

OUTCOME CRITERIA

- Urinary volume, specific gravity, and osmolality are normal.
- Thirst is reduced.
- Plasma osmolality and serum sodium level are normal.

NURSING INTERVENTIONS AND *RATIONALE*

1. Monitor the assessment parameters listed under "Defining Characteristics." Additionally, monitor for signs of critical volume deficits (i.e., hypotension, fall in pulmonary artery pressures, tachycardia).
2. With physician's collaboration, administer intravenous electrolyte replacement solutions *because critical electrolyte loss occurs along with water loss.* Replace losses milliliter for milliliter plus 50 ml/hr for insensible losses. Avoid replacement of losses with intravenous dextrose solutions *because of the risk of water intoxication.*
3. If patient is alert, encourage the patient to satisfy partially his or her replacement needs by drinking according to thirst. Caution should be observed regarding the patient's excessive ingestion of water (typically, the patient will crave iced water) *because of the risk of water intoxication.*
4. With physician's collaboration, administer vasopressin intravenously, intramuscularly, or per the nasal route.

NURSING MANAGEMENT PLAN OF CARE	FLUID VOLUME EXCESS

DEFINITION

State in which an individual experiences increased isotonic fluid retention.

Fluid Volume Excess Related to Increased Secretion of ADH

DEFINING CHARACTERISTICS

- Weight gain *without* edema
- Hyponatremia (dilutional)
- Decreased urinary output
  Urinary osmolality above normal, exceeding plasma osmolality
- Urinary specific gravity >1.030
- Evidence of water intoxication:
  Fatigue
  Headache
  Abdominal cramps
  Altered level of consciousness
  Diarrhea
  Seizures

OUTCOME CRITERIA

- Weight returns to baseline.
- Serum sodium is 135-145 mEq/L.
- Urinary output is >30 ml/hr.
- Urinary osmolality is 200-800 mOsm/kg.
- Urinary specific gravity is 1.005-1.030.
- Patient has no evidence of water intoxication.

NURSING MANAGEMENT PLAN OF CARE

FLUID VOLUME EXCESS—cont'd

NURSING INTERVENTIONS AND *RATIONALE*

1. Monitor the assessment parameters listed under "Defining Characteristics." In addition, monitor patient closely for evidence of cardiac decompensation caused by excessive preload (i.e., elevated pulmonary artery diastolic pressure [PADP] or pulmonary artery wedge pressure [PAWP], tachycardia, lung congestion).
2. Anticipate administration of demeclocycline, lithium carbonate, furosemide, and/or narcotic agonists.
3. With physician's collaboration, administer intravenous hypertonic sodium chloride *to temporarily correct hyponatremia.*
4. Weigh patient daily at same time in same clothing, preferably with same scale.
5. Maintain fluid restriction.
6. Monitor hydration status.
7. Initiate seizure precautions *because severe sodium deficit can result in seizures.*

NURSING MANAGEMENT RELATED TO TRAUMA

NURSING MANAGEMENT PLAN OF CARE	DYSREFLEXIA

DEFINITION

State in which an individual with a spinal cord injury at T7 or above experiences a life-threatening uninhibited sympathetic response of the nervous system to a noxious stimulus.

Dysreflexia Related to Excessive Autonomic Response to Certain Noxious Stimuli (e.g., Distended Bladder, Distended Bowel, Skin Irritation) Occurring in Patients with Cervical or High Thoracic (T7 or above) Spinal Cord Injury

DEFINING CHARACTERISTICS

NOTE: Anyone who has had dysreflexia knows how his or her body responds. Listen to the patient.

Major

- Paroxysmal hypertension (sudden periodic elevated blood pressure [BP] greater than 20 mm Hg above patient's normal BP); for many spinal cord injury patients, a normal BP may be only 90/60 mm Hg
- Bradycardia (most common; pulse rate <60 beats/minute) or tachycardia (pulse rate >100 beats/minute)
- Diaphoresis (above the injury)
- Facial flushing
- Pallor (below the injury)
- Pounding headache (a diffuse pain in different portions of the head and not confined to any nerve distribution area)

Minor

- Nasal congestion
- Engorgement of temporal and neck vessels
- Conjunctival congestion
- Chills without fever
- Pilomotor erection (goosebumps) below the injury
- Blurred vision
- Chest pain
- Metallic taste in mouth
- Horner's syndrome (constriction of the pupil, partial ptosis of the eyelid, enophthalmos, and sometimes loss of sweating over the affected side of the face)

OUTCOME CRITERIA

- BP has returned to patient's norm.
- Pulse rate is >60 or <100 beats/minute (or within patient's norm).
- Headache is absent.
- Nasal stuffiness, sweating, and flushing above level of injury are absent.

- Chills, goosebumps, and pallor below level of injury are absent.
- Patient verbalizes causes, prevention, symptoms, and treatment of condition.

NURSING INTERVENTIONS AND *RATIONALE*

1. Continue to monitor the assessment parameters listed under "Defining Characteristics."
2. Place patient on cardiac monitor, and assess for bradycardia, tachycardia, or other dysrhythmias. *Disturbances of cardiac rate and rhythm can occur because of autonomic dysfunction associated with dysreflexia.*
3. Do not leave patient alone. One nurse monitors the BP and patient status every 3 to 5 minutes while another provides treatment.
4. Place patient's head of bed to upright position *to decrease BP and promote cerebral venous return.*
5. Remove any support stockings or abdominal binder *to reduce venous return.*
6. Investigate for and remove offending cause of dysreflexia.
   a. Bladder
      - If catheter not in place, immediately catheterize patient.
      - Lubricate catheter with lidocaine jelly before insertion.
      - Drain 500 ml of urine, and recheck BP.
      - If BP still elevated, drain another 500 ml of urine.
      - If BP declines after the bladder is empty, serial BP must be monitored closely *because the bladder can go into severe contractions causing hypertension to recur.* With physician's collaboration, instill 30 ml tetracaine through the catheter *to decrease the flow of impulses from the bladder.*

NURSING MANAGEMENT PLAN OF CARE

DYSREFLEXIA—cont'd

NURSING INTERVENTIONS AND *RATIONALE*—cont'd

- If indwelling catheter is in place, check for kinks or granular sediment that may indicate occlusion.
- If plugged catheter is suspected, irrigate it gently with no more than 30 ml of sterile normal saline solution. If the bladder is in tetany, fluid will go in but will not drain out.
- If unable to irrigate catheter, remove it, and prepare to reinsert a new catheter: proceed with its lubrication, drainage, and observation as previously stated.
- Atropine is sometimes administered *to relieve bladder tetany.*

  b. Bowel
- Using glove lubricated with anesthetic ointment, check rectum for fecal impaction.
- If impaction is felt, *to decrease flow of impulses from bowel,* insert anesthetic ointment into rectum 10 minutes before manual removal of impaction.

- A low, hypertonic enema or a suppository may be given *to assist bowel evacuation.*

  c. Skin
- Loosen clothing or bed linens as indicated.
- Inspect skin for pimples, boils, pressure sores, and ingrown toenails and treat as indicated.

7. If symptoms of dysreflexia do not subside, have available the intravenous (IV) solutions and antihypertensive drugs of the physician's choosing (e.g., hydralazine, nifedipine, phentolamine, diazoxide, sodium nitroprusside). Administer medications and monitor their effectiveness. Assess BP, pulse, and subjective and objective signs and symptoms.

8. Instruct patient about causes, symptoms, treatment, and prevention of dysreflexia.

9. Encourage patient to carry medical bracelet or informational card to present to medical personnel in the event dysreflexia may be developing.

NURSING MANAGEMENT OF MULTIPLE ORGAN DYSFUNCTION SYNDROME

NURSING MANAGEMENT PLAN OF CARE	DECREASED CARDIAC OUTPUT

DEFINITION

State in which the blood pumped by an individual's heart is sufficiently reduced to the extent that it is inadequate to meet the needs of the body's tissues.

Decreased Cardiac Output Related to Sympathetic Blockade

DEFINING CHARACTERISTICS

- Decreased cardiac output (CO) and cardiac index (CI)
- Systolic blood pressure (SBP) <90 mm Hg or below patient's baseline
- Decreased right atrial pressure (RAP) and pulmonary artery wedge pressure (PAWP)
- Decreased systemic vascular resistance (SVR)
- Bradycardia
- Cardiac dysrhythmias
- Postural hypotension

OUTCOME CRITERIA

- CO and CI are within normal limits.
- SBP 90 mm Hg or returns to baseline.
- RAP and PAWP are within normal limits.
- SVR is within normal limits.
- Sinus rhythm.
- Dysrhythmias are absent.
- Fainting or dizziness with position change is absent.

NURSING INTERVENTIONS AND *RATIONALE*

1. Implement measures to prevent episodes of postural hypotension.
   - Change patient's position slowly *to allow the cardiovascular system time to compensate.*
   - Apply antiembolic stockings *to promote venous return.*
   - Perform range-of-motion exercises every 2 hours *to prevent venous pooling.*
   - Collaborate with the physician and physical therapist regarding the use of a tilt table *to progress the patient from supine to upright position.*
2. Collaborate with the physician regarding the administration of the following:
   - Crystalloids and/or colloids *to increase the patient's circulating volume, which increases stroke volume and subsequently cardiac output.*
   - Vasopressors if fluids are ineffective *to constrict the patient's vascular system, which increases resistance and subsequently blood pressure.*
3. Monitor cardiac rhythm for bradycardia and/or dysrhythmias, *which can further decrease cardiac output.*
4. Avoid any activity that can stimulate the vagal response *because bradycardia can result.*
5. Treat symptomatic bradycardia and symptomatic dysrhythmias according to unit's emergency protocol or Advanced Cardiac Life Support (ACLS) guidelines.

NURSING MANAGEMENT PLAN OF CARE	RISK FOR INFECTION

DEFINITION

State in which an individual is at increased risk for being invaded by pathogenic organisms.

RISK FACTORS

- Inadequate primary defenses (broken skin, traumatized tissue, decreased ciliary action, stasis of body fluids, change in pH secretions, altered peristalsis)
- Inadequate secondary defenses (decreased hemoglobin, leukopenia, suppressed inflammatory/immune response)
- Immunocompromise
- Inadequate acquired immunity

NURSING MANAGEMENT PLAN OF CARE   RISK FOR INFECTION—cont'd

RISK FACTORS—cont'd

- Tissue destruction and increased environmental exposure
- Chronic disease
- Invasive procedures
- Malnutrition
- Pharmacologic agents (antibiotics, steroids)

OUTCOME CRITERIA

- Total lymphocyte count is >1000 mm^3
- White blood cell count is within normal limits
- Temperature is within normal limits
- Blood, urine, wound, and sputum cultures are negative

NURSING INTERVENTIONS AND RATIONALE

1. Wash hands before and after patient care *to reduce the transmission of microorganisms.*
   - Wet hands.
   - Apply 5 ml of soap and thoroughly distribute over both hands.
   - Vigorously wash hands for 10 to 15 seconds.
   - Rinse and thoroughly dry hands.
2. Use aseptic technique for insertion or manipulation of invasive monitoring devices, intravenous lines, and urinary drainage catheters *to maintain sterility of environment.*
3. Stabilize all invasive lines and catheters *to avoid unintentional manipulation and contamination.*
4. Use aseptic technique for dressing changes *to prevent contamination of wounds or insertion sites.*
5. Change any line placed under emergent conditions within 24 hours *since aseptic technique is usually breeched during an emergency.*
6. Collaborate with the physician to change any dressing that is saturated with blood or drainage *since these are mediums for microorganism growth.*

7. Minimize use of stopcocks and maintain caps on all stopcock ports *to reduce the ports of entry for microorganisms.*
8. Avoid the use of nasogastric tubes, nasoendotracheal tubes, and nasopharyngeal suctioning in the patient with a suspected cerebrospinal fluid leak *to decrease the incidence of central nervous system infection.*
9. Change ventilator circuits with humidifiers no more than every 48 hours *to avoid introducing microorganisms into the system.*
10. Provide the patient with a clean manual resuscitation bag *to avoid cross-contamination between patients.*
11. Provide meticulous mouth care at least every shift and suction oropharyngeal secretions as needed *to avoid accumulation.*
12. Cleanse in-line suction catheters with sterile saline according to the manufacturer's instructions *to avoid accumulation of secretions within the catheter.*
13. Use disposable sterile scissors, forceps, and hemostats *to reduce the transmission of microorganisms.*
14. Maintain a closed urinary drainage system *to decrease incidence of urinary infections.*
15. Keep the urinary drainage tubing and bag below the level of the patient's bladder *to prevent the backflow of urine.*
16. Assess the urinary drainage tubing for kinks *to prevent stasis of urine.*
17. Protect all access device sites from potential sources of contamination (nasogastric reflux, draining wounds, ostomies, sputum).
18. Refrigerate parenteral nutrition solutions and open enteral nutrition formulas before use *to inhibit bacterial growth.*
19. Perform daily inspection of all invasive devices for signs of infection.

APPENDICES

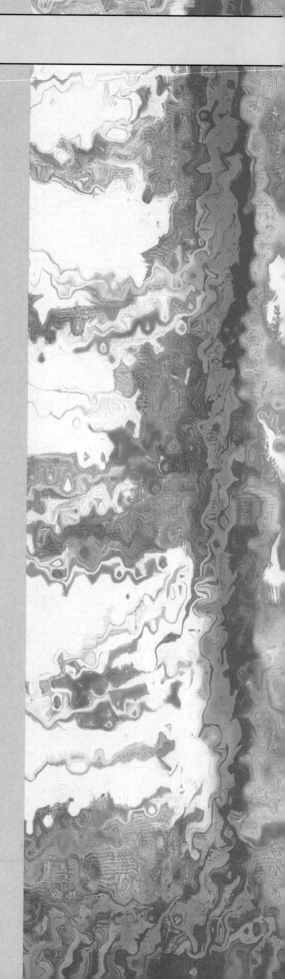

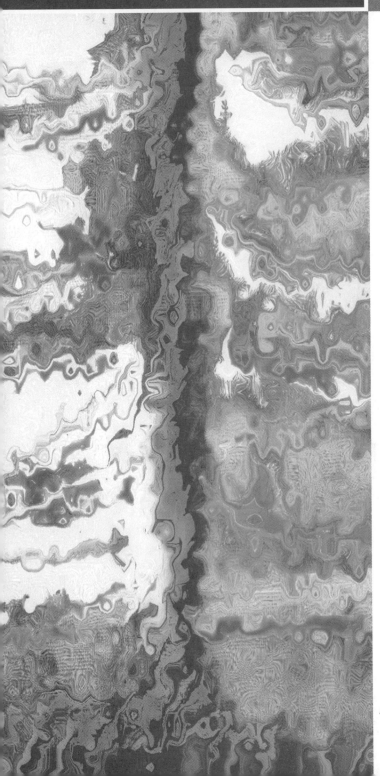

appendix
A

Advanced Cardiac
Life Support
(ACLS) Guidelines

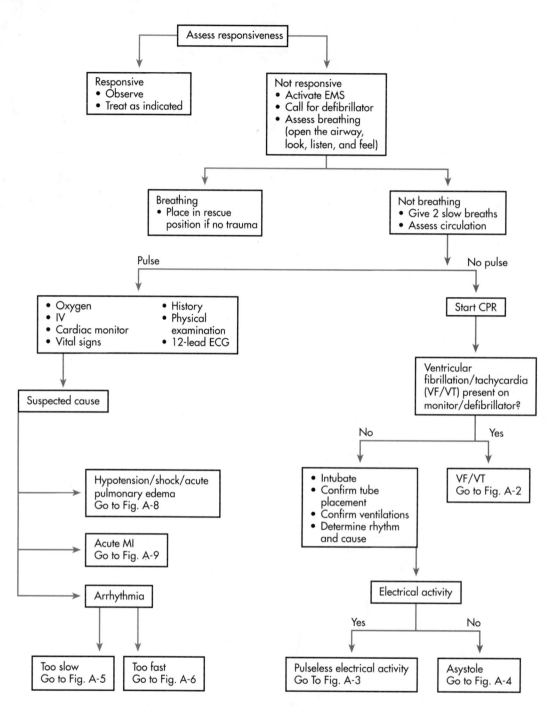

Fig. **A-1** Universal algorithm for adult emergency cardiac care (ECC). (From American Heart Association: *Advanced Cardiac Life Support,* Dallas, 1997, AHA.)

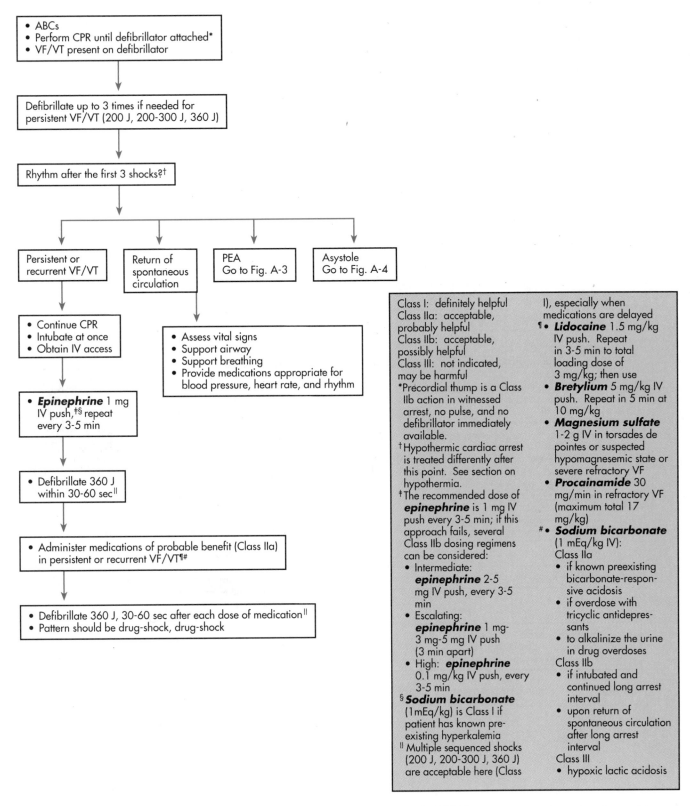

- ABCs
- Perform CPR until defibrillator attached*
- VF/VT present on defibrillator

↓

Defibrillate up to 3 times if needed for persistent VF/VT (200 J, 200-300 J, 360 J)

↓

Rhythm after the first 3 shocks?†

Persistent or recurrent VF/VT

Return of spontaneous circulation

PEA Go to Fig. A-3

Asystole Go to Fig. A-4

- Continue CPR
- Intubate at once
- Obtain IV access

↓

- Assess vital signs
- Support airway
- Support breathing
- Provide medications appropriate for blood pressure, heart rate, and rhythm

- **Epinephrine** 1 mg IV push,†§ repeat every 3-5 min

↓

- Defibrillate 360 J within 30-60 sec‖

↓

- Administer medications of probable benefit (Class IIa) in persistent or recurrent VF/VT¶#

↓

- Defibrillate 360 J, 30-60 sec after each dose of medication‖
- Pattern should be drug-shock, drug-shock

Class I: definitely helpful
Class IIa: acceptable, probably helpful
Class IIb: acceptable, possibly helpful
Class III: not indicated, may be harmful
*Precordial thump is a Class IIb action in witnessed arrest, no pulse, and no defibrillator immediately available.
† Hypothermic cardiac arrest is treated differently after this point. See section on hypothermia.
‡ The recommended dose of **epinephrine** is 1 mg IV push every 3-5 min; if this approach fails, several Class IIb dosing regimens can be considered:
- Intermediate: **epinephrine** 2-5 mg IV push, every 3-5 min
- Escalating: **epinephrine** 1 mg-3 mg-5 mg IV push (3 min apart)
- High: **epinephrine** 0.1 mg/kg IV push, every 3-5 min
§ **Sodium bicarbonate** (1mEq/kg) is Class I if patient has known pre-existing hyperkalemia
‖ Multiple sequenced shocks (200 J, 200-300 J, 360 J) are acceptable here (Class

I), especially when medications are delayed
¶ • **Lidocaine** 1.5 mg/kg IV push. Repeat in 3-5 min to total loading dose of 3 mg/kg; then use
- **Bretylium** 5 mg/kg IV push. Repeat in 5 min at 10 mg/kg
- **Magnesium sulfate** 1-2 g IV in torsades de pointes or suspected hypomagnesemic state or severe refractory VF
- **Procainamide** 30 mg/min in refractory VF (maximum total 17 mg/kg)
• **Sodium bicarbonate** (1 mEq/kg IV): Class IIa
- if known preexisting bicarbonate-responsive acidosis
- if overdose with tricyclic antidepressants
- to alkalinize the urine in drug overdoses
Class IIb
- if intubated and continued long arrest interval
- upon return of spontaneous circulation after long arrest interval
Class III
- hypoxic lactic acidosis

Fig. **A-2** Algorithm for ventricular fibrillation and pulseless ventricular tachycardia (VF/VT). (From American Heart Association: *Advanced Cardiac Life Support*, Dallas, 1997, AHA.)

PEA includes
- Electromechanical dissociation (EMD)
- Pseudo-EMD
- Idioventricular rhythms
- Ventricular escape rhythms
- Bradyasystolic rhythms
- Postdefibrillation idioventricular rhythms

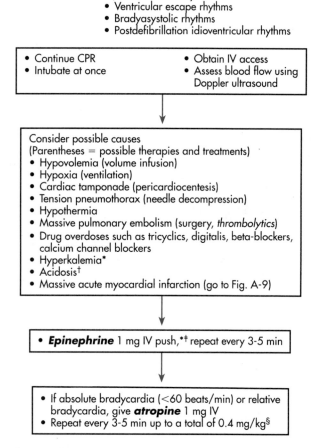

- Continue CPR
- Intubate at once
- Obtain IV access
- Assess blood flow using Doppler ultrasound

↓

Consider possible causes
(Parentheses = possible therapies and treatments)
- Hypovolemia (volume infusion)
- Hypoxia (ventilation)
- Cardiac tamponade (pericardiocentesis)
- Tension pneumothorax (needle decompression)
- Hypothermia
- Massive pulmonary embolism (surgery, *thrombolytics*)
- Drug overdoses such as tricyclics, digitalis, beta-blockers, calcium channel blockers
- Hyperkalemia*
- Acidosis†
- Massive acute myocardial infarction (go to Fig. A-9)

↓

- **Epinephrine** 1 mg IV push,*† repeat every 3-5 min

↓

- If absolute bradycardia (<60 beats/min) or relative bradycardia, give **atropine** 1 mg IV
- Repeat every 3-5 min up to a total of 0.4 mg/kg§

Class I: definitely helpful
Class IIa: acceptable, probably helpful
Class IIb: acceptable, possibly helpful
Class III: not indicated, may be harmful
*__Sodium bicarbonate__ 1mEq/kg is Class I if patient has known preexisting hyperkalemia.
†__Sodium bicarbonate__ 1 mEq/kg:
Class IIa
- if known preexisting bicarbonate-responsive acidosis
- if overdose with tricyclic antidepressants
- to alkalinize the urine in drug overdoses
Class IIb
- if intubated and long arrest interval
- upon return of spontaneous circulation after long arrest interval
Class III
- hypoxic lactic acidosis
†The recommended dose of **epinephrine** is 1 mg IV push every 3-5 min. If this approach fails, several Class IIb dosing regimens can be considered.
- Intermediate: **epinephrine** 2-5 mg IV push every 3-5 min
- Escalating: **epinephrine** 1 mg-3 mg-5 mg IV push (3 min apart)
- High: **epinephrine** 0.1 mg/kg IV push every 3-5 min
§Shorter **atropine** dosing intervals are possibly helpful in cardiac arrest (Class IIb).

Fig. **A-3** Algorithm for pulseless electrical activity (PEA) (electromechanical dissociation [EMD]). (From American Heart Association: *Advanced Cardiac Life Support,* Dallas, 1997, AHA.)

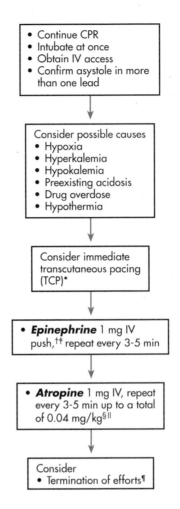

Fig. **A-4** Asystole treatment algorithm. (From American Heart Association: *Advanced Cardiac Life Support,* Dallas, 1997, AHA.)

Class I: definitely helpful
Class IIa: acceptable, probably helpful
Class IIb: acceptable, possibly helpful
Class III: not indicated, may be harmful
*TCP is a Class IIb intervention. Lack of success may be due to delays in pacing. To be effective TCP must be performed early, simultaneously with drugs. Evidence does not support routine use of TCP for asystole.
†The recommended dose of **epinephrine** is 1 mg IV push every 3-5 min. If this approach fails, several Class IIb dosing regimens can be considered:
• Intermediate: **epinephrine** 2-5 mg IV push every 3-5 min
• Escalating: **epinephrine** 1 mg-3 mg-5 mg IV push, (3 min apart)
• High: **epinephrine** 0.1 mg/kg IV push every 3-5 min
‡**Sodium bicarbonate** 1 mEq/kg is Class I if patient has known preexisting hyperkalemia.

§Shorter **atropine** dosing intervals are Class IIb in asystolic arrest.
‖**Sodium bicarbonate** 1 mEq/kg:
Class IIa
• if known preexisting bicarbonate-responsive acidosis
• if overdose with tricyclic antidepressants
• to alkalinize the urine in drug overdoses
Class IIb
• if intubated and continued long arrest interval
• upon return of spontaneous circulation after long arrest interval
Class III
• hypoxic lactic acidosis
¶If patient remains in asystole or other agonal rhythms after successful intubation and initial medications and no reversible causes are identified, consider termination of resuscitative efforts by a physician. Consider interval since arrest.

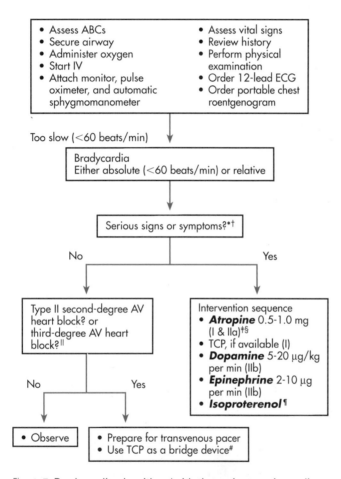

Too slow (<60 beats/min)

Bradycardia
Either absolute (<60 beats/min) or relative

Serious signs or symptoms?*†

No

Type II second-degree AV heart block? or third-degree AV heart block?‖

No   Yes

• Observe

• Prepare for transvenous pacer
• Use TCP as a bridge device#

Yes

Intervention sequence
• *Atropine* 0.5-1.0 mg (I & IIa)†§
• TCP, if available (I)
• *Dopamine* 5-20 µg/kg per min (IIb)
• *Epinephrine* 2-10 µg per min (IIb)
• *Isoproterenol*¶

*Serious signs or symptoms must be related to the slow rate. Clinical manifestations include:
symptoms (chest pains, shortness of breath, decreased level of consciousness) and
signs (low BP, shock, pulmonary congestion, CHF, acute MI)
†Do not delay TCP while awaiting IV access or for *atropine* to take effect if patient is symptomatic.
‡Denervated transplanted hearts will not respond to *atropine*. Go at once to pacing, *catecholamine* infusion, or both.
§*Atropine* should be given at repeat doses in 3-5 min up to total of 0.04 mg/kg. Consider shorter dosing intervals in severe clinical conditions. It has been suggested that atropine should be used with caution in atrioventricular (AV) block at the His-Purkinje level (type II AV block and new third-degree heart block with wide QRS complexes) (Class IIb)
‖Never treat third-degree heart block plus ventricular escape beats with *lidocaine.*
¶*Isoproterenol* should be used, if at all, with extreme caution. At low doses it is Class IIb (probably helpful); at higher doses it is Class III (harmful).
#Verify patient tolerance and mechanical capture. Use analgesia and sedation as needed.

Fig. **A-5** Bradycardia algorithm (with the patient not in cardiac arrest). (From American Heart Association: *Advanced Cardiac Life Support,* Dallas, 1997, AHA.)

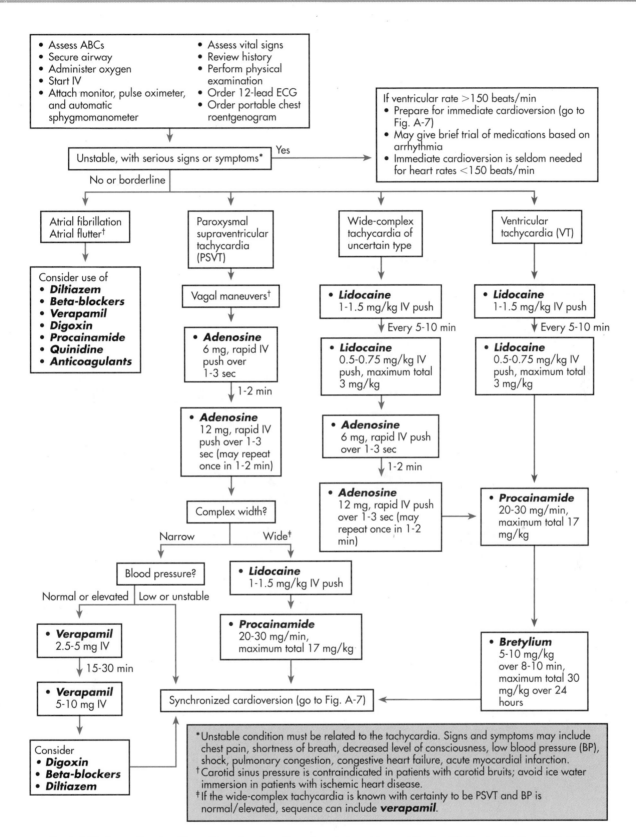

Fig. **A-6** Tachycardia algorithm. (From American Heart Association: *Advanced Cardiac Life Support,* Dallas, 1997, AHA.)

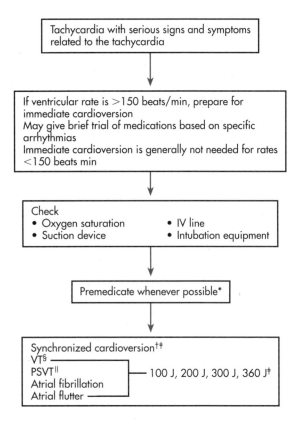

Tachycardia with serious signs and symptoms related to the tachycardia

If ventricular rate is >150 beats/min, prepare for immediate cardioversion
May give brief trial of medications based on specific arrhythmias
Immediate cardioversion is generally not needed for rates <150 beats min

Check
• Oxygen saturation
• Suction device
• IV line
• Intubation equipment

Premedicate whenever possible*

Synchronized cardioversion†‡
VT§
PSVT‖ —— 100 J, 200 J, 300 J, 360 J‡
Atrial fibrillation
Atrial flutter

*Effective regimens have included a sedative (e.g., **diazepam, midazolam, barbiturates, stomidate, ketamine, methohexital**) with or without an analgesic agent (e.g., **fentanyl, morphine, meperidine**). Many experts recommend anesthesia if service is readily available.
†Note possible need to resynchronize after each cardioversion.
‡If delays in synchronization occur and clinical conditions are critical, go to immediate unsynchronized shocks.
§Treat polymorphic VT (irregular form and rate) like VF: 200 J, 200-300 J, 360 J.
‖PSVT and atrial flutter often respond to lower energy levels (start with 50 J).

Fig. **A-7** Electrical cardioversion algorithm (with the patient not in cardiac arrest). (From American Heart Association: *Advanced Cardiac Life Support*, Dallas, 1997, AHA.)

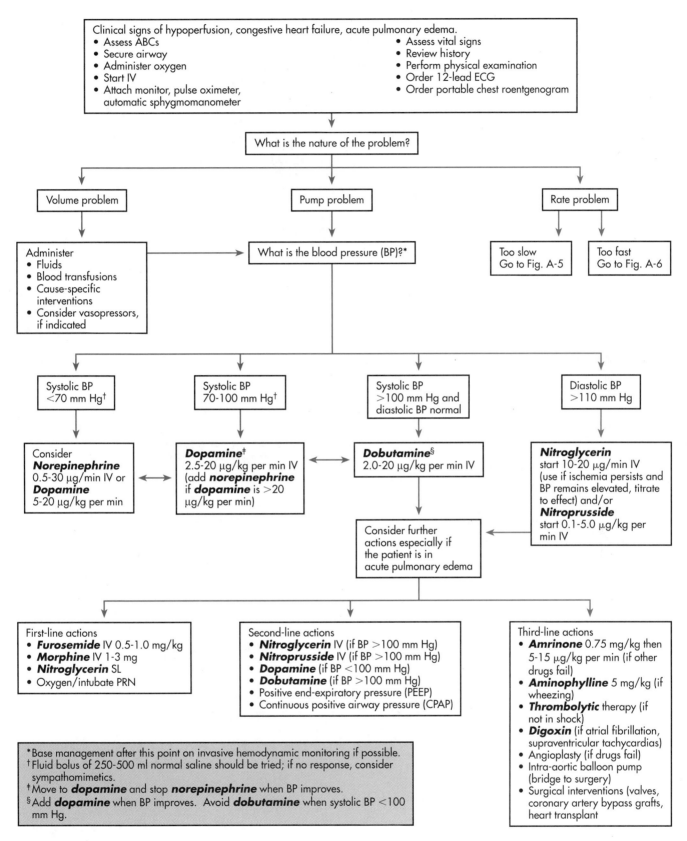

Fig. **A-8** Algorithm for hypotension, shock, and acute pulmonary edema. (From American Heart Association: *Advanced Cardiac Life Support*, Dallas, 1997, AHA.)

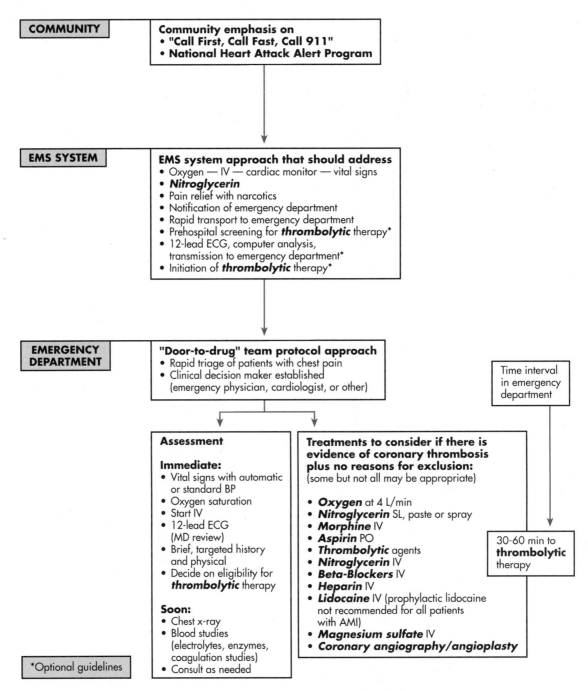

COMMUNITY

Community emphasis on
• "Call First, Call Fast, Call 911"
• National Heart Attack Alert Program

EMS SYSTEM

EMS system approach that should address
• Oxygen — IV — cardiac monitor — vital signs
• *Nitroglycerin*
• Pain relief with narcotics
• Notification of emergency department
• Rapid transport to emergency department
• Prehospital screening for *thrombolytic* therapy*
• 12-lead ECG, computer analysis, transmission to emergency department*
• Initiation of *thrombolytic* therapy*

EMERGENCY DEPARTMENT

"Door-to-drug" team protocol approach
• Rapid triage of patients with chest pain
• Clinical decision maker established (emergency physician, cardiologist, or other)

Time interval in emergency department

Assessment

Immediate:
• Vital signs with automatic or standard BP
• Oxygen saturation
• Start IV
• 12-lead ECG (MD review)
• Brief, targeted history and physical
• Decide on eligibility for *thrombolytic* therapy

Soon:
• Chest x-ray
• Blood studies (electrolytes, enzymes, coagulation studies)
• Consult as needed

Treatments to consider if there is evidence of coronary thrombosis plus no reasons for exclusion:
(some but not all may be appropriate)

• *Oxygen* at 4 L/min
• *Nitroglycerin* SL, paste or spray
• *Morphine* IV
• *Aspirin* PO
• *Thrombolytic* agents
• *Nitroglycerin* IV
• *Beta-Blockers* IV
• *Heparin* IV
• *Lidocaine* IV (prophylactic lidocaine not recommended for all patients with AMI)
• *Magnesium sulfate* IV
• *Coronary angiography/angioplasty*

30-60 min to **thrombolytic** therapy

*Optional guidelines

Fig. **A-9** Acute myocardial infarction algorithm. Recommendations for early management of patients with chest pain and possible AMI. (From American Heart Association: *Advanced Cardiac Life Support,* Dallas, 1997, AHA.)

✔ Detection
✔ Dispatch
✔ Delivery

EMS Treatment
Immediate assessments performed by
EMS system personnel, include
- *Cincinnati Prehospital Stroke Scale* (includes language abnormality, motor arm, facial droop)
- Alert hospital possible stroke patient
- Rapid transport to hospital

✔ **Door**

Immediate general assessment: <10 min from arrival	**Immediate neurologic assessment: <25 min from arrival**

- Assess ABCs, vital signs
- Provide oxygen by nasal cannula
- Obtain IV access; obtain blood samples (CBC, electrolytes, coagulation studies)
- Check blood sugar; treat if indicated
- Perform general neurologic screening assessment
- Alert Stroke Team: neurologist, radiologist, CT technician
	- Review patient history
	- Establish onset (<3 hours required for thrombolytics)
	- Perform physical examination
	- Perform neurologic examination:
	  ✔ Determine level of consciousness *(Glasgow Coma Scale)*
	  ✔ Determine level of stroke severity *(NIH Stroke Scale or Hunt and Hess Scale)*
	- Order urgent noncontrast CT scan (door-to–CT scan performed: goal <25 min from arrival)
	- Read CT scan (door-to–CT read: goal <45 min from arrival)
	- Perform lateral cervical spine x-ray (if patient comatose/history of trauma)

Does CT scan show intracerebral or subarachnoid hemorrhage?

✔ **Data**   **No**   **Yes**

Probable acute ischemic stroke
✔ Review CT exclusions: are any observed?
✔ Repeat neurologic exam: are deficits variable or rapidly improving?
✔ Review thrombolytic exclusions: are any observed?
✔ Review patient data: is symptom onset now >3 hours?

Consult neurosurgery

Blood on LP

No to All of Above

If high suspicion of subarachnoid hemorrhage remains despite negative findings on CT scan, perform lumbar puncture (lumbar puncture excludes use of thrombolytic therapy)

Initiate actions for acute hemorrhage
- Reverse any anticoagulants
- Reverse any bleeding disorder
- Monitor neurologic condition
- Treat hypertension in awake patients

No Blood on LP

✔ **Decision**

Patient remains candidate for thrombolytic therapy?   **No**

- Initiate supportive therapy as indicated
- Consider admission
- Consider anticoagulation
- Consider additional conditions needing treatment
- Consider alternative diagnoses

✔ **Drug**   **Yes**

- Review risks/benefits with patient and family: If acceptable —
Begin thrombolytic treatment (door-to-treatment goal <60 min):
- Monitor neurologic status: emergent CT if deterioration
- Monitor BP; treat as indicated
- Admit to Critical Care Unit
- No anticoagulants or antiplatelet treatment × 24 hours

Fig. **A-10** Algorithm for suspected stroke patients. (From American Heart Association: *Advanced Cardiac Life Support,* Dallas, 1997, AHA.)

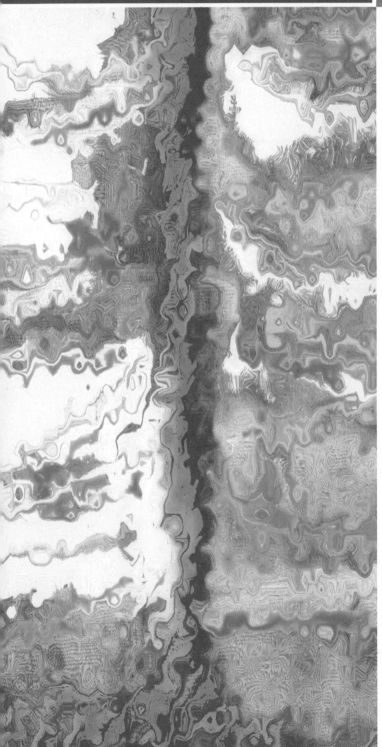

Physiologic Formulas for Critical Care

HEMODYNAMIC FORMULAS

Mean Arterial Pressure (MAP)

$$MAP = [SBP + (2 \times DBP)] \div 3$$

SBP = systolic blood pressure (measured via arterial line or blood pressure cuff)
DBP = diastolic blood pressure (measured via arterial line or blood pressure cuff)

Normal range is 70 to 100 mm Hg

Cardiac Index (CI)

$$CI = CO \div BSA$$

CO = cardiac output (measured via pulmonary artery catheter)
BSA = body surface area (calculated value)

Normal range is 2.5 to 4.0 L/min/m²

Stroke Volume (SV)

$$SV = (CO \div HR) \times 1000$$

CO = cardiac output (measured via pulmonary artery catheter)
HR = heart rate (measured via bedside electrocardiogram)

Normal range is 60 to 100 ml/beat

Stroke Volume Index (SVI)

$$SVI = (CI \div HR) \times 1000$$

CI = cardiac index (calculated value)
HR = heart rate (measured via bedside electrocardiogram)

Normal range is 33 to 47 ml/m²/beat

Systemic Vascular Resistance (SVR)

$$SVR = [(MAP - RAP) \div CO] \times 80$$

MAP = mean arterial pressure (measured via arterial line or calculated value)
RAP = right atrial pressure (measured via pulmonary artery catheter)
CO = cardiac output (measured via pulmonary artery catheter)

Normal range is 800 to 1200 dynes/sec/cm^{-5}

Pulmonary Vascular Resistance (PVR)

$$PVR = [(PAMP - PAWP) \div CO] \times 80$$

PAMP = pulmonary artery mean pressure (measured via pulmonary artery catheter)
PAWP = pulmonary artery wedge pressure (measured via pulmonary artery catheter)
CO = cardiac output (measured via pulmonary artery catheter)

Normal range is less than 250 dynes/sec/cm^{-5}

Left Ventricular Stroke Work Index (LVSWI)

$$LVSWI = (MAP - PAWP) \times SVI \times 0.0136$$

MAP = mean arterial pressure (measured via arterial line or calculated value)
PAWP = pulmonary artery wedge pressure (measured via pulmonary artery catheter
SVI = stroke volume index (calculated value)

Normal range is 50 to 62 g-m/m^2/beat

Right Ventricular Stroke Work Index (RVSWI)

$$RVSWI = (PAMP - RAP) \times SVI \times 0.0136$$

PAMP = pulmonary artery mean pressure (measured via pulmonary artery catheter)
RAP = right atrial pressure (measured via pulmonary artery catheter)
SVI = stroke volume (calculated value)

Normal range is 5.0 to 10.0 g-m/m^2/beat

Corrected QT Interval (Qtc)

$$Qtc = QT \div \sqrt{RR}$$

QT = QT interval
RR = R to R interval

Upper limit is 0.44 seconds

Body Surface Area (BSA)

To calculate (Fig. B-1):
1. Obtain patient's height and weight.
2. Mark height on the left scale and weight on the right scale.
3. Draw a straight line between the two points marked on each scale.

The number where the line crosses the middle scale is the BSA value

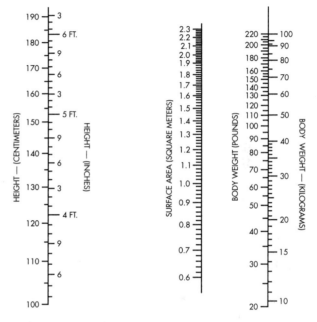

Fig. **B-1** Body surface area (BSA) nomogram.

PULMONARY FORMULAS

Calculation of the Shunt Equation (Qs/Qt)

$$\frac{Qs}{Qt} = \frac{Cco_2 - Cao_2}{Cco_2 - Cvo_2}$$

Cco$_2$ = capillary oxygen content (calculated value)
Cao$_2$ = arterial oxygen content (calculated value)
Cvo$_2$ = venous oxygen content (calculated value)

Normal range is less than 5%

Calculation of the Capillary Oxygen Content (Cco$_2$)

$$Cco_2 = (Hgb \times 1.34 \times Sco_2) + (Pco_2 \times 0.003)$$

Hgb = hemoglobin (measured via laboratory sample or arterial blood gas)
Sco$_2$ = pulmonary capillary oxygen saturation
Pco$_2$ = partial pressure of oxygen in capillary blood

Calculation of Arterial Oxygen Content (CaO$_2$)

$$CaO_2 = (Hgb \times 1.34 \times SaO_2) + (0.003 \times PaO_2)$$

Hgb = hemoglobin (measured via laboratory sample or arterial blood gas)
SaO$_2$ = arterial oxygen saturation (measured via arterial blood gas)
PaO$_2$ = partial pressure of oxygen in arterial blood (measured via arterial blood gas)

Normal range is 17 to 20 ml/100 ml

Calculation of Venous Oxygen Content (CvO$_2$)

$$CvO_2 = (Hgb \times 1.34 \times SvO_2) + (0.003 \times PvO_2)$$

Hgb = hemoglobin (measured via laboratory sample or arterial blood gas)
SvO$_2$ = mixed venous oxygen saturation (measured via mixed venous blood gas)
PvO$_2$ = partial pressure of oxygen in mixed venous blood (measured via mixed venous blood gas)

Normal range is 12 to 15 ml/100 ml

Calculation of Alveolar Pressure of Oxygen (PaO$_2$)

$$PaO_2 = FIO_2 \times (Pb - PH_2O) - PaCO_2/RQ$$

FIO$_2$ = fraction of inspired oxygen (obtained from oxygen settings)
Pb = barometric pressure (assumed to be 760 mm Hg as sea level)
PH$_2$O = water pressure in the lungs (assumed to be 47 mm Hg)
PaCO$_2$ = partial pressure of carbon dioxide in arterial blood (measured via arterial blood gas)
RQ = respiratory quotient (assumed to be 0.8)

Normal range is 60 to 100 mm Hg

Calculation of PaO$_2$/FIO$_2$ Ratio

$$PaO_2/FIO_2 \; Ratio = \frac{PaO_2}{FIO_2}$$

PaO$_2$ = partial pressure of oxygen in arterial blood (measured via arterial blood gas)
FIO$_2$ = fraction of inspired oxygen (obtained from oxygen settings)

Normal range is greater than 286

Calculation of Arterial/Alveolar Ratio

$$PaO_2/PAO_2 \; Ratio = \frac{PaO_2}{PAO_2}$$

PaO$_2$ = partial pressure of oxygen in arterial blood (measured via arterial blood gas)
PAO$_2$ = partial pressure of oxygen in alveoli (calculated value)

Normal range is greater than 60%

Calculation of Alveolar-Arterial Gradient

$$P(A-a)O_2 = PAO_2 - PaO_2$$

PAO$_2$ = partial pressure of oxygen in alveoli (calculated value)
PaO$_2$ = partial pressure of oxygen in arterial blood (measured via arterial blood gas)

Normal range is 0 to 20 mm Hg

Calculation of the Dead Space Equation (Vd/Vt)

$$\frac{Vd}{Vt} = \frac{PaCO_2 - PetCO_2}{PaCO_2}$$

PaCO$_2$ = partial pressure of carbon dioxide in arterial blood (measured via arterial blood gas)
PetCO$_2$ = partial pressure of carbon dioxide in exhaled gas (measured via end-tidal CO$_2$ monitor)

Normal range 0.2 to 0.4 (20% to 40%)

Calculation of Static Compliance (C$_{ST}$)
This value is calculated on mechanically ventilated patients.

$$C_{ST} = \frac{Vt}{PP - PEEP}$$

Vt = tidal volume (obtained from ventilator)
PP = plateau pressure (measured via ventilator)
PEEP = positive end-expiratory pressure (obtained from ventilator)

Normal value is greater than 50 ml/cm H$_2$O

Calculation of Dynamic Compliance (C$_{DY}$) (Also Called Characteristic)
This value is calculated on mechanically ventilated patients.

$$C_{DY} = \frac{Vt}{PIP - PEEP}$$

Vt = tidal volume (obtained from ventilator)
PIP = peak inspiratory pressure (obtained from ventilator)
PEEP = positive end-expiratory pressure (obtained from ventilator)

Normal value is 40 to 50 ml/cm H_2O

NEUROLOGIC FORMULAS

Calculation of Cerebral Perfusion Pressure (CPP)

$$CPP = MAP - ICP$$

MAP = mean arterial pressure (measured via arterial line or blood pressure cuff)
ICP = intracranial pressure (measured via intracranial pressure monitoring device)

Normal range is 60 to 150 mm Hg

ENDOCRINE FORMULAS

Serum Osmolality

$$Serum\ Osmolality = 2(Na^+ + K^+) + \frac{Glucose}{18} + \frac{BUN}{2.8}$$

Na^+ = sodium
K^+ = potassium
BUN = blood urea nitrogen

Normal range is 270 to 300 mOsm/kg of water

RENAL FORMULA

Clearance

$$Clearance = U \times \left(\frac{V}{P}\right)$$

U = concentration of substance in urine
V = time
P = concentration of substance in plasma

Normal range is dependent on substance measured

NUTRITIONAL FORMULAS*

Formulas for estimating caloric needs

Step 1. Calculate basal energy expenditure (BEE). This is the energy needed for basic life processes such as respiratory function and maintenance of body temperature.

Women: BEE = 795 + 7.18 × weight (kg)
Men: BEE = 879 + 10.20 × weight (kg)

Step 2. Multiply by an appropriate stress factor to meet the needs of the ill or injured patient (see the following table). If the patient has more than one stress present (e.g., burn and pneumonia), use only the stress factor for the highest level of stress.

TYPE OF STRESS	MULTIPLY THE VALUE OBTAINED IN STEP 2 BY
Fever	1 + 0.13/° C elevation above normal (or 0.07/° F)
Pneumonia	1.2
Major injury	1.3
Severe sepsis, burn of 15%-30% of body surface area (BSA)	1.5
Burn of 31%-49% BSA content (calculated value)	1.5-2.0
Burn ≥50% BSA	1.8-2.1

Estimating protein needs

Protein needs vary with degree of malnutrition and stress.

CONDITION	MULTIPLY DESIRABLE BODY WEIGHT (kg) BY
Healthy individual or well-nourished elective surgery patient	0.8-1.0 g protein
Malnourished or catabolic state (e.g., sepsis, major injury)	1.2 to 2+ g protein
Burns	
15%-30% BSA	1.5 g protein
31%-49% BSA	1.5-2.0 g protein
≥50% BSA	2.0-2.5 g protein

Example of calculation of calorie and protein needs

A 28-year-old female patient has a fracture of the left femur and burns of 40% of her BSA after an automobile accident. Her height is 1.65 m (5'5″) and her weight is 59.1 kg (130 lb).

Energy needs
1. BEE = 795 + 7.18 × 59.1 = 1219 calories/day
2. Energy needs for injury = 1219 calories × 1.75 = 2133 calories/day

Protein needs

Protein needs = 59.1 kg × 1.75 g = 103 g/day

---

*Deitch EA: *Crit Care Clin* 11:735, 1995; Owen OE, et al: *Am J Clin Nutr* 4:1, 1986; Owen OE, et al: *Am J Clin Nutr* 46:875, 1987; Garrel DR, Jobin N, de Jonge LH: *Nutr Clin Prac* 11:99, 1996.

INDEX

Hyperglycemia
    clinical manifestations of, *379*
    monitoring for, in diabetic ketoacidosis, 379
    signs of, observation for, 365-366
Hyperglycemic hyperosmolar nonketotic syndrome
        (HHNS), 381-385
    assessment of, 383
    description of, 381-382
    diabetic ketoacidosis compared with, 381t
    diagnosis of, 383
    etiology of, 381-382
    medical management of, 383-384
    nursing management of, 384-385
    pathophysiology of, 382-383
Hyperkalemia
    in acute renal failure, 319t
        management of, 322
    in cardiovascular assessment, 107
    clinical manifestations of, 380t
    monitoring for, in diabetic ketoacidosis, 379-380
Hyperlipidemia, coronary artery disease and, 147
Hypermagnesemia in acute renal failure, 319t
Hypermetabolism in multiple organ dysfunction
        syndrome, 432, 434
Hypernatremia in acute renal failure, 319t
Hyperoxia, 249-250
Hyperphosphatemia in acute renal failure, 320t
Hypersensitivity reaction, immediate, anaphylactic
        shock and, 422
Hypertension
    in cardiovascular disorders, 49t
    control of, in aortic aneurysm and dissection, 173
    coronary artery disease and, 147
    induced, in subarachnoid hemorrhage management,
        286
    intracranial; *see* Intracranial hypertension
    nutrition intervention for, 48, 50
    pulmonary, in acute respiratory distress syndrome,
        228
Hypertensive, hypervolemic, hemodilution (HHH)
        therapy for subarachnoid hemorrhage, 286
Hypertensive crisis, 173-175
Hyperthyroidism, signs and symptoms of, 369
Hypertrophic cardiomyopathy (HCM), 165
Hyperventilation, central neurogenic, 271t
Hypervolemia, induced, in subarachnoid hemorrhage
        management, 286
Hypoalbuminemia in acute renal failure, 320t
Hypocalcemia
    in acute renal failure, 319t
    in cardiovascular assessment, 108-109
Hypochloremia in acute renal failure, 320t
Hypoglycemia
    clinical manifestations of, *379*
    monitoring for, in diabetic ketoacidosis, 379

Hypokalemia
    in acute renal failure, 319t
    in cardiovascular assessment, 107-108
    clinical manifestations of, 380t
    monitoring for, in diabetic ketoacidosis, 379-380
Hypomagnesemia
    in acute renal failure, 319t
    in cardiovascular assessment, 109
Hyponatremia
    in acute renal failure, 319t
    dilutional, in acute renal failure, management of, 322
    monitoring for, in diabetic ketoacidosis, 380
    subarachnoid hemorrhage and, 286
Hypophosphatemia in acute renal failure, 320t
Hypotension
    algorithm for, *505*
    sepsis-induced, definition of, *427*
    in shock, 416
Hypothermia
    for cardiopulmonary bypass, 177-178
    complicating hemodynamic monitoring, 144t
    in neurogenic shock, management of, 426
Hypothyroidism, signs and symptoms of, 369
Hypoventilation
    in acute respiratory failure, preventing, 227
    alveolar
        in acute respiratory failure, 225
        gas exchange impairment from, nursing
            management plan of care for, 476-477
Hypovolemia in neurogenic shock, management of, 426
Hypovolemic shock, 418-419
Hypoxia
    in neurogenic shock, management of, 426
    tissue, in trauma patient, factors contributing to, *399*

I

IABP; *see* Intraaortic balloon pump (IABP)
Ibuprofen, impact of renal failure and dialysis on, 334t
ICD (implantable cardioverter defibrillator), 191-194
ICH (intracerebral hemorrhage), 286-288
ICHD (Inter-Society Commission for Heart Disease), 185
ICP; *see* Intracranial pressure (ICP)
IDH (intracerebral hematoma), 402
Idioventricular rhythm, *126*
Illness
    critical, stress and, 372-373
    undernutrition and, 46
ILV (independent lung ventilation), 259t
IMA (internal mammary artery) graft, 175, *176*
Imagery, guided, in pain management, 96
Imipenem, impact of renal failure and dialysis on, 332t
Immobility, prolonged, activity intolerance related to,
        nursing management plan of care for, 465-466
Immune system
    dysfunction of, clinical manifestations of, *433*
    gerontologic alterations in, 78-79

Paraplegia, 404
Paroxysmal nocturnal dyspnea in heart failure, 162-163
Paroxysmal supraventricular tachycardia (PSVT), *121*
Passy-Muir valve, 256-257
Patient(s)
  education of, 21-26; *see also* Education, patient and
      family
  high-risk, psychosocial alterations in, 32-34
Patient Self-Determination Act, 18-19
Patient-controlled analgesia (PCA) in pain
      management, 93
Patient-ventilator asynchrony complicating mechanical
      ventilation, 260
PCA (patient-controlled analgesia) in pain
      management, 93
PE; *see* Pulmonary embolism (PE)
Pectoriloquy, whispering, 216
Pectus carinatum, 212
Pectus excavatum, 212
PEEP; *see* Positive end-expiratory pressure (PEEP)
Pelvic injuries, 411
Penetrating trauma, 397
  abdominal, 409-410
  cardiac, 408-409
  spinal cord, 404
  thoracic, 406
Penicillin, impact of renal failure and dialysis on, 333t
Pentobarbital
  in intracranial hypertension management, 304
  sleep and, 40t
Peptic ulcer
  acute gastrointestinal hemorrhage from, 347
  bleeding control in, 349
Percussion
  in gastrointestinal assessment, 339-340
  in pulmonary assessment, 213-214
  in renal assessment, 309
Percussion tones, conditions associated with, 213t
Percutaneous transhepatic portography in
      gastrointestinal diagnosis, 344t
Percutaneous transluminal coronary angioplasty
      (PTCA), 194-195
Perfusion pressure, cerebral, intracranial pressure and,
      298
Pericardial friction rubs, identification of, 106
Pericardiocentesis in cardiovascular assessment, 112t
Pericarditis, myocardial infarction and, 159
Peripheral arteriography in cardiovascular assessment,
      112t
Peripheral nervous system in pathophysiology of pain,
      85
Peripheral vascular system, age-related changes in, 71-72
Peripheral venography in cardiovascular assessment,
      112t
Peritoneal dialysis, 329-331
Personal liability, 15

Personality type, coronary artery disease and, 148
PET; *see* Positron emission tomography (PET)
pH, urine, in renal assessment, 311
Pharmacodynamics, age-related changes in, 75
Pharmacokinetics, age-related changes in, 75
Pharyngeal airways, 250-251
Phenobarbital
  impact of renal failure and dialysis on, 334t
  sleep and, 40t
Phentolamine for cardiovascular disorders, 208
Phenylephrine, physiologic effects of, 206t
Phenytoin, impact of renal failure and dialysis on, 334t
Phlebitis, observation for signs of, 103
Phlegmon complicating acute pancreatitis, 353
Phonocardiography in cardiovascular assessment, 112t
Phosphate disturbances in acute renal failure, 320t
Phosphodiesterase inhibitors, 207
Phosphorus
  excess of, in renal disorders, 54t
  regulation of, in acute renal failure management, 322
Physical inactivity, coronary artery disease and, 148
Pigeon breast, 212
Piperacillin, impact of renal failure and dialysis on, 333t
Pitting edema, scale for, *103*
Pituitary gland
  assessment of, 367-369
  response of, during stress, 374t
PJC (premature junctional contraction), *123*
Planning in nursing process, 3
Plaque in coronary artery disease, 148-149; *see also*
      Atherosclerosis, plaque in
Plasmapheresis for Guillain-Barré syndrome, 289
Platelet activating factor (PAF) in multiple organ
      dysfunction syndrome, *432, 434, 435*
Pleural friction rub, 215t
Pneumoencephalography in neurologic diagnosis, 275t
Pneumonectomy, 240t
Pneumonia, 230-233
  aspiration, 233-235
  assessment of, 232
  community-acquired, 230
  complicating craniotomy, 292-293
  description of, 230-231
  diagnosis of, 232
  etiology of, 230-231
  hospital-acquired, 230
  medical management of, 232-233
  nosocomial, complicating mechanical ventilation, 260
  nursing management of, 233
  pathophysiology of, 231-232
  precipitating conditions of, 231t
  ventilator-associated, 230-231
Pneumothorax
  complicating hemodynamic monitoring, 144t
  open, 408
  tension, 407-408